Antioxidants in Foods

Antioxidants in Foods

Editors

Isabel Seiquer
José M. Palma

MDPI • Basel • Beijing • Wuhan • Barcelona • Belgrade • Manchester • Tokyo • Cluj • Tianjin

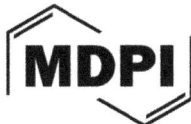

Editors
Isabel Seiquer
Estación Experimental del
Zaidín, CSIC
Spain

José M. Palma
Estación Experimental del
Zaidín, CSIC
Spain

Editorial Office
MDPI
St. Alban-Anlage 66
4052 Basel, Switzerland

This is a reprint of articles from the Special Issue published online in the open access journal *Antioxidants* (ISSN 2076-3921) (available at: https://www.mdpi.com/journal/antioxidants/special_issues/Antioxidants_Foods).

For citation purposes, cite each article independently as indicated on the article page online and as indicated below:

LastName, A.A.; LastName, B.B.; LastName, C.C. Article Title. *Journal Name* **Year**, *Volume Number*, Page Range.

ISBN 978-3-0365-0578-7 (Hbk)
ISBN 978-3-0365-0579-4 (PDF)

Cover image courtesy of Isabel Seiquer.

© 2021 by the authors. Articles in this book are Open Access and distributed under the Creative Commons Attribution (CC BY) license, which allows users to download, copy and build upon published articles, as long as the author and publisher are properly credited, which ensures maximum dissemination and a wider impact of our publications.

The book as a whole is distributed by MDPI under the terms and conditions of the Creative Commons license CC BY-NC-ND.

Contents

About the Editors ix

José M. Palma and Isabel Seiquer
To Be or Not to Be... An Antioxidant? That Is the Question
Reprinted from: *Antioxidants* **2020**, *9*, 1234, doi:10.3390/antiox9121234 1

José M. Palma, Fátima Terán, Alba Contreras-Ruiz, Marta Rodríguez-Ruiz and Francisco J. Corpas
Antioxidant Profile of Pepper (*Capsicum annuum* L.) Fruits Containing Diverse Levels of Capsaicinoids
Reprinted from: *Antioxidants* **2020**, *9*, 878, doi:10.3390/antiox9090878 7

Vidmantas Bendokas, Vidmantas Stanys, Ingrida Mažeikienė, Sonata Trumbeckaite, Rasa Baniene and Julius Liobikas
Anthocyanins: From the Field to the Antioxidants in the Body
Reprinted from: *Antioxidants* **2020**, *9*, 819, doi:10.3390/antiox9090819 27

Florinda Fratianni, Antonio d'Acierno, Autilia Cozzolino, Patrizia Spigno, Riccardo Riccardi, Francesco Raimo, Catello Pane, Massimo Zaccardelli, Valentina Tranchida Lombardo, Marina Tucci, Stefania Grillo, Raffaele Coppola and Filomena Nazzaro
Biochemical Characterization of Traditional Varieties of Sweet Pepper (*Capsicum annuum* L.) of the Campania Region, Southern Italy
Reprinted from: *Antioxidants* **2020**, *9*, 556, doi:10.3390/antiox9060556 45

Nawel Benbouguerra, Tristan Richard, Cédric Saucier and François Garcia
Voltammetric Behavior, Flavanol and Anthocyanin Contents, and Antioxidant Capacity of Grape Skins and Seeds during Ripening (*Vitis vinifera var. Merlot, Tannat,* and *Syrah*)
Reprinted from: *Antioxidants* **2020**, *9*, 800, doi:10.3390/antiox9090800 61

Giulia Costanzo, Maria Rosaria Iesce, Daniele Naviglio, Martina Ciaravolo, Ermenegilda Vitale and Carmen Arena
Comparative Studies on Different *Citrus* Cultivars: A Revaluation of Waste Mandarin Components
Reprinted from: *Antioxidants* **2020**, *9*, 517, doi:10.3390/antiox9060517 81

Danuta Zielińska and Marcin Turemko
Electroactive Phenolic Contributors and Antioxidant Capacity of Flesh and Peel of 11 Apple Cultivars Measured by Cyclic Voltammetry and HPLC–DAD–MS/MS
Reprinted from: *Antioxidants* **2020**, *9*, 1054, doi:10.3390/antiox9111054 93

Celia Vincent, Tania Mesa and Sergi Munne-Bosch
Identification of a New Variety of Avocados (*Persea americana* Mill. CV. Bacon) with High Vitamin E and Impact of Cold Storage on Tocochromanols Composition
Reprinted from: *Antioxidants* **2020**, *9*, 403, doi:10.3390/antiox9050403 111

Karolina Jakubczyk, Justyna Kałduńska, Joanna Kochman and Katarzyna Janda
Chemical Profile and Antioxidant Activity of the Kombucha Beverage Derived from White, Green, Black and Red Tea
Reprinted from: *Antioxidants* **2020**, *9*, 447, doi:10.3390/antiox9050447 125

José Ramón Acosta-Motos, Laura Noguera-Vera, Gregorio Barba-Espín, Abel Piqueras and José A. Hernández
Antioxidant Metabolism and Chlorophyll Fluorescence during the Acclimatisation to Ex Vitro Conditions of Micropropagated *Stevia rebaudiana* Bertoni Plants
Reprinted from: *Antioxidants* **2019**, *8*, 615, doi:10.3390/antiox8120615 . . . . **141**

Julián Lozano-Castellón, Anna Vallverdú-Queralt, José Fernando Rinaldi de Alvarenga, Montserrat Illán, Xavier Torrado-Prat and Rosa Maria Lamuela-Raventós
Domestic Sautéing with EVOO: Change in the Phenolic Profile
Reprinted from: *Antioxidants* **2020**, *9*, 77, doi:10.3390/antiox9010077 . . . . **157**

Valentina Melini, Francesca Melini and Rita Acquistucci
Phenolic Compounds and Bioaccessibility Thereof in Functional Pasta
Reprinted from: *Antioxidants* **2020**, *9*, 343, doi:10.3390/antiox9040343 . . . . **169**

Nabeelah Bibi Sadeer, Domenico Montesano, Stefania Albrizio, Gokhan Zengin and Mohamad Fawzi Mahomoodally
The Versatility of Antioxidant Assays in Food Science and Safety—Chemistry, Applications, Strengths, and Limitations
Reprinted from: *Antioxidants* **2020**, *9*, 709, doi:0.3390/antiox9080709 . . . . **199**

Muhammad Imran, Fereshteh Ghorat, Iahtisham Ul-Haq, Habib Ur-Rehman, Farhan Aslam, Mojtaba Heydari, Mohammad Ali Shariati, Eleonora Okuskhanova, Zhanibek Yessimbekov, Muthu Thiruvengadam, Mohammad Hashem Hashempur and Maksim Rebezov
Lycopene as a Natural Antioxidant Used to Prevent Human Health Disorders
Reprinted from: *Antioxidants* **2020**, *9*, 706, doi:0.3390/antiox9080706 . . . . **239**

Shlomit Odes-Barth, Marina Khanin, Karin Linnewiel-Hermoni, Yifat Miller, Karina Abramov, Joseph Levy and Yoav Sharoni
Inhibition of Osteoclast Differentiation by Carotenoid Derivatives through Inhibition of the NF-κB Pathway
Reprinted from: *Antioxidants* **2020**, *9*, 1167, doi:10.3390/antiox9111167 . . . . **267**

Xiao-Yu Xu, Jie Zheng, Jin-Ming Meng, Ren-You Gan, Qian-Qian Mao, Ao Shang, Bang-Yan Li, Xin-Lin Wei and Hua-Bin Li
Effects of Food Processing on In Vivo Antioxidant and Hepatoprotective Properties of Green Tea Extracts
Reprinted from: *Antioxidants* **2019**, *8*, 572, doi:10.3390/antiox8120572 . . . . **283**

Elena Lima-Cabello, Juan D. Alché, Sonia Morales-Santana, Alfonso Clemente and Jose C. Jimenez-Lopez
Narrow-Leafed Lupin (*Lupinus angustifolius* L.) Seeds Gamma-Conglutin is an Anti-Inflammatory Protein Promoting Insulin Resistance Improvement and Oxidative Stress Amelioration in PANC-1 Pancreatic Cell-Line
Reprinted from: *Antioxidants* **2020**, *9*, 12, doi:0.3390/antiox9010012 . . . . **297**

Taekil Eom, Ekyune Kim and Ju-Sung Kim
In Vitro Antioxidant, Antiinflammation, and Anticancer Activities and Anthraquinone Content from *Rumex crispus* Root Extract and Fractions
Reprinted from: *Antioxidants* **2020**, *9*, 726, doi:10.3390/antiox9080726 . . . . **317**

Md Badrul Alam, Arif Ahmed, Syful Islam, Hee-Jeong Choi, Md Abdul Motin, Sunghwan Kim and Sang-Han Lee
Phytochemical Characterization of *Dillenia indica* L. Bark by Paper Spray Ionization-Mass Spectrometry and Evaluation of Its Antioxidant Potential Against t-BHP-Induced Oxidative Stress in RAW 264.7 Cells
Reprinted from: *Antioxidants* **2020**, *9*, 1099, doi:10.3390/antiox9111099 331

Luana Izzo, Yelko Rodríguez-Carrasco, Severina Pacifico, Luigi Castaldo, Alfonso Narváez and Alberto Ritieni
Colon Bioaccessibility under In Vitro Gastrointestinal Digestion of a Red Cabbage Extract Chemically Profiled through UHPLC-Q-Orbitrap HRMS
Reprinted from: *Antioxidants* **2020**, *9*, 955, doi:10.3390/antiox9100955 347

Sabina Lachowicz, Michał Świeca and Ewa Pejcz
Improvement of Health-Promoting Functionality of Rye Bread by Fortification with Free and Microencapsulated Powders from *Amelanchier alnifolia* Nutt
Reprinted from: *Antioxidants* **2020**, *9*, 614, doi:10.3390/antiox9070614 365

Paulina Keska, Sascha Rohn, Michał Halagarda and Karolina M. Wójciak
Peptides from Different Carcass Elements of Organic and Conventional Pork—Potential Source of Antioxidant Activity
Reprinted from: *Antioxidants* **2020**, *9*, 835, doi:10.3390/antiox9090835 389

About the Editors

Isabel Seiquer is a senior researcher at Estación Experimental del Zaidín, a research center from the Spanish National Research Council (CSIC). Dr. Seiquer has more than 30 years of professional experinece dedicated to the study of diverse topics related to the areas of Nutrition and Food Science and Technology. Her research activity has been focused on the effects of food components on the metabolism of minerals and proteins, the bioavailability of nutrients and the antioxidant properties of new compounds formed during food processing and digestive processes. She has addressed different aspects related to oxidative stress, through in vitro, cell cultures and in vivo assays. Moreover, her research interest also deals with animal nutrition and the study of obtaining food products with high quality preserving the environment. She is coauthor of more than 100 publications in international peer-reviewed journals.

José M. Palma Palma is Research Professor of the Spanish National Research Council (CSIC), with expertise in antioxidants and free radicals in plant systems. With more than 150 peer-reviewed research papers published, he has also been editor of five books and several Special Issues of a number of international impact journals. At present, he is involved in the investigation of the interactions between nitric oxide, hydrogen sulfide and antioxidants during fruit ripening and pot-harvest. He leads the research group "Antioxidants, Free Radicals and Nitric Oxide in Biotechnology, Food and Agriculture" at Estación Experimental del Zaidín (EEZ), CSIC, Granada, Spain. He was also Deputy Director and Acting Director of the EEZ (CSIC) during the period 2007–2014.

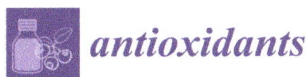

Editorial

To Be or Not to Be... An Antioxidant? That Is the Question

José M. Palma [1,*] and Isabel Seiquer [2,*]

[1] Department of Biochemistry, Cell and Molecular Biology of Plants, Estación Experimental del Zaidín, CSIC, 18008 Granada, Spain
[2] Department of Physiology and Biochemistry of Animal Nutrition, Estación Experimental del Zaidín, CSIC, Armilla, 18100 Granada, Spain
* Correspondence: josemanuel.palma@eez.csic.es (J.M.P.); isabel.seiquer@eez.csic.es (I.S.);
Tel.: +34-958-181600 (J.M.P.); +34-958-572757 (I.S.); Fax: +34-958-181609 (J.M.P.); +34-958-572753 (I.S.)

Received: 25 November 2020; Accepted: 2 December 2020; Published: 5 December 2020

The concept of antioxidants refers to a substance with the capacity to either directly scavenge or indirectly prevent the formation of pro-oxidant molecules, basically associated to the so called reactive oxygen species (ROS). Considering the cell/tissue target, the picture is quite different. Thus, in animal tissues, the main source for ROS production is the mitochondria, whereas in plants, chloroplast is the most important organelle to generate ROS, including singlet oxygen ($^1O_2$), superoxide radicals ($O_2^{\bullet-}$) or hydrogen peroxide (H_2O_2). Accordingly, and due to the respective peculiarities, each organelle/cell/tissue has its own antioxidant machinery to overcome the deleterious effects of their internal ROS levels and production.

The real situation is that our cells are continually threatened by ROS, that disturb their normal and pacific living. Oxidative stress arises from an augmented ROS generation, but also from a decay of the antioxidant defense system, leading to the imbalance between the occurrence of reactive species and the organism's ability to counteract them. Oxidative stress is responsible for cell damage, sometimes irrecoverable, which is further implicated in a cascade of degenerative diseases, cardiovascular diseases, cancer and aging. Therefore, in this dangerous situation, the endogenous defense system (which includes antioxidant enzymes and non-enzymatic compounds such as glutathione, vitamins, coenzyme Q and others) needs external help to lower/modulate the negative effects of excessive ROS. This exogenous help is represented by the dietary antioxidants, i.e., food antioxidants, most of them present in fruits and vegetables or other sources from the plant kingdom.

Oxidative stress is also suffered by plants, in which illumination conditions and excess of light may lead to ROS formation. Chloroplasts contain a well-equipped battery of both enzymatic and non-enzymatic antioxidants to reestablish the initial balanced state and to avoid a situation of oxidative stress. In this response mainly participate the molecular antioxidants α-tocopherol, carotenoids and ascorbate, the enzyme superoxide dismutase and the ascorbate glutathione cycle (AGC) which involves ascorbate, glutathione, NADPH and four redox enzymes. Some of these antioxidants, which in plants are required in great amounts to cope against the stressful conditions, have vitamin properties and may function as dietary antioxidants for animal and human beings. Thus, α-tocopherol is the chemical nature of vitamin E, whereas β-carotene is precursor of vitamin A once the plant carotene is assimilated by our metabolism; ascorbate is vitamin C, one of the most powerful antioxidants and has the ability to directly scavenge most ROS. Besides this antioxidant team, plants contain a huge amount of secondary metabolites with potential antioxidant activity.

As indicated above, the antioxidants are usually required in high quantities to neutralize the oxidative effects of ROS in plants. This is in contradiction with the concept of vitamins in the animal/human scenario, which is considered as an organic molecule that is essential in small quantities for the proper functioning of the organism's metabolism. Commonly, in animals and humans these essential micronutrients are insufficiently or not synthesized and they need to obtain them through the diet. Whereas in plant systems, α-tocopherol and carotenoids are basically used as singlet oxygen scavengers, thus protecting cells against this ROS, in animal cells vitamins A and E play important roles regulating the redox homeostasis in a series of physiological processes. Thus, vitamin A is crucial for vision, growth and development, and for protecting epithelium and mucus integrity in the respiratory, urinary and gastro intestinal tract. Likewise, vitamin E seems to prevent cardiovascular episodes, neurodegenerative disease, macular degeneration and cancer. Little amounts of such lipophilic substances are necessary to carry out their antioxidant role, but the excessive intake may lead to unwanted redox imbalances which may provoke some disorders, and their use as complements is sometimes under debate.

Ascorbic acid (vitamin C) is synthesized in the majority of living beings, excepting primates (including humans), guinea pigs, bats and some birds. This makes our dependency of external vitamin C provision (basically plant products) strictly necessary. In animals and humans, vitamin C stimulates enzymes involved in the biosynthesis of collagen, catecholamines, L-carnitine, cholesterol, and amino acids, as well as in the hormonal activation, histamine detoxification, and phagocytosis by leukocytes, among others. In addition, vitamin C is linked to the reduction of incidence of a series of pathologies related to cancer, blood pressure and cardiovascular diseases prevention, immunity dysfunction, tissue regeneration, nervous system, etc. A lack of vitamin C causes scurvy, which leads to fragility of blood vessels and damage of connective tissue. Then, a failure in the collagen production takes place that may end in death as a consequence of the general collapse.

In plants, ascorbate is synthesized in mitochondria but its main target as powerful antioxidant is the chloroplast, where besides scavenging diverse ROS, as referred above, it is integrated in the AGC for hydrogen peroxide removal. Besides, ascorbate can regenerate α-tocopherol and participates in the xanthophylls' cycle, one type of carotenoids. Thus, due to its functionality, ascorbate is necessary in high amounts (as α-tocopherol and carotenoids are), not only in chloroplasts but also in other plant organelles. An example of the dualism antioxidant/vitamin and regarding ascorbate is as follows: (i) one pepper fruit from the California type (about 250 g) contains 350–375 mg [1]; (ii) one pepper plant is able to yield about 10 Kg fruits, which means around 14 g vitamin C, only in fruits, without considering leaves and other organs (pepper is a factory for vitamin C production); (iii) however, our daily requirements are about 80 mg of this vitamin; (iv) thus, one such pepper plant can satisfy the daily requirements of about 175 people. Why such a difference? The common physiological conditions imposed by light in plants, from an antioxidant-consuming perspective, are much more stressful than those operating in the majority of our physiological dysfunctions and diseases.

Following this rationale about the different viewpoints depending on the target organism, either human, animal or plant, this Special Issue will cover the same question posed in the title and developed on above for antioxidant/vitamin concepts. Thus, the concept of antioxidants in the transition from the field to the body, either human or animal, is exemplified using antocyanins as the case study [2]. Several plant materials have been used as vehicle to provide antioxidants for our diet. Thus, pepper fruits have been shown as one of the most important ascorbate sources, although the global provision of vitamin C upon the pepper intake depends on the variety and the ripening stage of fruits [1,3]. Moreover, in some cases, this antioxidant provision is also complemented by some functional compounds which, in the case of pepper, includes capsaicin, an alkaloid exclusive of this species with diverse therapeutic properties [1]. Variety and ripening are also relevant cues in the antioxidant content (ascorbate, polyphenols, flavonoids) of other noteworthy fruits in our diet, such as the *Citrus* species (Mandarin, Kumquat and Clementine), apples and grapes, and this antioxidant capacity is extensive to any of their parts, either pulp, seeds and peel/skin [4–6]. Likewise, fruits are also sources of other important antioxidants, i.e., α-tocopherol (vitamin E) and tocochromanols. It was proved that avocados are very rich in these compounds, always depending on the variety and the storage conditions [7]. Plants are also used to brew antioxidant-enriched beverages like tea. The type of tea, either white, green, black and red has been found to be essential for the preparation of Kombucha, a beverage obtained from fermented tea [8].

Many plant products are used for the food industry, giving rise to a huge diversity of manufactured goods undergoing a series of processes, which do not necessarily imply transformation. This is the case for stevia, which is a sweetener directly extracted from the original plant without any transformation. In this Special Issue, it is reported that the antioxidant metabolism of stevia is influenced by the acclimation of plants when they are exposed to ex vitro conditions [9].

Virgin olive oil deserves a special mention as a particular source of antioxidants [10], greatly attributed to its high content in polyphenols. Although the phenolic profile of extra virgin olive oil (EVOO) is modified when cooking, EVOO maintains its nutritional parameters and properties within the EU's health claims [11].

In the chapter of transformed products, pasta is one of the most paradigmatic foods obtained from wheat. Pasta can be used as a functional product since it is often consumed and it contains certain levels of phenolic compounds. Studies of bioaccesibility and bioavailability of such antioxidants can help formulating pasta where by-products could be even used as functional ingredients after the application of some pre-processing technologies [12].

Undoubtedly, all screening and quantification assays of antioxidants contained in natural or manufactured foods should be updated to gain accuracy, liability and reproducibility, so the nutritional standards can be fit through the use of consensual methods and approaches. Such a critical review of existing assays and a prospect analysis has been achieved in this Special Issue [13].

This volume also includes a series of articles focused on the role of food antioxidants in the prevention of chronic diseases and health disorders. Thus, the relevance of lycopene, a carotenoid which is abundant in tomato, has been highlighted in certain diseases including diabetes mellitus, cardiac complications, cancer insurgences, oxidative stress-mediated malfunctions, inflammatory, skin and bone diseases, as well as reproductive, hepatic and neural disorders [14]. It has been also reported that carotenoid derivatives inhibit osteoclast differentiation through the partial inhibition of the NF-ßB pathway. Additionally, they can synergistically inhibit osteoclast differentiation as well in the presence of curcumin and carnosic acid [15].

This goodness of natural food for our health is in some cases undermined by processing. Thus, in the analysis of the antioxidant activity of green tea once it was processed, it was found that food processing does not always have positive effect on products destined for human consumption [16]. In this line, a gamma-conglutin found in narrow-leafed lupin showed anti-inflammatory properties through the promotion of insulin resistance and amelioration of the potential oxidative stress underwent in PANC-1 pancreatic cells [17]. Likewise, using Raw 264.7 murine, it was found that root cell extracts from curly dock (*Rumex crispus*) displayed anti-inflammatory and anticancer activities, possibly due to the anthraquinone present in this plant material [18]. In the same animal model, it was also demonstrated the antioxidant potential of elephant apple (*Dillenia indica* L.) bark against *tert*-butyl-hydroperoxide)-induced oxidative stress [19].

Strategies of (micro)encapsulation of materials and how they can contribute to benefit human health are another trend which is gaining attention nowadays. The use of encapsulating red cabbage extracts to improve the bioaccesibility of their polyphenols has been reported to be a good choice to counteract the diseases associated to oxidative stress episodes [20]. Similarly, it was reported that microencapsulation of Saskatoon Berry fruit (*Amelanchier alnifolia*) might be a promising practice with positive impact in the functionality of rye bread [21].

Research on antioxidant capacity of foods coming from animal sources has been also included in this Special Issue. By making comparisons of the meat origin, either conventional or organic, from selected elements of the pork carcass (ham, loin and shoulder), it was observed that meat products from conventional rearing systems had the best antioxidant properties with respect to antioxidant peptides. This discovery could be addressed to the human health field but also to the related industry [22].

Globally, this volume compiles a series of articles focused on the potential contribution of consuming certain food products for the human welfare. The basis of such benefits is mainly related to the antioxidant contribution of those products, but their content of other health promoting compounds cannot be discarded. This drives our attention to investigate those products and their chemical composition to convert them into functional foods with nutraceutical properties. Much research is necessary to understand the specific mechanisms by which many secondary plant metabolites act over our physiology in a beneficial manner and how they interact to prevent a number of human disorders.

Funding: This research received no external funding.

Conflicts of Interest: The authors declare no conflict of interest

References

1. Palma, J.M.; Terán, F.; Contreras-Ruiz, A.; Rodríguez-Ruiz, M.; Corpas, F.J. Antioxidant profile of pepper (*Capsicum annuum* L.) fruits containing diverse levels of capsaicinoids. *Antioxidants* **2020**, *9*, 878. [CrossRef] [PubMed]
2. Bendokas, V.; Stanys, V.; Mažeikienė, I.; Trumbeckaite, S.; Baniene, R.; Liobikas, J. Anthocyanins: From the field to the antioxidants in the body. *Antioxidants* **2020**, *9*, 819. [CrossRef] [PubMed]
3. Fratianni, F.; d'Acierno, A.; Cozzolino, A.; Spigno, P.; Riccardi, R.; Raimo, F.; Pane, C.; Zaccardelli, M.; Tranchida Lombardo, V.; Tucci, M.; et al. Biochemical characterization of traditional varieties of sweet pepper (*Capsicum annuum* L.) of the Campania region, Southern Italy. *Antioxidants* **2020**, *9*, 556. [CrossRef] [PubMed]
4. Nawel Benbouguerra, N.; Richard, T.; Saucier, C.; Garcia, F. Voltammetric behavior, flavanol and anthocyanin contents, and antioxidant capacity of grape skins and seeds during ripening (*Vitis vinifera* var. Merlot, Tannat, and Syrah). *Antioxidants* **2020**, *9*, 800. [CrossRef] [PubMed]
5. Costanzo, G.; Iesce, M.R.; Naviglio, D.; Ciaravolo, M.; Vitale, E.; Arena, C. Comparative studies on different citrus cultivars: A revaluation of waste mandarin components. *Antioxidants* **2020**, *9*, 517. [CrossRef] [PubMed]
6. Zielińska, D.; Turemko, M. Electroactive phenolic contributors and antioxidant capacity of flesh and peel of 11 apple cultivars measured by Cyclic Voltammetry and HPLC-DAD5 MS/MS. *Antioxidants* **2020**, *9*, 1054. [CrossRef]
7. Vincent, C.; Mesa, T.; Munné-Bosch, S. Identification of a new variety of avocados (*Persea americana* Mill. CV. Bacon) with high vitamin E and impact of cold storage on tocochromanols composition. *Antioxidants* **2020**, *9*, 403. [CrossRef]
8. Jakubczyk, K.; Kałduńska, J.; Kochman, J.; Janda, K. Chemical profile and antioxidant activity of the Kombucha beverage derived from white, green, black and red tea. *Antioxidants* **2020**, *9*, 447. [CrossRef]
9. Acosta-Motos, J.R.; Noguera-Vera, L.; Barba-Espín, G.; Piqueras, A.; Hernández, J.A. Antioxidant metabolism and chlorophyll fluorescence during the acclimatisation to ex vitro conditions of micropropagated *Stevia rebaudiana* bertoni plants. *Antioxidants* **2019**, *8*, 615. [CrossRef]
10. Borges, T.H.; Serna, A.; López, L.C.; Lara, L.; Nieto, R.; Seiquer, I. Composition and antioxidant properties of Spanish extra virgin olive oil regarding cultivar, harvest year and crop stage. *Antioxidants* **2019**, *8*, 217. [CrossRef]
11. Lozano-Castellón, J.; Vallverdú-Queralt, A.; Rinaldi de Alvarenga, J.F.; Illán, M.; Torrado-Prat, X.; Lamuela-Raventós, R.M. Domestic sautéing with EVOO: Change in the phenolic profile. *Antioxidants* **2020**, *9*, 77. [CrossRef] [PubMed]
12. Melini, V.; Melini, F.; Acquistucci, R. Phenolic compounds and bioaccessibility thereof in functional pasta. *Antioxidants* **2020**, *9*, 343. [CrossRef] [PubMed]
13. Sadeer, N.B.; Montesano, D.; Albrizio, S.; Zengin, G.; Mahomoodally, M.F. The versatility of antioxidant assays in food science and safety—Chemistry, applications, strengths, and limitations. *Antioxidants* **2020**, *9*, 709. [CrossRef] [PubMed]
14. Imran, M.; Ghorat, F.; Ul-Haq, I.; Ur-Rehman, H.; Aslam, F.; Heydari, M.; Shariati, M.A.; Okuskhanova, E.; Yessimbekov, Z.; Thiruvengadam, M.; et al. Lycopene as a natural antioxidant used to prevent human health disorders. *Antioxidants* **2020**, *9*, 706. [CrossRef]
15. Odes-Barth, S.; Khanin, M.; Linnewiel-Hermoni, K.; Miller, Y.; Abramov, K.; Levy, J.; Sharoni, Y. Inhibition of osteoclast differentiation by carotenoid derivatives through inhibition of the NF-ƙB pathway. *Antioxidants* **2020**, *9*, 1167. [CrossRef]

16. Xu, X.Y.; Zheng, J.; Meng, J.M.; Gan, R.Y.; Mao, Q.Q.; Shang, A.; Li, B.Y.; Wei, X.L.; Li, H.B. Effects of food processing on in vivo antioxidant and hepatoprotective properties of green tea extracts. *Antioxidants* **2019**, *8*, 572. [CrossRef]
17. Lima-Cabello, E.; Alché, J.D.; Morales-Santana, S.; Clemente, A.; Jimenez-Lopez, J.C. Narrow-leafed lupin (*Lupinus angustifolius* L.) seeds gamma-conglutin is an anti-inflammatory protein promoting insulin resistance improvement and oxidative stress amelioration in PANC-1 pancreatic cell-line. *Antioxidants* **2020**, *9*, 12. [CrossRef]
18. Eom, T.; Kim, E.; Kim, J.S. In vitro antioxidant, antiinflammation, and anticancer activities and anthraquinone content from *Rumex crispus* root extract and fractions. *Antioxidants* **2020**, *9*, 726. [CrossRef]
19. Alam, M.B.; Islam, S.; Ahmed, A.; Choi, H.J.; Motin, M.D.; Kim, S.; Lee, S.H. Phytochemical characterization of *Dillenia indica* L. bark by paper spray ionization mass spectrometry and evaluation of its antioxidant potential against t-BHP-induced oxidative stress. *Antioxidants* **2020**, *9*, 1099. [CrossRef]
20. Izzo, L.; Rodríguez-Carrasco, Y.; Pacifico, S.; Castaldo, L.; Narváez, A.; Ritieni, A. Colon bioaccessibility under in vitro gastrointestinal digestion of a red cabbage extract chemically profiled through UHPLC-Q-Orbitrap HRMS. *Antioxidants* **2020**, *9*, 955. [CrossRef]
21. Lachowicz, S.; Świeca, M.; Pejcz, E. Improvement of health-promoting functionality of rye bread by fortification with free and microencapsulated powders from *Amelanchier alnifolia* Nutt. *Antioxidants* **2020**, *9*, 614. [CrossRef] [PubMed]
22. Kęska, P.; Rohn, S.; Halagarda, M.; Wójciak, K.M. Peptides from different carcass elements of organic and conventional pork—Potential source of antioxidant activity. *Antioxidants* **2020**, *9*, 835. [CrossRef] [PubMed]

Publisher's Note: MDPI stays neutral with regard to jurisdictional claims in published maps and institutional affiliations.

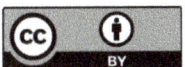

© 2020 by the authors. Licensee MDPI, Basel, Switzerland. This article is an open access article distributed under the terms and conditions of the Creative Commons Attribution (CC BY) license (http://creativecommons.org/licenses/by/4.0/).

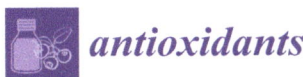

Article

Antioxidant Profile of Pepper (*Capsicum annuum* L.) Fruits Containing Diverse Levels of Capsaicinoids

José M. Palma [1,*], Fátima Terán [1,2], Alba Contreras-Ruiz [1,3], Marta Rodríguez-Ruiz [4] and Francisco J. Corpas [1]

1. Group of Antioxidant, Free Radical and Nitric Oxide in Biotechnology, Food and Agriculture, Department Biochemistry, Cell and Molecular Biology of Plants, Estación Experimental del Zaidín, CSIC, 18008 Granada, Spain; fatimateca26@gmail.com (F.T.); acontreras@iata.csic.es (A.C.-R.); javier.corpas@eez.csic.es (F.J.C.)
2. Department Agricultural and Environmental Sciences, Universitat Jaume I, 12071 Castelló de la Plana, Spain
3. Instituto de Agroquímica y Tecnología de Alimentos, IATA-CSIC, 46980 Paterna, Valencia, Spain
4. Laboratório de Fisiologia do Desenvolvimento Vegetal, Instituto de Biociências, Universidade de São Paulo, Cidade Universitária, São Paulo 05508-900, SP, Brazil; martarodriguezruiz@usp.br
* Correspondence: josemanuel.palma@eez.csic.es; Tel.: +34-958-181600; Fax: +34-958-181609

Received: 30 July 2020; Accepted: 14 September 2020; Published: 17 September 2020

Abstract: *Capsicum* is the genus where a number of species and varieties have pungent features due to the exclusive content of capsaicinoids such as capsaicin and dihydrocapsaicin. In this work, the main enzymatic and non-enzymatic systems in pepper fruits from four varieties with different pungent capacity have been investigated at two ripening stages. Thus, a sweet pepper variety (Melchor) from California-type fruits and three autochthonous Spanish varieties which have different pungency levels were used, including Piquillo, Padrón and Alegría riojana. The capsaicinoids contents were determined in the pericarp and placenta from fruits, showing that these phenyl-propanoids were mainly localized in placenta. The activity profiles of catalase, total and isoenzymatic superoxide dismutase (SOD), the enzymes of the ascorbate–glutathione cycle (AGC) and four NADP-dehydrogenases indicate that some interaction with capsaicinoid metabolism seems to occur. Among the results obtained on enzymatic antioxidants, the role of Fe-SOD and the glutathione reductase from the AGC is highlighted. Additionally, it was found that ascorbate and glutathione contents were higher in those pepper fruits which displayed the greater contents of capsaicinoids. Taken together, all these data indicate that antioxidants may contribute to preserve capsaicinoids metabolism to maintain their functionality in a framework where NADPH is perhaps playing an essential role.

Keywords: ascorbate; ascorbate–glutathione cycle; capsaicin; catalase; dihydrocapsaicin; glutathione; NADP-dehydrogenases; superoxide dismutase

1. Introduction

Pepper (*Capsicum annuum* L.) fruits are one of the most consumed vegetables worldwide. Pepper fruits are mainly characterized by their high vitamin C and A and mineral contents [1–8]. Thus, about 60–80 g intake of fruits per day can provide 100 and 25% of recommended daily amounts of vitamin C and A, respectively [5,9]. Besides, this horticultural product contains important levels of other health-promoting substances with antioxidant capacity, and they include carotenoids, flavonoids and other polyphenols, among others [1,10–12].

The diversity of pepper varieties is quite high and they are basically differentiated by shape, size, pulp (pericarp) thickness and final color at the ripe stages. This diversity is also mirrored by the number of common names to designate pepper fruits which, in most cases, are used very locally. From culinary and gastronomic points of view, pepper fruits are mainly classified as sweet and hot depending on the absence or presence of capsaicin, respectively [4,5,12,13]. Within the sweet pepper (also amply known as bell pepper) varieties, three main types are distinguished according to their shape and size: California, Lamuyo and Dulce italiano. Hot peppers include the highest number of varieties and names including chili, habanero, jalapeño, paprika, chipotle and the Spanish Alegría riojana, Padrón and Piquillo used in this work, among others.

Capsaicin is exclusive to the genus *Capsicum* and is responsible for the pungency trait. According to the pungent level, pepper fruits are ranked on the so-called Scoville scale which assigns a score to each fruit variety. In this scale, the highest value for the most pungent pepper fruit variety is around 3×10^6, pure capsaicin being 16×10^6 [14–18]. Capsaicin is an alkaloid with a phenyl-propanoid nature which has given rise to a family of capsaicinoids composed of at least 22 primary compounds. Out of them, capsaicin and dihydrocapsaicin contribute to about 90–95% of total capsaicinoids present in most hot pepper varieties [19,20]. These compounds are mainly localized in the epidermal vacuoles of the placenta and the septum from fruits, and they can be separated and identified through the use of high-performance liquid chromatography associated with electrospray ionization mass spectrometry (HPLC-ESI/MS) [19,21,22]. Capsaicin is useful for pepper plants to avoid biting by insects and other animals since this chemical has repellent/insecticide capacity [23–27]. From a pharmacological perspective, the research carried out so far has shown that capsaicinoids, particularly capsaicin, have a diversity of biological and physiological functions in vitro, so they play roles as antioxidants, stimulants of the energetic metabolism, fat accumulating suppressors, anti-inflammatories, neurostimulants and apoptosis-alleviating agents in neurodegenerative disorders [20,28–30]. Regarding the mechanism of action, capsaicinoids act on a family of ion channels known as transient receptor potential (TRP) channels which, in mammals, are framed within the subtype TRP Vanilloid (TRPV1) [31,32]. It has been also found that in many types of cancers, the proapoptotic activity of capsaicin is also mediated by this TRPV, and the activation of the p53 tumor suppressing protein by a phosphorylation process is induced by capsaicin [33,34].

Another relevant feature of pepper fruits is the ripening process, visibly characterized by a shift in the fruit color from green to red, yellow, orange or purple depending on the variety. This event implies chlorophyll breakdown and synthesis of new carotenoids and anthocyanins, emission of organic volatiles, new protein synthesis and cleavage of existing ones and cell wall softening, among others [5,7,35–39]. Relevant differences between the transcriptomes from green immature and ripe pepper fruits have been also reported, involving thousands of genes [8,40] and references therein. From a redox viewpoint, it has been found that reactive oxygen species (ROS) metabolism is also affected during fruit ripening, leading to major changes in total soluble reducing equivalents and the antioxidant capacity in fruits [41]. The profile of the major non-enzymatic antioxidants, including ascorbate, glutathione, carotenoids and polyphenols, has been followed during ripening in pepper fruits [4,11,12,42–46], but less is known on how enzymatic antioxidants evolve with this physiological process. These enzyme systems basically include superoxide dismutase (SOD), catalase (CAT) and the ascorbate–glutathione cycle as the primary defense barriers against ROS, and some NADP-dehydrogenases as a secondary system to help the antioxidative enzymatic block. The profile of these enzymes throughout fruit ripening has been mostly carried out in sweet pepper [4,11,45,46], but scarce references have been reported on how those antioxidant enzymatic systems behave in the ripening of hot varieties [47–49]. Accordingly, using pepper varieties containing increasing capsaicin and dihydrocapsaicin contents, this work was aimed at characterizing the profile of the main antioxidants and their potential interaction with capsaicinoids during fruit ripening. This could provide a biochemical support and an added value for the particular features of each Spanish autochthonous cultivar that is included in the European Register of protected designations of origin for these horticultural products.

2. Materials and Methods

2.1. Plant Material

Fruits from four pepper (*Capsicum annuum* L.) varieties were used in this work: California-type (sweet), obtained from plants grown in plastic-covered greenhouses (Zeraim Iberica/Syngenta Seeds, Ltd., El Ejido, Almería, Spain); Padrón (mild hot), provided by the Regulatory Council of Denomination of Origin "Pemento de Herbón" (Herbón, Coruña, Spain) and Piquillo (slightly hot) and Alegría riojana (quite hot), both provided by the Regulatory Council of Denomination of Origin "Pimiento del Piquillo-Lodosa" (Navarra, Spain). Padrón, Piquillo and Alegría riojana (onwards Alegría) fruits were obtained from plants grown in orchards under the local conditions. In all varieties, fruits at both green and red ripe stages were analyzed. Both stages were set according to marketing and consuming preferences as indicated by the growers. Green fruits did not show any ripening symptoms, mainly color shift, and they were totally green. Red fruits were harvested after several days they underwent the color change *in planta*. In all cases, fruits did not display any apparent damages. Figure 1A shows representative pictures of the different varieties used in this work, and in Table 1, comparative data on the mean fresh weight (g) of each type of fruit are given. Fresh weight data were obtained from 10 fruits of each variety at both maturation stages. After harvesting, in all fruits set for analyses, the pericarp and placenta (once seeds were discarded) were separated (Figure 1B), and each one was cut into small cubes (approximately 3–5 mm/side), frozen under liquid nitrogen and then stored at −80 °C until use. All biochemical parameters were determined thrice from 5 fruits in each variety and at the two ripening stages. As a whole, each mean was obtained from 15 assays.

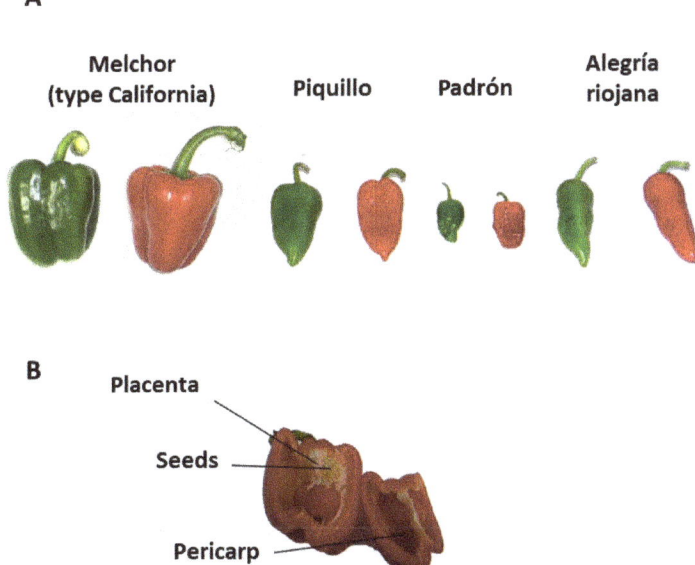

Figure 1. Representative pictures of plant materials used in this work. (**A**) Fruits from the four varieties at two ripening stages: green and ripe red. Melchor is a variety of California-type sweet pepper fruit. Piquillo Padrón and Alegría riojana contain different levels of capsaicin with the sequence Piquillo <<< Padrón < Alegría riojana. (**B**) Different parts of the pepper fruit.

Table 1. Fresh weight (FW) of whole fruits from four pepper varieties at two ripening stages.

Variety	FW Green (g)	FW Ripe Red (g)
Melchor	245.22 ± 13.41	212.05 ± 12.45
Piquillo	43.50 ± 2.62	40.91 ± 6.69
Padrón	16.19 ± 1.91	24.37 ± 1.58
Alegría	43.78 ± 1.94	36.13 ± 2.38

Data are the means ± SEM of ten fruits from each variety and ripening stage.

2.2. Determination of Capsaicin and Dihydrocapsaicin by High-Performance Liquid Chromatography-Electrospray Mass Spectrometry (HPLC-ES/MS)

Samples were ground into a powder under liquid N_2 and using an IKA® A11 Basic mill (IKA Laboratories Inc., Tirat Carmel, Israel). For each sample, three extractions were made as follows. Plant materials (0.5 g powder) were suspended into 2.0 mL acetonitrile (AcN) containing 100 ppm N-[(3,4-dimethoxyphenyl)methyl]-4-methyl-octanamide (DMBMO), as an internal standard. Mixtures were incubated in the following sequence: 1 h at room temperature and darkness with continuous shaking; 65 °C and darkness for 1 h and short shakings every 15 min; and 1 h at room temperature in the dark. Then, samples were centrifuged at 16,000× *g* and room temperature for 15 min. Supernatants were passed through 0.22 μm pore size polyvinylidene fluoride filters and were used for analysis through HPLC-ESI/MS with mode multiple reaction monitoring (MRM). An XBridge 2.1 × 10 mm pre-column and an XBridge 2.1 × 100 mm C18 3.5 μm column (Waters Corporation, Milford, MA, USA) were used connected to an Alliance 2695 HPLC system coupled to a Micromass Quattro micro API triple quadrupole mass spectrometer both obtained from the Waters Corporation. The chromatography was run at a flux of 0.3 mL/min with temperatures of 35 °C for the column and 5 °C for the auto-injector, with 5 μL being injected per sample. The gradient used was: 6 min with AcN:H_2O (60:40) containing 0.1% (*v/v*) formic acid; 10 + 5 min with AcN:H_2O (90:10); and 20 + 4 min with AcN:H_2O (60:40). Standard curves were prepared using pure capsaicin and dihydrocapsaicin (Cayman Chemical, Ann Arbor, MI, USA). Under these conditions, the retention time for capsaicin and dihydrocapsaicin was 1.88 and 2.24 min, respectively. The concentration of capsaicinoids was expressed as $\mu g\ g^{-1}$ of fresh weight (FW).

2.3. Detection and Quantification of Ascorbate, GSH and GSSG by High-Performance Liquid Chromatography-Electrospray Mass Spectrometry (LC-ES/MS)

Pericarps and placentas were ground under liquid N_2 with a pestle and a mortar. Then, 0.4 g of powdered tissues was suspended into 1 mL of 0.1 M HCl and spun for 20 min at 15,000× *g* and 4 °C. Supernatants were passed through polyvinylidene fluoride filters (0.22-μm pore size) and analyzed immediately. All procedures were performed at 4 °C with protection from light to prevent potential degradation of the metabolites. Samples were analyzed by liquid chromatography–electrospray/mass spectrometry (LC-ES/MS) using the HPLC system and mass spectrometer indicated above. HPLC runs were performed with an Atlantis® T3 3 μm 2.1 × 100 mm column (Waters Corporation). The MassLynx 4.1 software package (Waters Corporation) was used for the instrument control and collection, analysis and management of data. With this method, the simultaneous detection and quantification of ascorbate, reduced (GSH), and oxidized (GSSG) glutathione is achieved [7,50]. The analytes concentration was calculated with the use of external standards and expressed with reference to fresh weight (FW).

2.4. Preparation of Crude Extracts for Enzyme Activity

Protein extracts from pericarps and placentas were powdered under liquid nitrogen and then suspended in 0.1 M Tris-HCl buffer, pH 8.0, containing 1 mM EDTA, 0.1% (*v/v*) Triton X-100 and 10% (*v/v*) glycerol, in a final 1:1 (*w:v*) plant material/buffer ratio. Crude extracts were centrifuged at 15,000× *g* for 30 min and the supernatants were used for enzymatic assays.

2.5. Enzyme Activity Assays

All enzyme activities were determined using an Evolution 201 UV–visible spectrophotometer (Thermo Fisher Scientific, Waltham, MA, USA). Catalase (EC 1.11.1.6) activity was determined by following the H_2O_2 breakdown at 240 nm [51]. Ascorbate peroxidase (APX; EC 1.11.1.11) was monitored at 290 nm by plotting the initial ascorbate oxidation by H_2O_2 [52]. Monodehydroascorbate reductase (MDAR; EC 1.6.5.4) activity was assayed by following the monodehydroascorbate-dependent NADH oxidation. In these assays, monodehydroascorbate was generated through the ascorbate/ascorbate oxidase system as reported earlier [53]. The monodehydroascorbate-independent NADH oxidation rate (without ascorbate oxidase and ascorbate) was deducted from the monodehydroascorbate-dependent reaction. Dehydroascorbate reductase (DHAR, EC 1.8.5.1) activity was measured by monitoring at 265 nm the increase in ascorbate formation, with the use of a N_2-saturated buffer. The reaction rate was corrected by the non-enzymatic dehydroascorbate reduction through reduced glutathione (GSH). A 0.98 factor was also considered, due to the little contribution to the absorbance by oxidized glutathione (GSSG) [54]. Glutathione reductase (GR; EC 1.6.4.2) activity was analyzed by following at 340 nm the NADPH oxidation associated with the reduction of GSSG to GSH [55]. The GR reaction rate was corrected for the very small, non-enzymatic NADPH oxidation by GSSG.

Total SOD (EC 1.15.1.1) activity was determined by the ferricytochrome c reduction method, with the system xanthine/xanthine oxidase as a superoxide radical ($O_2^{·-}$) source. One activity unit was defined as the amount of protein necessary to inhibit 50% of the cytochrome c reduction [56]. For the analysis of the SOD isoenzyme profile, proteins from crude extracts were separated by vertical non-denaturing PAGEs on 10% acrylamide gels, using a Mini-Protean III Tetra Cell system (Bio-Rad Laboratories, Hercules, CA, USA). SOD isozymes were detected in the gels as acromatic bands over a purple background by a specific staining based in the photochemical reduction method of nitroblue tetrazolium (NBT) [57]. For the identification of the different SOD isozymes, before the staining procedure, pre-incubation of gels was carried out in the presence of specific inhibitors, either 5 mM KCN or 5 mM H_2O_2. Copper- and zinc-containing SODs (CuZn-SODs) are inhibited by both KCN and H_2O_2; iron-containing SODs (Fe-SODs) are inactivated by H_2O_2; and Mn-SODs are resistant to both inhibitors [58,59].

NADP-dependent dehydrogenase (NADP-DHs) activities were determined by recording the NADPH formation at 340 nm and 25 °C. The assay was performed in a reaction medium containing 50 mM HEPES [(4-(2-hydroxyethyl)-1-piperazineethanesulfonic acid)], pH 7.6, 2 mM $MgCl_2$ and 0.8 mM NADP. Each enzymatic reaction was initiated by the addition of the respective specific substrates [46]. For the glucose-6-phosphate dehydrogenase (G6PDH, EC 1.1.1.49) activity, the reaction started after the addition of 5 mM glucose-6-phosphate. To monitor 6-phosphogluconate dehydrogenase (6PGDH, EC 1.1.1.44) activity, 5 mM 6-phosphogluconate was used as the substrate. NADP-isocitrate dehydrogenase (NADP-ICDH, EC 1.1.1.42) activity was triggered with 10 mM 2R,3S-isocitrate [60,61]. For the NADP-malic enzyme (NADP-ME, EC 1.1.1.40) activity, the reaction was initiated with 1 mM L-malate [62].

Protein concentration in samples was determined by the Bradford method [63], using the Bio-Rad protein assay solution (Bio-Rad Laboratories) and bovine serum albumin as the standard.

2.6. Immunoblot Analysis

Proteins separated by native-PAGE (10% acrylamide) and SDS-PAGE (12% acrylamide) were transferred onto polyvinylidene difluoride (PVDF) membranes, using a Trans-Blot SD equipment (Bio-Rad Laboratories). The transfer buffer used was 10 mM N-cyclohexyl-3-aminopropanesulfonic acid (CAPS), pH 11.0, 10% (v/v) methanol. Runs were developed at 1.5 mA/cm^2 membrane for 2 h [64]. After the protein transfer, membranes were processed for further blotting assays. An antibody against Fe-SOD from pepper fruits (dilution 1:5000) was used. The antibody-recognizing proteins were visualized using the ClarityTM Western ECL Substrate kit (Thermo Fisher Scientific) following the manufacturer's instructions.

2.7. Statistical Analysis

One-way ANOVA was used for the comparisons between means of capsaicin and dihydrocapsaicin contents using the Statgraphics Centurion program (Statgraphics Technologies, Inc., Madrid, Spain). For other parameters, the t-student test was used to detect differences between the two ripening stages of each variety. In both the ANOVA and t-student, values for $p < 0.05$ were considered different with statistical significance.

3. Results

In this work, pepper fruits from four varieties with different pungency tastes were investigated. Thus, the concentration of the main capsaicinoids, capsaicin and dihydrocapsaicin, was analyzed. As shown in Table 2, Melchor, which is a sweet variety, did not contain any of the capsaicinoids, and Piquillo only displayed little values both in green and red fruits, with placenta being the tissue where both metabolites were present in higher amounts. Regarding Padrón and Alegría, both varieties showed high capsaicinoid contents, with less amounts in the pericarp and the major levels being clearly observed in the placenta. In these two last varieties, the concentration of capsaicin and dihydrocapsaicin was remarkably increased in ripe red fruits.

Table 2. Content of capsaicin and dihydrocapsaicin in pericarp and placenta from fruits of four pepper varieties at two ripening stages.

Variety	Ripening Stage	Tissue	Capsaicin (µg/g FW)	Dihydrocapsaicin (µg/g FW)	Capsaicin + Dihydrocapsaicin (µg/g FW)
Melchor	Green	Pericarp	0 k	0 k	0 l
		Placenta	0 k	0 k	0 l
	Red	Pericarp	0 k	0 k	0 l
		Placenta	0 k	0 k	0 l
Piquillo	Green	Pericarp	0.40 ± 0.01 i	0.56 ± 0.01 i	0.96 ± 0.02 j
		Placenta	1.35 ± 0.63 gh	0.24 ± 0.13 j	1.59 ± 0.76 hijk
	Red	Pericarp	0.25 ± 0.02 j	0.54 ± 0.01 i	0.79 ± 0.03 k
		Placenta	0.59 ± 0.03 h	0.61 ± 0.01 h	1.20 ± 0.04 i
Padrón	Green	Pericarp	2.11 ± 0.08 g	0.03 ± 0.02 k	2.14 ± 0.10 gh
		Placenta	244.09 ± 34.85 c	33.10 ± 4.31 d	277.19 ± 39.16 c
	Red	Pericarp	22.45 ± 2.26 e	3.02 ± 0.19 f	25.47 ± 2.45 e
		Placenta	553.47 ± 29.59 b	166.96 ± 5.00 b	720.43 ± 34.59 b
Alegría	Green	Pericarp	8.91 ± 1.69 f	1.55 ± 0.21 g	10.46 ± 1.90 f
		Placenta	205.23 ± 9.46 c	72.96 ± 3.42 c	278.19 ± 12.88 c
	Red	Pericarp	51.06 ± 0.55 d	7.25 ± 0.35 e	58.31 ± 0.90 d
		Placenta	766.26 ± 37.00 a	269.44 ± 27.77 a	1035.70 ± 64.77 a

Placenta tissue was used once seeds were discarded. Data are the means ± SEM of three replicates determined from five fruits of the four varieties and at the two ripening stages. Different letters after each value indicate that differences were statistically significant (ANOVA, $p < 0.05$). FW, fresh weight.

As shown in Figure 2, the higher ascorbate concentration was found in Melchor, and this parameter only changed due to ripening in the two varieties with higher capsaicinoid levels, Padrón and Alegría. In both, ascorbate was significantly enhanced after fruits ripened. Likewise, this tendency also occurred with GSH, which only increased significantly in Padrón and Alegría after ripening, whereas it lowered in Melchor after this physiological process took place (Figure 3A). The oxidized form of glutathione (GSSG) diminished in Melchor and Piquillo ripened fruits and no changes were observed in Padrón and Alegría. As indicated in Table 3, total glutathione content (GSH + GSSG) increased in Padrón and Alegría and lowered in Melchor after ripening. The ratio GSH/GSSG was enhanced by ripening in the four varieties, thus indicating a shift to a higher reducing environment (Table 3).

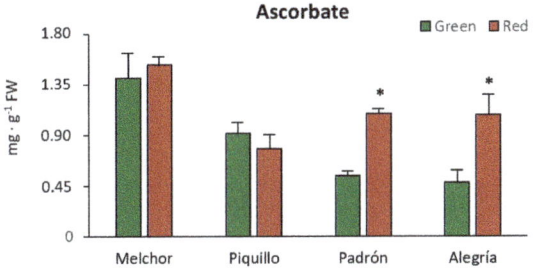

Figure 2. Ascorbate content in pericarp from fruits of four pepper varieties at two ripening stages. Data are the means ± SEM of three replicates determined from five fruits of the four varieties and at the two ripening stages. Asterisks indicate significant differences of red fruits with respect to green fruits for each variety (*t*-student, $p < 0.05$). FW, fresh weight.

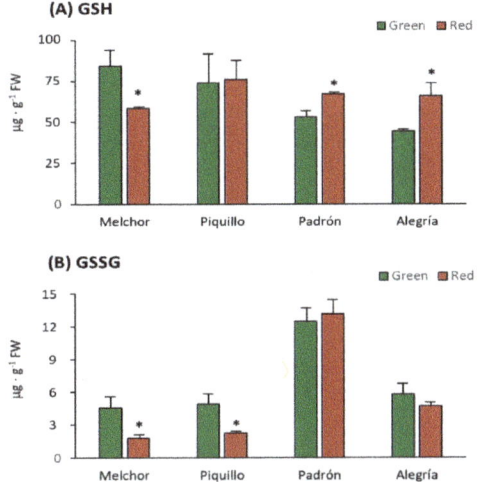

Figure 3. Reduced (GSH) and oxidized (GSSG) glutathione contents in pericarp from fruits of four pepper varieties at two ripening stages. (**A**) GSH. (**B**) GSSG. Data are the means ± SEM of three replicates determined from five fruits of the four varieties and at the two ripening stages. Asterisks indicate significant differences of red fruits with respect to green fruits for each variety (*t*-student, $p < 0.05$). FW, fresh weight.

Table 3. Total glutathione (GSH + GSSG) and the ratio GSH/GSSG from fruits of four pepper varieties at two ripening stages.

Variety	Ripening Stage	GSH + GSSG ($\mu g \cdot g^{-1}$ FW)	GSH/GSSG
Melchor	Green	88.93 ± 12.84	18.55
Melchor	Red	60.12 ± 1.38 *	32.02 *
Piquillo	Green	78.83 ± 21.43	15.04
Piquillo	Red	78.84 ± 13.10	33.71 *
Padrón	Green	65.24 ± 8.57	4.24
Padrón	Red	80.07 ± 5.75 *	5.08 *

Table 3. *Cont.*

Variety	Ripening Stage	GSH + GSSG ($\mu g \cdot g^{-1}$ FW)	GSH/GSSG
Alegría	Green	50.08 ± 2.08	7.62
Alegría	Red	70.43 ± 4.16 *	13.89 *

GSH, reduced glutathione. GSSG, oxidized glutathione. Data are the means ± SEM of three replicates determined from five fruits of the four varieties and at the two ripening stages. Asterisks indicate significant differences of red fruits with respect to green fruits for each variety (*t*-student, $p < 0.05$). FW, fresh weight.

The activity of the main enzymatic antioxidants was studied. Catalase was significantly lower in ripe fruits from all varieties except for Padrón, where the activity increased after ripening (Figure 4A). SOD activity increased as a consequence of ripening but only significantly in Padrón and Alegría. No changes were observed in the Piquillo variety at the two stages (Figure 4B). This SOD activity pattern was partially confirmed by the analysis of the isoenzymatic profile. Thus, in the Padrón variety, no Fe-SOD activity was detected in green fruits, whereas this isozyme appeared in red fruits (Figure 5A). Additionally, CuZn-SOD I and II were also higher in ripe fruits than in green ones. Regarding the Alegría variety, it was observed that Fe-SOD and CuZn-SOD II were more prominent in red fruits than in green fruits (Figure 5A). To seek for the possible reason of the absence of Fe-SOD activity in the Padrón variety, immunoblot assays were performed under native and denaturing conditions. Thus, after native PAGE and Western blotting analysis using an antibody against an Fe-SOD from pepper fruits, no cross-reacting bands were observed in green fruits from the Padrón variety. Additionally, the use of this approach confirmed that the activity pattern observed in Alegría was due to a higher Fe-SOD protein amount in red fruits (Figure 5B). To further check that Padrón did not contain the Fe-SOD protein, SDS-PAGE and Western blotting was achieved. In all samples, a cross-reacting band, characteristic of the plant Fe-SOD monomeric size (23 kDa), was detected, including green fruits from the Padrón variety, although with a very low quantity (Figure 5C). This indicates that this isozyme is present in this variety, but in such a little amount that its contribution to the total SOD activity is possibly irrelevant.

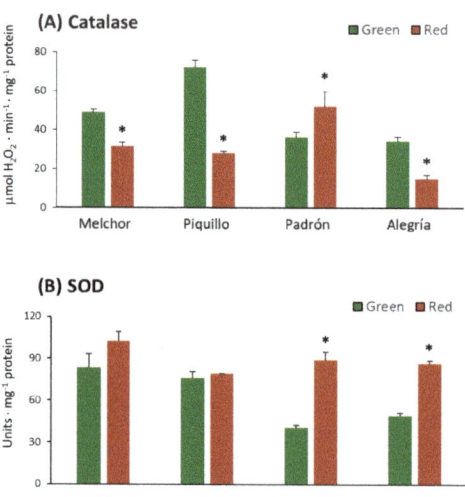

Figure 4. Catalase and superoxide dismutase (SOD) activity in pericarp from fruits of four pepper varieties at two ripening stages. (**A**), catalase. (**B**), SOD. Data are the means ± SEM of three replicates determined from five fruits of the four varieties and at the two ripening stages. Asterisks indicate significant differences of red fruits with respect to green fruits for each variety (*t*-student, $p < 0.05$).

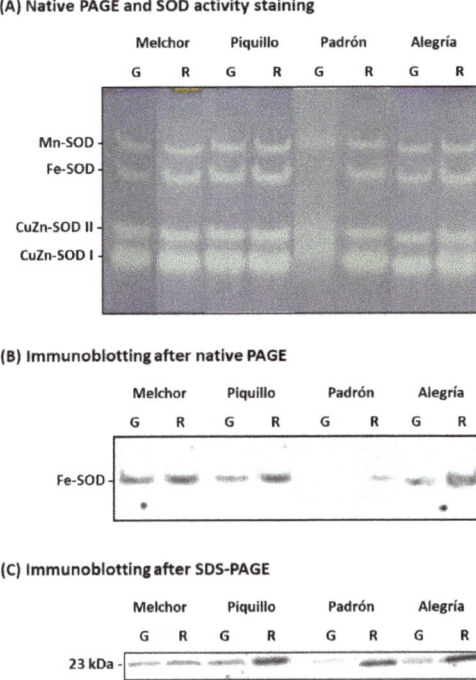

Figure 5. Isoenzymatic superoxide dismutase (SOD) pattern in pericarp from fruits of four pepper varieties at two ripening stages. (**A**) Native PAGE on 10% acrylamide gels and further in-gel SOD activity staining by the NBT reduction method; 34 µg protein per well was loaded. (**B**) Immunoblotting after native PAGE on 10% acrylamide gels. (**C**) Immunoblotting after SDS-PAGE on 12% acrylamide gels. In both immunoblotting assays, an antibody against Fe-SOD from pepper fruits (dilution 1:5000) was used. In panel B, the mobility of the detected bands was similar to the one observed for Fe-SOD in panel A. The monomeric molecular size of the cross-reacting bands (23 kDa) is indicated on the left in panel C. Data are representative of at least three independent experiments where different samples from each variety and ripening stage were used. G, green fruits. R, red fruits.

The enzymatic side of the AGC was analyzed, following the activity of APX, MDAR, DHAR and GR. APX was little, but significantly enhanced in ripe fruits with respect to green fruits in Melchor and Piquillo, and lower in red fruits from Padrón (Figure 6A). Regarding MDAR, this enzyme did not show significant changes upon ripening in the four varieties (Figure 6B). DHAR was only significantly lower in red fruits from those varieties with a high capsaicinoid content, Padrón and Alegría (Figure 6C). Finally, all varieties displayed significant enhanced GR activity after ripening (Figure 6D).

Regarding the activity profile of NADP-dependent dehydrogenases (NADP-DHs), four eznymes were studied: G6PDH, 6PGDH, NADP-ICDH and NADP-ME. G6PDH and NADP-ICDH displayed parallel profiles with lower activities in red than in green fruits in the varieties Melchor and Alegría, but enhanced activity after fruits from the Padrón variety ripened (Figure 7A,C). No changes in those enzymatic systems were observed in fruits from the Piquillo variety. With respect to 6PGDH, this activity only changed in Padrón, with enhancement after ripening (Figure 7B). NADP-ME showed disparate evolution depending on the varieties. Thus, it increased in Melchor and Piquillo upon ripening and lowered in Padrón, with no changes in Alegría (Figure 7D).

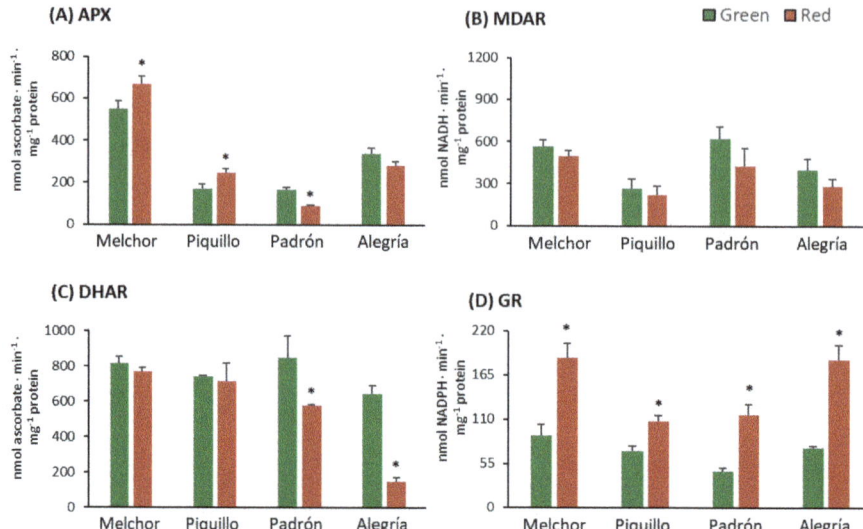

Figure 6. Activity of enzymes from the ascorbate—glutathione cycle in pericarp from fruits of four pepper varieties at two ripening stages. (**A**) Ascorbate peroxidase (APX). (**B**) Monodehydroascorbate reductase (MDAR). (**C**) Dehydroascorbate reductase (DHAR). (**D**) Glutathione reductase (GR). Data are the means ± SEM of three replicates determined from five fruits of the four varieties and at the two ripening stages. Asterisks indicate significant differences of red fruits with respect to green fruits for each variety (*t*-student, $p < 0.05$).

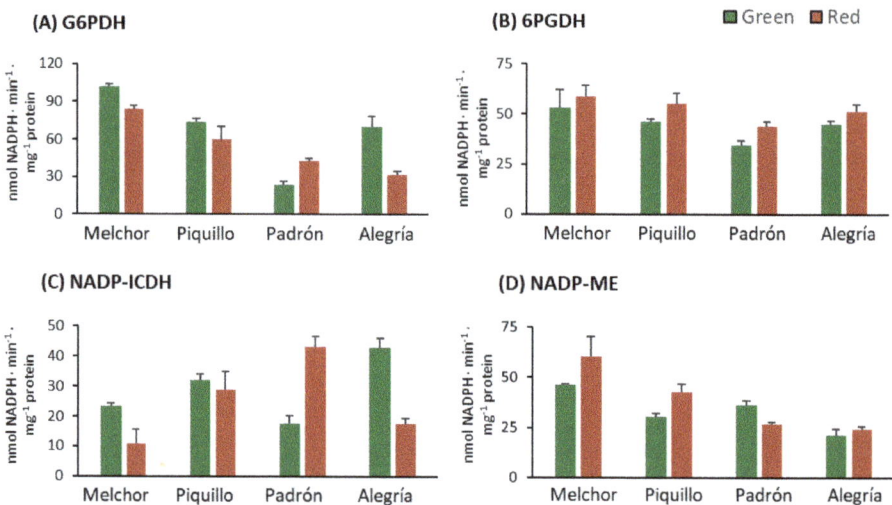

Figure 7. Activity of NADP-dehydrogenases in pericarp from fruits of four pepper varieties at two ripening stages. (**A**) Glucose-6-phosphate dehydrogenase (G6PDH). (**B**) 6-Phosphogluconate dehydrogenase (6PGDH). (**C**) NADP-dependent isocitrate dehydrogenase (ICDH). (**D**) NADP-dependent malic enzyme (ME). Data are the means ± SEM of three replicates determined from five fruits of the four varieties and at the two ripening stages.

4. Discussion

4.1. The Experimental Design Provided a Gradual Capsaicin Concentration Depending on the Pepper Variety and the Ripening Stage

Pepper varieties used in this work were selected because of their different pungency levels according to consumers taste, which is the basis where the Scoville scale resides. All four varieties are common in Spanish food markets and their culinary uses are diverse. Melchor is a type of sweet pepper characterized by its consistency and appropriateness for different purposes. This variety, along with other sweet pepper varieties, provides the high production figures in Spain. Its tasting features in either green or red frame this variety in the non-pungent fruits' group. Piquillo is an autochthonous variety from northern Spain and its main phenotypic feature is its triangle shape with a sharp-peaked extreme. Upon intake, it is characterized by a very slight pleasant pungency, but it is only consumed in its ripe red stage. Padrón is characteristic of and originally from northwestern Spain, although lately it is also cultivated in many other lands in the Mediterranean area. These fruits are small, and they are usually consumed as green after cooking. Commonly, in the green stage, they show a very slight spicy taste, but it is in the red stage that it is not consumed due to its strong pungency. Finally, Alegría riojana (which might be translated as Riojan joy) is also autochthonous from northern Spain and it is usually used as spice in the red stage. Both green and red, but mainly red, fruits from this variety are extremely pungent.

With this tasting background and considering the antioxidant quality attributed to capsaicinoids [20,28,29], we aimed, in this work, to investigate the potential influence of these compounds (capsaicin plus dihydrocapsaicin; Cap+DiCap) in the profile of the main enzymatic and non-enzymatic antioxidants of pepper fruits containing different levels of these alkaloids. Our experimental design established a gradual scale from null values of Cap+DiCap, both in green and red ripe stages (Melchor), to red Alegría which contained high levels of the two capsaicinoids. The content of the Cap+DiCap couple matched with the tasting scale and the higher values, as expected, were found in the placenta in the three pungent varieties. Based on these data, we found quite the appropriate selection of these varieties and ripening stages to target our objective.

Except for Alegría which has been scarcely used for research purposes so far, reports on the other three varieties can be found in the literature. Thus, the Melchor variety has been used to decipher the mechanisms involved in fruit ripening [18,38,65,66], where some of their antioxidant systems have been reported to be involved [67]. The Piquillo variety was used as a model to address the effects triggered by infection with *Verticillum* [68–71] and how to protect pepper plants against it through diverse practices [72,73], as well as to investigate the effect of sanitized sewage sludge on the growth, yield, fruit quality, soil microbial community and physiology of pepper plants [74,75]. On the other hand, the Padrón variety was set, for example, to investigate either how wounding induces local resistance but systemic susceptibility to *Botrytis cinerea* in pepper plants [76], as a reference to assess real-time PCR as a method for determining the presence of *Verticillium dahliae* in distinct solanaceae species [77], or to study the virulence and pathogenesis issues of *Phytophthora capsici* [78], among others.

4.2. The Ripening Stage and the Capsaicinoids Content Alter the Metabolism of Enzymatic Antioxidants

The profile of antioxidant enzymes during the ripening process has been investigated in pepper fruits previously but, to our knowledge, no comparisons have been made between varieties with different capsaicinoid contents. Thus, for example, in California-type pepper fruits, it has been reported that the catalase activity decreases as the fruit ripens [79,80] and this event is due to the post-translational modification (PTMs) underwent by the enzyme and promoted by ROS and reactive nitrogen species (RNS) derived from nitric oxide (NO) [41,81]. In fact, it has been proved that the ripening of pepper fruits is controlled by NO [8,40,80]. This inhibitory effect of ripening in the catalase activity also occurred in the same California-type fruits subjected to storage at 20 °C [80], in other sweet pepper varieties from Lamuyo and Dulce italiano types [4], and during the ripening of hot pepper Kulai [49]. Our data on the Melchor, Piquillo and Alegría varieties confirm this activity pattern of the catalase activity, although, interestingly, this profile is opposite in the Padrón variety where catalase activity increases in ripe fruits. This same increasing catalase activity was reported in hot pepper varieties either under saline stress conditions [47] or in preventing seed browning during low-temperature storage [48].

Regarding SOD, the total activity was higher in ripe fruits from those varieties which contained a higher capsaicinoids content, namely Padrón and Alegría. In Alegría, this higher activity seems basically to be due to an enhancement of the isozymes Fe-SOD and CuZn-SOD II, whereas in Padrón, the presence of Fe-SOD (nearly absent in green fruits) and the higher activity of both CuZn-SODs could be responsible for such changes. Due to this interesting behavior of the Fe-SOD isozyme in the Padrón variety, complementary immunoblot analyses were performed using an antibody against the isozyme from pepper fruits. Thus, by Western blotting after both non-denaturing- and SDS-PAGEs, it was confirmed that the negligible Fe-SOD activity in ripe Padrón fruits was due to the little amounts of its corresponding protein, whose monomer (23 kDa) could only be detected after SDS-PAGE. This issue needs to be further investigated at the molecular level (gene and protein expression) since it means that it might be an identity feature of this pepper variety. The SOD activity has been also studied earlier in pepper varieties including some of those included in the present work. So, recently, it has been reported that the SOD isoenzyme pattern and gene expression of California-type pepper fruits are regulated by ripening and NO [67], and this enzymatic system from sweet pepper is also involved in the response against low temperatures [4] and the storage of fruits at 20 °C [79], as well as in the "accommodation" of fruits to nitrogen deprivation during plant growth [82]. The isoenzymatic SOD pattern was also investigated in the plastid population from sweet pepper fruits of different California-type varieties, and a protective role of these organelles by the different SOD internal isozymes during ripening was reported [45]. In the Piquillo variety, it was found that SOD is involved in the association of pepper plants with arbuscular mycorrhizal fungi (AMF) to avoid the negative effects promoted by *Verticillum* [73]. A number of studies have reported the involvement of SOD from hot pepper in diverse processes including ripening and post-harvest [49,83], salt stress [47,84], storage at low temperature [48] and iodine bio-fortification practices to improve fruit quality [85].

The activity of the four enzymes of the ascorbate–glutathione cycle (AGC), APX, MDAR, DHAR and GR, were analyzed in this work. APX is responsible for the direct scavenging of hydrogen peroxide (H_2O_2) using ascorbate as the electron donor, whereas MDAR and DHAR restore the reduced status of ascorbate using NAD(P)H and GSH, respectively. The last step of the AGC is carried out by GR, an enzyme which converts the oxidized form of glutathione (GSSG) to the reduced form (GSH) with the use of NADPH as the reducing power. In our experimental design, the most remarkable response of this cycle was found at the GR side which was significantly enhanced in ripe fruits from all four varieties. The profile of these AGC enzymes has been investigated in pepper fruits from diverse varieties, both sweet and hot, and different trends have been reported depending on the experimental conditions, including ripening, post-harvest, salt stress, defense mechanisms or bioremediation practices [4,11,45,49,75,82,83,86]. In our case, it is remarkable that APX behaved oppositely in sweet and hot varieties, with the activity increasing in ripe fruits from Melchor and Piquillo and decreasing in hot ripe fruits from Padrón and Alegría. MDAR and DHAR shared a similar trend with lower values in ripe fruits, but only significant in MDAR from Padrón and Alegría. According to the activity profile of APX, MDAR and DHAR from green to red stages, it could be hypothesized that the cycle seems to be operative in the first steps which involve direct ascorbate metabolism, but more research at different levels is necessary to obtain a whole picture of this antioxidant metabolic pathway. According to our results, it seems that hot peppers have less capacity to recycle ascorbate but all varieties showed a great potentiality to provide GSH.

The activity pattern displayed by the NADP-dehydrogenases (NADP-DHs) can be framed in three main features: (i) the behavior of the two varieties with less Cap+DiCap levels (Melchor and Piquillo) was quite similar with slight, although not strongly significant, decreases in G6PDH and little, although not significant enough, decreases in 6PGDH and NADP-ME in ripe fruits; (ii) except for NADP-ME, all other NADP-DHs rose after ripening in the Padrón variety (high capsaicinoids content), and this suggests a higher NADPH availability for different purposes in ripe fruits from this variety; and (iii) interestingly, the behavior of these enzymatic systems in the other variety with high capsaicinoids content was different to that showed by Padrón. Thus, green fruits from Alegría seemed to have higher capacity to generate NADPH. To our knowledge, no reports on NADP-DHs from hot pepper fruits have been published previously, and the only data concerning these NADP/NADPH systems in pepper refer to sweet varieties. Our data mostly confirm those previously found for other California-type pepper varieties [46]. Recent data report that pepper fruit NADP-DHs are not only influenced by ripening in the Melchor variety [8], but also by NO through diverse PTMs [87,88]. Moreover, it was also found that NADP-DHs are involved in the response of sweet pepper plants to stress exerted by high Cd levels [89].

4.3. The Higher Capsaicinoids Level the Higher Ascorbate and Glutathione Content

Capsaicinoids, specially capsaicin, have been reported to have, among others, antioxidant properties [20,28–30]. In pepper fruits containing these alkaloids, this feature is quite interesting since these horticultural products are one of those with the highest ascorbate levels [5], with ascorbate being perhaps the most paradigmatic molecular antioxidant for living beings. In fact, ascorbate is one of the parameters which is commonly determined in (sweet and hot) pepper fruit research including either ripening and post-harvest, any type of stress (biotic, abiotic and environmental) or culture practices [4,5,7,11,14,18,45,47,49,75,84,90]. As an appraisal of the potential roles attributed to ascorbate in pepper fruits, it was proposed that in the sweet varieties, ascorbate functions as a redox buffer to balance the great metabolic changes which undergo during ripening [5,7]. Regarding the hottest varieties (Padrón and Alegría), the pattern observed in this work, where ascorbate levels increased in those fruits, was also reported earlier for diverse hot pepper varieties [14,18,49,90]. Perhaps, the redox stabilizing role of ascorbate indicated above for sweet pepper could be also applicable to hot varieties to assure the capsaicinoids level. In fact, it was proved that during the capsaicinoids oxidation catalyzed by peroxidases, capsaicinoid radicals are formed, and ascorbate rapidly reduces capsaicinoid radicals, this being an important cue for capsaicinoid content and preservation in pepper fruits [91].

Glutathione is a ubiquitous and powerful antioxidant in eukaryotes [92]. In spite of its relevant role in many biological processes, this tripeptide has been less investigated in pepper fruits, mainly associated to ripening, or bioremediation purposes [49,75,82,93]. However, not much information is available on glutathione metabolism in capsaicinoids-containing pepper varieties. This work provides the first comparison of the levels of both GSH and GSSG in different pepper varieties containing gradual amounts of capsaicinoids. It is noteworthy that, whereas the total glutathione content (GSH + GSSG) did not change or decrease after ripening in the varieties with no or very few capsaicinoids (Merlchor and Piquillo), in the hot varieties, this parameter augmented in mature fruits. This was due to the evolution of the reduced form of GSH during those physiological processes. This higher content of GSH in ripe fruits found in the hottest pepper varieties could be due to an enhanced GR activity. In these cases, the enzyme GR is perhaps playing a role not linked to the AGC. GSH could be used, in cooperation with ascorbate, to preserve the capsaicinoids functionality in these hot varieties. However, more research is necessary to bring light to this emerging subject. Besides, GSH could be also driven to signaling processes by either glutathionylation events (another PTM), or as S-nitrosoglutathione, a chemical form which allows transporting NO among cells and tissues [50,94–96]. GR uses NADPH to achieve the reduction of glutathione. NADPH is also essential in intermediate steps of capsaicin biosynthesis [97]. These eventualities point towards the necessity of investigating the interaction capsaicinoids–ascorbate–glutathione–NADPH in more detail, especially after the perspective of considering NADPH as a quality footprint in horticultural crops, as it has been proposed recently [98].

5. Conclusions and Future Prospects

The obtained data in this work point towards a close relationship among capsaicinoids and the antioxidant systems in pepper fruits. This interaction seems to maintain a redox and functional homeostasis to preserve the role of capsaicinoids with the cooperation of antioxidants, basically ascorbate and glutathione. However, some antioxidant enzymatic systems are also involved. The exclusivity of capsaicinoid metabolism in *Capsicum* species makes this research more attractive to look for an exclusive model that could provide interesting information at the plant physiological level, but also considering the pharmacological and nutraceutical uses of hot pepper fruits, based mainly on the content of capsaicinoids but also on vitamins C and A. On the other hand, another interesting cue is opened. The role of Fe-SOD needs to be investigated in pepper fruit physiology due to the diverse behavior of this isozyme among varieties. Fe-SOD has been localized in peroxisomes from pepper fruits [5,99] and lately its gene expression profile has been reported in sweet pepper during ripening and under NO treatment. Overall, the interaction of NO in pungent pepper fruits is another issue that deserves to be investigated. Furthermore, this characterization contributes to providing a biochemical antioxidant pattern for each pepper cultivar which could be part of the particular features of these cultivars that are included in the European Register of protected designations of origin for these Spanish agricultural products. Besides, this provides an added value to these autochthonous products and may have some incidence at the marketing and economical levels in their respective producing sectors.

Author Contributions: F.T., A.C.-R. and M.R.-R. carried out all biochemical experiments. F.J.C. and J.M.P. designed the work, drove and coordinated the tasks and wrote the manuscript. All authors have read and agreed to the published version of the manuscript.

Funding: This work was supported by the ERDF-cofinanced grants AGL2015-65104-P from MINECO, PID2019-103924GB-I00 from MICIT, and P18-FR-1359 from the Plan Andaluz de Investigación, Desarrollo e Innovación, Spain.

Acknowledgments: The technical support of the Scientific Instrumental Service from the Estación Experimental del Zaidín (CSIC, Granada, Spain) is acknowledged. The valuable assistance of Carmelo Ruiz-Torres, Tamara Molina-Márquez and María Jesús Campos is also appreciated. Authors are thankful to the different companies and Regulatory Councils of Denomination of Origin for their valuable and generous collaboration providing the different pepper cultivars: Melchor by the Zeraim Iberica/Syngenta Seeds, Ltd., El Ejido, Almería, Spain; Padrón by the Regulatory Council of Denomination of Origin "Pemento de Herbón" (Herbón, A Coruña, Spain), and Piquillo and Alegría riojana, both provided by the Regulatory Council of Denomination of Origin "Pimiento del Piquillo-Lodosa" (Navarra, Spain).

Conflicts of Interest: The authors declare no conflict of interest.

References

1. Howard, L.R.; Talcott, S.T.; Brenes, C.H.; Villalon, B. Changes in phytochemical and antioxidant activity of selected pepper cultivars (*Capsicum* species) as influenced by maturity. *Food Chem.* **2000**, *48*, 1713–1720. [CrossRef] [PubMed]
2. Proteggente, A.R.; Pannala, A.S.; Paganga, G.; Van Buren, L.; Wagner, E.; Wiseman, S.; Van De Put, F.; Dacombe, C.; Rice-Evans, C.A. The antioxidant activity of regularly consumed fruit and vegetables reflects their phenolic and vitamin C composition. *Free Rad. Res.* **2002**, *36*, 217–233. [CrossRef] [PubMed]
3. Mariko, N.; Hassimoto, A.; Genovese, M.I.; Lajolo, F.M. Antioxidant capacity of Brazilian fruit, vegetables and commercially-frozen fruit pulps. *J. Food Comp. Anal.* **2009**, *22*, 394–396.
4. Mateos, R.M.; Jiménez, A.; Román, P.; Romojaro, F.; Bacarizo, S.; Leterrier, M.; Gómez, M.; Sevilla, F.; Del Río, L.A.; Corpas, F.J.; et al. Antioxidant systems from pepper (*Capsicum annuum* L.): Involvement in the response to temperature changes in ripe fruits. *Int. J. Mol. Sci.* **2013**, *14*, 9556–9580. [CrossRef] [PubMed]
5. Palma, J.M.; Sevilla, F.; Jiménez, A.; Del Río, L.A.; Corpas, F.J.; Álvarez de Morales, P.; Camejo, D.M. Physiology of pepper fruit and the metabolism of antioxidants: Chloroplasts, mitochondria and peroxisomes. *Ann. Bot.* **2015**, *116*, 627–636. [CrossRef]

6. Palma, J.M.; Corpas, F.J.; Ruiz, C.; Molina, T.; Campos-Ramos, M.J.; Juanena, A.; Torreira, J.R. Los pimientos de las variedades Padrón, Piquillo y Alegría riojana: Una buena fuente de macro y microelementos para nuestra dieta. *Horticultura* **2016**, *323*, 60–64.
7. Rodríguez-Ruiz, M.; Mateos, R.M.; Codesido, V.; Corpas, F.J.; Palma, J.M. Characterization of the galactono-1,4-lactone dehydrogenase from pepper fruits and its modulation in the ascorbate biosynthesis. Role of nitric oxide. *Redox Biol.* **2017**, *12*, 171–181. [CrossRef]
8. Corpas, F.J.; Freschi, L.; Rodríguez-Ruiz, M.; Mioto, P.T.; González-Gordo, S.; Palma, J.M. Nitro-oxidative metabolism during fruit ripening. *J. Exp. Bot.* **2018**, *69*, 3449–3463. [CrossRef]
9. Song, W.; Derito, C.M.; Liu, M.K.; He, H.J.; Dong, M.; Hai Liu, R. Cellular antioxidant activity of common vegetables. *J. Agric. Food Chem.* **2010**, *58*, 6621–6629. [CrossRef]
10. Palma, J.M.; Corpas, F.J.; Del Río, L.A. Proteome of plant peroxisomes: New perspectives on the role of these organelles in cell biology. *Proteomics* **2009**, *9*, 2301–2312. [CrossRef]
11. Martí, M.C.; Camejo, D.; Vallejo, F.; Romojaro, F.; Bacarizo, S.; Palma, J.M.; Sevilla, F.; Jiménez, A. Influence of fruit ripening stage and harvest period on the antioxidant content of sweet pepper cultivars. *Plant Foods Hum. Nut.* **2011**, *66*, 416–423. [CrossRef] [PubMed]
12. Fratianni, F.; D'Acierno, A.; Cozzolino, A.; Spigno, P.; Riccardi, R.; Raimo, F.; Pane, C.; Zaccardelli, M.; Lombardo, V.T.; Tucci, M.; et al. Biochemical characterization of traditional varieties of sweet pepper (*Capsicum annuum* L.) of the Campania Region, Southern Italy. *Antioxidants* **2020**, *9*, 556. [CrossRef] [PubMed]
13. Basu, S.K.; De, A.K. *Capsicum*: Historical and Botanical Perspectives. In *Capsicum. The Genus Capsicum*; De, A.K., Ed.; Taylor & Francis: London, UK, 2003; pp. 1–15, ISBN 0-415-29991-8.
14. Topuz, A.; Ozdemir, F. Assessment of carotenoids, capsaicinoids and ascorbic acid composition of some selected pepper cultivars (*Capsicum annuum* L.) grown in Turkey. *J. Food Comp. Anal.* **2007**, *20*, 596–602. [CrossRef]
15. Roy, A. Bhut jolokia (*Capsicum chinense* jaqc): A review. *Int. J. Pharm. Sci. Res.* **2016**, *7*, 882–889.
16. Aguiar, A.C.; Coutinho, J.P.; Fernández-Barbero, G.; Godoy, H.T.; Martinez, J. Comparative study of capsaicinoid composition in capsicum peppers grown in Brazil. *Int. J. Food Prop.* **2016**, *19*, 1292–1302. [CrossRef]
17. Parvez, G.M.M. Current advances in pharmacological activity and toxic effects of various *Capsicum* species. *Int. J. Pharm. Sci. Res.* **2017**, *8*, 1900–1912.
18. Kopta, T.; Sekara, A.; Pokluda, R.; Ferby, V.; Caruso, G. Screening of chilli pepper genotypes as a source of capsaicinoids and antioxidants under conditions of simulated drought stress. *Plants* **2020**, *9*, 364. [CrossRef]
19. Ishikawa, K. Biosynthesis of capsaicinoids in *Capsicum*. In *Capsicum. The Genus Capsicum*; De, A.K., Ed.; Taylor & Francis: London, UK, 2003; pp. 87–95, ISBN 0-415-29991-8.
20. Reyes-Escogido, M.L.; González-Mondragón, E.G.; Vázquez-Tzompantzi, E. Chemical and pharmacological aspects of capsaicin. *Molecules* **2011**, *16*, 1253–1270. [CrossRef]
21. Garcés-Claver, A.; Arnedo-Andrés, M.S.; Abadía, J.; Gil-Ortega, R.; Álvarez-Fernández, A. Determination of capsaicin and dihydrocapsaicin in *Capsicum* fruits by Liquid Chromatography–Electrospray/Time-of-Flight Mass Spectrometry. *J. Agric. Food Chem.* **2007**, *54*, 9303–9311. [CrossRef]
22. Al Othman, Z.A.; Ahmed, Y.B.; Habila, M.A.; Ghafar, A.A. Determination of capsaicin and dihydrocapsaicin in Capsicum fruit samples using high performance liquid chromatography. *Molecules* **2011**, *16*, 8919–8929. [CrossRef]
23. Liu, X.; Lin, Y. The bioactivity of capsaicin on peach aphid and its combination with several insecticides. *J. Pest Sci.* **2003**, *52*, 94–96.
24. Jin, M.S.; Liu, S.W.; Gu, Z.M.; Wei, S.H.; Wang, Y.Z. Repellent activity of capsaicin and its effects on glutathione-S-transferase and Na^+, K^+- ATPase activity in *Plutella xylostella* (*Lepidoptera: Plutellidae*). *Acta Entomol. Sin.* **2008**, *51*, 1039–1043.
25. Aley, J.P.; Adams, N.J.; Ladyman, R.J.; Fraser, D.L. The efficacy of capsaicin as an equine repellent for chewing wood. *J. Veter Behav. Clin. App. Res.* **2015**, *10*, 243–247. [CrossRef]
26. Dickens, J.C.; Bohbot, J.D. Neuromolecular basis of repellent action. In *Insect Repellents Handbook*, 2nd ed.; Debboun, M., Frances, S.P., Strickman, D.A., Eds.; CRC Press: Boca Raton, FL, USA, 2015; pp. 31–42.
27. Li, B.; Yang, M.; Shi, R.; Ye, M. Insecticidal activity of natural capsaicinoids against several agricultural insects. *Nat. Prod. Commun.* **2019**. [CrossRef]

28. Sancho, R.; Lucena, C.; Macho, A.; Calzado, M.A.; Blanco-Molina, M.; Minassi, A.; Appendino, G.; Muñoz, E. Immunosuppressive activity of capsaicinoids: Capsiate derived from sweet peppers inhibits NF-kappa activation and is a potent antiinflammatory compound in vivo. *Eur. J. Immunol.* **2002**, *32*, 1753–1763. [CrossRef]
29. Materska, M.; Perucka, I. Antioxidant activity of the main phenolic compounds isolated from hot pepper fruit (*Capsicum annuum* L). *J. Agric. Food Chem.* **2005**, *53*, 1750–1756. [CrossRef] [PubMed]
30. Liu, J.; Liu, H.; Zhao, Z.; Wang, J.; Guo, D.; Liu, Y. Regulation of Actg1 and Gsta2 is possible mechanism by which capsaicin alleviates apoptosis in cell model of 6-OHDA-induced Parkinson's disease. *Biosci. Rep.* **2020**, *40*, BSR20191796. [CrossRef]
31. Tabrizi, M.A.; Baraldi, P.G.; Baraldi, S.; Gessi, S.; Merighi, S.; Borea, P.A. Medicinal chemistry, pharmacology, and clinical implications of TRPV1 receptor antagonists. *Med. Res. Rev.* **2017**, *37*, 936–983. [CrossRef] [PubMed]
32. Yang, F.; Zheng, J. Understand spiciness: Mechanism of TRPV1 channel activation by capsaicin. *Protein Cell* **2017**, *8*, 169–177. [CrossRef]
33. Chapa-Oliver, A.M.; Mejía-Teniente, L. Capsaicin: From plants to a cancer-suppressing agent. *Molecules* **2016**, *21*, 931. [CrossRef]
34. Clark, R.; Ho Lee, S. Anticancer properties of capsaicin against human cancer. *Anticancer Res.* **2016**, *36*, 837–844. [PubMed]
35. Klie, S.; Osorio, S.; Tohge, T.; Drincovich, M.F.; Fait, A.; Giovannoni, J.J.; Fernie, A.R.; Nikoloski, Z. Conserved changes in the dynamics of metabolic processes during fruit development and ripening across species. *Plant Physiol.* **2014**, *164*, 55–68. [CrossRef] [PubMed]
36. Palma, J.M.; Corpas, F.J.; Del Río, L.A. Proteomics as an approach to the understanding of the molecular physiology of fruit development and ripening. *J. Proteom.* **2011**, *74*, 1230–1243. [CrossRef] [PubMed]
37. Barsan, C.; Zouine, M.; Maza, E.; Bian, W.; Egea, I.; Rossignol, M.; Bouyssie, D.; Pichereaux, C.; Purgatto, E.; Bouzayen, M.; et al. Proteomic analysis of chloroplast to chromoplast transition in tomato reveals metabolic shifts coupled with disrupted thylakoid biogenesis machinery and elevated energy-production components. *Plant Physiol.* **2012**, *160*, 708–725. [CrossRef] [PubMed]
38. Corpas, F.J.; Palma, J.M. Nitric oxide on/off in fruit ripening. *Plant Biol.* **2018**, *20*, 805–807. [CrossRef]
39. Zhang, L.; Zhu, M.; Ren, L.; Li, A.; Chen, G.; Hu, Z. The SlFSR gene controls fruit shelf-life in tomato. *J. Exp. Bot.* **2018**, *69*, 2897–2909. [CrossRef]
40. González-Gordo, S.; Bautista, R.; Claros, M.G.; Cañas, A.; Palma, J.M.; Corpas, F.J. Nitric oxide-dependent regulation of sweet pepper fruit ripening. *J. Exp. Bot.* **2019**, *70*, 4557–4570. [CrossRef]
41. Rodríguez-Ruiz, M.; González-Gordo, S.; Cañas, A.; Campos, M.J.; Paradela, A.; Corpas, F.J.; Palma, J.M. Sweet pepper (Capsicum annuum L.) fruits contain an atypical peroxisomal catalase that is modulated by reactive oxygen and nitrogen species. *Antioxidants* **2019**, *8*, 374. [CrossRef]
42. Hamed, M.; Kalita, D.; Bartolo, M.E.; Jayanty, S.S. Capsaicinoids, polyphenols and antioxidant activities of *Capsicum annuum*: Comparative study of the effect of ripening stage and cooking methods. *Antioxidants* **2019**, *8*, 364. [CrossRef]
43. Cisternas-Jamet, J.; Salvatierra-Martínez, R.; Vega-Gálvez, A.; Stoll, A.; Uribe, E.; Goñi, M.G. Biochemical composition as a function of fruit maturity stage of bell pepper (*Capsicum annum*) inoculated with Bacillus amyloliquefaciens. *Sci. Hortic.* **2020**, *263*, 109107. [CrossRef]
44. Ribes-Moya, A.M.; Adalid, A.M.; Raigón, M.D.; Hellín, P.; Fita, A.; Rodríguez-Burruezo, A. Variation in flavonoids in a collection of peppers (*Capsicum* sp.) under organic and conventional cultivation: Effect of the genotype, ripening stage, and growing system. *J. Sci. Food Agric.* **2020**, *100*, 2208–2223. [CrossRef]
45. Martí, M.C.; Camejo, D.; Olmos, E.; Sandalio, L.M.; Fernández-García, N.; Jiménez, A.; Sevilla, F. Characterisation and changes in the antioxidant system of chloroplasts and chromoplasts isolated from green and mature pepper fruits. *Plant Biol.* **2009**, *11*, 613–624. [CrossRef] [PubMed]
46. Mateos, R.M.; Bonilla-Valverde, D.; Del Río, L.A.; Palma, J.M.; Corpas, F.J. NADP-dehydrogenases from pepper fruits: Effect of maturation. *Physiol. Plant.* **2009**, *135*, 130–139. [CrossRef]
47. Ramírez-Serrano, R.; Larrinaga-Mayoral, J.A.; Murillo-Amador, B.; Hernández-Saavedra, N.Y.; Fujiyama, H. ntioxidant enzymatic response of hot pepper (*Capsicum annuum* L.) under saline stress conditions. *Interciencia* **2008**, *33*, 377–383.

48. Boonsiri, K.; Ketsa, S.; Van Doorn, W.G. Seed browning of hot peppers during low temperature storage. *Postharvest Biol. Technol.* **2007**, *45*, 358–365. [CrossRef]
49. Tan, C.K.; Ali, Z.M.; Zainal, Z. Changes in ethylene production, carbohydrase activity and antioxidant status in pepper fruits during ripening. *Sci. Hortic.* **2012**, *142*, 23–31. [CrossRef]
50. Airaki, M.; Sánchez-Moreno, L.; Leterrier, M.; Barroso, J.B.; Palma, J.M.; Corpas, F.J. Detection and quantification of S-nitrosoglutathione (GSNO) in pepper (*Capsicum annuum* L.) plant organs by LC-ES/MS. *Plant Cell Physiol.* **2011**, *52*, 2006–2015. [CrossRef]
51. Aebi, H. Catalase in vitro. *Methods Enzym.* **1984**, *105*, 121–126.
52. Hossain, M.A.; Asada, K. Inactivation of ascorbate peroxidase in spinach chloroplasts on dark addition of hydrogen peroxide: Its protection by ascorbate. *Plant Cell Physiol.* **1984**, *25*, 1285–1295.
53. Hossain, M.A.; Nakano, Y.; Asada, K. Monodehydroascorbate reductase in spinach chloroplast and its participation in regeneration of ascorbate for scavenging of hydrogen peroxide. *Plant Cell Physiol.* **1984**, *25*, 385–395.
54. Dalton, D.A.; Baird, L.M.; Langeberg, L.; Taugher, C.Y.; Anyan, W.R.; Vance, C.P.; Sarath, G. Subcellular localization of oxygen defense enzymes in soybean (*Glycine max* [L.] Merr.) root nodules. *Plant Physiol.* **1993**, *102*, 481–489. [CrossRef]
55. Edwards, E.A.; Rawsthone, S.; Mullineaux, P.M. Subcellular distribution of multiple forms of glutathione reductase in leaves of pea (*Pisum sativum* L.). *Planta* **1990**, *180*, 278–284. [CrossRef] [PubMed]
56. McCord, J.M.; Fridovich, I. Superoxide dismutase: An enzymic function for erythrocuprein. *J. Biol. Chem.* **1969**, *244*, 6049–6055. [PubMed]
57. Beauchamp, C.; Fridovich, I. Superoxide dismutase: Improved assays and an assay applicable to acrylamide gels. *Anal. Biochem.* **1971**, *44*, 276–287. [CrossRef]
58. Houmani, H.; Rodríguez-Ruiz, M.; Palma, J.M.; Abdelly, C.; Corpas, F.J. Modulation of superoxide dismutase (SOD) isozymes by organ development and high long-term salinity in the halophyte *Cakile maritima*. *Protoplasma* **2016**, *253*, 885–894. [CrossRef]
59. Pinilla, M.; Iglesias-Moya, J.; Campos, M.J.; Corpas, F.J.; Palma, J.M. Pomegranate (*Punica granatum* L.) Fruits: Characterization of the main enzymatic antioxidants (peroxisomal catalase and SOD isozymes) and the NADPH-regenerating system. *Agronomy* **2019**, *9*, 338. [CrossRef]
60. Leterrier, M.; Airaki, M.; Palma, J.M.; Chaki, M.; Barroso, J.B.; Corpas, F.J. Arsenic triggers the nitric oxide (NO) and S-nitrosoglutathione (GSNO) metabolism in Arabidopsis. *Environ. Pollut.* **2012**, *166*, 136–143. [CrossRef] [PubMed]
61. Leterrier, M.; Barroso, J.B.; Palma, J.M.; Corpas, F.J. Cytosolic NADP-isocitrate dehydrogenase in Arabidopsis leaves and roots. *Biol. Plant.* **2012**, *56*, 705–710. [CrossRef]
62. Barroso, J.B.; Peragon, J.; Contreras-Jurado, C.; Garcia-Salguero, L.; Corpas, F.J.; Esteban, F.J.; Peinado, M.A.; De la Higuera, M.; Lupiáñez, J.A. Impact of starvation-refeeding on kinetics and protein expression of trout liver NADPH-production systems. *Am. J. Physiol.* **1998**, *274*, R1578–R1587. [CrossRef]
63. Bradford, M.M. A rapid and sensitive method for the quantitation of microgram quantities of protein utilizing the principle of protein-dye binding. *Anal. Biochem.* **1976**, *72*, 248–254. [CrossRef]
64. Corpas, F.J.; Barroso, J.B.; Sandalio, L.M.; Distefano, S.; Palma, J.M.; Lupiáñez, J.A.; Del Río, L.A. A dehydrogenase-mediated recycling system of NADPH peroxisomes. *Biochem. J.* **1998**, *330*, 777–784. [CrossRef] [PubMed]
65. Palma, J.M.; Freschi, L.; Rodríguez-Ruiz, M.; González-Gordo, S.; Corpas, F.J. Nitric oxide in the physiology and quality of fleshy fruits. *J. Exp. Bot.* **2019**, *70*, 4405–4417. [CrossRef]
66. Chu-Puga, Á.; González-Gordo, S.; Rodríguez-Ruiz, M.; Palma, J.M.; Corpas, F.J. NADPH oxidase (Rboh) activity is up regulated during sweet pepper (*Capsicum annuum* L.) fruit ripening. *Antioxidants* **2019**, *8*, 9. [CrossRef]
67. González-Gordo, S.; Rodríguez-Ruiz, M.; Palma, J.M.; Corpas, F.J. Superoxide radical metabolism in sweet pepper (*Capsicum annuum* L.) fruits is regulated by ripening and by a NO-enriched environment. *Front. Plant Sci.* **2020**, *11*, 485. [CrossRef]
68. Goicoechea, N.; Aguirreola, J.; Cenoz, S.; García-Mina, J.M. *Verticillium dahliae* modifies the concentrations of proline, soluble sugars, starch, soluble protein and abscisic acid in pepper plants. *Eur. J. Plant Pathol.* **2000**, *106*, 19–25. [CrossRef]

69. Goicoechea, N.; Aguirreolea, J.; Cenoz, S.; García-Mina, J.M. Gas exchange and flowering in Verticillium-wilted pepper plants. *J. Phytopathol.* **2001**, *149*, 281–286. [CrossRef]
70. Goicoechea, N.; Aguirreolea, J.; García-Mina, J.M. Alleviation of verticillium wilt in pepper (*Capsicum annuum* L.) by using the organic amendment COACH of natural origin. *Sci. Hortic.* **2004**, *101*, 23–37. [CrossRef]
71. Pascual, I.; Azcona, I.; Morales, F.; Aguirreolea, J.; Sánchez-Díaz, M. Photosynthetic response of pepper plants to wilt induced by Verticillium dahliae and soil water déficit. *J. Plant Physiol.* **2010**, *167*, 701–708. [CrossRef]
72. Garmendia, I.; Goicoechea, N.; Aguirreolea, J. Effectiveness of three Glomus species in protecting pepper (*Capsicum annuum* L.) against verticillium wilt. *Biol. Control.* **2004**, *31*, 296–305. [CrossRef]
73. Goicoechea, N.; Garmendia, I.; Sánchez-Díaz, M.; Aguirreolea, J. Arbuscular mycorrhizal fungi (AMF) as bioprotector agents against wilt induced by *Verticillium* spp. in pepper. *Span. J. Agric. Res.* **2010**, *8*, S25–S42. [CrossRef]
74. Pascual, I.; Avilés, M.; Aguirreolea, J.; Sánchez-Díaz, M. Effect of sanitized and non-sanitized sewage sludge on soil microbial community and the physiology of pepper plants. *Plant Soil* **2008**, *310*, 41. [CrossRef]
75. Pascual, I.; Azcona, I.; Aguirreolea, J.; Morales, F.; Corpas, F.J.; Palma, J.M.; Rellán-Álvarez, R.; Sánchez-Díaz, M. Growth, yield, and fruit quality of pepper plants amended with two sanitized sewage sludges. *J. Agric. Food Chem.* **2010**, *58*, 6951–6959. [CrossRef] [PubMed]
76. García, T.; Gutiérrez, J.; Veloso, J.; Gago-Fuentes, R.; Díaz, J. Wounding induces local resistance but systemic susceptibility to Botrytis cinerea in pepper plants. *J. Plant Pathol.* **2015**, *176*, 202–209. [CrossRef]
77. Gayoso, C.; De la Ilarduya, O.M.; Pomar, F.; Merino, F. Assessment of real-time PCR as a method for determining the presence of Verticillium dahliae in different Solanaceae cultivars. *Eur. J. Plant Pathol.* **2007**, *118*, 199–209. [CrossRef]
78. Silvar, C.; Merino, F.; Díaz, J. Diversity of *Phytophthora capsici* in northwest Spain: Analysis of virulence, metalaxyl response, and molecular characterization. *Plant Dis.* **2006**, *90*, 1135–1142. [CrossRef]
79. Jiménez, A.; Romojaro, F.; Llanos, M.R.; Gómez, J.M.; León, A.; Sevilla, F. Antioxidant systems and their relationship with the response of pepper fruits to storage at 20 °C. *J. Agric. Food Chem.* **2003**, *51*, 6293–6299. [CrossRef]
80. Chaki, M.; Álvarez de Morales, P.; Ruiz, C.; Begara-Morales, J.C.; Barroso, J.B.; Corpas, F.J.; Palma, J.M. Ripening of pepper (*Capsicum annuum*) fruit is characterized by an enhancement of protein tyrosine nitration. *Ann. Bot.* **2015**, *116*, 637–647. [CrossRef]
81. Palma, J.M.; Mateos, R.M.; López-Jaramillo, J.; Rodríguez-Ruiz, M.; González-Gordo, S.; Lechuga-Sancho, A.M.; Corpas, F.J. Plant catalases as NO and H_2S targets. *Redox Biol.* **2020**, *34*, 101525. [CrossRef]
82. Tortosa, G.; González-Gordo, S.; Ruiz, C.; Bedmar, E.J.; Palma, J.M. "Alperujo" compost improves the ascorbate (Vitamin C) content in pepper (*Capsicum annuum* L.) fruits and influences their oxidative metabolism. *Agronomy* **2018**, *8*, 82. [CrossRef]
83. Tan, C.K.; Ali, Z.M.; Zainal, Z. MnSOD and 9-LOX gene expression along with antioxidant changes of *Capsicum annuum* cv. Kulai during postharvest treatment. *Sci. Hortic.* **2016**, *213*, 403–409. [CrossRef]
84. Azuma, R.; Ito, N.; Nakayama, N.; Suwa, R.; Nguyen, T.N.; Larrinaga-Mayoral, J.A.; Esaka, M.; Fujiyama, H.; Saneoka, H. Fruits are more sensitive to salinity than leaves and stems in pepper plants (*Capsicum annuum* L.). *Sci. Hortic.* **2010**, *125*, 171–178. [CrossRef]
85. Li, R.; Li, D.W.; Liu, H.P.; Hong, C.L.; Song, M.Y.; Dai, Z.X.; Liu, J.W.; Zhou, J.; Weng, H.X. Enhancing iodine content and fruit quality of pepper (*Capsicum annuum* L.) through biofortification. *Sci. Hortic.* **2017**, *214*, 165–173. [CrossRef]
86. Padilha, H.K.M.; Madruga, N.D.; Aranha, B.C.; Hoffmann, J.F.; Lopes Crizel, R.L.; Barbieri, R.L.; Chaves, F.C. Defense responses of *Capsicum* spp. genotypes to post-harvest *Colletotrichum* sp. inoculation. *Phytoparasitica* **2019**, *47*, 557–573. [CrossRef]
87. Muñoz-Vargas, M.A.; González-Gordo, S.; Cañas, A.; López-Jaramillo, J.; Palma, J.M.; Corpas, F.J. Endogenous hydrogen sulfide (H2S) is up-regulated during sweet pepper (*Capsicum annuum* L.) fruit ripening. In vitro analysis shows that NADP-dependent isocitrate dehydrogenase (ICDH) activity is inhibited by H_2S and NO. *Nitric Oxide* **2018**, *81*, 36–45. [CrossRef]
88. Muñoz-Vargas, M.A.; González-Gordo, S.; Palma, J.M.; Corpas, F.J. Inhibition of NADP-malic enzyme activity by H_2S and NO in sweet pepper (*Capsicum annuum* L.) fruits. *Physiol. Plant.* **2020**, *168*, 278–288.

89. León, A.M.; Palma, J.M.; Corpas, F.J.; Gómez, M.; Romero-Puertas, M.C.; Chatterjee, D.; Mateos, R.M.; Del Río, L.A.; Sandalio, L.M. Antioxidative enzymes in cultivars of pepper plants with different sensitivity to cadmium. *Plant Physiol. Biochem.* **2002**, *40*, 813–820.
90. Kopta, T.; Slosar, M.; Andrejiova, A.; Jurica, M.; Pokluda, R. The influence of genotype and season on the biological potential of chilli pepper cultivars. *Folia Hortic.* **2019**, *31*, 365–374. [CrossRef]
91. Goodwin, D.C.; Hertwig, K.M. Peroxidase-catalyzed oxidation of capsaicinoids: Steady-state and transient-state kinetic studies. *Arch. Biochem. Biophys.* **2003**, *417*, 18–26. [CrossRef]
92. Díaz-Vivancos, P.; De Simone, A.; Kiddle, G.; Foyer, C.H. Glutathione—Linking cell proliferation to oxidative stress. *Free Radic. Biol. Med.* **2015**, *89*, 1154–1164. [CrossRef]
93. Mateos, R.M.; León, A.M.; Sandalio, L.M.; Gómez, M.; Del Río, L.A.; Palma, J.M. Peroxisomes from pepper fruits (*Capsicum annuum* L): Purification, characterization and antioxidant activity. *J. Plant Physiol.* **2003**, *160*, 1507–1516. [CrossRef]
94. Broniowska, K.A.; Diers, A.R.; Hogg, N. S-nitrosoglutathione. *Biochim. Biophys. Acta* **2013**, *1830*, 3173–3181. [CrossRef]
95. Corpas, F.J.; Alché, J.D.; Barroso, J.B. Current overview of S-nitrosoglutathione (GSNO) in higher plants. *Front. Plant Sci.* **2013**, *4*, 126. [CrossRef]
96. Belcastro, E.; Gaucher, C.; Corti, A.; Leroy, P.; Lartaud, I.; Pompella, A. Regulation of protein function by S-nitrosation and S-glutathionylation: Processes and targets in cardiovascular pathophysiology. *Biol. Chem.* **2017**, *398*, 1267–1293. [CrossRef] [PubMed]
97. Mazourek, M.; Pujar, A.; Borovsky, Y.; Paran, I.; Mueller, L.; Jahn, M.M. A dynamic interface for capsaicinoid systems biology. *Plant Physiol.* **2009**, *150*, 1806–1821. [CrossRef]
98. Aghdam, M.S.; Palma, J.M.; Corpas, F.J. NADPH as quality footprinting in horticultural crops marketability. *Trends Food Sci. Technol.* **2020**, *168*, 111244. [CrossRef]
99. Palma, J.M.; Álvarez de Morales, P.; Del Río, L.A.; Corpas, F.J. The proteome of fruit peroxisomes: Sweet pepper (*Capsicum annuum* L.) as a model. *Subcell Biochem.* **2018**, *89*, 323–341.

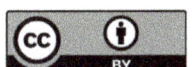

© 2020 by the authors. Licensee MDPI, Basel, Switzerland. This article is an open access article distributed under the terms and conditions of the Creative Commons Attribution (CC BY) license (http://creativecommons.org/licenses/by/4.0/).

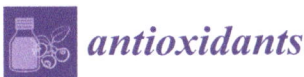

Review

Anthocyanins: From the Field to the Antioxidants in the Body

Vidmantas Bendokas [1],*, Vidmantas Stanys [1], Ingrida Mažeikienė [1], Sonata Trumbeckaite [2,3], Rasa Baniene [2,4] and Julius Liobikas [2,4],*

1. Institute of Horticulture, Lithuanian Research Centre for Agriculture and Forestry, 54333 Babtai, Lithuania; Vidmantas.stanys@lammc.lt (V.S.); ingrida.mazeikiene@lammc.lt (I.M.)
2. Laboratory of Biochemistry, Neuroscience Institute, Lithuanian University of Health Sciences, 44307 Kaunas, Lithuania; sonata.trumbeclaite@lsmuni.lt (S.T.); rasa.baniene@lsmuni.lt (R.B.)
3. Department of Pharmacognosy, Medical Academy, Lithuanian University of Health Sciences, 44307 Kaunas, Lithuania
4. Department of Biochemistry, Medical Academy, Lithuanian University of Health Sciences, 44307 Kaunas, Lithuania
* Correspondence: vidmantas.bendokas@lammc.lt (V.B.); julius.liobikas@lsmuni.lt or julius.liobikas@outlook.com (J.L.)

Received: 22 July 2020; Accepted: 29 August 2020; Published: 2 September 2020

Abstract: Anthocyanins are biologically active water-soluble plant pigments that are responsible for blue, purple, and red colors in various plant parts—especially in fruits and blooms. Anthocyanins have attracted attention as natural food colorants to be used in yogurts, juices, marmalades, and bakery products. Numerous studies have also indicated the beneficial health effects of anthocyanins and their metabolites on human or animal organisms, including free-radical scavenging and antioxidant activity. Thus, our aim was to review the current knowledge about anthocyanin occurrence in plants, their stability during processing, and also the bioavailability and protective effects related to the antioxidant activity of anthocyanins in human and animal brains, hearts, livers, and kidneys.

Keywords: anthocyanin metabolites; antioxidants; cardioprotection; hepatoprotection; nephroprotection; neuroprotection

---

1. Introduction

Anthocyanins are pigments belonging to the flavonoid group, which is widely distributed in plants. They are responsible for blue, purple, and red colors in flowers, fruits, and vegetables and protect plants from environmental stresses such as high sunlight irradiance [1] or low nitrogen [2]. Chemically, anthocyanins are produced when anthocyanidins are glycosylated. The most abundant anthocyanidin in plants is cyanidin. Other anthocyanidins are less abundant, and their frequency decreases in this order: delphinidin, peonidin, pelargonidin, petunidin, and malvidin [3]. Anthocyanidins are flavylium ion derivatives that vary in terms of their substituent groups: –H, –OH, or –OCH$_3$. Usually, anthocyanidins are glycosylated at the C3 or C3 and C5 sites, but the glycosylation of other sites has also been reported [4]. The biological activity of anthocyanins depends on their structure; however, all samples, including those with different compositions and amounts of anthocyanins, extracted from various berries and vegetables, are biologically active [5]. Azevedo et al. [6] established that the radical scavenging activity and reducing properties of anthocyanins strongly depend on the chemical structures of particular anthocyanins; this effect increases with the presence of catechol and pyrogallol groups in ring B of cyanidin-3-glucosides and the respective aglycones. Some studies have shown that delphinidin has the highest antioxidant activity compared with the other five anthocyanidins due to the three hydroxyl groups on the B-ring [5,7]. An increasing body of evidence shows that anthocyanin intake can have a protective effect on human and animal brains, hearts, livers, and kidneys, and many of the therapeutic effects may be purported to the antioxidant activities of anthocyanins and their metabolites [8–12]. The antioxidant activity of these compounds manifests through direct and indirect methods of action. Thus, anthocyanins can directly scavenge reactive oxygen species (ROS) [13,14], whereas the indirect pathways involve stimulation of the synthesis or activity of antioxidant enzymes (catalase, superoxide dismutase (SOD), glutathione peroxidase) [15]; inhibition of ROS-forming enzymes, such as nicotinamide adenine dinucleotide phosphate (NADPH) oxidase and others [16,17]; or even mild uncoupling of mitochondrial respiration preventing ROS generation [9,18]. It can also be assumed that for effective therapeutic action of anthocyanins, both the ROS scavenging activity and the modulation of cellular antioxidant systems are required [14]. Here, we review the current knowledge about anthocyanin occurrence in plants, their stability during processing, and the health benefits to humans and animals.

2. Natural Sources of Anthocyanins

Anthocyanins are natural, water-soluble plant pigments that are responsible for blue, red, or purple colors in plants. Plant genotypes, agro-climatic conditions, and fruit or vegetable maturity are significant factors in the composition and quantity of anthocyanins [19]. Therefore, the main sources of anthocyanins in human diet are fruits and vegetables, which accumulate anthocyanins in both the peel and flesh; however, their content varies greatly (Table 1).

Table 1. Maximum amount of anthocyanins (mg 100 g^{-1} of fresh weight (FW)) in fruits and vegetables.

Source	Anthocyanin Amount mg 100 g^{-1} FW	Dominant Anthocyanins	References
Bilberry	772.4	Dp3gal, Dp3glc, Dp3ara, Mv3glc, Cy3gal, Cy3glc, Cy3ara	[20]
Blackcurrant	478.6	Dp3rut, Cy3rut, Dp3glc, Cy3glc	
Golden currant	615.5	Cy3rut, Cy3glc, Pn3rut	[21,22]
Redcurrant	66.7	Cy3glc, Cy3rut, Cy3sam	
Elderberry	580.0	Cy3sam, Cy3glc	[19]
Grapes	116.4	Mv3glc, Cy3glc, Dp3glc, Pt3glc, Pn3glc	[23]
Sour cherry	147.0	Cy3rut	[24]
Sweet cherry	244.0	Cy3rut, Pn3rut	[25]
Wild strawberry	10.0	Pg3glc, Cy3glc	[26]
Black carrot	126.4	Cy3xylglcgal, Cy3xylgal	[27]
Eggplant	8.7	Dp3glc, Dp3rut,	[28,29]
Red cabbage	23.4	Cy3glc, Cy3rut, Dp3glc, Dp3rut, Cy3diglc5glc	[30,31]
Red chicory	39.2	Cy3glc	[29]
Purple wheat	23.5	Cy3glc	[32]

Cy—cyanidin; Dp—delphinidin; Mv—malvidin; Pg—pelargonidin; Pn—peonidin; Pt—petunidin; ara—arabinoside; gal—galactoside; glc—glucoside; rut—rutinoside; sam—sambubioside; xyl—xyloside.

Fruits, especially dark blue berries, accumulate a large total amount of anthocyanins, while vegetables tend to have lower anthocyanin concentrations. One of the highest anthocyanin concentrations was identified in bilberries, with delphinidins being the dominant anthocyanins making up over 57.6% of the total, with cyanidins representing 23.7% and malvidins representing 14.1% of the total [20]. Berries of the golden currant cultivar 'Corona' are the richest in anthocyanins among *Ribes* spp., with cyanidins being the dominant type [21]. Blackcurrants have a higher proportion of delphinidins, ranging from 66.7% to 70.2%, as shown in various studies [20,21]. In contrast, cyanidins dominate in redcurrant, elderberry, sweet cherry, and sour cherry, and sometimes, they are the only anthocyanins [11,20,22,23] (Mikulic-Petkovsek et al., 2014; Veberic et al., 2015; Bendokas et al., 2017; Blackhall et al., 2018). Malvidins are the main anthocyanin in grapes with a relative content ranging from 35.8% to 67.1% [25].

In terms of vegetables, red chicory has been shown to have the highest concentration of anthocyanins; however, it is 2–20 times lower than that in berries. Cyanidins are major anthocyanins in most vegetables; however, eggplant only accumulates delphinidins.

The consumption of anthocyanins varies from 9 mg/day on average in the United States to 19 mg/day in Europe, but daily consumption may reach 28 mg in some European countries [33]. The main sources of anthocyanins are berries (39% in the US and 43% in Europe), wine (18% in the US and 22% in Europe), and fruits (9% in the US and 19% in Europe), with other sources being vegetables and other foods [34].

3. Stability of Anthocyanins in Foods and Beverages

Anthocyanins are natural plant compounds that are increasingly being used in the food and pharmaceutical industry due to their effects on human health. However, the low stability of anthocyanins is still an obstacle to their use [35]. The stability of anthocyanins depends on the pH, temperature, light, presence of solvents and oxygen, and other factors [36]. Anthocyanins are more stable under acidic conditions. At a pH of 1.0, flavylium cations are the predominant species and contribute to the development of purple and red pigments, while at pH 2.0–4.0, the blue quinoidal species predominates. When the pH value reaches 7.0, anthocyanins are usually degraded [36]. The storage temperature affects the concentration of anthocyanins in extracts; for instance, 11% of rosella anthocyanins were lost after storage for 60 days at 4 °C, while 99% of anthocyanins were degraded in the same extracts stored at 37 °C for the same period [37].

The stability of anthocyanins from various *Ribes* species was reported to depend on their composition and storage conditions [24]. Anthocyanins in redcurrant berry extract have been shown to be more stable at room temperature and in the presence of light than extracts from berries of golden currant and gooseberry. After the storage of anthocyanin extracts under dark and cold conditions (+4 °C) for 84 days, up to 90% of redcurrant, 80% of gooseberry and golden currant, and up to 50% of blackcurrant anthocyanins remained intact [24].

Thermal food processing negatively affects the nutritional value of anthocyanin-rich juices as it results in anthocyanin degradation [38]. Thermal processing is responsible for the loss of up to 35% of anthocyanins. Even short-term thermal treatment (5 s at 85 °C) resulted in a loss of 9% of anthocyanins from strawberry juice, while pasteurization for 15 min resulted in a loss of 21% [39]. Boiling of red cabbage resulted in a loss of 41.2% of anthocyanins, while the anthocyanin concentration remained the same after steaming or stir-frying. Possibly, as highly water-soluble pigments, anthocyanins may be lost by leaching in the case of boiling [30].

Various anthocyanin stabilization methods are being developed. For instance, the improvement of anthocyanin thermal stability by yeast mannoproteins at pH 7.0 has been studied. The complexes were found to effectively protect anthocyanins from degradation during heating at 80 and 126 °C [40]. Mixing of clarified acerola juice with montmorillonite resulted in 50% more anthocyanins, regardless of time or pH changes [41]. Copigmentation is another natural tool that can be used to enhance anthocyanin stability. The most studied copigments are phenolic acids such as hydroxycinnamic and hydroxybenzoic acids [42]. Babaloo and Jamei [43] established that caffeic acid provides more stability for anthocyanins than benzoic, tannic, and coumaric acids. Encapsulation with polysaccharides, such as β-cyclodextrin, maltodextrin, or Arabic gum, is also important for the stabilization of anthocyanins. The protective effect of β-cyclodextrin was evident for all blackberry anthocyanins after thermal treatment at 90 °C for 2 h [44].

Novel techniques for phenolic compound isolation from natural products that avoid the degradation of these compounds have been developed. Block freeze concentration has been employed to extract anthocyanins from strawberries and enrich yogurt with the obtained concentrated strawberry juice. As a result, yogurt with a high anthocyanin content and greater antioxidant activity was produced; however, it had a short shelf life [45]. The foam mat drying technique is now considered to be an effective dehydration method to produce powder from juices or pulp. Only a small reduction in anthocyanins (7–9%) was observed after the storage of jambolana juice powder produced by foam mat drying for 150 days [46]. When foam-mat freeze-drying was used for powder production from blueberry juice, 80–100% of anthocyanins remained after processing; the most stable was Cy3glc [47].

4. Bioavailability of Anthocyanins

The beneficial health effects of anthocyanins strongly depend on their bioavailability, as only a small fraction of anthocyanins is absorbed by human body [48,49]. The concentration of anthocyanins in the plasma reaches a maximum value within 0.5–2 h after the consumption of anthocyanin-rich foods [50]. A low concentration of anthocyanins in plasma and urine has been observed in several studies. Less than 2% of original anthocyanins may be found in the plasma or urine after consumption; however, anthocyanins go through several transformations in the small and large intestines; thus, only a small fraction of the anthocyanins remains nonmetabolized or catabolized [51]. Mueller et al. [52] stated that a complex mixture of anthocyanin metabolites in the plasma rather than a single type of anthocyanins may cause beneficial effects in humans.

Gamel et al. [32] evaluated the absorption of anthocyanin metabolites after the consumption of purple wheat crackers and bars. They established that the total concentration of anthocyanin metabolites in urine peaked at 0–2 and 2–4 h, with 18–22 ng/mL excreted on average. For both products, the total amount of accumulated anthocyanins reached 13 µg in 24 h, representing 0.19%. A significant difference between male and female participants was also observed: males excreted 17.1 µg, while females excreted 11.6 µg of anthocyanin metabolites in a 24-h period. Krga and Milenkovic [53] conducted a comprehensive analysis of 20 studies on the anthocyanin concentration in human plasma after the ingestion of food, extracts, and drinks. They found that anthocyanin adsorption was the fastest after drinking red wine and red grape juice. The maximum concentration in the plasma was reached in 0.3 and 0.5 h, respectively, while the maximum concentration of anthocyanins from blueberry powder was reached in 4 h. Interestingly, the maximum anthocyanin concentration in plasma varied from 1.4 to 591.7 nM and did not depend on the administered dose, which was possibly due to differences in the anthocyanin composition in various foods. Recently, a human pilot study was performed by Röhrig and colleagues [54] on five healthy male volunteers who were consuming anthocyanin-rich blackcurrant extract. They studied the kinetics of the dominant anthocyanins—Dp3rut and Cy3rut—in plasma and urine after the consumption of blackcurrant extract. The peak concentrations of both anthocyanins in plasma were reached within 2 h after consumption. The maximum concentrations were 8.6 ± 5.8 nmol/L for Dp3rut and 9.8 ± 3.1 nmol/L for Cy3rut, which later gradually decreased. Similarly, urinary excretion rates of both studied anthocyanins peaked within 0–2 h of ingestion and reached 20.0 ± 2.6 nmol/h (Dp3rut) and 21.2 ± 3.8 nmol/h (Cy3rut). The total excreted amount was calculated: 0.040% (Dp3rut) and 0.048% (Cy3rut) of the ingested doses. In addition, after consumption of the anthocyanin-rich extract, the concentration of the main metabolite, protocatechuic acid, increased significantly [54].

In humans, anthocyanins consumed with food may be digested in the gastrointestinal tract, absorbed into the blood, and later metabolized [55]. Some studies have stated that minute amounts of anthocyanins are absorbed in the small intestine. The majority of ingested anthocyanins reach the large intestine where they are metabolized [56] and where structural modifications (deglycolysation, degradation, hydroxylation, etc.) take place due to the changing physiological conditions. Anthocyanins can also be further modified by various enzymes in the small intestine before entering the bloodstream [57]. Twenty-two metabolites of Cy3glc were identified using an isotopic approach [58]. Among them, phloroglucinaldehyde, 3,4-dihydroxybenzaldehyde, and hydroxybenzoic acid were found to be produced as phase I metabolites, while the phase II metabolites identified were mainly glucuronidated and methylated cyanidins. Colonic anthocyanin metabolites included hydroxybenzoic acid, hippuric acid, phenylpropenoic acid, ferulic acid, and phase II protocatechuic acid conjugates [58–60]. Bresciani and colleagues [61] analyzed the catabolism of anthocyanin-rich elderberry extract with different gut microbial strains in vitro and established that their metabolic pathways were different. Some common metabolites were found among all studied strains; however, each of them had several phenolic metabolites produced specifically by that strain. These in vitro results could provide new knowledge of the variability in anthocyanin metabolism in different organisms. After absorption, the fast transport of anthocyanins and their metabolites to the liver, heart, lungs, brain, and kidneys may be observed [55,62].

Sandoval-Ramírez and colleagues [63] summarized studies on the anthocyanin concentration in various animal tissues and stated that in short-term experiments, after a single dose of bilberry extract, the highest concentration of cyanidin-3-O-glucoside (40.46 pmol/g) was found in the brain after 0.25 min [62]. In addition, Cy3glc was identified in other tissues, such as the gastrointestinal tract (8×10^5 pmol/g), lungs (5.19×10^4 pmol/g), and prostate (4×10^4 pmol/g), with peak concentrations occurring at different times after a single oral dose of the extract [63,64]. In long-term studies, the highest concentration of Mv3glc (4.43 pmol/g) was established in the brains of pigs, while the concentration of Pt3glc reached 6.66 pmol/g [63]. Cy3ara from tart cherry was identified in the hearts, brains, livers, kidneys, and bladders of Wistar rats; however, its concentration was low and ranged from 2.28×10^{-4} to 1.16×10^{-3} pmol/g [65]. In general, Cy3glcand its metabolites are the most abundant anthocyanins in animal tissues, and Cy3glcmay be one of the most promising bioactive molecules for human health [63]. It is also worth noting that care is needed to avoid artefacts when studying and evaluating antioxidant effects of bioavailable anthocyanins in model organisms and the human body, as findings can depend on the chosen marker, the sensitivity of method to detect ROS and to measure oxidative damage, or even on the changes in plasma urate concentrations [66]). It is not the aim of the present review to analyze the suitability of methods to evaluate the antioxidant activity of anthocyanins; thus, for the complexity of the matter, one could consult several excellent reviews [66–70].

5. Biological Effects Related to the Antioxidant Activity of Anthocyanins—In Vivo Studies in Model Organisms

5.1. Neuroprotection

At the animal level, oral administration of anthocyanin-rich berry extract of *Vaccinium myrtillis* L. (100 mg/kg for 7 days) has been shown to suppress psychological stress-induced cerebral oxidative stress and dopamine abnormalities in distressed mice [71]. Anthocyanins extracted from black soybeans have also been demonstrated to reverse D-galactose- or lipopolysaccharide (LPS)-induced oxidative stress, neuroinflammation, and neurodegeneration in adult murine models [72–74]. Likewise, the same anthocyanins were shown to reduce elevation of the ROS level and consequent oxidative stress induced by the amyloid beta oligomer (Aβ 1-42) through stimulating the intracellular antioxidant system (the transcription factor E2-related factor 2 (Nrf2) and heme oxygenase-1 (HO-1) pathways). These anthocyanins also prevented apoptosis and neurodegeneration by suppressing the apoptotic and neurodegenerative markers in the amyloid precursor protein/presenilin-1 (APP/PS1) mouse model of Alzheimer's disease (AD) [75].

Positive findings have also been reported by Qin et al. [76] in Cy3glc-treated (10 mg/kg for 30 days) rats injected with Aβ 1-42, which showed an attenuation of Aβ- and oxidative stress-induced GSK-3β hyperactivation and hyperphosphorylation of the tau protein. These findings are in agreement with a study in which rats were injected with Aβ 1-42 bilaterally into the hippocampal CA1 area in order to produce an animal model of AD [77]. It was observed that the memory impairment was reduced in rats that received 80 mg/kg of *Lycium ruthenicum* Murr. anthocyanin-rich extract in comparison to other AD model rats. Moreover, the anthocyanin extract enhanced the activities of total SOD and catalase and increased the glutathione concentration in serum and brain tissues.

Chen et al. [78] also confirmed that *Lycium ruthenicum* Murr. anthocyanins can exert neuroprotective effects in D-galactose (D-gal)-treated rats. Anthocyanins reduce the level of receptor for advanced glycation end products (RAGE), suppress oxidative stress, and reduce levels of inflammation markers such as nuclear factor kappa B (NF-κB), interleukin-1-β (IL-1β), cyclooxygenase-2 (COX-2), and tumor necrosis factor-α (TNF-α), among others. Sustained levels of antioxidant enzymes (SOD and catalase), a decreased concentration of the lipid peroxidation product malondialdehyde, and significantly decreased expression of aging-associated monoamine oxidase-B in D-gal-treated mice were also demonstrated after the administration (30 mg/kg and 60 mg/kg) of black rice anthocyanins [79]. Anthocyanins from fruits of *Aronia melanocarpa* (Michx.) Elliot (30 mg/kg) retained the levels of total SOD and glutathione peroxidase and inhibited the excessive accumulation of inflammatory cytokines in the brain tissue of D-gal-treated mice [80]. Furthermore, recently, a study using a model of streptozotocin-induced dementia of sporadic AD [81] proposed that pretreatment with a commercial anthocyanin extract from grape skins (200 mg/kg for 25 days) can prevent behavioral alterations and protect against the changes in ROS and antioxidant enzyme (SOD, catalase, and glutathione peroxidase) levels.

Notably, purified anthocyanins and anthocyanidins have also been found to exert neuroprotective activities. For instance, pre-treatment with pelargonidin (Pg) (20 mg/kg) significantly suppressed the formation of thiobarbituric acid reactive substances, indicating reduced lipid peroxidation in 6-hydroxydopamine-lesioned rats (an experimental model or Parkinson's disease) [82]. Furthermore, orally consumed Cy3glc (2 mg/kg) reduced brain superoxide levels, infarct size, and improved neurological functions, thus revealing a neuroprotective effect in the cerebral artery occlusion model of ischemia in mice [83]. A recent report [84] also showed that an intravenous injection of Cy3gal and Cy3glc (0.025 mg/kg and 0.05 mg/kg), but not Cy3rut, in rats protected against ischemia-induced caspase-3 activation and necrotic cell death, as well as reducing the infarct size in the cerebral cortex and cerebellum. In contrast, 0.025 mg/kg of Pg3glc had no effect of the activity of caspase-3 but reduced the infarct size. The effects of anthocyanins have been found to correlate with the cytochrome c reducing capacity, and Pg3glc has been shown to have the smallest effect among tested anthocyanins. Thus, authors have proposed that under certain conditions, such as ischemic brain damage, the reducing properties rather than antioxidant properties of anthocyanins might be important in providing neuroprotection.

5.2. Cardioprotection

Since it is known that bilberries and blackcurrant berries are rich in anthocyanins, Brader et al. [85] investigated the effects of a berry-enriched diet (5 g of berry powder containing 172 mg of anthocyanins per day) on lipid profiles and other biomarkers in Zucker diabetic fatty rats. The results after eight weeks of supplementation demonstrated reduced levels of total and LDL-cholesterol, which was partly due to the altered expression of hepatic liver X receptor-α. Using an in vivo model of coronary occlusion and reperfusion, another study showed that the infarct size was reduced in the hearts of rats that received a long-term purple maize anthocyanin-enriched diet (with Cy and Pg glycosides as the main components) [86]. The authors proposed that the observed cardioprotection could be associated with increased myocardial glutathione levels and thus an improved endogenous cardiac antioxidant defense system. Moreover, Ziberna et al. [87] demonstrated that bilberry anthocyanins could exert concentration-dependent responses on whole rat hearts under ischemia–reperfusion (I-R) conditions. Thus, at low concentrations (0.01–1 mg/L, expressed as Cy3glc equivalents), the extent of I-R injury was significantly reduced, whereas at 5–50 mg/L, anthocyanins showed cardiotoxic activity despite having an intracellular antioxidant capability that increased in a concentration-dependent manner.

In addition, recent evidence from an LPS-induced myocardial injury model in mice [88] showed that pure anthocyanins such as Cy3glc could restore the activity of the mitochondrial electron transport chain (namely, the activity of complexes I and II) and thus significantly attenuate ROS production. Furthermore, the anthocyanins ameliorated cardiac injury, cell death, and improved cardiac function. It is worth noting that Cy3glc also suppressed the expression of endotoxin-induced pro-inflammatory cytokines and the level of protein nitration while elevating the intracellular level of reduced glutathione.

In general, these observations suggest that the cardioprotective activities of anthocyanins may not be solely attributed to their antioxidant properties; therefore, a broader view should be implemented [18,87,89,90].

5.3. Hepatoprotection

The liver plays an important role in the metabolic elimination of drugs and toxic compounds known to cause injury and reduce the function of the liver. Arjinajarn et al. [91] observed that rice bran extract (250–1000 mg/kg) rich in Cy3glc and Pn3glc (13.24 and 5.33 mg/g of crude extract, respectively) significantly prevented gentamicin-induced intoxication of the liver. It has been shown that an anthocyanin-rich extract significantly reduced the hepatic malondialdehyde level (a biomarker for oxidized lipids), increased expression of the antioxidant enzyme SOD, and prevented elevation of levels of liver injury markers, namely alanine and aspartate aminotransferase. These effects were related to the suppression of both the oxidative pathway regulated by the transcription factor Nrf2 and the inflammatory pathway regulated by NF-κB. The authors proposed that Cy3glc, the major anthocyanin in this extract, is responsible for these antioxidant and anti-inflammatory properties [91]. Moreover, Hou et al. found that black rice bran extract, which is rich in anthocyanins (mainly Cy3glc and Pn3glc), protected mice liver intoxicated with carbon tetrachloride (CCl_4) [87]. It was found that mice treated with black rice extract (200–800 mg/kg) showed increased SOD and glutathione peroxidase activities and increased levels of reduced glutathione as compared with a CCl_4-intoxicated model group [92]. Similar results about the protective effects of blueberry anthocyanin extract (anthocyanin content up to 25%) on CCl_4-induced liver injury in mice in vivo were presented by [93]. The extract had reduced concentrations of alanine aminotransferase, aspartate aminotransferase, and malondialdehyde in a dose-dependent manner, while the activities of SOD, catalase, and glutathione reductase increased [93]. Blackberry fruit extract was similarly shown to attenuate lipid peroxidation and to recover the activity of antioxidant enzymes in CCl_4-treated rats [94]. Recently, Sun et al. observed that anthocyanins from blueberry (100 mg/kg and 200 mg/kg per day) protected mouse liver from CCl_4-induced hepatic fibrosis [95]. It was detected that blueberry anthocyanins reduced ROS generation and tissue oxidative damage, decreased inflammation, and suppressed the activity of hepatic stellate cells. Interestingly, the activity of mitochondrial electron transport chain complexes I and II was also restored after treatment with anthocyanins [95].

It is also known that liver inflammation and an excessive accumulation of lipids play critical roles in the pathogenesis of alcoholic liver diseases. Accordingly, in a recent study, Cy3glc extracted from *Lonicera caerulea* L. was shown to exert a hepatoprotective effect on alcoholic steatohepatitis in mice [96]. Zuo et al. detected substantial decreases in serum aminotransferases and triglycerides and found increased albumin levels after treatment. In addition, anthocyanidins significantly suppressed the expression of SREBP1 (a transcription factor involved in lipogenesis) and enhanced the phosphorylation of AMPK as compared with chronic ethanol administration. Cy-3-g suppressed inflammasome activation, thereby preventing activated macrophages from producing pro-inflammation cytokines [96]. Moreover, another study demonstrated that a phenolic fraction of *Lonicera caerulea* L. ameliorated inflammation and lipid peroxidation by upregulating Nrf2 and SOD and downregulating the transcription factor forkhead box protein O1 and HO-1 in a mouse model of nonalcoholic steatohepatitis (NASH) induced by a high-fat diet in combination with CCl_4 [97]. Prokop et al. also showed in vivo that a blue grain bread wheat-based diet (genotype UC66049, containing 121 mg of Cy3glc per kg of wheat) increased the activity of the microsomal xenobiotic-metabolizing system cytochrome P450 by 20–50% in rats after 72 days of intake. In addition, an anthocyanin-rich diet significantly increased the antioxidant power of plasma as shown by a FRAP assay and the level of total –SH groups in plasma when compared with the control [98].

5.4. Nephroprotective Effects

Anthocyanins are considered to be a functional food factor and to play an important role in the prevention of kidney diseases. For example, a recent study [99] investigated the effects of anthocyanin-rich bilberry extract (200 mg/kg daily) on the antioxidant status of animals intoxicated with CCl_4. Rats received the extract orally for 7 days, and on the last day, a single dose of CCl_4 was intraperitoneal (i.p.) injected. It was found that pretreatment with the anthocyanin-rich extract resulted in a significant reduction in pro-oxidative (H_2O_2, oxidized glutathione, xanthine oxidase) and pro-inflammatory markers (myeloperoxidase, nitric oxide, and TNF-α), and a substantial increase of antioxidant enzyme levels (catalase, SOD, glutathione peroxidase, and S-transferase). Moreover, the anthocyanins significantly reduced the degree of damage to the proximal and distal tubules in the kidney cortex [99].

Positive findings have also been reported by another study [100]. It showed that the administration of *Malva sylvestris* L. extract (200 or 400 mg/kg) rich in anthocyanins reduced the renal toxicity induced by gentamicin and thus led to (i) an improvement in kidney function, (ii) a decrease in the expression levels of pro-inflammatory markers (TNF-α), (iii) a reduction in oxidative stress (levels of malondialdehyde and total antioxidant capacity), and (iv) a decrease in tissue injuries.

Similar beneficial effects of the bilberry diet (100 mg/kg daily) on the levels of serum malondialdehyde, catalase, and advanced oxidation protein products were demonstrated in a rat model of gentamicin-induced nephrotoxicity, and the effects correlated well with the antioxidant activity (assessed in vivo and in vitro) as well as with high anthocyanin levels [101]. It is worth noting that anthocyanin-rich fruits of *Panax ginseng* Meyer have also been shown to attenuate cisplatin-induced elevations in blood urea nitrogen and creatinine levels as well as the prevalence of histopathological injuries in mice [102]. The positive outcomes are related to reduced levels of malondialdehyde, HO-1, cytochrome P450 E1, 4-hydroxynonenal, TNF-α, and IL-1β, as well as concomitantly increased levels of reduced glutathione, catalase, and SOD.

In addition, Lee et al. [103] recently revealed that intravenously administered pure Pg (0.4 mg/kg) could modulate renal function in a mouse model of sepsis. Treatment with Pg reduced renal tissue injury, plasma nitrite and nitrate production, and TNF-α, IL-6, myeloperoxidase, and malondialdehyde levels. The total glutathione content as well as the activity of antioxidant enzymes such as SOD, glutathione peroxidase, and catalase in kidney tissues were also found to be restored after Pg injection.

6. Biological Effects Related to the Antioxidant Activity of Anthocyanins—In Vivo Studies in Humans

Epidemiological and clinical studies suggest that an anthocyanin-enriched diet may lower levels of certain oxidative stress biomarkers in humans, and this could be associated with reduced risk of cognitive decline and the development of neurodegenerative and cardiovascular diseases, as well as having sustained hepatic function and kidney protecting activities [12,104–115].

6.1. Antioxidant and Anti-Atherosclerogenic Effects

A randomized clinical trial [116] evaluated the effects of a standardized maqui berry (*Aristotelia chilensis* (Mol.) Stuntz) extract (containing 162 mg of anthocyanins) on products of lipid peroxidation in healthy, overweight, and smoker adults. The results suggested that supplementation with the extract can be related to a limited term (max for 40 days) reduction in oxidized low-density lipoprotein (LDL) levels and a decrease in urinary F2-isoprostanes. Another study [117] concluded that the acute consumption of anthocyanin-rich red *Vitis labrusca* L. grape juices could be related to decreased levels of thiobarbituric acid reactive substances and lipid peroxides in the serum of healthy subjects. It has also been demonstrated that regular (for 30 days) anthocyanin-rich sour cherry consumption could suppress the formation of ROS by circulating phagocytes and decrease the risk of systemic imbalance between oxidants and antioxidants [118]. It is worth noting that a portion (300 g) of blueberries, the dietary source of anthocyanins provided to young volunteers involved in a randomized cross-over study, significantly reduced H_2O_2-induced DNA damage in blood mononuclear cells [119]. In another human pilot intervention study, the consumption of anthocyanin-rich bilberry (*Vaccinium myrtillius* L.) pomace extract was found to modulate transcription factor E2-related factor 2 (Nrf2)-dependent gene expression in peripheral blood mononuclear cells [120].

A single-blind randomized placebo-controlled intervention trial, which lasted for 8 weeks and involved 72 unmedicated subjects, revealed that the administration of various berries (including bilberries, chokeberries, and blackcurrants) increased both the concentration of high-density lipoprotein (HDL) cholesterol and the plasma antioxidant capacity [121]. Higher dietary anthocyanin and flavan-3-ol intake was associated with anti-inflammatory effects in 2375 Framingham Heart Study Offspring Cohort participants [122]. Interestingly, the consumption of 300 mL of red wine (a total dose of anthocyanins was 304 µM, which was the highest amount among detected compounds) with a meal was shown to prevent the postprandial increases in plasma lipid hydroperoxides and cholesterol oxidation products and therefore protect against a potential pro-atherosclerogenic effect [123]. Similar findings were obtained in a randomized cross-over trial, which concluded that a moderate consumption of red wine decreases erythrocyte SOD activity [124]. In another randomized double-blind trial, 150 subjects with hypercholesterolemia consumed a purified anthocyanin mixture derived from bilberries and blackcurrants (320 mg/day) for 24 weeks [125]. It was found that anthocyanin consumption significantly decreased the levels of inflammatory biomarkers (C-reactive protein, soluble vascular cell adhesion molecule-1, and plasma IL-1β) and increased the HDL cholesterol level. Recently, it was shown that a daily intake of 150 g of anthocyanin-rich blueberries resulted in clinically relevant improvements in endothelial function and systemic arterial stiffness, which was probably due to the improved nitric oxide bioactivity and HDL status [126].

6.2. Hepatoprotective Benefits

Nonalcoholic fatty liver disease (NAFLD), defined by excessive lipid accumulation in the liver, is the hepatic manifestation of insulin resistance and metabolic syndrome. NAFLD encompasses a wide spectrum of liver diseases ranging from simple uncomplicated steatosis to steatohepatitis, cirrhosis, and hepatocellular carcinoma [106]. Zhang et al. [127] reported that anthocyanins extracted from bilberry and blackcurrant (320 mg/day) and administered for 12 weeks ameliorated liver injury in patients with NAFLD. It was observed that a so-called "anthocyanin group" exhibited significant decreases in the plasma alanine aminotransferase, cytokeratin-18 M30 fragment, and myeloperoxidase levels. It was also found that consumption of *Myrica rubra* Sieb. and Zucc. juice (250 mL for 4 weeks) protected young adults (18–25 years old) against NAFLD by improving the plasma antioxidant status and inhibiting the inflammatory and apoptotic responses involved in this disease [128].

6.3. Nephroprotection

In another study, red fruit juice (40% red grape juice, 20% blackberry juice, 15% sour cherry juice, 15% blackcurrant juice, and 10% elderberry juice) with high polyphenol and anthocyanin contents was tested for its preventive potential in hemodialysis patients [129]. For this purpose, 21 subjects consumed 200 mL/day of juice according to the following protocols: 3-week run-in; 4-week juice uptake; 3-week wash-out. The results revealed a significant decrease in DNA oxidation damage and protein and lipid peroxidation and an increase in the reduced glutathione level; the effects were attributed to the high anthocyanin and polyphenol contents of the juice [129]. Another study [130] demonstrated that the regular consumption of concentrated red grape juice by hemodialysis patients could be associated with the reduced neutrophil NADPH oxidase activity and plasma concentrations of oxidized LDL and inflammatory biomarkers.

7. Concluding Remarks

In conclusion, anthocyanins are valuable biomolecules with a broad variety of biological effects on human health, and we suggest adding more anthocyanin rich fruits, vegetables, and their products to the daily diet. Numerous studies indicate that bilberry, blackcurrant, elderberry, and other berries have the highest total concentrations of anthocyanins; therefore, the consumption of fresh berries and their processed products may have greater beneficial effects on humans. Various anthocyanin stabilization methods have been developed e.g., copigmentation with other phenolic acids, encapsulation with polysaccharides, block freeze concentration, and powder production using the foam mat drying technique. All of them enable anthocyanins to be preserved during processing, thus increasing their bioavailability and delivery to target tissues in the human body. However, long-term studies on the impacts of anthocyanin-rich product consumption on human health are still rare. Further studies could focus on the identification and tracking of individual anthocyanin metabolites and on the determination of the exact dosage and delivery platforms sustaining the antioxidant properties of anthocyanins in vivo. In addition, as an alternative to natural sources, synthesis of the most bioactive anthocyanins in bioreactors should be considered.

Author Contributions: Original idea and conceptualization V.S. and J.L., original draft preparation V.B., V.S., I.M., S.T., R.B. and J.L., review and editing V.B., I.M. and J.L. All authors have read and agreed to the published version of the manuscript.

Funding: This research was funded by the Research Council of Lithuania (V.B., V.S. and J.L.; No. SVE-11-008). J.L. was supported by the COST Action FA0602 «Bioactive food components, mitochondrial function and health». J.L. and S.T. are supported by the program «2014-2020 Investment of EU Funds in Lithuania: Intellect. Common Scientific and Business Projects» (project No J05-LVPA–K-03-0117).

Conflicts of Interest: The authors declare no conflict of interest.

References

1. Landi, M.; Tattini, M.; Gould, K.S. Multiple functional roles of anthocyanins in plant-environment interactions. *Environ. Exp. Bot.* **2015**, *119*, 4–17. [CrossRef]
2. Liang, J.; He, J. Protective role of anthocyanins in plants under low nitrogen stress. *Biochem. Biophys. Res. Commun.* **2018**, *498*, 946–953. [CrossRef] [PubMed]
3. Cody, R.B.; Tamura, J.; Downard, K.M. Quantitation of anthocyanins in elderberry fruit extracts and nutraceutical formulations with paper spray ionization mass spectrometry. *J. Mass Spectrom.* **2018**, *53*, 58–64. [CrossRef] [PubMed]
4. Zhao, C.L.; Chen, Z.J.; Bai, X.S.; Ding, C.; Long, T.J.; Wei, F.G.; Miao, K.R. Structure–activity relationships of anthocyanidin glycosylation. *Mol. Divers.* **2014**, *18*, 687–700. [CrossRef] [PubMed]
5. Blando, F.; Calabriso, N.; Berland, H.; Maiorano, G.; Gerardi, C.; Carluccio, M.A.; Andersen, Ø.M. Radical Scavenging and Anti-Inflammatory Activities of Representative Anthocyanin Groupings from Pigment-Rich Fruits and Vegetables. *Int. J. Mol. Sci.* **2018**, *19*, 169. [CrossRef]
6. Azevedo, J.; Fernandes, I.; Faria, A.; Oliveira, J.; Fernandes, A.; de Freitas, V.; Mateus, N. Antioxidant properties of anthocyanidins, anthocyanidins 3-glucosides and respective portisins. *Food Chem.* **2010**, *119*, 518–523. [CrossRef]
7. Ali, M.H.; Almagribi, W.; Al-Rashidi, M.N. Antiradical and reductant activities of anthocyanidins and anthocyanins, structure-activity relationship and synthesis. *Food Chem.* **2016**, *194*, 1275–1282. [CrossRef]
8. Pojer, E.; Mattivi, F.; Johnson, D.; Stockley, C.S. The Case for Anthocyanin Consumption to Promote Human Health: A Review. *Compr. Rev. Food Sci. Food Saf.* **2013**, *12*, 483–508. [CrossRef]
9. Liobikas, J.; Skemiene, K.; Trumbeckaite, S.; Borutaite, V. Anthocyanins in Cardioprotection: A Path through Mitochondria. *Pharmacol. Res.* **2016**, *113*, 808–815. [CrossRef]
10. Kalt, W. Anthocyanins and Their C_6-C_3-C_6 Metabolites in Humans and Animals. *Molecules* **2019**, *24*, 4024. [CrossRef]
11. Bendokas, V.; Skemiene, K.; Trumbeckaite, S.; Stanys, V.; Passamonti, S.; Borutaite, V.; Liobikas, J. Anthocyanins: From Plant Pigments to Health Benefits at Mitochondrial Level. *Crit. Rev. Food Sci. Nutr.* **2019**, In Press. [CrossRef] [PubMed]
12. Kalt, W.; Cassidy, A.; Howard, L.R.; Krikorian, R.; Stull, A.J.; Tremblay, F.; Zamora-Ros, R. Recent Research on the Health Benefits of Blueberries and Their Anthocyanins. *Adv. Nutr.* **2020**, *11*, 224–236. [CrossRef] [PubMed]
13. Miguel, M.G. Anthocyanins: Antioxidant and/or anti-inflammatory activities. *J. Appl. Pharm. Sci.* **2011**, *1*, 7–15.
14. Ereminas, G.; Majiene, D.; Sidlauskas, K.; Jakstas, V.; Ivanauskas, L.; Vaitiekaitis, G.; Liobikas, J. Neuroprotective Properties of Anthocyanidin Glycosides Against H_2O_2-induced Glial Cell Death Are Modulated by Their Different Stability and Antioxidant Activity In Vitro. *Biomed. Pharmacother.* **2017**, *94*, 188–196. [CrossRef]

15. Aboonabi, A.; Singh, I. Chemopreventive Role of Anthocyanins in Atherosclerosis via Activation of Nrf2-ARE as an Indicator and Modulator of Redox. *Biomed. Pharmacother.* **2015**, *72*, 30–36. [CrossRef]
16. Lim, T.G.; Jung, S.K.; Kim, J.; Kim, Y.; Lee, H.J.; Jang, T.S.; Lee, K.W. NADPH Oxidase Is a Novel Target of Delphinidin for the Inhibition of UVB-induced MMP-1 Expression in Human Dermal Fibroblasts. *Exp. Dermatol.* **2013**, *22*, 428–430. [CrossRef]
17. Reis, J.F.; Monteiro, V.V.S.; de Souza Gomes, R.; do Carmo, M.M.; da Costa, G.V.; Ribera, P.C.; Monteiro, M.C. Action Mechanism and Cardiovascular Effect of Anthocyanins: A Systematic Review of Animal and Human Studies. *J. Transl. Med.* **2016**, *14*, 315. [CrossRef]
18. Skemiene, K.; Rakauskaite, G.; Trumbeckaite, S.; Liobikas, J.; Brown, G.C.; Borutaite, V. Anthocyanins block ischemia-induced apoptosis in the perfused heart and support mitochondrial respiration potentially by reducing cytosolic cytochrome c. *Int. J. Biochem. Cell Biol.* **2013**, *45*, 23–29. [CrossRef]
19. Mikulic-Petkovsek, M.; Schmitzer, V.; Slatnar, A.; Todorovic, B.; Veberic, R.; Stampar, F.; Ivancic, A. Investigation of anthocyanin profile of four elderberry species and interspecific hybrids. *J. Agric. Food Chem.* **2014**, *62*, 5573–5580. [CrossRef]
20. Veberic, R.; Slatnar, A.; Bizjak, J.; Stampar, F.; Mikulic-Petkovsek, M. Anthocyanin composition of different wild and cultivated berry species. *LWT* **2015**, *60*, 509–517. [CrossRef]
21. Stanys, V.; Bendokas, V.; Rugienius, R.; Sasnauskas, A.; Frercks, B.; Mažeikienė, I.; Šikšnianas, T. Management of anthocyanin amount and composition in genus *Ribes* using interspecific hybridisation. *Sci. Hortic.* **2019**, *247*, 123–129. [CrossRef]
22. Siksnianas, T.; Bendokas, V.; Rugienius, R.; Sasnauskas, A.; Stepulaitiene, I.; Stanys, V. Anthocyanin content and stability in *Ribes* species and interspecific hybrids. *Rural Dev.* **2013**, *6*, 258–261.
23. Dimitrovska, M.; Bocevska, M.; Dimitrovski, D.; Murkovic, M. Anthocyanin composition of Vranec, Cabernet Sauvignon, Merlot and Pinot Noir grapes as indicator of their varietal differentiation. *Eur. Food Res. Technol.* **2011**, *32*, 591–600. [CrossRef]
24. Bendokas, V.; Stepulaitiene, I.; Stanys, V.; Siksnianas, T.; Anisimoviene, N. Content of anthocyanin and other phenolic compounds in cherry species and interspecific hybrids. *Acta Hortic.* **2017**, *1161*, 587–592. [CrossRef]
25. Blackhall, M.L.; Berry, R.; Davies, N.W.; Wallsa, J.T. Optimized extraction of anthocyanins from Reid Fruits' *Prunus avium* 'Lapins' cherries. *Food Chem.* **2018**, *256*, 280–285. [CrossRef]
26. Rugienius, R.; Bendokas, V.; Kazlauskaitė, E.; Siksnianas, T.; Stanys, V.; Kazanaviciute, V.; Sasnauskas, A. Anthocyanin content in cultivated Fragaria vesca berries under high temperature and water deficit stress. *Acta Hortic.* **2016**, *1139*, 639–644. [CrossRef]
27. Algarra, M.; Fernandes, A.; Mateus, N.; de Freitas, V.; da Silva, J.C.G.; Casado, E.J. Anthocyanin profile and antioxidant capacity of black carrots (*Daucus carota* L. ssp. *sativus* var. *atrorubens* Alef.) from Cuevas Bajas, Spain. *J. Food Compost. Anal.* **2014**, *33*, 71–76. [CrossRef]
28. Liu, Y.; Tikunov, Y.; Schouten, R.E.; Marcelis, L.F.M.; Visser, R.G.F.; Bovy, A. Anthocyanin Biosynthesis and Degradation Mechanisms in Solanaceous Vegetables: A Review. *Front. Chem.* **2018**, *6*, 52. [CrossRef]
29. Frond, A.D.; Iuhas, C.I.; Stirbu, I.; Leopold, L.; Socaci, S.; Andreea, S.; Ayvaz, H.; Andreea, S.; Mihai, S.; Diaconeasa, Z.; et al. Phytochemical Characterization of Five Edible Purple-Reddish Vegetables: Anthocyanins, Flavonoids, and Phenolic Acid Derivatives. *Molecules* **2019**, *24*, 1536. [CrossRef]
30. Murador, D.C.; Mercadante, A.Z.; de Rosso, V.V. Cooking techniques improve the levels of bioactive compounds and antioxidant activity in kale and red cabbage. *Food Chem.* **2016**, *196*, 1101–1107. [CrossRef]
31. Tong, T.; Niu, Y.H.; Yue, Y.; Wu, S.-C.; Ding, H. Beneficial effects of anthocyanins from red cabbage (*Brassica oleracea* L. var. *capitata* L.) administration to prevent irinotecaninduced mucositis. *J. Funct. Foods* **2017**, *32*, 9–17. [CrossRef]
32. Gamel, T.H.; Wright, A.J.; Tucker, A.J.; Pickard, M.; Rabalski, I.; Podgorski, M.; Di Ilio, N.; O'Brien, C.; Abdel-Aal, E.M. Absorption and metabolites of anthocyanins and phenolic acids after consumption of purple wheat crackers and bars by healthy adults. *J. Cereal Sci.* **2019**, *86*, 60–68. [CrossRef]
33. Vogiatzoglou, A.; Mulligan, A.A.; Lentjes, M.A.H.; Luben, R.N.; Spencer, J.P.E.; Schroeter, H.; Khaw, K.-T.; Kuhnle, G.G.C. Flavonoid Intake in European Adults (18 to 64 Years). *PLoS ONE* **2015**, *10*, e0128132. [CrossRef] [PubMed]
34. Kim, K.; Vance, T.M.; Chun, O.K. Estimated intake and major food sources of flavonoids among US adults: Changes between 1999–2002 and 2007–2010 in NHANES. *Eur. J. Nutr.* **2016**, *55*, 833–843. [CrossRef]

35. Tan, C.; Selig, M.J.; Lee, M.C.; Abbaspourrad, A. Polyelectrolyte microcapsules built on $CaCO_3$ scaffolds for the integration, encapsulation, and controlled release of copigmented anthocyanins. *Food Chem.* **2018**, *246*, 305–312. [CrossRef]
36. Castañeda-Ovando, A.; Pacheco-Hernández, M.L.; Páez-Hernández, M.E.; Rodríguez, J.A.; Galán-Vidal, C.A. Chemical studies of anthocyanins: A review. *Food Chem.* **2009**, *113*, 859–871. [CrossRef]
37. Sinela, A.; Rawat, N.; Mertz, C.; Achir, N.; Fulcrand, H.; Dornier, M. Anthocyanins degradation during storage of Hibiscus sabdariffa extract and evolution of its degradation products. *Food Chem.* **2017**, *214*, 234–241. [CrossRef]
38. Wang, Z.; Zhang, M.; Wu, Q. Effects of temperature, pH, and sunlight exposure on the color stability of strawberry juice during processing and storage. *LWT* **2015**, *60*, 1174–1178. [CrossRef]
39. Weber, F.; Larsen, L.R. Influence of fruit juice processing on anthocyanin stability. *Food Res. Int.* **2017**, *100*, 354–365. [CrossRef]
40. Wu, J.; Guan, Y.; Zhong, Q. Yeast mannoproteins improve thermal stability of anthocyanins at pH 7.0. *Food Chem.* **2015**, *172*, 121–128. [CrossRef]
41. Ribeiro, H.L.; de Oliveira, A.V.; de Brito, E.S.; Ribeiro, P.R.V.; Filho, M.M.S.; Azeredo, H.M.C. Stabilizing effect of montmorillonite on acerola juice anthocyanins. *Food Chem.* **2018**, *245*, 966–973. [CrossRef] [PubMed]
42. Bimpilas, A.; Panagopoulou, M.; Tsimogiannis, D.; Oreopoulou, V. Anthocyanin copigmentation and color of wine: The effect of naturally obtained hydroxycinnamic acids as cofactors. *Food Chem.* **2016**, *197*, 39–46. [CrossRef] [PubMed]
43. Babaloo, F.; Jamei, R. Anthocyanin pigment stability of Cornus mas–Macrocarpa under treatment with pH and some organic acids. *Food Sci. Nutr.* **2018**, *6*, 168–173. [CrossRef] [PubMed]
44. Fernandes, A.; Rocha, M.A.A.; Santos, L.M.N.B.F.; Brás, J.; Oliveira, J.; Mateus, N.; de Freitas, V. Blackberry anthocyanins: β-Cyclodextrin fortification for thermal and gastrointestinal stabilization. *Food Chem.* **2018**, *245*, 426–431. [CrossRef]
45. Jaster, H.; Arend, G.D.; Rezzadori, K.; Chaves, V.C.; Reginatto, F.H.; Petrus, J.C.C. Enhancement of antioxidant activity and physicochemical properties of yogurt enriched with concentrated strawberry pulp obtained by block freeze concentration. *Food Res. Int.* **2018**, *104*, 119–125. [CrossRef]
46. de Carvalho Tavares, I.M.; Sumere, B.R.; Gómez-Alonso, S.; Gomes, E.; Hermosín-Gutiérrez, I.; Da-Silva, R.; Lago-Vanzela, E.S. Storage stability of the phenolic compounds, color and antioxidant activity of jambolan juice powder obtained by foam mat drying. *Food Res. Int.* **2020**, *128*, 108750. [CrossRef]
47. Darniadi, S.; Ifie, I.; Ho, P.; Murray, B.S. Evaluation of total monomeric anthocyanin, total phenolic content and individual anthocyanins of foam-mat freeze-dried and spray-dried blueberry powder. *J. Food Meas. Charact.* **2019**, *13*, 1599–1606. [CrossRef]
48. Faria, A.; Pestana, D.; Azevedo, J.; Martel, F.; de Freitas, V.; Azevedo, I.; Mateus, N.; Calhau, C. Absorption of anthocyanins through intestinal epithelial cells – putative involvement of GLUT2. *Mol. Nutr. Food Res.* **2009**, *53*, 1430–1437. [CrossRef]
49. Braga, A.R.C.; Murador, D.C.; de S Mesquita, L.M.; De Rosso, V.V. Bioavailability of anthocyanins: Gaps in knowledge, challenges and future research. *J. Food Composit. Anal.* **2018**, *68*, 31–40. [CrossRef]
50. Fang, J. Bioavailability of anthocyanins. *Drug Metab. Rev.* **2014**, *46*, 508–520. [CrossRef]
51. Eker, M.E.; Aaby, K.; Budic-Leto, I.; Rimac Brnčić, S.; El, S.N.; Karakaya, S.; Simsek, S.; Manach, C.; Wiczkowski, W.; de Pascual-Teresa, S. A Review of Factors Affecting Anthocyanin Bioavailability: Possible Implications for the Inter-Individual Variability. *Foods* **2020**, *9*, 2. [CrossRef] [PubMed]
52. Mueller, D.; Jung, K.; Winter, M.; Rogoll, D.; Melcher, R.; Richling, E. Human intervention study to investigate the intestinal accessibility and bioavailability of anthocyanins from bilberries. *Food Chem.* **2017**, *231*, 275–286. [CrossRef]
53. Krga, I.; Milenkovic, D. Anthocyanins: From Sources and Bioavailability to Cardiovascular-Health Benefits and Molecular Mechanisms of Action. *J. Agric. Food Chem.* **2019**, *67*, 1771–1783. [CrossRef] [PubMed]
54. Röhrig, T.; Kirsch, V.; Schipp, D.; Galan, J.; Richling, E. Absorption of Anthocyanin Rutinosides after Consumption of a Blackcurrant (*Ribes nigrum* L.) Extract. *J. Agric. Food Chem.* **2019**, *67*, 6792–6797. [CrossRef]
55. Han, F.; Yang, P.; Wang, H.; Fernandes, I.; Mateus, N.; Liu, Y. Digestion and absorption of red grape and wine anthocyanins through the gastrointestinal tract. *Trends Food Sci. Technol.* **2019**, *83*, 211–224. [CrossRef]

56. Kay, C.D.; Pereira-Caro, G.; Ludwig, I.A.; Clifford, M.N.; Crozier, A. Anthocyanins and Flavanones Are More Bioavailable than Previously Perceived: A Review of Recent Evidence. *Annu. Rev. Food Sci. Technol.* **2017**, *8*, 155–180. [CrossRef]
57. Sandhu, A.K.; Miller, M.G.; Thangthaeng, N.; Scott, T.M.; Shukitt-Hale, B.; Edirisinghe, I.; Burton-Freeman, B. Metabolic fate of strawberry polyphenols after chronic intake in healthy older adults. *Food Funct.* **2018**, *9*, 96–106. [CrossRef]
58. Czank, C.; Cassidy, A.; Zhang, Q.; Morrison, D.J.; Preston, T.; Kroon, P.A.; Botting, N.P.; Kay, C.D. Human metabolism and elimination of the anthocyanin, cyanidin-3-glucoside: A 13C-tracer study. *Am. J. Clin. Nutr.* **2013**, *97*, 995–1003. [CrossRef]
59. De Ferrars, R.M.; Czank, C.; Zhang, Q.; Botting, N.P.; Kroon, P.A.; Cassidy, A.; Kay, C.D. The pharmacokinetics of anthocyanins and their metabolites in humans. *Br. J. Pharmacol.* **2014**, *171*, 3268–3282. [CrossRef]
60. Xie, L.; Lee, S.G.; Vance, T.M.; Wang, Y.; Kim, B.; Lee, J.Y.; Chun, O.K.; Bolling, B.W. Bioavailability of anthocyanins and colonic polyphenol metabolites following consumption of aronia berry extract. *Food Chem.* **2016**, *211*, 860–868. [CrossRef]
61. Bresciani, L.; Angelino, D.; Vivas, E.I.; Kerby, R.L.; García-Viguera, C.; Del Rio, D.; Rey, F.E.; Mena, P. Differential Catabolism of an Anthocyanin-Rich Elderberry Extract by Three Gut Microbiota Bacterial Species. *J. Agric. Food Chem.* **2020**, *68*, 1837–1843. [CrossRef] [PubMed]
62. Fornasaro, S.; Ziberna, L.; Gasperotti, M.; Tramer, F.; Vrhovšek, U.; Mattivi, F.; Passamonti, S. Determination of cyanidin 3-glucoside in rat brain, liver and kidneys by UPLC/MS-MS and its application to a short-term pharmacokinetic study. *Sci. Rep.* **2016**, *6*, 1–11. [CrossRef] [PubMed]
63. Sandoval-Ramírez, B.A.; Catalán, Ú.; Fernández-Castillejo, S.; Rubio, L.; Macia, A.; Sola, R. Anthocyanin tissue bioavailability in animals: Possible implications for human health: A systematic review. *J. Agric. Food Chem.* **2018**, *66*, 11531–11543. [CrossRef]
64. Marczylo, T.H.; Cooke, D.; Brown, K.; Steward, W.P.; Gescher, A.J. Pharmacokinetics and Metabolism of the Putative Cancer Chemopreventive Agent Cyanidin-3-Glucoside in Mice. *Cancer Chemother. Pharmacol.* **2009**, *64*, 1261–1268. [CrossRef] [PubMed]
65. Kirakosyan, A.; Seymour, E.M.; Wolforth, J.; McNish, R.; Kaufman, P.B.; Bolling, S.F. Tissue Bioavailability of Anthocyanins from Whole Tart Cherry in Healthy Rats. *Food Chem.* **2015**, *171*, 26–31. [CrossRef]
66. Halliwell, B.; Rafter, J.; Jenner, A. Health promotion by flavonoids, tocopherols, tocotrienols, and other phenols: Direct or indirect effects? Antioxidant or not? *Am. J. Clin. Nutr.* **2005**, *81* (Suppl. 1), 268S–276S. [CrossRef]
67. Halliwell, B.; Whiteman, M. Measuring reactive species and oxidative damage in vivo and in cell culture: How should you do it and what do the results mean? *Br. J. Pharmacol.* **2004**, *142*, 231–255. [CrossRef]
68. Tang, S.Y.; Halliwell, B. Medicinal plants and antioxidants: What do we learn from cell culture and Caenorhabditis elegans studies? *Biochem. Biophys. Res. Commun.* **2010**, *394*, 1–5. [CrossRef]
69. Apak, R.; Özyürek, M.; Güçlü, K.; Çapanoğlu, E. Antioxidant Activity/Capacity Measurement. 1. Classification, Physicochemical Principles, Mechanisms, and Electron Transfer (ET)-Based Assays. *J. Agric. Food Chem.* **2016**, *64*, 997–1027. [CrossRef]
70. Gulcin, I. Antioxidants and antioxidant methods: An updated overview. *Arch. Toxicol.* **2020**, *94*, 651–715. [CrossRef]
71. Rahman, M.M.; Ichiyanagi, T.; Komiyama, T.; Sato, S.; Konishi, T. Effects of Anthocyanins on Psychological Stress-Induced Oxidative Stress and Neurotransmitter Status. *J. Agric. Food Chem.* **2008**, *56*, 7545–7550. [CrossRef]
72. Khan, M.S.; Ali, T.; Kim, M.W.; Jo, M.H.; Chung, J.I.; Kim, M.O. Anthocyanins Improve Hippocampus-Dependent Memory Function and Prevent Neurodegeneration via JNK/Akt/GSK3β Signaling in LPS-Treated Adult Mice. *Mol. Neurobiol.* **2019**, *56*, 671–687. [CrossRef]
73. Khan, M.S.; Ali, T.; Kim, M.W.; Jo, M.H.; Jo, M.G.; Badshah, H.; Kim, M.O. Anthocyanins Protect Against LPS-induced Oxidative Stress-Mediated Neuroinflammation and Neurodegeneration in the Adult Mouse Cortex. *Neurochem. Int.* **2016**, *100*, 1–10. [CrossRef] [PubMed]
74. Rehman, S.U.; Shah, S.A.; Ali, T.; Chung, J.I.; Kim, M.O. Anthocyanins Reversed D-Galactose-Induced Oxidative Stress and Neuroinflammation Mediated Cognitive Impairment in Adult Rats. *Mol. Neurobiol.* **2017**, *54*, 255–271. [CrossRef] [PubMed]

75. Ali, T.; Kim, T.; Rehman, S.U.; Khan, M.S.; Amin, F.U.; Khan, M.; Ikram, M.; Kim, M.O. Natural Dietary Supplementation of Anthocyanins via PI3K/Akt/Nrf2/HO-1 Pathways Mitigate Oxidative Stress, Neurodegeneration, and Memory Impairment in a Mouse Model of Alzheimer's Disease. *Mol. Neurobiol.* **2018**, *55*, 6076–6093. [CrossRef] [PubMed]

76. Qin, L.; Zhang, J.; Qin, M. Protective Effect of Cyanidin 3-O-glucoside on Beta-Amyloid Peptide-Induced Cognitive Impairment in Rats. *Neurosci. Lett.* **2013**, *534*, 285–288. [CrossRef] [PubMed]

77. Wu, X.L.; Li, X.X.; Jis, S.L.; Gao, Z.L.; Lu, Z.; Dai, X.L.; Sun, Y.X. Memory Enhancing and Antioxidant Activities of Lycium ruthenicum Murray Anthocyanin Extracts in an Aβ 42-Induced Rat Model of Dementia. *Xiandai Shipin Keji* **2017**, *33*, 29–34.

78. Chen, S.; Zhou, H.; Zhang, G.; Meng, J.; Deng, K.; Zhou, W.; Wang, H.; Wang, Z.; Hu, N.; Suo, Y. Anthocyanins From Lycium Ruthenicum Murr. Ameliorated d-Galactose-Induced Memory Impairment, Oxidative Stress, and Neuroinflammation in Adult Rats. *J. Agric. Food Chem.* **2019**, *67*, 3140–3149. [CrossRef]

79. Lu, X.; Zhou, Y.; Wu, T.; Hao, L. Ameliorative Effect of Black Rice Anthocyanin on Senescent Mice Induced by D-galactose. *Food Funct.* **2014**, *5*, 2892–2897. [CrossRef]

80. Wei, J.; Zhang, G.; Zhang, X.; Xu, D.; Gao, J.; Fan, J.; Zhou, Z. Anthocyanins From Black Chokeberry (Aroniamelanocarpa Elliot) Delayed Aging-Related Degenerative Changes of Brain. *J. Agric. Food Chem.* **2017**, *65*, 5973–5984. [CrossRef]

81. Pacheco, S.M.; Soares, M.S.P.; Gutierres, J.M.; Gerzson, M.F.B.; Carvalho, F.B.; Azambuja, J.H.; Schetinger, M.R.C.; Stefanello, F.M.; Spanevello, R.M. Anthocyanins as a Potential Pharmacological Agent to Manage Memory Deficit, Oxidative Stress and Alterations in Ion Pump Activity Induced by Experimental Sporadic Dementia of Alzheimer's Type. *J. Nutr. Biochem.* **2018**, *56*, 193–204. [CrossRef] [PubMed]

82. Roghani, M.; Niknam, A.; Jalali-Nadoushan, M.-R.; Kiasalari, Z.; Khalili, M.; Baluchnejadmojarad, T. Oral Pelargonidin Exerts Dose-Dependent Neuroprotection in 6-hydroxydopamine Rat Model of Hemi-Parkinsonism. *Brain Res. Bull.* **2010**, *82*, 279–283. [CrossRef] [PubMed]

83. Min, J.; Yu, S.-W.; Baek, S.-H.; Nair, K.M.; Bae, O.-N.; Bhatt, A.; Kassab, M.; Nair, M.G.; Majid, A. Neuroprotective Effect of cyanidin-3-O-glucoside Anthocyanin in Mice With Focal Cerebral Ischemia. *Neurosci. Lett.* **2011**, *500*, 157–161. [CrossRef]

84. Skemiene, K.; Pampuscenko, K.; Rekuviene, E.; Borutaite, V. Protective Effects of Anthocyanins against Brain Ischemic Damage. *J. Bioenerg. Biomembr.* **2020**, *52*, 71–82. [CrossRef] [PubMed]

85. Brader, L.; Overgaard, A.; Christensen, L.P.; Jeppesen, P.B.; Hermansen, K. Polyphenol-Rich Bilberry Ameliorates Total Cholesterol and LDL-Cholesterol when Implemented in the Diet of Zucker Diabetic Fatty Rats. *Rev. Diabet. Stud.* **2013**, *10*, 270–282. [CrossRef]

86. Toufektsian, M.C.; de Lorgeril, M.; Nagy, N.; Salen, P.; Donati, M.B.; Giordano, L.; Mock, H.P.; Peterek, S.; Matros, A.; Petroni, K.; et al. Chronic Dietary Intake of Plant-Derived Anthocyanins Protects the Rat Heart Against Ischemia-Reperfusion Injury. *J. Nutr.* **2008**, *138*, 747–752. [CrossRef]

87. Ziberna, L.; Lunder, M.; Moze, S.; Vanzo, A.; Tramer, F.; Passamonti, S.; Drevensek, G. Acute Cardioprotective and Cardiotoxic Effects of Bilberry Anthocyanins in Ischemia-Reperfusion Injury: Beyond Concentration-Dependent Antioxidant Activity. *Cardiovasc. Toxicol.* **2010**, *10*, 283–294. [CrossRef]

88. Li, F.; Lang, F.; Wang, Y.; Zhai, C.; Zhang, C.; Zhang, L.; Hao, E. Cyanidin ameliorates endotoxin-induced myocardial toxicity by modulating inflammation and oxidative stress through mitochondria and other factors. *Food Chem. Toxicol.* **2018**, *120*, 104–111. [CrossRef]

89. Skemiene, K.; Jablonskiene, G.; Liobikas, J.; Borutaite, V. Protecting the Heart Against Ischemia/Reperfusion-Induced Necrosis and Apoptosis: The Effect of Anthocyanins. *Medicina (Kaunas)* **2013**, *49*, 84–88.

90. Skemiene, K.; Liobikas, J.; Borutaite, V. Anthocyanins as Substrates for Mitochondrial Complex I—Protective Effect against Heart Ischemic Injury. *FEBS J.* **2015**, *282*, 963–971. [CrossRef]

91. Arjinajarn, P.; Chueakula, N.; Pongchaidecha, A.; Jaikumkao, K.; Chatsudthipong, V.; Mahatheeranont, S.; Norkaew, O.; Chattipakorn, N.; Lungkaphin, A. Anthocyanin-rich Riceberry Bran Extract Attenuates Gentamicin-Induced Hepatotoxicity by Reducing Oxidative Stress, Inflammation and Apoptosis in Rats. *Biomed. Pharmacother.* **2017**, *92*, 412–420. [CrossRef] [PubMed]

92. Hou, F.; Zhang, R.; Zhang, M.; Su, D.; Wei, Z.; Deng, Y.; Zhang, Y.; Chi, J.; Tang, X. Hepatoprotective and Antioxidant Activity of Anthocyanins in Black Rice Bran on Carbon Tetrachloride-Induced Liver Injury in Mice. *J. Funct. Foods* **2013**, *5*, 1705–1713. [CrossRef]

93. Chen, J.; Sun, H.; Sun, A.; Lin, Q.; Wang, Y.; Tao, X. Studies of the Protective Effect and Antioxidant Mechanism of Blueberry Anthocyanins in a CC14-Induced Liver Injury Model in Mice. *Food Agric. Immunol.* **2012**, *23*, 352–362. [CrossRef]
94. Cho, B.O.; Ryu, H.W.; Jin, C.H.; Choi, D.S.; Kang, S.Y.; Kim, D.S.; Byun, M.-W.; Jeong, I.Y. Blackberry Extract Attenuates Oxidative Stress through Up-Regulation of Nrf2-dependent Antioxidant Enzymes in Carbon Tetrachloride-Treated Rats. *J. Agric. Food Chem.* **2011**, *59*, 11442–11448. [CrossRef]
95. Sun, J.; Wu, Y.; Long, C.; He, P.; Gu, J.; Yang, L.; Liang, Y.; Wang, Y. Anthocyanins Isolated From Blueberry Ameliorates CCl4 Induced Liver Fibrosis by Modulation of Oxidative Stress, Inflammation and Stellate Cell Activation in Mice. *Food Chem. Toxicol.* **2018**, *120*, 491–499. [CrossRef]
96. Zuo, A.; Wang, S.; Liu, L.; Yao, Y.; Guo, J. Understanding the Effect of Anthocyanin Extracted from *Lonicera caerulea* L. On Alcoholic Hepatosteatosis. *Biomed. Pharmacother.* **2019**, *117*, 109087. [CrossRef]
97. Wu, S.; Yano, S.; Hisanaga, A.; He, X.; He, J.; Sakao, K.; Hou, D.-X. Polyphenols from *Lonicera caerulea* L. Berry Attenuate Experimental Nonalcoholic Steatohepatitis by Inhibiting Proinflammatory Cytokines Productions and Lipid Peroxidation. *Mol. Nutr. Food Res.* **2017**, *61*, 1600858. [CrossRef]
98. Prokop, J.; Anzenbacher, P.; Mrkvicová, E.; Pavlata, L.; Zapletalová, I.; Šťastník, O.; Martinek, P.; Kosina, P.; Anzenbacherová, E. In Vivo Evaluation of Effect of Anthocyanin-Rich Wheat on Rat Liver Microsomal Drug-Metabolizing Cytochromes P450 and on Biochemical and Antioxidant Parameters in Rats. *Food Chem. Toxicol.* **2018**, *122*, 225–233. [CrossRef]
99. Popović, D.; Kocić, G.; Katić, V.; Jović, Z.; Zarubica, A.; Janković Veličković, L.; Nikolić, V.; Jović, A.; Kundalić, B.; Rakić, V.; et al. Protective Effects of Anthocyanins From Bilberry Extract in Rats Exposed to Nephrotoxic Effects of Carbon Tetrachloride. *Chem. Biol. Interact.* **2019**, *304*, 61–72. [CrossRef]
100. Yarijani, Z.M.; Najafi, H.; Shackebaei, D.; Madani, S.H.; Modarresi, M.; Jassemi, S.V. Amelioration of Renal and Hepatic Function, Oxidative Stress, Inflammation and Histopathologic Damages by Malva Sylvestris Extract in Gentamicin Induced Renal Toxicity. *Biomed. Pharmacother.* **2019**, *112*, 108635. [CrossRef]
101. Veljković, M.; Pavlović, D.R.; Stojiljković, N.; Ilić, S.; Jovanović, I.; Poklar Ulrih, N.; Rakić, V.; Veličković, L.; Sokolović, D. Bilberry: Chemical Profiling, in vitro and in vivo Antioxidant Activity and Nephroprotective Effect Against Gentamicin Toxicity in Rats. *Phytother. Res.* **2017**, *31*, 115–123. [CrossRef] [PubMed]
102. Qi, Z.-L.; Wang, Z.; Li, W.; Hou, J.-G.; Liu, Y.; Li, X.-D.; Li, H.-P.; Wang, Y.-P. Nephroprotective Effects of Anthocyanin from the Fruits of Panax Ginseng (GFA) on Cisplatin-Induced Acute Kidney Injury in Mice. *Phytother. Res.* **2017**, *31*, 1400–1409. [CrossRef] [PubMed]
103. Lee, I.-C.; Bae, J.-S. Pelargonidin Protects Against Renal Injury in a Mouse Model of Sepsis. *J. Med. Food* **2019**, *22*, 57–61. [CrossRef] [PubMed]
104. Suda, I.; Ishikawa, F.; Hatakeyama, M.; Miyawaki, M.; Kudo, T.; Hirano, K.; Ito, A.; Yamakawa, O.; Horiuchi, S. Intake of Purple Sweet Potato Beverage Affects on Serum Hepatic Biomarker Levels of Healthy Adult Men With Borderline Hepatitis. *Eur. J. Clin. Nutr.* **2008**, *62*, 60–67. [CrossRef]
105. Gao, X.; Cassidy, A.; Schwarzschild, M.A.; Rimm, E.B.; Ascherio, A. Habitual intake of dietary flavonoids and risk of Parkinson disease. *Neurology* **2012**, *78*, 1138–1145. [CrossRef]
106. Valenti, L.; Riso, P.; Mazzocchi, A.; Porrini, M.; Fargion, S.; Agostoni, C. Dietary Anthocyanins as Nutritional Therapy for Nonalcoholic Fatty Liver Disease. *Oxid. Med. Cell. Longev.* **2013**, *2013*, 145421. [CrossRef]
107. Vendrame, S.; Del Bo, C.; Ciappellano, S.; Riso, P.; Klimis-Zacas, D. Berry Fruit Consumption and Metabolic Syndrome. *Antioxidants* **2016**, *5*, 34. [CrossRef]
108. Oki, T.; Kano, M.; Ishikawa, F.; Goto, K.; Watanabe, O.; Suda, I. Double-blind, Placebo-Controlled Pilot Trial of Anthocyanin-Rich Purple Sweet Potato Beverage on Serum Hepatic Biomarker Levels in Healthy Caucasians With Borderline Hepatitis. *Eur. J. Clin. Nutr.* **2017**, *71*, 290–292. [CrossRef]
109. Fairlie-Jones, L.; Davison, K.; Fromentin, E.; Hill, A.M. The Effect of Anthocyanin-Rich Foods or Extracts on Vascular Function in Adults: A Systematic Review and Meta-Analysis of Randomised Controlled Trials. *Nutrients* **2017**, *9*, 908. [CrossRef]
110. Godos, J.; Vitale, M.; Micek, A.; Ray, S.; Martini, D.; Del Rio, D.; Riccardi, G.; Galvano, F.; Grosso, G. Dietary Polyphenol Intake, Blood Pressure, and Hypertension: A Systematic Review and Meta-Analysis of Observational Studies. *Antioxidants* **2019**, *8*, 152. [CrossRef]
111. Ullah, R.; Khan, M.; Shah, S.A.; Saeed, K.; Kim, M.O. Natural Antioxidant Anthocyanins-A Hidden Therapeutic Candidate in Metabolic Disorders With Major Focus in Neurodegeneration. *Nutrients* **2019**, *11*, 1195. [CrossRef] [PubMed]

112. Winter, A.N.; Bickford, P.C. Anthocyanins and Their Metabolites as Therapeutic Agents for Neurodegenerative Disease. *Antioxidants* **2019**, *8*, 333. [CrossRef] [PubMed]
113. Krikorian, R.; Kalt, W.; McDonald, J.E.; Shidler, M.D.; Summer, S.S.; Stein, A.L. Cognitive performance in relation to urinary anthocyanins and their flavonoid-based products following blueberry supplementation in older adults at risk for dementia. *J. Funct. Foods* **2020**, *64*, 103667. [CrossRef]
114. Cásedas, G.; Les, F.; López, V. Anthocyanins: Plant Pigments, Food Ingredients or Therapeutic Agents for the CNS? A Mini-Review Focused on Clinical Trials. *Curr. Pharm. Des.* **2020**, *26*, 1790–1798. [CrossRef]
115. Danielewski, M.; Matuszewska, A.; Nowak, B.; Kucharska, A.Z.; Sozański, T. The Effects of Natural Iridoids and Anthocyanins on Selected Parameters of Liver and Cardiovascular System Functions. *Oxid. Med. Cell. Longev.* **2020**, *2020*, 2735790. [CrossRef]
116. Davinelli, S.; Bertoglio, J.C.; Zarrelli, A.; Pina, R.; Scapagnini, G. A Randomized Clinical Trial Evaluating the Efficacy of an Anthocyanin-Maqui Berry Extract (Delphinol®) on Oxidative Stress Biomarkers. *J. Am. Coll. Nutr.* **2015**, *34*, 28–33. [CrossRef]
117. Toaldo, I.M.; Cruz, F.A.; de Lima Alves, T.; de Gois, J.S.; Borges, D.L.G.; Cunha, H.P.; da Silva, E.L.; Bordignon-Luiz, M.T. Bioactive Potential of Vitis Labrusca L. Grape Juices from the Southern Region of Brazil: Phenolic and Elemental Composition and Effect on Lipid Peroxidation in Healthy Subjects. *Food Chem.* **2015**, *173*, 527–535. [CrossRef]
118. Bialasiewicz, P.; Prymont-Przyminska, A.; Zwolinska, A.; Sarniak, A.; Wlodarczyk, A.; Krol, M.; Markowski, J.; Rutkowski, K.P.; Nowak, D. Sour Cherries but Not Apples Added to the Regular Diet Decrease Resting and fMLP-Stimulated Chemiluminescence of Fasting Whole Blood in Healthy Subjects. *J. Am. Coll. Nutr.* **2018**, *37*, 24–33. [CrossRef]
119. Del Bó, C.; Riso, P.; Campolo, J.; Møller, P.; Loft, S.; Klimis-Zacas, D.; Brambilla, A.; Rizzolo, A.; Porrini, M. A Single Portion of Blueberry (*Vaccinium corymbosum* L) Improves Protection against DNA Damage but Not Vascular Function in Healthy Male Volunteers. *Nutr. Res.* **2013**, *33*, 220–227. [CrossRef]
120. Kropat, C.; Mueller, D.; Boettler, U.; Zimmermann, K.; Heiss, E.H.; Dirsch, V.M.; Rogoll, D.; Melcher, R.; Richling, E.; Marko, D. Modulation of Nrf2-dependent Gene Transcription by Bilberry Anthocyanins in vivo. *Mol. Nutr. Food Res.* **2013**, *57*, 545–550. [CrossRef]
121. Erlund, I.; Koli, R.; Alfthan, G.; Marniemi, J.; Puukka, P.; Mustonen, P.; Mattila, P.; Jula, A. Favorable Effects of Berry Consumption on Platelet Function, Blood Pressure, and HDL Cholesterol. *Am. J. Clin. Nutr.* **2008**, *87*, 323–331. [CrossRef] [PubMed]
122. Cassidy, A.; Rogers, G.; Peterson, J.J.; Dwyer, J.T.; Lin, H.; Jacques, P.F. Higher Dietary Anthocyanin and Flavonol Intakes Are Associated With Anti-Inflammatory Effects in a Population of US Adults. *Am. J. Clin. Nutr.* **2015**, *102*, 172–181. [CrossRef] [PubMed]
123. Natella, F.; Macone, A.; Ramberti, A.; Forte, M.; Mattivi, F.; Matarese, R.M.; Scaccini, C. Red Wine Prevents the Postprandial Increase in Plasma Cholesterol Oxidation Products: A Pilot Study. *Br. J. Nutr.* **2011**, *105*, 1718–1723. [CrossRef] [PubMed]
124. Estruch, R.; Sacanella, E.; Mota, F.; Chiva-Blanch, G.; Antúnez, E.; Casals, E.; Deulofeu, R.; Rotilio, D.; Andres-Lacueva, C.; Lamuela-Raventos, R.M.; et al. Moderate Consumption of Red Wine, but Not Gin, Decreases Erythrocyte Superoxide Dismutase Activity: A Randomised Cross-Over Trial. *Nutr. Metab. Cardiovasc. Dis.* **2011**, *21*, 46–53. [CrossRef]
125. Zhu, Y.; Ling, W.; Guo, H.; Song, F.; Ye, Q.; Zou, T.; Li, D.; Zhang, Y.; Li, G.; Xiao, Y.; et al. Anti-inflammatory Effect of Purified Dietary Anthocyanin in Adults With Hypercholesterolemia: A Randomized Controlled Trial. *Nutr. Metab. Cardiovasc. Dis.* **2013**, *23*, 843–849. [CrossRef]
126. Curtis, P.J.; van der Velpen, V.; Berends, L.; Jennings, A.; Feelisch, M.; Umpleby, A.M.; Evans, M.; Fernandez, B.O.; Meiss, M.S.; Minnion, M.; et al. Blueberries Improve Biomarkers of Cardiometabolic Function in Participants With Metabolic Syndrome-Results From a 6-month, Double-Blind, Randomized Controlled Trial. *Am. J. Clin. Nutr.* **2019**, *109*, 1535–1545. [CrossRef]
127. Zhang, P.-W.; Chen, F.-X.; Li, D.; Ling, W.-H.; Guo, H.-H. A CONSORT-compliant, Randomized, Double-Blind, Placebo-Controlled Pilot Trial of Purified Anthocyanin in Patients with Nonalcoholic Fatty Liver Disease. *Medicine (Baltimore)* **2015**, *94*, e758. [CrossRef]
128. Guo, H.; Zhong, R.; Liu, Y.; Jiang, X.; Tang, X.; Li, Z.; Xia, M.; Ling, W. Effects of Bayberry Juice on Inflammatory and Apoptotic Markers in Young Adults with Features of Non-Alcoholic Fatty Liver Disease. *Nutrition* **2014**, *30*, 198–203. [CrossRef]

129. Spormann, T.M.; Albert, F.W.; Rath, T.; Dietrich, H.; Will, F.; Stockis, J.-P.; Eisenbrand, G.; Janzowski, C. Anthocyanin/polyphenolic-rich Fruit Juice Reduces Oxidative Cell Damage in an Intervention Study with Patients on Hemodialysis. *Cancer Epidemiol. Biomark. Prev.* **2008**, *17*, 3372–3380. [CrossRef]
130. Castilla, P.; Dávalos, A.; Teruel, J.L.; Cerrato, F.; Fernández-Lucas, M.; Merino, J.L.; Sánchez-Martín, C.C.; Ortuño, J.; Lasunción, M.A. Comparative Effects of Dietary Supplementation With Red Grape Juice and Vitamin E on Production of Superoxide by Circulating Neutrophil NADPH Oxidase in Hemodialysis Patients. *Am. J. Clin. Nutr.* **2008**, *87*, 1053–1061. [CrossRef]

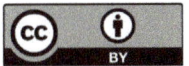

© 2020 by the authors. Licensee MDPI, Basel, Switzerland. This article is an open access article distributed under the terms and conditions of the Creative Commons Attribution (CC BY) license (http://creativecommons.org/licenses/by/4.0/).

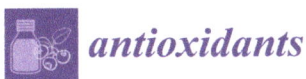

Article

Biochemical Characterization of Traditional Varieties of Sweet Pepper (*Capsicum annuum* L.) of the Campania Region, Southern Italy

Florinda Fratianni [1,*], Antonio d'Acierno [1,*], Autilia Cozzolino [2], Patrizia Spigno [3], Riccardo Riccardi [3], Francesco Raimo [4], Catello Pane [4], Massimo Zaccardelli [4], Valentina Tranchida Lombardo [5], Marina Tucci [5], Stefania Grillo [5], Raffaele Coppola [2] and Filomena Nazzaro [1]

1. Institute of Food Science, CNR-ISA, Via Roma 64, 83100 Avellino, Italy; filomena.nazzaro@isa.cnr.it
2. Department of Agricultural, Environmental and Food Sciences (DiAAA)-University of Molise, Via de Sanctis snc, 86100 Campobasso, Italy; autilia.cozzolino@unimol.it (A.C.); coppola@unimol.it (R.C.)
3. Cooperativa "ARCA 2010", Via Varignano 7, 8100 Acerra (NA), Italy; patspigno@hotmail.com (P.S.); ricc.riccardi@libero.it (R.R.)
4. Horticulture Research Center (CRA-ORT), Via Cavalleggeri 25, 84098 Pontecagnano Faiano (SA), Italy; francesco.raimo@crea.gov.it (F.R.); catello.pane@crea.gov.it (C.P.); massimo.zaccardelli@crea.gov.it (M.Z.)
5. Institute of Biosciences and Bioresources, CNR-IBBR, O.U. of Portici (NA), Via Università 100, 80055 Portici (NA), Italy; valentinatranchida@tiscali.it (V.T.L.); mtucci@unina.it (M.T.); grillo@unina.it (S.G.)
* Correspondence: florinda.fratianni@isa.cnr.it (F.F.); dacierno.a@isa.cnr.it (A.d.); Tel. +39-082-529-9110 (F.F.); +39-082-529-9509 (A.d.)

Received: 18 May 2020; Accepted: 24 June 2020; Published: 26 June 2020

Abstract: Bioactive compounds of different Campania native sweet pepper varieties were evaluated. Polyphenols ranged between 1.37 mmol g^{-1} and 3.42 mmol g^{-1}, β-carotene was abundant in the red variety "Cazzone" (7.05 µg g^{-1}). Yellow and red varieties showed a content of ascorbic acid not inferior to 0.82 mg g^{-1}, while in some green varieties the presence of ascorbic acid was almost inconsistent. Interrelationships between the parameters analyzed and the varieties showed that ascorbic acid could represent the factor mostly influencing the antioxidant activity. Polyphenol profile was different among the varieties, with a general prevalence of acidic phenols in yellow varieties and of flavonoids in red varieties. Principal Component Analysis, applied to ascorbic acid, total polyphenols and β-carotene, revealed that two of the green varieties ("Friariello napoletano" and "Friariello Sigaretta") were well clustered and that the yellow variety "Corno di capra" showed similarity with the green varieties, in particular with "Friariello Nocerese". This was confirmed by the interrelationships applied to polyphenol composition, which let us to light on a clustering of several red and yellow varieties, and that mainly the yellow "Corno di capra" was closer to the green varieties of "Friariello".

Keywords: biodiversity; *Capsicum annuum* L.; antioxidant activity; β-carotene; ascorbic acid; polyphenols; statistical analysis

1. Introduction

Sweet pepper (*Capsicum annuum* L.), belonging to the Solanaceae family, is one of five cultivated species of the genus *Capsicum*, including sweet and hot peppers. It is a component present in the diet of many populations in the world; as such, therefore it represents an important source of income for farmers and operators in the agro-industrial sector. *C. annuum* L., originated from Central and South America and arrived in Europe in the sixteenth century with the Spanish and Portuguese expeditions to the lands of the New World. Once introduced in cultivation, pepper soon became a very common vegetable in the kitchens of all the countries of Europe. Today, *C. annuum* L. is cultivated in a large number of varieties all over the world, reaching a cultivated area that exceeds 1.5 million hectares. Italy is one of the most important countries in the world for this crop. The commercial produce of sweet pepper is the fruit, having different forms and size, as well as several colors, which range from yellow to red, from intense purple to dark green to black, depending on cultivar, maturity, growing conditions, and postharvest manipulation. Sweet pepper represents an excellent source of several antioxidant molecules, in particular carotenoids [1,2] ascorbic acid, and polyphenols, such as quercetin [3], which received huge interest for to their antioxidant properties [4]. A considerable weight of evidence suggests that consumption of fruit and vegetables is beneficial for human health and may help in preventing several chronic diseases [5]. Since last decades, secondary metabolites of vegetables have come into light for their presumed role in fighting cancer and cardiovascular diseases [6,7] as well as in slowing down aging and atherosclerosis [8].

Campania is among the most prominent regions of Europe in terms of production and number of varieties of fruit and vegetables [9]. Over the millennia, indigenous plant varieties, in a sort of ideal symbiosis with the territory, have managed to express their quality and nutritional value at the best. Several of these varieties are still widespread, while others are cultivated as niche products, or have been abandoned, supplanted by commercial varieties, which are more productive but often have lower quality. Pepper is one of the most important crops for this area and several varieties have become traditional of the Campania region, giving very worthy inputs to its rich cultivated biodiversity. Plant biodiversity includes the enormous amount of vegetal germplasm differentiated in the course of the long history of biological evolution of species. In agriculture, biodiversity is also the work of human selection from a "wild" gene pool to obtain breeds and varieties adapted to various ecological, economic and social conditions. Phytochemicals of sweet peppers undoubtedly arouse great interest mainly act as antioxidant agents. They represent also important element for human health and can prevent the occurrence of disease linked to oxidative stress, including cardiovascular and neurodegenerative diseases, and cancer [10]. Certain green, red, orange, and yellow pepper showed interesting capacity to inhibit some key enzymes linked to Alzheimer disease [acetylcholinesterase (AChE), butyrylcholinesterase (BChE), and β-secretase (BACE1)] [11]. Due to the broad biochemical and nutritional variations existing among the different varieties within each plant species, the identification of the best genotypes assumes a particular importance for both breeders and consumers, which thereby can select and consume products with high nutritional quality, respectively. Keeping this in view, the present study focused on the following objectives: (a) to analyze the contents of bioactive compounds of native pepper varieties from the Campania region, Southern Italy, including β-carotene, total phenolics, phenolic profiles, ascorbic acid; (b) to determine their in vitro antioxidant activities through the DPPH radical-scavenging activity; (c) to correlate the antioxidant activity of the varieties to total phenolics, ascorbic acid and carotenoids, with the aim of identifying the main factors influencing the antioxidant properties of the product. Interrelationships between the parameters analyzed and the different varieties were investigated by principal component analysis (PCA).

2. Materials and Methods

2.1. Chemicals

Caffeic, ferulic, p-coumaric, gallic, chlorogenic acids, epicatechin, rutin, quercetin, 2,2-diphenyl-1-picrylhydrazyl (DPPH), β-carotene, ascorbic acid, HPLC-grade methanol, sulphuric, metaphosphoric, acetic and formic acids, acetonitrile, petroleum ether, ethanol and acetone were purchased from Sigma-Aldrich (Milano, Italy). Apigenin was purchased from Extrasynthese (Genay, France). The Folin–Ciocalteu reagent was purchased from BIO-RAD (Milano, Italy). Water was distilled and filtered through a Milli-Q apparatus (Millipore, Milano, Italy) before use.

2.2. Plant Material

Plant material (Figure 1) included seven types of yellow and red sweet pepper, (*Capsicum annuum* L.) ("Papaccella napoletana", "Papaccella liscia", "Corno Marconi", "Corno di capra", "Cornetto di Acerra", "Cazzone", "Sassaniello"), corresponding to fourteen varieties, and three varieties of green sweet pepper ("Friariello napoletano", "Friariello nocerese", "Friariello a sigaretta") listed by the Official Bulletin of the Campania Region (B.U.R.C. n°42, 145, 2009), grown and collected in the farm of the "Cooperativa ARCA 2010" sited in Acerra (NA), Italy. Acerra (40.9441° N, 14.3714° E) is characterized by a Mediterranean climate with an average of air temperature (T), humidity (U) and rainy days (R) T = 22.7 °C; U = 63.8%; R = 6.6 during the growing season [12]. The seeds of the varieties of pepper are stored and preserved by the gene bank "banca del germoplasma" at the "Consorzio Arca 2010" on behalf of the Campania region. Seedlings were transplanted in three rows with 60 plants ("Cazzone" and "Sassaniello"); 100 plants ("Friariello"); 83 plants ("Papaccella napoletana", "Papaccella napoletana liscia", "Corno di capra"). Cultivation techniques included stakes (1.2 m) as support and twine threads to tie the plants. Microirrigation was used as technique of irrigation. Replicates were 3. Each replicate included 10 plants collected for the determination of marketable production. Four harvests were generally performed from the beginning of August to the beginning of October. Before analysis, fruits were gently cleaned. Peduncles and seeds of pepper fruits were removed; the comestible portion was cut and immediately stored at −26 °C.

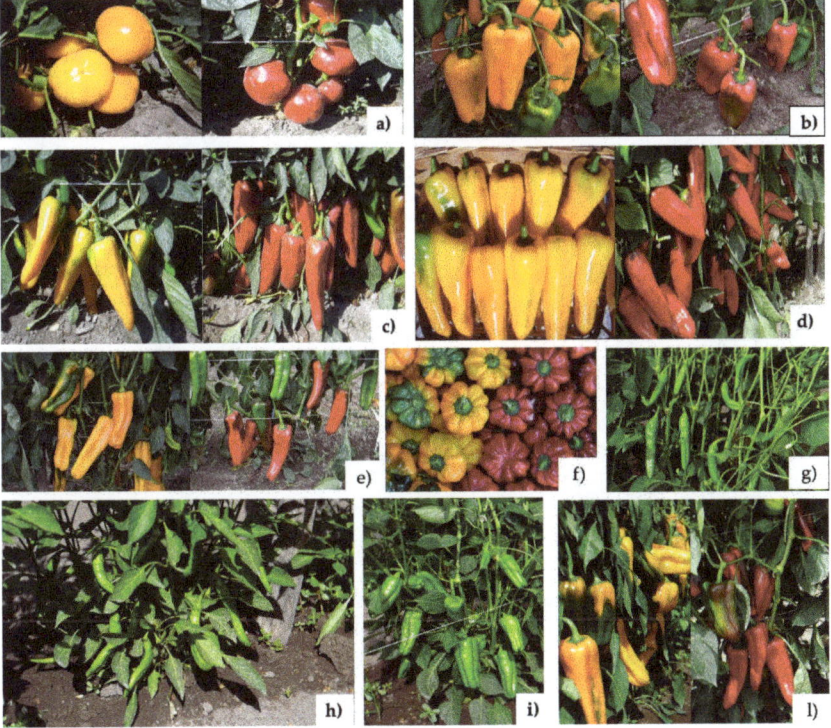

Figure 1. Traditional sweet pepper varieties of the Campania region analyzed in the present work. Legend: (**a**) Papaccella liscia; (**b**) Sassaniello; (**c**) Cornetto di Acerra; (**d**) Corno di capra; (**e**) Corno Marconi (**f**) Papaccella Napoletana; (**g**) Friariello a sigaretta; (**h**) Friariello Napoletano; (**i**) Friariello Nocerese; (**l**) Cazzone. The photos were made by the authors.

2.3. Dosage of Ascorbic Acid

Dosage of ascorbic acid was performed following the method of Nazzaro et al. [13]. All samples were cut, squeezed and incubated in three volumes of metaphosphoric acid (4%) and maintained for 1 h at 4 °C, avoiding the exposition to the light. Extracts were subjected to centrifugation (11,600× g for 10 min at 4 °C, Biofuge, Beckman Italia, Cassina de' Pecchi, Milano, Italy), and filtration (0.45 μm mesh, Millipore, Milano, Italy) to recovery the supernatant. A Gold System chromatograph equipped with an UV detector (Beckman Italia, Cascina dè Pecchi MI, Italy) and a Khromasil KR 100-5 C_{18} column (25 cm × 4.6 mm) was used to assess, through RP-HPLC, the amount of ascorbic acid present in the samples (run condition = mobile phase: sulphuric acid 0.001 M in HPLC-grade water; injection volume: 20 μL; flow rate: 1.0 mL min^{-1}; detection wavelength: 245 nm; Temperature: room temperature). Ascorbic acid, previously dissolved in the mobile phase, was used as standard to generate the standard curve.

2.4. Carotene Content

Extraction was carried out according to the method described by Nazzaro et al. [13], modified as follows: fresh sample was cut and squeezed in ethanol (1:1 w/v), and then petroleum ether was added (1.5:1 v/v). The mixture was vigorously shaken; the supernatant was recovered by centrifugation (11,600× g, 15 min; Biofuge, Beckman Italia, Milano, Italy). The steps were repeated until the complete disappearance of the color, then the supernatants were put together. The amount of carotenoids was evaluated at 450 nm with petroleum ether as blank, and using the extinction coefficient $\varepsilon = 2592$, using the spectrophotometer Cary 50 Uv/Vis (Varian-Agilent Italia, Cernusco sul Naviglio, Italy).

2.5. Total Polyphenols and Antioxidant Activity

Samples were cut and squeezed (1:3 w/v) in methanol (containing acetic acid 1%) overnight at 4 °C. After centrifugation (11,600× g, 15 min; Biofuge, Beckman Italia), supernatants were recovered and the polyphenols amount and profile as well as the antioxidant activity was evaluated. The content of total polyphenols was spectrophotometrically evaluated (Cary 50 Varian-Agilent Italia) at $\lambda = 760$ nm, following the method described by Singleton and Rossi [14] with Folin Ciocalteau reagent. Gallic acid was used as standard. Results were indicated as mMol gallic acid equivalent g^{-1} of fresh sample. Radical-scavenging activity was assayed through the use of the stable radical 2,2-diphenyl-1-picrylhydrazyl (DPPH assay) following the method of Ombra et al. [15]. The analysis was performed in microplates by adding 15 μL of extract to 300 μL of a methanol- DPPH solution (6×10^{-5} M). The absorbance was measured at $\lambda = 517$ nm (Cary 50 MPR Varian-Agilent Italia). The scavenging activity was expressed in terms of EC_{50}, indicating the amount of sample amount (mg) necessary to inhibit DPPH radical activity by 50% for the duration of 60 min of incubation.

The experiments were performed in triplicate. Results were expressed as the mean values ± standard deviation.

2.6. Chromatographic Analysis

Ultra-high-performance liquid chromatography (UPLC) analysis was made using the ACQUITY Ultra Performance LC^{TM} system (Waters, Milford, MA, USA) connected to a PDA 2996 photodiode array detector (Waters), characterized by a low dispersion with enlargement of the band lower than 10 μL; automatic control of the temperature; technology Smart-Start for the gradient, to perform a controlled mixing of the solvents until pressure = 15,000 psi; controlled degassing and automatized firmness of the solvents; direct setting of gradients in terms of pH, molarity and/or organic composition. Detector PDA: linear answer in the interval of wavelength ranging between 190 nm and 500 nm and for values of absorbance until 2.0 AU: Deviation of 1.3% at 2.0 AU; Deviation at 5.0% at 2.8 AU. The acquisition and processing of the relative data, as well as the control of the instruments was performed through the Empower software. The analysis was performed following the method described by Fratianni et al. [16]

and Pane et al. [17]. All the extracts and standards were dissolved in methanol, and filtered through Whatman 0.45 µm (Waters, Milford, MA, USA). The analyses were performed at 30 °C. Running conditions = Injection volume: 5 µL. Mobile phase: solvent A (7.5 mMol acetic acid) and solvent B (acetonitrile); flow rate: 250 µL min^{-1}; column: reversed phase column (BEH C_{18}, 1.7 µm, 2.1 × 100 mm Waters, based on ethyl bridge silanes, stable in a range of pH between 2 and 12 and temperatures up to 90 °C). The analysis was performed with a gradient elution (5% B for 0.8 min; 5–20% B over 5.2 min; 20% B for 0.5 min; 20–30% B for 1 min; 30% B for 0.2 min, 30–50% B over 2.3 min, 50–100% B over 1 min, 100% B for 1 min; 100–5% B over 0.5 min). Finally, the column was restored to the initial conditions for 2.5 min. Conditions of the apparatus= Pressure ranging from 6000–8000 psi; Scanning range of LC detector: 210–400 nm, resolution: 1.2 nm).

2.7. Statistical Analysis

Data were expressed as mean ± standard deviation of triplicate measurements. The PC software "Excel Statistics" was used for the calculations. Interrelationships between the parameters analyzed and the different varieties were investigated by principal component analysis (PCA), following the method of Fratianni et al. [18] and using the software package MATLAB.

3. Results and Discussion

3.1. Ascorbic Acid Content

Ascorbic acid, β-carotene, total polyphenols contents and antioxidant activity are shown in Table 1.

Table 1. Content of ascorbic acid, β-carotene, total polyphenols and antioxidant activity exhibited by the yellow, red and green traditional varieties of sweet pepper of the Campania region. Data represent the average (± SD) of three independent experiments. For details, see the Section Materials and Methods.

Table 1	Ascorbic Acid mg g^{-1} ± SD	β-Carotene µg g^{-1} SD	Total Polyphenols mMol g^{-1} ± SD	Antioxidant Activity mg EC$_{50}$ ± SD
Yellow varieties				
Cazzone giallo	1.13 ± 0.13	5.79 ± 1.24	3.14 ± 0.43	2.74 ± 0.51
Papaccella Napoletana gialla	1.12 ± 0.15	3.84 ± 0.73	3.42 ± 0.40	2.10 ± 0.21
Papaccella liscia gialla	0.95 ± 0.15	4.33 ± 0.93	2.80 ± 0.05	2.88 ± 0.24
Corno Marconi giallo	1.72 ± 0.22	2.55 ± 0.09	2.79 ± 0.40	1.97 ± 0.22
Corno di capra giallo	1.33 ± 0.10	3.20 ± 0.12	2.03 ± 0.15	2.70 ± 0.24
Cornetto di Acerra giallo	1.35 ± 0.14	2.99 ± 0.47	3.18 ± 0.21	2.06 ± 0.16
Sassaniello giallo	0.80 ± 0.17	4.56 ± 0.47	3.02 ± 0.19	2.56 ± 0.38
Red varieties				
Cazzone rosso	1.02 ± 0.17	7.05 ± 0.79	2.66 ± 0.35	2.93 ± 0.42
Papaccella Napoletana rossa	1.13 ± 0.16	5.38 ± 1.59	3.13 ± 0.29	2.26 ± 0.28
Papaccella liscia rossa	0.82 ± 0.08	6.25 ± 1.35	2.21 ± 0.06	3.64 ± 0.76
Corno Marconi rosso	1.20 ± 0.12	5.31 ± 0.58	3.36 ± 0.14	2.11 ± 0.14
Corno di capra rosso	0.93 ± 0.07	4.94 ± 1.19	3.07 ± 0.26	2.84 ± 0.08
Cornetto di Acerra rosso	1.19 ± 0.38	5.24 ± 0.49	3.15 ± 0.38	2.22 ± 0.43
Sassaniello rosso	0.91 ± 0.05	3.96 ± 0.80	2.98 ± 0.26	2.91 ± 0.23
Green varieties				
Friariello Napoletano	0.05 ± 0.01	1.64 ± 0.45	1.44 ± 0.09	9.57 ± 1.50
Friariello Nocerese	0.35 ± 0.22	2.24 ± 0.59	2.26 ± 0.48	7.27 ± 1.65
Friariello sigaretta	0.10 ± 0.09	1.54 ± 0.49	1.37 ± 0.11	13.18 ± 5.09

Among the yellow varieties, the amount of ascorbic acid ranged between 0.80 mg g^{-1} ("Sassaniello") and 1.72 mg g^{-1} ("Corno Marconi") of fresh product. We observed a less wide situation in red varieties, where the concentration of ascorbic acid ranged between 0.82 mg g^{-1} ("Papaccella liscia") to 1.20 mg g^{-1} ("Corno Marconi"). Both in yellow and red varieties, "Corno Marconi" showed the highest amount of ascorbic acid. Among the red varieties is to remark also the high amount of ascorbic acid in the "Cornetto di Acerra" (1.19 mg g^{-1} of fresh product). The three green varieties showed the smallest content of ascorbic acid. "Friariello nocerese" contained a slightly higher content of ascorbic acid than "Friariello Napoletano" and "Friariello sigaretta". For the most of the analyzed varieties, the amount of ascorbic acid was also higher than that reported by Howard et al. [19], and in some cases it was similar (in the case of yellow "Cazzone" or slightly inferior (red "Cazzone" and yellow "Corno di capra") than reported by Mennella et al. [20]. Considering a portion of 100 g of raw pepper, all varieties of sweet pepper analyzed, with the exception of the two green varieties "Friariello Napoletano" and "Friariello a sigaretta", reached a concentration of vitamin C at least two-fold the recommended daily dosage suggested by different international committees (WHO, the USA National Academy of Sciences, the USA Ministry of Health), and the *Codex alimentarius*, which indicate a minimum of 30 mg/die of ascorbic acid in human diet [21].

3.2. β-Carotene

β-Carotene or pro-vitamin-A is an abundant carotenoid present, as stable all-trans isomer, in many vegetal tissues including those of pepper. Due to its nutritional and coloring properties, it is used for several purposes, such as food coloring and preserving agent, in pharmaceuticals, as drug or drug ingredient that help to counteract vitamin A deficiency (VAD), thus preventing anomalies in growth, development, vision and immune function and cosmetics, for example as protective skin agent [22]. Pepper represents one of the primary dietary sources of pro-vitamin A [23] and generally, β-carotene is more abundant in fresh hot pepper than in sweet cultivars [23,24]. β-Carotene concentration is directly correlated to the total carotenoid content, being the precursor for the predominant orange and red carotenoids of pepper [25]. The data about the content of β-carotene present in the varieties of sweet pepper analyzed are shown in Table 1. In the yellow varieties, it ranged between 2.55 µg g^{-1} "(Corno Marconi") and 5.79 µg g^{-1} of fresh product ("Cazzone giallo"); on the other hand, the red varieties exhibited always a content of β-carotene higher than the analogous yellow varieties, with values ranging from 3.96 µg g^{-1} (Sassaniello that therefore was the only variety to show a content of β-carotene inferior to the corresponding yellow "Sassaniello") to 7.05 µg g^{-1} of fresh product (in the variety "Cazzone rosso"). Such values could be considered superior, for instance, respect to those reported by Thuphairo et al. [11], who indicated high values of carotenoids but considering the dry weight of the product. Respect to the shape of the varieties of peppers analyzed, we could say that the round red varieties of sweet pepper ("Papaccella napoletana" and "Papaccella napoletana liscia") almost always had a higher β-carotene content than the analogous yellow varieties and that among the elongated varieties, "Cazzone" had a slightly greater β-carotene content respect to the others. The green varieties "Friariello a sigaretta" and "Friariello Napoletano" showed a lower content of β-carotene. Also in this case, "Friariello nocerese" exhibited a different behavior, with 2.24 µg of β-carotene g^{-1}.

3.3. Total Polyphenol Content and Antioxidant Activity

Total polyphenol (TP) content ranged between 1.37 mmol g^{-1} (in the variety "Friariello sigaretta") and 3.42 mmol g^{-1} (observed in the yellow "Papaccella napoletana") of fresh product (Table 1). Such values were lower respect to those reported by Moktar et al. [26] and Hallmann and Rembiałkowska [27], but in some cases similar to those observed by Nazzaro et al. in elongated yellow and red varieties of sweet pepper cultivated in the Sicilia region [13] or to those cultivated in Romania, in different conditions of growth [28]. On the other hand, they resulted in some cases higher than those reported by Shotorbani et al. [29]. This indicates that such an important biochemical parameter might be related not only to the variety but also to the different geo-climatic conditions and to methods of treatment applied for their extraction. Among the round varieties of "Papaccella Napoletana", the yellow type showed slightly higher content of TPs than the red type (3.42 and 3.13 mmol g^{-1} of fresh product, respectively); on the other hand, the difference of total polyphenols was more marked between the two "Papaccella liscia", whose yellow type exhibited a TPs content 21.08% higher than the correspondent red type (2.80 mmol g^{-1} and 2.21 mmol g^{-1} of fresh product, respectively). Among the elongated varieties, the trend was different. Thus, while the red type of "Cazzone" contained less total polyphenols than the corresponding yellow type (2.66 mmol g^{-1} and 3.14 mmol g^{-1}, respectively), the red "Corno Marconi" showed higher total polyphenols than the yellow type (3.36 mmol g^{-1} and 2.79 mmol g^{-1} of fresh product, respectively). A much more marked difference was observed within the variety "Corno di capra", whose red type contained 1 mmol g^{-1} of total polyphenols more than the corresponding yellow type. Instead, the two varieties "Cornetto di Acerra" and "Sassaniello" showed almost the same amount of total polyphenols in both red and yellow types, with a very slight predominance in the yellow ones. The unusual difference between red and yellow "Corno di capra" was also observed in a genetic survey of the same set of traditional Campania peppers analyzed in the present study. The survey showed that the two varieties belong to two different and unrelated genetic groups according to Simple Sequence Repeats (SSR) DNA molecular markers (Tranchida-Lombardo et al., in prep.). Indeed, the "Corno di capra" yellow type is more related to the three green peppers, while the "Corno di capra" red type is more associated to "Cornetto di Acerra" (Tranchida-Lombardo et al., in prep.). The three green varieties of sweet pepper showed a much lower content of total polyphenols than those red and yellow. "Friariello nocerese" represented an exception, with total polyphenol similar to the yellow "Corno di capra" However, this did not correspond to a similar antioxidant activity, which resulted less effective (EC_{50}: 7.27 versus 2.70, respectively) in "Friariello nocerese" than the "Corno di capra" that therefore exhibited higher amounts of β-carotene and ascorbic acid. Its content of TPs was also higher than that of the red "Papaccella liscia". However, also in this case, to a higher amount of total polyphenols did not correspond a similar antioxidant activity; on the contrary, the antioxidant activity of red "Papaccella liscia" was two-time stronger respect to that of "Friariello nocerese" (EC_{50}: 7.27 versus 3.64, respectively). The other two green peppers, "Friariello a sigaretta" and "Friariello Napoletano", which showed the lowest values of all three parameters (ascorbic acid, β-carotene and total polyphenols) had the lowest effective antioxidant activity (EC_{50} = 9.57 mg and EC_{50} = 13.18 mg, respectively). Interestingly, the biochemical relationships observed among green peppers were also confirmed by SSR markers analysis, which showed that "Friariello nocerese" is less related to the two other green peppers ("Friariello sigaretta" and "Friariello napoletano") and more related to the "Corno Marconi" variety (red and yellow types) (Tranchida-Lombardo et al. in prep.).

Statistical analysis, performed taking into account these biochemical parameters, allowed us to potentially identify the contribution of ascorbic acid, β-carotene and total polyphenols on the antioxidant activity. Thus, as shown in Figure 2, although all three parameters concurred to affect the antioxidant activity of the varieties of sweet pepper, the content of total polyphenols and ascorbic acid seemed better correlated with the antioxidant activity (corr = −0.75 and corr = −0.81, respectively) than the β-carotene (corr = −0.51).

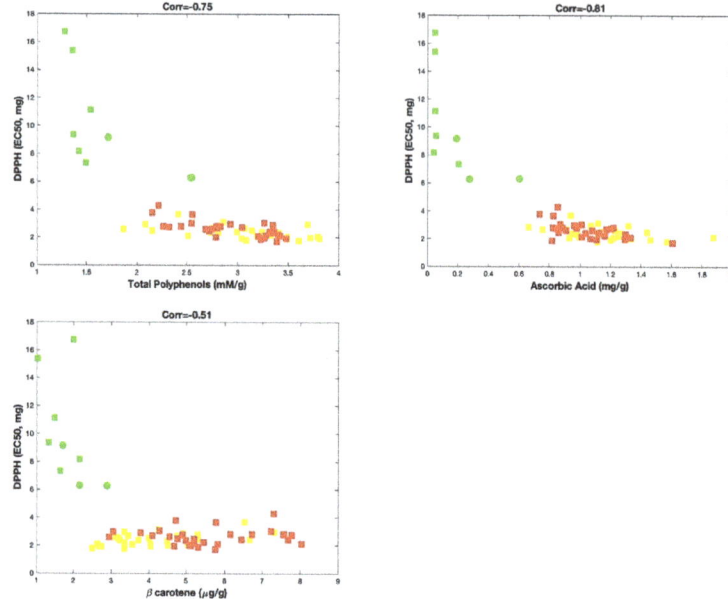

Figure 2. Correlation analysis. Red and yellow varieties are indicated with red and yellow squares, respectively. Green varieties are represented with green squares, except samples of "Friariello Nocerese", represented by green circles, to highlight that at least two (of three samples) resulted very similar to red and yellow samples.

In any case, for all analyses of correlation, we always observed a group formed by the red and yellow varieties and another distinct group formed by the green varieties. For this last group, the exception was represented by the "Friariello Nocerese", which seemed most moved towards the red and yellow varieties. Therefore, the sweet pepper 'Friariello', widely cultivated in the Campania region, is also one of the most common Italian varieties [30], for which distinct group types were ascertained by Parisi et al. [31], on the basis of the genetic, morphological traits and some qualitative traits.

Principal Component Analysis, obtained using MATLAB and applied to ascorbic acid, total polyphenols and β-carotene, revealed that the first principal component accounted for 66% of the total variance, while the first two components accounted for about 89% of the total variance of data (Figure 3). Interestingly, two of the green varieties ("Friariello napoletano" and "Friariello Sigaretta", indicated as green squares) are well clustered and completely located near the PCA1 axis. On the other hand, we observed a significant overlapping between red and yellow varieties. The green variety "Friariello Nocerese" -indicated in the Figure 3 with green circled- showed, once again, greater similarity with the complex group of yellow and red varieties, in particular with the yellow "Corno di capra" than with the other two green varieties of sweet pepper.

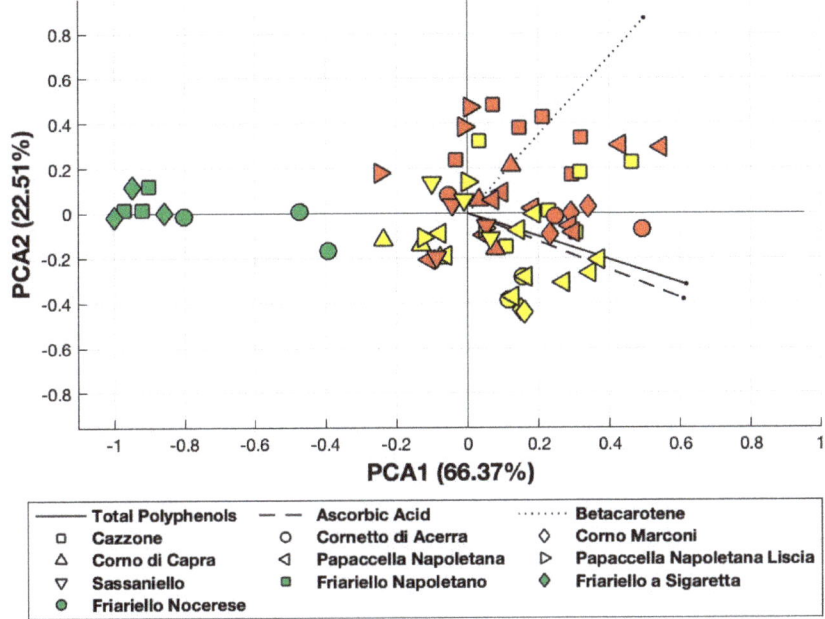

Figure 3. PCA obtained considering β-carotene, ascorbic and total polyphenols. Yellow and red-colored symbols indicate the yellow and red varieties, respectively.

3.4. Polyphenol Profile

Polyphenol profile, from qualitative and quantitative point of view, may vary in relation to genetic variation but also to different growth and geographic conditions. Obtaining as much information as possible on the polyphenolic composition becomes crucial for identifying the best varieties, from a qualitative and health-nutritional point of view, existing in a given territory. As far as we know, there are no studies that have characterized such a large number of traditional Campania varieties from a biochemical point of view. In particular, there are no scientific studies reporting the analysis of the qualitative and quantitative profile of the polyphenols present in many of the traditional sweet pepper varieties of the Campania region. This study was carried out using UPLC, an analytical approach that proved to be a powerful method for the analysis of individual polyphenols in a few minutes (in our case in an analysis time not exceeding 15′) and capable of providing a detailed analysis of the phenolic molecules and, above all, of their concentration, contained in the varieties. All data, reported as $\mu g\ g^{-1}$ respect to the metabolites identified through UPLC are shown in Table 2.

Table 2. Polyphenol composition of the yellow, red and green traditional varieties of sweet pepper of the Campania region, obtained by UPLC analysis, expressed as $\mu g\ g^{-1}$ ± Standard Deviation.

	GAL	CHL	CAF	CUM	FER	CAT	EPI	QUE	RUT	API	NAR
CG	127.81 ± 20.85	98.66 ± 26.13	19.46 ± 5.12	0 ± 0.00	0 ± 0.00	98.93 ± 7.20	112.09 ± 12.65	0 ± 0.00	49.91 ± 5.22	0 ± 0.00	0 ± 0.00
PNG	100.16 ± 21.20	97.79 ± 27.77	23.13 ± 5.48	0 ± 0.00	7.01 ± 1.63	95.51 ± 4.59	27.91 ± 2.71	76.38 ± 2.51	46.56 ± 3.65	4.71 ± 0.78	0 ± 0.00
PLG	109.83 ± 2.10	114.88 ± 2.20	51.47 ± 0.98	0 ± 0.00	22.78 ± 0.44	130.68 ± 2.50	145.96 ± 2.79	0 ± 0.00	0 ± 0.00	0 ± 0.00	0 ± 0.00

Table 2. Cont.

	GAL	CHL	CAF	CUM	FER	CAT	EPI	QUE	RUT	API	NAR
CAG	70.96 ± 4.64	31.00 ± 2.03	12.51 ± 0.82	0 ± 0.00	7.54 ± 0.49	44.10 ± 2.88	2.33 ± 0.33	0 ± 0.00	0 ± 0.0)	0 ± 0.00	0 ± 0.00
SG	100.13 ± 6.44	115.29 ± 7.41	29.16 ± 1.87	6.29 ± 0.40	23.44 ± 1.51	107.05 ± 6.88	0 ± 0.00	0 ± 0.00	0 ± 0.00	0 ± 0.00	0 ± 0.00
CCG	97.17 ± 7.19	127.05 ± 9.40	77.11 ± 5.71	0 ± 0.00	24.58(± 1.82	145.94 ± 10.80	0 ± 0.00	0 ± 0.00	0 ± 0.00	13.58 ± 1.01	22.97 ± 1.70
CMG	185.70 ± 27.89	103.93 ± 15.05	15.48 ± 2.24	0 ± 0.00	18.73 ± 2.71	0 ± 0.00	92.56 ± 13.40	17.23 ± 2.50	0 ± 0.00	7.82 ± 1.13	0 ± 0.00
CR	96.94 ± 20.85	97.79 ± 27.77	3.09 ± 0.73	0 ± 0.00	14.09 ± 1.68	129.18 ± 13.08	110.84 ± 15.15	0 ± 0.00	101.55 ± 18.69	8.32 ± 1.33	0 ± 0.00
PNR	112.27 ± 17.05	119.74 ± 20.11	15.69 ± 1.68	0 ± 0.00	10.37 ± 1.22	130.37 ± 11.53	92.47 ± 4.97	50.70 ± 2.23	33.02 ± 4.95	0 ± 0.00	0 ± 0.00
PLR	44.80 ± 1.13	58.54 ± 1.48	0 ± 0.00	0 ± 0.00	0.44 ± 0.01	0 ± 0.00	36.81 ± 0.93	0 ± 0.00	0 ± 0.00	0 ± 0.00	0 ± 0.00
CAR	93.74 ± 11.29	81.01 ± 9.70	3.82 ± 0.46	0 ± 0.00	11.10 ± 1.33	52.46 ± 6.28	64.03 ± 7.67	104.35 ± 12.50	77.24 ± 9.25	0 ± 0.00	0 ± 0.00
SR	101.18 ± 9.01	103.51 ± 9.22	4.49 ± 0.40	0 ± 0.00	10.02 ± 0.89	166.68 ± 14.84	121.93 ± 10.86	0 ± 0.00	64.41 ± 5.74	29.61 ± 2.64	5.44 ± 0.48
CCR	85.87 ± 7.39	65.53 ± 5.64	29.31 ± 2.52	0 ± 0.00	6.16 ± 0.53	133.93 ± 11.52	52.68 ± 4.53	7.36 ± 0.63	0 ± 0.00)	4.05 ± 0.35	0 ± 0.00
CMR	90.80 ± 3.83	108.05 ± 4.56	0 ± 0.00	0 ± 0.00	7.35 ± 0.31	119.05 ± 5.03	99.16 ± 4.19	124.86 ± 5.27	109.27 ± 4.61	0 ± 0.00	0 ± 0.00
FNAP	69.26 ± 4.19	112.93 ± 6.84	97.10 ± 5.88	8.06 ± 0.49	29.62 ± 1.79	244.37 ± 14.80	67.86 ± 4.11	0 ± 0.00	9.46 ± 0.57	0 ± 0.00	0 ± 0.00
FNOC	117.34 ± 24.94	273.57 ± 28.15	55.66 ± 1.83	2.71 ± 0.58	30.85 ± 2.56	170.79 ± 16.30	0 ± 0.00	0 ± 0.00	0 ± 0.00	0 ± 0.00	23.19 ± 1.93
FSIG	65.95 ± 5.20	124.66 ± 9.88	44.88 ± 3.56	0 ± 0.00	25.97 ± 2.06	216.03 ± 17.13	0 ± 0.00	0 ± 0.00	52.47 ± 4.17	0 ± 0.00	0 ± 0.00

Legend: molecules = GAL: gallic acid; CHL: chlorogenic acid; CAF: caffeic acid; CUM: *p*-coumaric acid; FER: ferulic acid; CAT: catechin; EPI: epicatechin; QUE: quercetin; RUT: rutin; NAR: naringenin; API: apigenin; Varieties = CG: Cazzone, yellow; PNG: Papaccella napoletana, yellow; PLG: Papaccella liscia, yellow; CAG: Cornetto di Acerra, yellow; SG: Sassaniello, yellow; CCG: Corno di Capra, yellow; CMG: Corno Marconi, yellow; CR: Cazzone, red; PNR: Papaccella napoletana, red; PLR: Papaccella liscia, red; CAR: Cornetto di Acerra, red; SR: Sassaniello, red; CCR: Corno di Capra, red; CMR: Corno Marconi, red; FNAP: Friariello Napoletano, green; FNOC: Friariello Nocerese, green; FSIG: Friariello Sigaretta, green.

Gallic acid and chlorogenic acid were the most abundant phenolic acids in all varieties. Among the yellow and red varieties, gallic acid ranged between 44.80 µg g^{-1} (in the red "Papaccella liscia") and 185.70 µg g^{-1} (found in the yellow type of "Corno Marconi"). "Friariello Nocerese" showed a content of gallic acid more similar, in terms of concentration, to some of yellow and red varieties (such as to the red variety of "Papaccella napoletana" (117.34 µg g^{-1} and 112.27 µg g^{-1}, respectively), than to the other two green varieties of Friariello, which content did not exceed 69.26 µg g^{-1} ("Friariello napoletano"). In general, almost all the traditional varieties analyzed exhibited a content of gallic acid undoubtedly superior if compared to that present in some commercial varieties such as Roberta or Berceo [27,32], but similar to such varieties for the high content of chlorogenic acid, the low amount of caffeic acid and for the negligible quantity of apigenin, therefore present only in very few varieties. Chlorogenic acid showed a sharped distribution along the varieties. It is to highlight that the green variety "Friariello Nocerese" contained the highest amount of this metabolite (273 µg g^{-1}); on the contrary, we observed that the yellow type of "Cornetto di Acerra" showed a ninth of chlorogenic acid respect to "Friariello Nocerese". Probably in the "Cornetto di Acerra" other metabolites, not recognized with the available standards, were also present, justifying the amount of polyphenols that, in the yellow "Cornetto di Acerra", was 1mmol higher than "Friariello Nocerese". Caffeic acid was much less abundant both in yellow and red varieties, not exceeding 77.11 µg g^{-1} (in the yellow "Corno di Capra"), while it was enough abundant in the three varieties of green pepper, reaching also 97.10 µg g^{-1} in the "Friariello napoletano". p-Coumaric acid was absent in all varieties, except two green varieties ("Friariello Napoletano and "Friariello Nocerese"), which content of this metabolite did not exceeded 8.06 µg g^{-1}. The trend of caffeic acid and chlorogenic acid was in agreement with Blanco-Rios et al. [33], which, analyzing different varieties of Mexican sweet pepper, found a higher amount of caffeic acid and chlorogenic acid in the green varieties, with a decreasing quantity starting from the red varieties, and following towards the orange and yellow ones. The almost complete absence of p-coumaric acid, observed only in the green varieties of "Friariello" is in agreement with Dimitriu et al. [34], which led to an increase of this metabolite at to 0.0487 mg GAE in 100 g FW only under microorganism fertilization in cultivars of pepper where it was not detected. Among flavonoids, catechin was detected in all varieties (except in the yellow "Corno Marconi" and in the red "Papaccella liscia") reaching also 166.68 µg g^{-1} (in the red "Sassaniello"). Its isomer epicatechin was slightly less abundant than catechin (121.93 µg g^{-1} as the highest concentration, in the red "Sassaniello"). The content of catechin observed by us was certainly higher than that reported by Ghasemnezhad et al. [35] in some varieties of sweet pepper, which contained a concentration of this metabolite ranging between 3.2 µg g^{-1} FW and 15.54 µg g^{-1} FW. The presence of such an important amount of catechin and epicatechin in some varieties of sweet pepper is very important. Catechins can reduce the risk of occurrence and development of some diseases. These metabolites can concur to regulate the glucose/insulin and lipid metabolism [36]; they have also neuroprotective [37], hearth protective [38], and anti-inflammatory effects [39]. Catechin can also protect from eye macula [40]. Catechin has also antibacterial activity. Nazzaro et al. found a strict correlation between the presence of catechin in extra virgin olive oil (EVO) and antibacterial activity exhibited by the EVO extract against *Staphylococcus aureus* [41]. Recently, catechin extracted from green tea-based polyphenol was also associated to rare earth (RE) metal ions to prepare catechin–RE complexes that showed significant anti-biofilm properties against *Pseudomonas aeruginosa*, *Staphylococcus sciuri* and *Aspergillus niger*, acting through the damage of microbial cell membrane [42]. Epicatechin and its metabolites can enhance muscle performance, improve symptoms of cardiovascular and cerebrovascular diseases, and support human health preventing diabetes and protecting the nervous system [43]. The presence of a so high amount of catechins and epicatechin in the varieties of sweet pepper resulted still more interesting, taking into account that, in some cases, flavonoid contents of pepper extracts can be enhanced with thermal process, such as by increasing temperature to 65 °C [29].

Quercetin was detected in the varieties "Papaccella napoletana" (both yellow and red), "Corno Marconi" (both yellow and red, 17.23 µg g^{-1} and 124.86 µg g^{-1}, respectively), in the red "Cornetto di Acerra" (104.35 µg g^{-1}) and in the red "Corno di Capra" (that showed 7.36 µg g^{-1}). Also in this case, our results, at least for the green varieties, were in agreement with Blanco-Rois et al. [33]; however, unlike these last, we found a certain amount of quercetin also in some varieties of red and yellow sweet peppers. Quercetin is one of the metabolites with the most known healthy effects. Recently Pingili et al. [44] ascertained an important role of quercetin as liver protective agent against different drugs and toxic agents. Therefore, due to its healthy properties [45], quercetin has been also used in the formulation of novel functional foods, such as quercetin-fortified bread [46]. Yellow "Papaccella napoletana" exhibited a content of quercetin also superior respect to that observed by Ghasemnezhad et al. in the variety Arona [35]. Rutin was detected in some varieties, such as "Cazzone" (both yellow and red), "Papaccella napoletana" (both yellow and red), and in the red types of "Cornetto di Acerra" and "Sassaniello". It was also identified and quantified in the two green varieties of sweet pepper "Friariello napoletano" and "Friariello sigaretta" that, on the other hand did not contain naringenin, present only in the third variety of green pepper "Friariello nocerese" and detected also in other two varieties, the yellow "Corno di capra" and the red "Sassaniello".

From a global analysis of polyphenolic profile, we could observe that the red "Sassaniello" and the yellow "Papaccella napoletana" showed almost all metabolites, except p-coumaric acid and quercetin in the "Sassaniello" and p-coumaric acid and naringenin in the "Papaccella napoletana". Therefore, the red type "Papaccella liscia" missed even seven polyphenols, in particular caffeic acid among the phenolic acids, and almost all flavonoids except epicatechin. This clearly shows in general a different metabolic pathway between the varieties of sweet pepper, which affects the presence and amount of these secondary metabolites.

PCA applied to the polyphenol composition of all varieties of sweet pepper analyzed, revealed that the first principal component accounted for 34.31% of the total variance, while the first two components accounted for about 52% of the total variance (Figure 4).

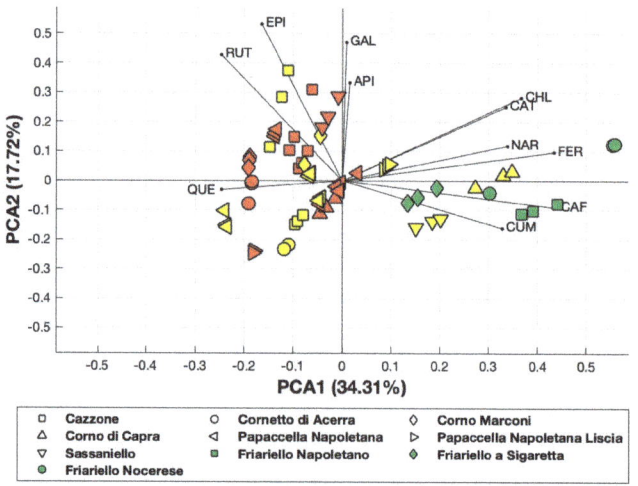

Figure 4. PCA obtained considering polyphenol composition. Yellow and red-colored symbols indicate the yellow and red varieties, respectively.

Although PCA covered 52% of the total variance, it allowed us to observe the clustering of several yellow and red varieties and that the yellow varieties "Corno di capra" and "Sassaniello" were close to the green varieties of "Friariello".

Calculating the percentages of the individual polyphenols with respect to the sum of the polyphenols recognized by the chromatographic analysis, and assembling phenolic acids and flavonoids in two groups, we could observe the general distribution of acidic phenols and flavonoids among the varieties of sweet pepper. Results are shown in Figure 5.

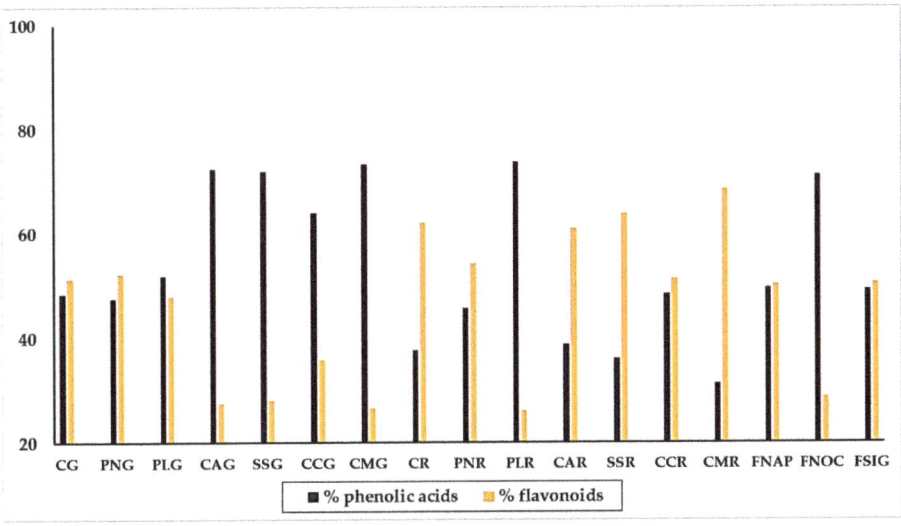

Figure 5. Distribution of phenolic acids and flavonoids and phenolic acids, respect to the molecules recognized by UPLC, in yellow, red and green traditional varieties of sweet pepper of the Campania Region. Varieties = CG: Cazzone, yellow; PNG: Papaccella napoletana, yellow; PLG: Papaccella liscia, yellow; CAG: Cornetto di Acerra, yellow; SG: Sassaniello, yellow; CCG: Corno di Capra, yellow; CMG: Corno Marconi, yellow; CR: Cazzone, red; PNR: Papaccella napoletana, red; PLR: Papaccella liscia, red; CAR: Cornetto di Acerra, red; SR: Sassaniello, red; CCR: Corno di Capra, red; CMR: Corno Marconi, red; FNAP: Friariello Napoletano, green; FNOC: Friariello Nocerese, green; FSIG: Friariello Sigaretta, green.

By the whole, the composition exhibited by the yellow and red varieties was quite different. Thus, we found that the majority of yellow varieties contained much more phenolic acids than flavonoids, in particular "Corno Marconi" (73.34% phenolic acids and 26.66% flavonoids), "Cornetto di Acerra" (72.5% phenolic acids and 27.5% flavonoids), "Sassaniello" (71.9% phenolic acids and 28.1% flavonoids) and "Corno di capra" (64.1% phenolic acids and 35.9% flavonoids). In the varieties "Cazzone" and" Papaccella liscia" the percentage of phenolic acids and flavonoids was almost equal, with a slightly preponderance of flavonoids. The trend was completely opposite in the red varieties, which contained generally much more flavonoids than phenolic acids. This was the behavior of "Corno Marconi (68.9% flavonoids and 31.31% phenolic acids), "Sassaniello" (containing 63.91% flavonoids and 36.09% phenolic acids) and "Cazzone" (62.68% flavonoids and 37.72% phenolic acids). Two red varieties, "Papaccella napoletana" and "Corno di capra" showed a similar content of phenolic acids and flavonoids. Only "Papaccella liscia" contained much more phenolic acids (73.81%) than flavonoids (26.19%). The three varieties of "Friariello" behaved completely different from each other. Thus, while the "Friariello Nocerese" showed a trend more similar to that of the yellow varieties, in particular "Cornetto di Acerra" and "Sassaniello", with a content of acid phenols (71.22%) much higher than that of the flavonoids (28.78%). The "Friariello napoletano" and the "Friariello a sigaretta" instead practically the same percentage of acid phenols (49.63% and 49.33%, respectively) and flavonoids (50.36% and 50.67% respectively). The behavior of "Friariello Nocerese", which in general showed highest values of phenolic acids and flavonoids than the other two green varieties, was in agreement with the results of Mennella et al. [20], which found similarities between 'Friariello Nocerese' and some yellow varieties of sweet pepper, in spite of the clear differences that the two varieties show as regard their morphological traits and color at maturation.

4. Conclusions

Breeding for high-value vegetables is an increasingly preferred ambition and the enhancement of crop bioactive compounds might be strategic to encounter the actual ideas of the market and consumers indeed. As far as we know, this is the first time that a similar study was performed on different yellow, red and green traditional varieties of sweet pepper of the Campania region, grown at the same conditions and collected in the same period, so to avoid as more as possible all those variables that could affect the metabolic pathway of these products [47]. Our results suggest the great potential of these landraces in terms of phytochemicals of health interest. The interrelationships between the parameters analyzed and the different varieties let us to light on a clustering of several red and yellow varieties, and that mainly the yellow "Corno di capra" was closer to the green varieties of "Friariello". This could contribute in the exploitation and improvement of both cultivation and breeding programs at regional, national and international level, with the aims to safeguard the crop biodiversity, taking into account the health of consumers and without forgetting that an increase in the cultivation of these traditional varieties could rise the farmers' income.

Author Contributions: Conceptualization, F.F. and F.N.; Funding acquisition, P.S., R.R. and M.Z.; Investigation, F.F., A.d.A., A.C., P.S., R.R., F.R., M.Z., V.T.L., M.T., S.G. and F.N.; Methodology, F.F., A.d.A., C.P., R.C. and F.N.; Software, A.d.A.; Supervision, F.N.; Writing—original draft, F.N., M.T. and A.d.A.; Writing—review & editing, F.N., M.T., V.T.L., S.G. and A.d.A. All authors have read and agreed to the published version of the manuscript.

Funding: The work was partially supported by the Campania regional Projects "SALVE" and "AGRIGENET" PSR 2007-2013, az. f2. The authors are really grateful to Mario Parisi, which support contributed to enrich the discussion of the work.

Conflicts of Interest: The authors declare no conflict of interest.

References

1. Haytowitz, D.B.; Matthews, R.H. Composition of foods: Vegetables and vegetable products: Raw, processed, prepared. In *Agriculture Handbook*; U.S. Department of Agriculture: Washington, DC, USA, 1984; pp. 8–11.
2. Matsufuji, H.; Nakamura, H.; Chino, M.; Takeda, M. Antioxidant activity of capsanthin and the fatty acid esters in paprika (*Capsicum annuum*). *J. Agric. Food Chem.* **1998**, *9*, 3468–3472. [CrossRef]
3. Hasler, C.M. Functional foods: Their role in disease prevention and health. *Food Technol.* **1998**, *52*, 63–69.
4. Ou, B.; Huang, D.; Hampschwoodwill, M.; Flanagan, T.A.; Deemer, E.K. Analysis of antioxidant activities of common vegetables employing oxygen radical absorbance capacity and FRAP assays: A comparative study. *J. Agric. Food Chem.* **2002**, *50*, 3122–3128.
5. FAO. Fruit and Vegetables for Health. 2004. Available online: http://www.fao.org/3/a-y5861e (accessed on 18 May 2020).
6. Duthie, S.J.; Jenkinson, A.M.; Crozier, A.; Mullen, W.; Pirie, L.; Kyle, J.; Yap, L.S.; Christen, P.; Duthie, G.G. The effects of cranberry juice consumption on antioxidant status and biomarkers relating to heart disease and cancer in healthy human volunteers. *Eur. J. Nutr.* **2006**, *45*, 113–122. [CrossRef]
7. World Health Organization. *Anon Joint WHO/FAO Expert Consultation on Diet, Nutrition and the Prevention of Chronic Diseases*; WHO Technical Report Series; World Health Organization: Geneva, Switzerland, 2002; p. 916.
8. Grassi, D.; Desideri, G.B.; Ferri, C. Flavonoids: Antioxidants Against Atherosclerosis. *Nutrients* **2010**, *2*, 889–902. [CrossRef]
9. Prodotti Vegetali Allo Stato Naturale o Trasformati. Available online: http://agricoltura.regione.campania.it/Tipici/tradizionali-vegetali.htm (accessed on 23 April 2020).
10. Serrano, M.; Zapata, P.J.; Castillo, S.; Guillén, F.; Martínez-Romero, D.; Valero, D. Antioxidant and nutritive constituents during sweet pepper development and ripening are enhanced by nitrophenolate treatments. *Food Chem.* **2010**, *118*, 497–503. [CrossRef]
11. Thuphairo, K.; Sornchan, P.; Suttisansanee, U. Bioactive compounds, antioxidant activity and inhibition of key enzymes relevant to Alzheimer's disease from sweet pepper (*Capsicum annuum*) extracts. *Prev. Nutr. Food Sci.* **2019**, *24*, 327–337. [CrossRef] [PubMed]
12. Archivio Meteo Storico. Available online: http://www.ilmeteo (accessed on 18 May 2020).

13. Nazzaro, F.; Caliendo, G.; Arnesi, G.; Veronesi, A.; Sarzi, P.; Fratianni, F. Comparative content of some bioactive compounds in two varieties of *Capsicum annuum* L. Sweet pepper and evaluation of their antimicrobial and mutagenic activities. *J. Food Biochem.* **2009**, *33*, 852–868. [CrossRef]
14. Singleton, V.L.; Rossi, J.A. Colorimetry of Total Phenolics with Phosphomolybdic Phosphotungstic Acid Reagents. *Am. J. Enol. Vitic.* **1965**, *16*, 144–158.
15. Ombra, M.N.; d'Acierno, A.; Nazzaro, F.; Riccardi, R.; Spigno, P.; Zaccardelli, M.; Pane, C.; Maione, M.; Fratianni, F. Phenolic composition and antioxidant and antiproliferative activities of the extracts of twelve common bean (*Phaseolus vulgaris* L.) endemic ecotypes of Southern Italy before and after cooking. *Oxidative Med. Cell. Longev.* **2016**, *2016*, 1398298. [CrossRef]
16. Fratianni, F.; Cardinale, F.; Cozzolino, A.; Granese, T.; Pepe, S.; Riccardi, R.; Spigno, P.; Coppola, R.; Nazzaro, F. Polyphenol Composition and Antioxidant Activity of Two Autochthonous Brassicaceae of the Campania Region, Southern Italy. *Food Nutr. Sci.* **2014**, *5*, 1–5. [CrossRef]
17. Pane, C.; Fratianni, F.; Parisi, M.; Nazzaro, F.; Zaccardelli, M. Control of Alternaria post-harvest infections on cherry tomato fruits by wild pepper phenolic-rich extracts. *Crop Prot.* **2016**, *84*, 81–87. [CrossRef]
18. Fratianni, F.; Cozzolino, R.; Martignetti, A.; Malorni, L.; d'Acierno, A.; De Feo, V.; Cruz, A.G.; Nazzaro, F. Biochemical composition and antioxidant activity of three extra virgin olive oils from the Irpinia province, Southern Italy. *Food Sci. Nutr.* **2019**, *7*, 3233–3243. [CrossRef] [PubMed]
19. Howard, L.R.; Talcott, S.T.; Brenes, C.H.; Villalon, B. Changes in phytochemical and antioxidant activity of selected pepper cultivars (*Capsicum* species) as influenced by maturity. *J. Agric. Food Chem.* **2000**, *48*, 1713–1720. [CrossRef] [PubMed]
20. Mennella, G.; D'Alessandro, A.; Francese, G.; Fontanella, D.; Parisi, M.; Tripodi, P. Occurrence of variable levels of health-promoting fruit compounds in horn-shaped Italian sweet pepper varieties assessed by a comprehensive approach. *J. Sci. Food Agric.* **2018**, *98*, 3280–3289. [CrossRef]
21. Codexalimentarius.com. Available online: www.codexalimentarius.net (accessed on 23 April 2020).
22. Zhang, Y.; Navarro, E.; Cánovas-Márquez, J.T.; Almagro, L.; Chen, H.; Chen, Y.Q.; Zhang, H.; Torres-Martínez, S.; Chen, W.; Garre, V. A new regulatory mechanism controlling carotenogenesis in the fungus *Mucor circinelloides* as a target to generate β-carotene over-producing strains by genetic engineering. *Microb. Cell Fact.* **2016**, *15*, 99. [CrossRef]
23. Perucka, I.; Materska, M. Antioxidant vitamin contents of *Capsicum annuum* fruit extracts as affected by processing and varietal factors. *ACTA Sci. Pol. Technol. Aliment.* **2007**, *6*, 67–74.
24. Tomlekova, N.B.; White, P.J.; Thompson, J.A.; Penchev, E.A.; Nielen, S. Mutation increasing β-carotene concentrations does not adversely affect concentrations of essential mineral elements in pepper fruit. *PLoS ONE* **2017**, *12*, e0172180.
25. Mohd Hassan, N.; Yusof, N.A.; Yahaya, A.F.; Mohd Rozali, N.N.; Othman, R. Carotenoids of *Capsicum* fruits: Pigment profile and health-promoting functional attributes. *Antioxidants* **2019**, *8*, 469. [CrossRef]
26. Mokhtar, M.; Soukup, J.; Donato, P.; Cacciola, F.; Dugo, P.; Riazi, A.; Jandera, P.; Mondello, L. Determination of the polyphenolic content of a *Capsicum annuum* L. extract by liquid chromatography coupled to photo diode array and mass spectrometry detection and evaluation of its biological activity. *J. Sep. Sci.* **2015**, *38*, 171–178.
27. Hallmann, E.; Rembiałkowska, E. Characterisation of antioxidant compounds in sweet bell pepper (*Capsicum annuum* L.) under organic and conventional growing systems. *J. Sci. Food Agric.* **2012**, *92*, 2409–2415.
28. Caruso, G.; Stoleru, V.V.; Munteanu, N.C.; Sellitto, V.M.; Teliban, G.C.; Burducea, M.; Tenu, I.; Morano, G.; Butnariu, M. Quality performances of sweet pepper under farming management. *Not. Bot. Horti Agrobot. Cluj-Napoca* **2019**, *47*, 458–464. [CrossRef]
29. Shotorbani, N.Y.; Jamei, R.; Heidari, R. Antioxidant activities of two sweet pepper *Capsicum annuum* L. varieties phenolic extracts and the effects of thermal treatment. *Avicenna J. Phytomedicine* **2013**, *3*, 25–34.
30. Caruso, G.; Villari, A.; Impembo, M. Effect of nutritive solution EC and shading on berry chemical composition of NFT-grown "Friariello" pepper. *Acta Hortic. (ISHS)* **2004**, *659*, 783–790. [CrossRef]
31. Parisi, M.; Di Dato, F.; Ricci, S.; Mennella, G.; Cardi, T.; Tripodi, P. A multi-trait characterization of the 'Friariello' landrace: A Mediterranean resource for sweet pepper breeding. *Plant Genet. Resour. Charact. Util.* **2015**, 1–12. [CrossRef]

32. Hallmann, E.; Marszałek, K.; Lipowski, J.; Jasińska, U.; Kazimierczak, R.; Średnicka-Tober, D.; Rembiałkowska, E. Polyphenols and carotenoids in pickled bell pepper from organic and conventional production. *Food Chem.* **2019**, *278*, 254–260. [CrossRef] [PubMed]
33. Blanco-Ríos, A.K.; Medina-Juárez, L.A.; González-Aguilar, G.A.; Gámez-Meza, N. Antioxidant Activity of the Phenolic and Oily Fractions of Different Sweet Bell Peppers. *J. Mex. Chem. Soc.* **2013**, *57*, 137–143. [CrossRef]
34. Dimitriu, D.C.; Stoleru, V.; Corciovă, A.; Vlase, L.; Stan, T.; Jităreanu, A.; Munteanu, N.; Rotaru, L.; Patraş, A. p-Coumaric acid content in sweet pepper under farming methods. *Environ. Eng. Manag. J. (EEMJ)* **2016**, *15*, 1841–1848.
35. Ghasemnezhad, M.; Sherafati, M.; Gholam Ali Payvast, G.A. Variation in phenolic compounds, ascorbic acid and antioxidant activity of five coloured bell pepper (*Capsicum annum*) fruits at two different harvest times. *J. Funct. Foods* **2011**, *3*, 44–49. [CrossRef]
36. Spínola, V.; Pinto, J.; Llorent-Martínez, E.J.; Tomas, H.; Castilho, P.C. Evaluation of *Rubus grandifolius* L. (wild blackberries) activities targeting management of type-2 diabetes and obesity using in vitro models. *Food Chem. Toxicol.* **2019**, *123*, 443–452.
37. Ortiz López, L.; Márquez Valadez, B.; Gómez Sánchez, A.; Silva-Lucero, M.D.C.; Ortiz-López, L.; Márquez-Valadez, B.; Gómez-Sánchez, A. Green tea compound epigallo cathechin 3 gallate (EGCG) increases neuronal survival in adult hippocampal neurogenesis in vivo and in vitro. *Neuroscience* **2016**, *322*, 208–220.
38. Oyama, J.; Shiraki, A.; Nishikido, T.; Maeda, T.; Komoda, H.; Shimizu, T.; Makino, N.; Node, K. EGCG, a green tea catechin, attenuates the progression of heart failure induced by the heart/muscle specific deletion of MnSOD in mice. *J. Cardiol.* **2017**, *69*, 417–427. [CrossRef]
39. Kapoor, M.P.; Sugita, M.; Nishimura, A.; Sudo, S.; Okubo, T. Influence of acute ingestion and regular intake of green tea catechins on resting oxidative stress biomarkers assays in a paralleled randomized controlled crossover supplementation study in healthy men. *J. Funct. Foods* **2018**, *45*, 381–391. [CrossRef]
40. Moine, E.; Brabet, P.; Guillou, L.; Durand, T.; Vercauteren, J.; Crauste, C. New lipophenol antioxidants reduce oxidative damage in retina pigment epithelial cells. *Antioxidants* **2018**, *7*, 197. [CrossRef]
41. Nazzaro, F.; Fratianni, F.; Cozzolino, R.; Martignetti, A.; Malorni, L.; De Feo, V.; Cruz, A.G.; d'Acierno, A. Antibacterial activity of three extra virgin olive oils of the Campania region, Southern Italy, related to their polyphenol content and composition. *Microorganisms* **2019**, *7*, 321. [CrossRef]
42. Liu, L.; Xiao, X.; Li, K.; Li, X.; Shi, B.; Liao, X. Synthesis of catechin rare earth complex with efficient and broad spectrum anti biofilm activity. *Chem. Biodivers.* **2020**, in press. [CrossRef]
43. Qu, Z.; Liu, A.; Li, P.; Liu, C.; Xiao, W.; Huang, J.; Liu, Z.; Zhang, S. Advances in physiological functions and mechanisms of (−)-epicatechin. *Crit. Rev. Food Sci. Nutr.* **2020**, 1–23.
44. Pingili, R.B.; Challa, S.R.; Pawar, A.K.; Toleti, V.; Kodali, T.; Koppula, S. A systematic review on hepatoprotective activity of quercetin against various drugs and toxic agents: Evidence from preclinical studies. *Phytoterapy Res.* **2020**, *34*, 5–32. [CrossRef]
45. Cai, X.; Fang, Z.; Dou, J.; Yu, A.; Zhai, G. Bioavailability of quercetin: Problems and promises. *Curr. Med. Chem.* **2013**, *20*, 2572–2582. [CrossRef]
46. Lin, J.; Teo, L.M.; Leong, L.P.; Zhou, W. In vitro bio accessibility and bioavailability of quercetin from the quercetin-fortified bread products with reduced glycemic potential. *Food Chem.* **2019**, *286*, 629–635. [CrossRef] [PubMed]
47. Mateos, R.M.; Jiménez, A.; Román, P.; Romojaro, F.; Bacarizo, S.; Leterrier, M.; Gómez, M.; Sevilla, F.; Del Río, L.A.; Corpas, F.J.; et al. Antioxidant systems from pepper (*Capsicum annuum* L.): Involvement in the response to temperature changes in ripe fruits. *Inter. J. Mol. Sci.* **2013**, *14*, 9556–9580.

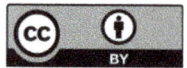

© 2020 by the authors. Licensee MDPI, Basel, Switzerland. This article is an open access article distributed under the terms and conditions of the Creative Commons Attribution (CC BY) license (http://creativecommons.org/licenses/by/4.0/).

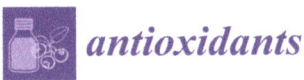

Article

Voltammetric Behavior, Flavanol and Anthocyanin Contents, and Antioxidant Capacity of Grape Skins and Seeds during Ripening (*Vitis vinifera* var. *Merlot*, *Tannat*, and *Syrah*)

Nawel Benbouguerra [1], Tristan Richard [2], Cédric Saucier [1] and François Garcia [1,*]

1. SPO, Université de Montpellier, INRAE, Montpellier SupAgro, 34000 Montpellier, France; nawel.benbouguerra@etu.umontpellier.fr (N.B.); cedric.saucier@umontpellier.fr (C.S.)
2. MIB, Unité de Recherche Oenologie, EA4577, USC 1366 INRA, ISVV, Université de Bordeaux, 33882 Villenave d'Ornon, France; tristan.richard@u-bordeaux.fr
* Correspondence: francois.garcia@umontpellier.fr; Tel.: +33-680733386

Received: 29 July 2020; Accepted: 25 August 2020; Published: 27 August 2020

Abstract: Skin and seed grape extracts of three red varieties (Merlot, Tannat, and Syrah) at different stages of ripening were studied for their total phenolic content (TPC) by using the Folin-Ciocalteu assay and for their total antioxidant capacity (TAC) by using spectrophotometric and electrochemical assays. Flavanol and anthocyanin compositions were also investigated using Ultra Performance Liquid Chromatography coupled with Mass Spectrometry (UPLC-MS). Results showed that seeds had the highest phenolic content and the highest antioxidant potential compared to skins at all stages of ripening. The highest TPC and TAC values were measured in seeds at close to veraison and veraison ripening stages. In skins, the highest values were found at the green stage, it was in accordance with the flavanols content. The voltammetric measurements were carried out using disposable single walled carbon nanotubes modified screen-printed carbon electrodes (SWCNT-SPCE). Three peaks on voltammograms were obtained at different oxidation potentials. The first anodic peak that oxidized at a low potential describes the oxidation of ortho-dihydroxy phenols and gallate groups, the second peak corresponds to the malvidin anthocyanins oxidation and the second oxidation of flavonoids. The third voltammetric peak could be due to phenolic acids such as *p*-coumaric acid and ferulic acid or the second oxidation of malvidin anthocyanins. The high linear correlation was observed between antioxidant tests and flavanols in skins ($0.86 \leq r \leq 0.94$), while in seeds, 'r' was higher between electrochemical parameters and flavanols ($0.64 \leq r \leq 0.8$).

Keywords: skins; seeds; *Vitis vinifera*; antioxidant activity; cyclic voltammetry; phenolic compounds

1. Introduction

Vitis vinifera is the most economically important species of grape vine in the world with 78 million tons of grapes production in 2018 (see http://www.oiv.int/en/oiv-life/oiv-2019-report-on-the-world-vitivinicultural-situation). Grapes consumed as fresh fruits, juices, and other processed products, contain many phenolic compounds which are mostly located in seeds and skins [1]. These compounds are synthesized in response to various biotic and abiotic stress such as fungal invasion, UV irradiations, ozone, and heavy metal ions [2]. Their content changes depending on the grape variety, soil, climatic conditions, and the ripening stages [3].

Polyphenols are commonly present in the plant kingdom and they bring more and more interest [4]. Phenolic compounds can be divided in two groups, flavonoids and non-flavonoids, according to their carbon skeleton [4]. The flavonoids (C6-C3-C6) are located in both skins and seeds and the anthocyanins and flavanols are the most abundant compounds [5]. The non-flavonoids such as stilbenes and phenolic acids are found in the skins [6]. The synergy between the various classes of polyphenols increases sample efficiency and activity [7]. Polyphenols protect plants against biotic and abiotic stresses and they are involved in organoleptic and qualitative properties of food and beverages derived from these plants [8]. Many studies have reported their biological activities. They have potent antioxidant capacity [7,9–18]. They may prevent diabetes [19,20], obesity [21–23], cardiovascular [24,25], and neurodegenerative diseases [25,26].

Radical scavenging capacity (DPPH and ABTS) and ferric reducing capacity, which are spectrophotometric assays, are usually used in order to determine the antioxidant capacity of foods and beverages [13]. In the last years, electrochemical techniques have been more widely used as alternative methods due to their sensitivity, rapidity, ease of use, and due to their minimal environmental effects [27]. Among these electrochemical techniques, cyclic voltammetry (CV) was the first and the most commonly used to characterize and determine the total polyphenols and the total antioxidant capacity [27]. The main CV (anodic curve) parameters are:

- The peak current which is proportional to the concentration of antioxidant.
- The peak potential which indicates the type of reductant (the more the oxidation potential is low, the more the reductant is strong and easy to oxidize).
- The charge (area under the curve) is in accordance with the antioxidant capacity of samples [28].

Electrode made of glassy carbon electrode is widely used but recently, carbon nanotubes electrode have become one of the most promising material [29]. This electrode is classified into two categories depending on the number of layers on multi-walled carbon nanotubes (MWCNTs) and single-walled nanotubes (SWCNTs) [29,30]. Actually, disposable screen-printed carbon electrodes modified with carbon nanotubes attract the attention of many researchers because of their numerous advantages including disposability [31], reproducibility, practicality, high sensitivity, the ability to be miniaturized to minimize the consumption of samples, and the low detection limits [32,33].

The aims of this work were:

- To determine the polyphenol content of skin and seed extracts (Merlot, Tannat, and Syrah) during ripening.
- To measure the antioxidant capacity (DPPH, ABTS, and FRAP) of these extracts.
- To determine the cyclic voltammetry behavior of these extracts by using disposable single walled carbon nanotubes electrodes for electrochemical tests.
- To determine the correlations of electrochemical parameters with the other antioxidant assays as well as with the phenolic contents.

2. Materials and Methods

2.1. Chemicals and Reagents

Folin-Ciocalteu reagent, sodium carbonate, 2,2'-azino-bis(3-ethylbenzothiazoline-6-sulfonic acid) diammonium salt (ABTS), persulfate de potassium, 1,1-diphenyl-2-picrylhydrazyl free radical (DPPH), sodium acetate trihydrate, ferric chlorure, 2,4,6-tri(2-pyridyl)-s-triazine (TPTZ), iron(II) sulfate heptahydrate, phloroglucinol, ascorbic acid, sodium acetate, tartaric acid, sodium hydroxide, gallic acid, trolox, catechin, caffeic acid, *trans-* resveratrol, hydrochloric acid, and glacial acetic acid were purchased from Sigma-Aldrich (Saint-Quentin Fallavier, France). Oenin chloride was obtained from Extrasynthese (Genay, France). Acetonitrile, methanol, and water UPLC-MS were purchased from Biosolve Chimie (Dieuze, France) and trifluoroacetic acid from Carlo Erba Reagents (Peypin, France).

2.2. Samples

Three *V. vinifera* varieties (Merlot, Tannat, and Syrah) were harvested on 2017 at different stages of ripening: Green stage (GS), close to veraison (CV), veraison (V), and maturity (M) (Supplementary

Data, Table S1) from INRAe experimental vineyard (Montpellier, France) (coordinates: 43°37′02.7″ N 3°51′22.3″ E, average annual temperature: 15.85 °C, average annual precipitation: 629 mm (the weather was quite dry), and soil: Gravels and river sand). The whole grapes were stored at −80 °C in plastic bags until polyphenols extraction.

2.3. Samples Preparation

Seeds and skins of thirty Merlot, Tannat, and Syrah berries were manually removed from the pulp. The polyphenols were extracted with 100 mL of acetone/water (70/30 v/v) deoxygenated with nitrogen for 5 min. The solutions were filtered through a 0.45 µm filter paper after stirring during 18 h in the dark, and they evaporated in a rotavapor under low pressure at 37 °C. The resulting products were freeze-dried and stored at −20 °C until their use in antioxidant and other analytical assays [34]. Three biological replicates were done. After extraction, skin and seed extracts were weighted (dry weight: DW) and they were stored at −20 °C between 5 and 12 months before being used in the experiments.

2.4. Determination of Phenolic Composition

2.4.1. Flavanols

The assay on flavanols was performed as described by [35]. Briefly, a solution of 0.1 N HCl in MeOH, containing 50 g/L phloroglucinol and 10 g/L ascorbic acid was prepared. Seed and skin grape extracts were dissolved in methanol and reacted for 20 min at 50 °C in this solution, and then combined with five volumes of 40 mM aqueous sodium acetate to stop the reaction.

The UPLC system was a Waters Acquity (Saint-Quentin-en-Yvelines, France), with a photodiode array detector (PDA), LC pump, and an auto sampler. The column used was a reversed phase UPLC with an Acquity UPLC BEH C18 column (2.1 × 50 mm, 1.7 µm particle size) (Saint-Quentin-en Yvelines, France). The method used a binary gradient with mobile phases: Mobile phase A containing 1% v/v aqueous trifluoroacetic acid and mobile phase B containing acetonitrile. The 20 min elution method at flow 0.45 mL/min was 0 min 2% B, 8 min 6% B, 14 min 20% B, 14.1 min 99% B, 16 min 99% B, 16.1 min 2% B, and 20 min 2% B. The column temperature was 40 °C. Eluting peaks were monitored at 280 nm. The catechin calibration curve was used. Results were expressed as mg/g of DW.

2.4.2. Anthocyanins

Skin grape extracts were solubilized in MeOH/water (80/20 v/v) at an appropriate concentration then injected directly after filtration as described previously with some modifications [36].

The conditions of the chromatographic apparatus are the same as those mentioned in experimental Section 2.4.1. The column temperature was set at 50 °C. The 40 min elution method at flow 0.25 mL/min was 0 min 1% B, 5 min 8.8% B, 30 min 20.6% B, 30.5 min 96% B, 34 min 96% B, 34.1 min 1% B, and 40 min 1% B. The detection was monitored at 520 nm. The malvidin-3-O-glucoside calibration curve was used. Results were expressed as mg malvidin-3-O-glucoside equivalent (M3GE)/g of DW.

2.5. Determination of Total Phenolic Content

Skin and seed grape extracts (dry weight) were solubilized in methanol at a concentration of 5 g/L. The same solution was used to determine the total phenolic content (TPC) and total antioxidant capacity (TAC) assays. To measure the absorbance, an Agilent Cary 60 UV-Vis spectrophotometer (Santa Clara, CA, USA) connected to the Cary win UV software was used.

The Folin-Ciocalteu method was used to determine the total phenolic content (TPC) [3,13,37]. Twenty µL of the diluted extract (see Section 2.5) and 100 µL of Folin-Ciocalteu reagent were added to 1.58 mL of water. After 30 s, 300 µL of sodium carbonate solution (20%) were added; the reaction mixture was thoroughly shaken and left for 120 min in the dark at room temperature (20 °C). Then, the absorbance was measured at 700 nm against the blank (sample was replaced by the methanol).

The gallic acid calibration curve was used to determine the concentration of phenolic compounds in samples. The results were expressed as mg gallic acid equivalent (GAE)/g DW.

2.6. Determination of Antioxidant Capacities

2.6.1. Radical Scavenging Activity: DPPH• Assay

DPPH antioxidant capacity was determined according to a published protocol [38]. Fifty µL of diluted extract (see Section 2.5) was added to 1.95 mL of a DPPH (6×10^{-5} M) methanolic solution. After 30 min of incubation in the dark at room temperature (20 °C), the absorbance was measured at 515 nm. The trolox calibration curve was used. The results were expressed as µmol TE/g DW.

2.6.2. Radical Scavenging Activity: ABTS Assay

ABTS antioxidant capacity was determined according to [39]. To generate ABTS• radical, 20 mL of ABTS solution (7 mM) was added to 20 mL of a potassium persulfate solution (2.45 mM). The mixture was incubated at room temperature in the dark all night. The stock solution was diluted with water/ethanol (50/50 v/v) to an absorbance of 0.7 ± 0.02 at 734 nm. One hundred µL of diluted extract (see Section 2.5) was mixed with 1 mL of ABTS• solution. After 10 min, the absorbance was measured at 735 nm. The trolox calibration curve was used. Results were expressed as µmol TE/g DW.

2.6.3. Ferric-Reducing Antioxidant Power: FRAP Assay

FRAP antioxidant capacity was determined according to reference [40]. Fifty µL of diluted extract (see Section 2.5) and 150 µL of distilled water were added to 1.5 mL freshly prepared FRAP reagent (mixture of 10 volumes of a 300 mmol/L acetate buffer pH 3.6 with 1 volume of 10 mmol/L TPTZ in 40 mmol/L hydrochloric acid and 1 volume of 20 mmol/L ferric chloride). The solution was incubated at 37 °C for 4 min. Absorbance was measured at 593 nm. The $FeSO_4 \cdot 7H_2O$ calibration curve was used. Results were expressed as mmol Fe^{+2}E/g DW.

2.6.4. Electrochemical Apparatus and Measurements

Electrochemical measurements were carried out with potentiostat/galvanostat, Autolab PGSTAT 302N controlled by the Nova 2.1.3 software (Metrohm, Switzerland) in the personal computer (Supplementary Data, Figure S1). Tartaric acid buffer (3.3 mM tartaric acid adjusted with 1 M NaOH to obtain a pH 3.6) was used to prepare standard phenolic compounds solutions as well as diluted extracts (see Section 2.5) at appropriate concentrations (100 mg/L for skins and 20 mg/L for seeds). The scan rate was 100 mV/s.

Disk Electrode

Voltammetric measurements were carried out in a standard three-electrode electrochemical cell using an Ag/AgCl (KCl, 3 M) reference electrode, platinum counter electrode, and a glassy carbon electrode (GCE) of 3 mm diameter (Metrohm, Switzerland) as working electrode. Before each test, the working electrode surface was carefully polished with 3 µm alumina powder, then washed with purified water and cleaned for 5 min in an ultrasonic bath.

Disposable Single-Walled Carbon Nanotubes Electrodes

Single-walled carbon nanotubes electrodes (4 mm diameter, Dropsens, Spain) were also used in a three-electrode configuration comprising single-walled carbon nanotubes (SWCNTs-SPCE) with a silver reference electrode and carbon counter electrode. An aliquot of 200 µL of a solution of standard polyphenols or samples was cast onto the surface of the electrode, and the electrochemical measurements were performed immediately.

2.7. Statistical Analysis

The ANOVA and correlation tests were calculated by using the XLSTAT software (Addinsoft version 19.02, Paris, France). A Tukey test was carried out and where p-values < 0.05 was considered as significant. Pearson's correlation coefficient was carried out for the determination of correlations between the different antioxidant assays (spectrophotometric and electrochemistry) and between the antioxidant assays and phenolic composition (anthocyanins and flavanols).

3. Results and Discussion

3.1. Flavanol and Anthocyanin Content of Skin and Seed Grape Extracts during Ripening

The results of the evolution of total flavanols and anthocyanins content in skin and seed grape extracts are presented in Table 1.

Table 1. Phenolic composition of skin and seed grape extracts of the studied varieties at different stages of ripening.

	Skins		Seed
	Flavanols (mg/g DW)	Anthocyanins (mg M3GE/g DW)	Flavanols (mg/g DW)
Merlot			
Green stage	199 ± 19 [a]	ND	545 ± 9 [a]
Close to veraison	124 ± 16 [b]	2 ± 1 [c]	598 ± 30 [a]
Veraison	45 ± 9 [c]	17 ± 1 [b]	437 ± 17 [b]
Maturity	42 ± 2 [c]	22 ± 1 [a]	329 ± 24 [c]
Tannat			
Green stage	224 ± 40 [a]	ND	424 ± 27 [bc]
Close to veraison	166 ± 74 [a]	ND	530 ± 16 [a]
Veraison	31 ± 5 [b]	10 ± 3 [b]	469 ± 21 [b]
Maturity	19 ± 2 [b]	36 ± 2 [a]	382 ± 23 [c]
Syrah			
Green stage	198 ± 34 [a]	ND	496 ± 19 [ab]
Close to veraison	100 ± 26 [b]	3 ± 1 [c]	532 ± 21 [a]
Veraison	40 ± 7 [c]	28 ± 1 [a]	439 ± 32 [b]
Maturity	18 ± 1 [c]	14 ± 1.0 [b]	201 ± 41 [c]

Values represent means of triplicate determination ± SD. Different letters indicate the significant differences between stages according to Tukey's test, $p < 0.05$. DW: Dry Weight; MG3E: Malvidin-3-O-Glucoside Equivalent.

3.1.1. Flavanols

Skins

For the three varieties, the highest flavanol content was determined at the green stage then it decreased significantly until maturity. It declined from 224 mg/g DW at the green stage to 19 mg/g DW at maturity in Tannat grape extracts. A similar evolution was shown in the literature [41,42]. On the opposite, an increase of flavanols content during ripening was also observed in other study [43].

Seeds

The highest content of flavanols was reached at close to veraison compared to the green stage and the maturity for all varieties. It increased from 424 mg/g DW at the green stage to 530 mg/g DW at close to veraison, then it declined significantly to 382 mg/g DW at maturity in seed Tannat grape extracts. This evolution was in accordance with a previous study [41]. The decline of flavanols content was explained by the oxidation of these compounds after veraison [44].

Flavanols are present in both skins and seeds at all stages of ripening with an abundance in seeds [27,45]. It has been shown that in Syrah skins at maturity the content was about 250 mg/g DW and about 455 mg/g DW in seeds [46]. There is an important variability in the literature concerning the phenolic composition content due to the extraction solutions, methods, and unit used to express results.

3.1.2. Anthocyanins

The anthocyanin synthesis started at close to veraison and they accumulated until maturity in Merlot and Syrah skins, in Tannat skins, the anthocyanin synthesis started at veraison. The content increased from 2 mg M3GE/g DW to 22 mg M3GE/g DW at maturity in skin Merlot extracts. A similar evolution was reported in the literature [41–43,47–50]. In the case of Syrah, the anthocyanins content decreased at maturity from 28 to 14 mg M3GE/g DW, this decline may be due to the degradation of anthocyanins by the peroxidases and glycosidases present in skins [47].

Anthocyanins, the pigmented compounds, are present only in skin red grapes. As flavanols, the anthocyanins content differs considerably in the literature. It increases from 1.80 to 3.81 mg/g DW in Tannat skins [51] and it is about 86.68 mg/g DW at maturity in another study [16]. As mentioned previously, the anthocyanins content is also greatly affected by weather, climatic conditions, soil conditions, cultivars, irrigation [49], temperature, and light [52].

3.2. Electrochemical Behavior of Polyphenol Standards and Skin and Seed Extracts for Various Cultivars at Different Stages of Ripening

3.2.1. Electrochemical Behavior of Standard Polyphenols

Cyclic voltammograms of polyphenol standards in tartaric acid buffer (pH 3.6) at glassy carbon electrode (GCE) in a potential range from 0 to 1100 mV (vs. Ag/AgCl-KCl 3M) and at single-walled nanotubes (SWCNT) in a potential range from 0 to 800 mV (vs. Ag) are illustrated in Figure 1 and peak potentials are given in Table 2. For caffeic acid, only one anodic peak was present. This peak corresponds to the oxidation of the *ortho*-diphenols to form the corresponding o-quinone. The potential values for the concentration 0.1 mM are 445 mV (vs. Ag/AgCl-KCl 3M) for GCE and 139 mV (vs. Ag) for SWCNT. Two peaks were observed for catechin and gallic acid at 0.1 mM. With GCE (vs. Ag/AgCl-KCl 3M), the voltage values were 483/826 mV for gallic acid and 472/766 mV for catechin. With SWCNT (vs. Ag), the voltage values were 132/468 mV and 122/465 mV for catechin and gallic acid, respectively. For both catechin and gallic acid, the first anodic peak correspond to the oxidation of the hydroxyl groups on the B-ring to quinone [53]. This oxidation was reversible generating cathodic peak in the negative scan for caffeic acid and catechin. The second peak corresponds to the oxidation of the hydroxyl group on the C-ring of catechin and can also correspond to the oxidation of the third phenol group adjacent to the ortho-diphenol group in gallic acid which is in agreement with previous results [54]. Other phenolic standards characterized corresponding to the anthocyanins and the flavonols are present mostly in skin grapes. Oenin chloride and rutin at 0.1 mM presented two anodic peaks at 377/669 mV and at 201/460 mV with SWCNT (vs. Ag), respectively, and at 652/987 mV and at 260/898 mV with GCE (vs. Ag/AgCl-KCl 3M), respectively (Figure 1).

The classification obtained considering only the first peak potential for the studied standards at the same concentration (0.1 mM) by increasing potential was: Gallic acid 122 (mV) < catechin (132 mV) < caffeic acid (139 mV) < rutin (201 mV) < oenin chloride (377 mV) was found [55] since catechin, caffeic, and gallic acid oxidized at lower potential.

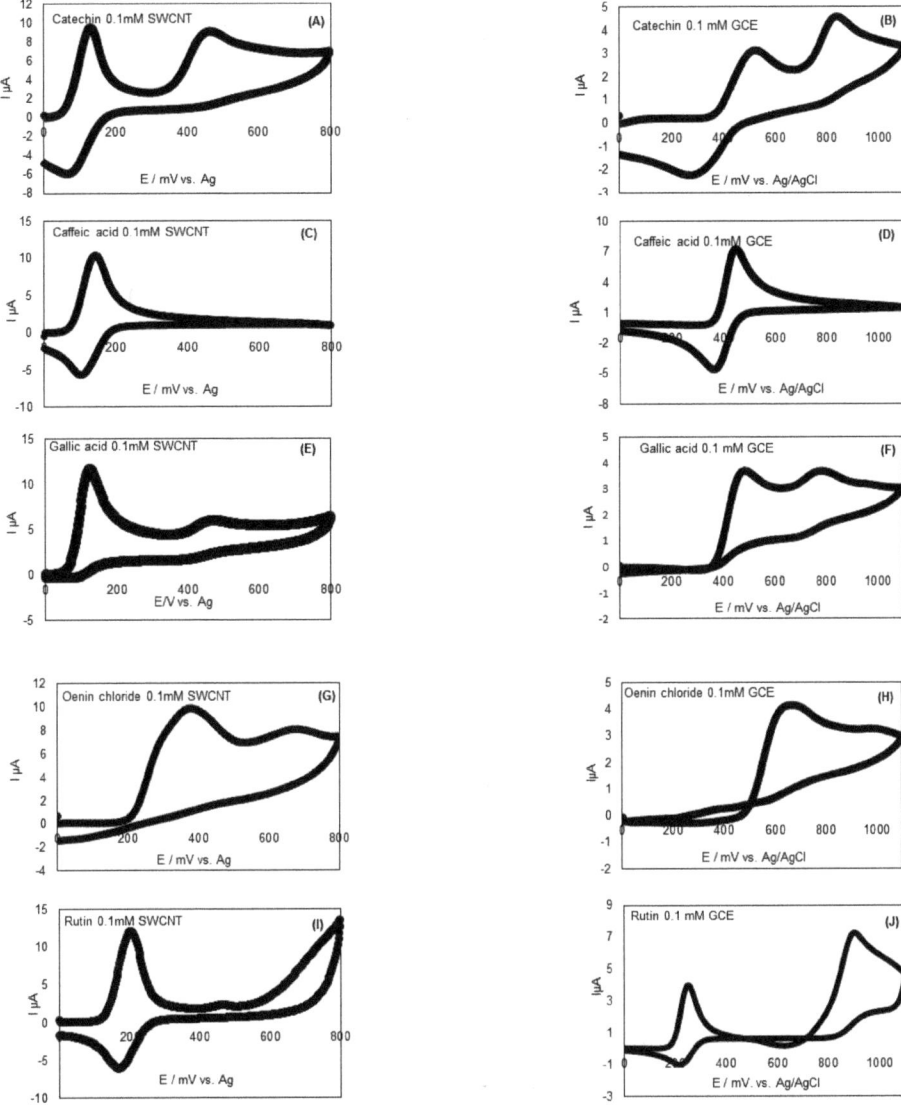

Figure 1. Cyclic voltammograms of catechin with SWCNT (**A**) and GCE (**B**), caffeic acid with SWCNT (**C**) and GCE (**D**), gallic acid with SWCNT (**E**) and GCE (**F**), oenin chloride with SWCNT(**G**) and GCE (**H**), rutin with SWCNT (**I**) and with GCE (**J**) at a concentration of 0.1 mM (blank subtracted). GCE: Glassy Carbon Electrode; SWCNT-SPCE: Single Walled Carbon Nanotubes modified Screen Printed Carbon Electrodes.

Table 2. Voltammetric behavior of the studied standard polyphenols in tartaric acid buffer (pH 3.6) with SWCNT-SPCE and GCE for a concentration of 0.1 mM.

Standards	Potential (mV)			
	SWCNT-SPCE (vs. Ag)		GCE (vs. Ag/AgCl-KCl 3M)	
	$E_{p,a1}$	$E_{p,a2}$	$E_{p,a1}$	$E_{p,a2}$
Catechin	132	468	483	826
Caffeic acid	139	/	445	/
Gallic acid	122	465	472	766
Oenin chloride	377	669	652	987
Rutin	201	460	260	898

GCE: Glassy Carbon Electrode; SWCNT-SPCE: Single Walled Carbon Nanotubes modified Screen Printed Carbon Electrodes.

3.2.2. Electrochemical Characterization of Skins and Seeds

Voltammetric measurements were performed on the extracts of each variety. For all varieties, cyclic voltammograms had three anodic peaks at different potentials depending on grape part (skins or seeds) (Figure 2) and the ripening stage. Syrah grape seed extracts were studied with both types of electrodes, as with SWCNT, three anodic peaks were also obtained with GCE (Figure 2).

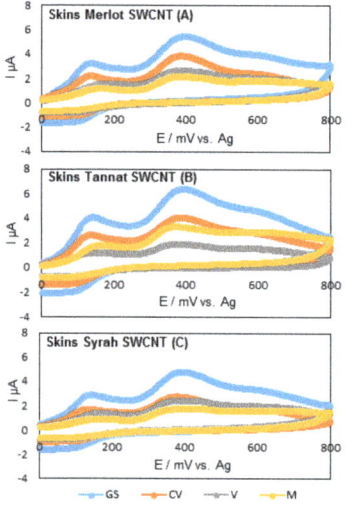
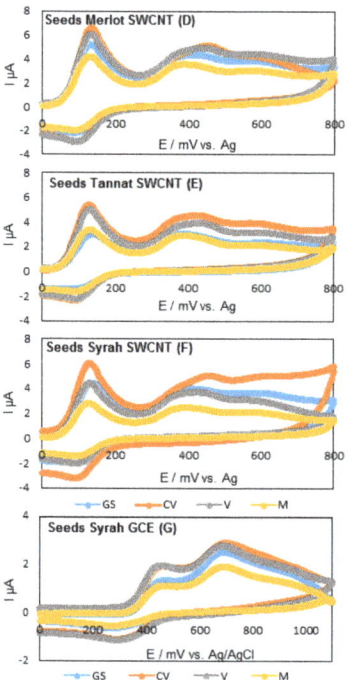

Figure 2. Cyclic voltammograms of skin (**A–C**) and seed grape extracts (**D–F**) with SWCNT and those of Syrah seed grape extract (**G**) with GCE at different stages of ripening (blank subtracted). GS: Green Stage; CV: Close to Veraison; V: Veraison; M: Maturity.

For skin Merlot grape extracts, the first anodic peak was measured at 137, 134, 159, and 157 mV at the green stage, close to veraison, veraison, and maturity, respectively. This peak corresponds to the more oxidizable compounds that oxidized at a low potential as catechin-type flavonoids, including larger oligomeric and polymeric molecules, gallic acid, caffeic acid, and flavonols. The second anodic peak appeared at 391, 383, 363, and 370 mV at the green stage, close to veraison, veraison, and maturity, respectively. This peak may result from the oxidation of malvidin anthocyanins and stilbene derivatives overlapped with the second oxidation of the catechin flavonoids [56]. The third peak close to 600 mV corresponds to the phenolic acids such as vanillic and *para*-coumaric acid or the second oxidation of malvidin anthocyanins [54]. The same behavior was observed for the two other varieties.

In grape seed extracts, the first anodic peak was obtained at the same potential in all stages of ripening, it was around 130 mV. For Syrah grape extracts for example, the first peak appeared at 136 mV, 127, 129, and 126 mV at the green stage, close to veraison, veraison, and maturity, respectively. The second peak followed the same trend of the first potential with the following potential values for Syrah at 396, 438, 409, and 391 mV for the different stages of ripening. This peak could be attributed to the oxidation of the hydroxyl group on the C-ring of catechin derivatives. The third anodic peak corresponds to the higher oxidation potential compound which produces a peak at around 600 mV [57].

3.3. Total Phenolic Content and Total Antioxidant Capacity by Spectrophotometric and Electrochemical Assays

3.3.1. Total Phenolic Content and Total Antioxidant Capacity by Spectrophotometric Assays

The total phenolic content and the antioxidant capacity of skin and seed grape extracts during ripening were determined using different spectrophotometric methods: Folin-Ciocalteu, DPPH, ABTS as well as FRAP assays, respectively. The results were summarized in Table 3.

Skins

The highest total phenolic content was detected at the green stage of ripening then it decreased significantly at maturity in the three varieties. For example, in Syrah grape extracts, the total phenolic content (TPC) was 212 mg GAE/g DW at the green stage then declined to 63 mg GAE/g DW at maturity.

The antioxidant capacities were measured using a single electron transfer (DPPH, ABTS, and FRAP). The highest total antioxidant capacity (TAC) was found in the green stage compared with maturity. The same evolution was obtained with the three assays on the three varieties. For example, in the skin Syrah grape extract, DPPH values decreased significantly from 853 at the green stage to 557 μmol TE/g DW at maturity, ABTS values from 843 to 357 μmol TE/g DW, and FRAP values from 2159 to 780 mmol Fe^{+2}E/g DW.

Seeds

The TPC in seed grape extracts increased before veraison then decreased after veraison with the highest content at close to veraison for both seed Tannat and Syrah grape extracts, whereas for seed Merlot grape extract, the content decreased significantly from 867 at the green stage to 571 mg GAE/g DW at maturity.

The antioxidant capacity of seed grape extracts followed the same trend with the three antioxidant assays. The antioxidant capacity at close to veraison was higher than that found at the green stage and maturity. Among the samples tested, for seed Syrah grape extracts, the DPPH values increased from 2677 to 2915 μmol TE/g DW then decreased to 1991 μmol TE/g DW. ABTS values raised from 1171 to 1325 then declined to 590 μmol TE/g DW. FRAP values increased from 3979 to 5386 mmol Fe^{+2}E/g DW then decreased to 3460 mmol Fe^{+2}E/g DW.

Several methods were used to determine total phenolic content and antioxidant capacity of samples to take into account not only the composition of the extracts but also the mode of action and the specificity of the antioxidant [58,59]. Due to its ease of use, the Folin-Ciocalteu assay is the common used method to determine the TPC. The principle is the transfer of electrons from phenolic compounds to phosphomolybdic/phosphotungstic complexes [60]. The weakness of this method is the overestimation of the phenolic content due to the lack of specificity [55,60,61] which can react with other compounds particularly aromatic amines, ascorbic acids, and sugars [61]. In addition, the phenolic compounds react with the Folin-Ciocalteu reagent only under the basic conditions [61]. The three colorimetric methods used to determine the antioxidant capacity DPPH, ABTS, and FRAP are considered as assays based on the electron transfer [58,61]. DPPH assay is an easy method widely used to determine the antioxidant capacity of natural extracts. The drawback of this method is the variation of reaction time with different phenolic compounds. Caffeic acid, for example, reacts quickly with DPPH whereas the catechin reacts slowly. The results obtained with this method differ depending on the time of readings (from 16 min to some hours) [55]. The FRAP assay is a simple, fast, and robust method used in the determination of the concentration of the most easily oxidized compounds [61]. It is based on the ability to reduce Fe^{3+} to Fe^{2+} quantified at 593 nm. Fe(III)/TPTZ reagent is more stable than DPPH• and gives results in shorter times [55]. The ABTS assay is based on the reduction by an antioxidant of the generated blue/green $ABTS^+$ [62]. DPPH and ABTS assays are the easiest to implement and yield the most reproducible results [58]. FRAP and DPPH methods are still used as they are the easy and accurate methods to measure the antioxidant activity [60].

The results of this work confirm that the total phenolic content in skins were lower than in seeds [13]. In skins, the highest antioxidant capacity was found at the green stage but a previous study [48] found the highest TAC at maturity. This difference may depend on the extraction method used but also on the protocol of the test. The total polyphenolic content increased when the berry weight decreased in accordance with previous studies [51].

Table 3. TPC and antioxidant capacities of skin and seed grape extracts of the three studied varieties at different stages of ripening by spectrophotometric methods.

	Skins			
	TPC (mg GAE/g DW)	DPPH (μmol TE/g DW)	ABTS (μmol TE/g DW)	FRAP (mmol Fe^{+2}E/g DW)
Merlot				
Green stage	280 ± 39 [a]	763 ± 67 [a]	804 ± 37 [a]	2781 ± 186 [a]
Close to veraison	138 ± 12 [b]	575 ± 46 [b]	748 ± 41 [a]	1925 ± 81 [b]
Veraison	82 ± 11 [b]	349 ± 24 [c]	424 ± 11 [b]	1036 ± 114 [c]
Maturity	76 ± 9 [b]	403 ± 28 [c]	527 ± 80 [b]	1180 ± 16 [c]
Tannat				
Green stage	258 ± 21 [a]	932 ± 120 [a]	1211 ± 120 [a]	2704 ± 431 [a]
Close to veraison	188 ± 44 [b]	647 ± 123 [b]	1109 ± 188 [a]	2322 ± 537 [a]
Veraison	72 ± 14 [c]	409 ± 54 [b]	696 ± 79 [b]	805 ± 8 [b]
Maturity	111 ± 9 [c]	528 ± 48 [b]	612 ± 36 [b]	1219 ± 39 [b]
Syrah				
Green stage	212 ± 39 [a]	853 ± 94 [a]	843 ± 124 [a]	2159 ± 432 [a]
Close to veraison	103 ± 21 [b]	674 ± 10 [ab]	687 ± 141 [ab]	1239 ± 251 [b]
Veraison	85 ± 8 [b]	639 ± 22 [b]	529 ± 88 [ab]	851 ± 29 [b]
Maturity	63 ± 8 [b]	557 ± 29 [b]	357 ± 14 [b]	780 ± 62 [b]
	Seeds			
Merlot				
Green stage	867 ± 60 [a]	3855 ± 413 [a]	1681 ± 302 [ab]	6047 ± 612 [a]
Close to veraison	834 ± 7 [a]	3998 ± 317 [a]	1846 ± 123 [a]	6006 ± 9928 [a]
Veraison	805 ± 92 [b]	3675 ± 172 [a]	1663.92 ± 89 [ab]	5436 ± 391 [a]
Maturity	571 ± 23 [b]	2876 ± 300 [b]	1340.8 ± 67 [b]	4683 ± 492 [a]
Tannat				
Green stage	586 ± 57 [ab]	3608 ± 201 [ab]	1467 ± 266 [ab]	4651 ± 726 [ab]
Close to veraison	712 ± 69 [a]	3875 ± 118 [a]	1697 ± 45 [a]	5557 ± 503 [a]
Veraison	676 ± 18 [a]	3706 ± 302 [a]	1656 ± 137 [a]	4201 ± 903 [ab]
Maturity	489 ± 55 [b]	3114 ± 127 [b]	1240.95 ± 47 [b]	3266 ± 300 [b]
Syrah				
Green stage	556 ± 52 [ab]	2677 ± 216 [ab]	1171 ± 91 [a]	3979 ± 2115 [a]
Close to veraison	615 ± 21 [a]	2915 ± 467 [a]	1325 ± 46 [a]	5386 ± 742 [a]
Veraison	467 ± 6 [b]	2366 ± 105 [ab]	1079 ± 159 [a]	4719 ± 639 [a]
Maturity	454 ± 96 [b]	1991 ± 211 [b]	590 ± 186 [b]	3460 ± 1065 [a]

Values represent means of triplicate determination ± SD. Different letters indicate the significant differences between stages according to Tukey's test, $p < 0.05$. TPC: Total Phenolic Content; DPPH: 1,1-diphenyl-2-picrylhydrazyl free radical; ABTS: 2,2'-azino-bis(3-ethylbenzothiazoline-6-sulfonic acid)diammonium salt; FRAP: Ferric Reducing Antioxidant Potential; DW: Dry Weight; GAE: Gallic Acid Equivalent; TE: Trolox Equivalent; Fe^{+2}E: Fe^{+2} Equivalent.

3.3.2. Antioxidant Capacity by Electrochemical Method of Skin and Seed Grape Extracts

Different parameters shown in Table 4 allowed the estimation of the antioxidant capacity of extracts by cyclic voltammetry. The total charge Q_{800mV} corresponds to all oxidizable phenolic compounds that will contribute to the total antioxidant capacity of the extract. Q_{240mV} represents the electrochemically of the easily oxidizable polyphenols that have consequently the highest antioxidant capacity. Q_{520mV} estimates the most antioxidant compounds which oxidize until 520 mV (until the second peak of the voltammogram). Q_{520mV}-Q_{240mV} corresponds to the compounds that have the lesser antioxidant capacity that oxidize until 520 mV. Finally, Q_{240mV}/Q_{800mV} ratio indicates the contribution of the most antioxidant compounds to the total antioxidant capacity of extract.

Skins

Q_{800mV}, Q_{240mV}, and Q_{520mV} values presented the same evolution for all grape skin extracts. They declined from the green stage to maturity. For example, in Merlot, Q_{800mV} values decreased from 262 to 118 µC/g DW, Q_{240mV} from 44 to 22 µC/g DW, and the antioxidant capacity until 520 mV diminished from 153 to 75 µC/g DW. The contribution of the most antioxidant compounds to the total antioxidant capacity was also determined. It followed the same evolution of the other parameters except for Merlot grape extracts where the percentage increased from 17 to 22% then decreased to 19%.

Seeds

Electrochemical parameters of seed grape extracts have the same evolution in the three varieties. They raised from the green stage to close to veraison and veraison then declined until maturity. In Merlot, Q_{800mV} values increased from 1232 to 1471 µQ/g DW then decreased to 1036 µC/g DW at maturity. The antioxidant capacity at 240 mV was about 358 µC/g DW at the green stage, 379 µC/g DW of extract at veraison, and 252 µC/g DW at maturity. Antioxidant capacity of seed extracts until 520 mV has the same trend than the other parameters, it stated from 905 µC/g DW at the green stage then increased to 944 µC/g DW at veraison, and declined to 639 µC/g DW at maturity. The most antioxidant compounds almost contribute with the same percent at all stages of ripening except for Merlot where the percent of Q_{240mV}/Q_{800mV} decreased from 30% to 24% at maturity.

Electrochemical parameters in both skins and seeds have the same trend than TPC, TAC values, and flavanol content. The higher TPC and TAC were found in seed grape extracts compared with skin grape extracts, in agreement with the literature [3,45,63]. The percent of Q_{240mV}/Q_{800mV} in seed grape extracts was more important than in skin grape extracts. It follows the same evolution of the other parameters in skins except for Merlot, in seeds there is no among differences between stages. At the charge Q_{240mV} corresponding to the oxidation of flavanols, this result suggests the abundance of these compounds in seeds compared with skins.

3.4. Correlation between TPC, Antioxidant Capacity, and Phenolic Composition

Table 5 shows the Pearson correlation coefficients between TPC, electrochemical parameters, antioxidant assays, and phenolic composition for which: $r < 0.39$ weak correlation, $0.4 < r < 0.69$ moderate correlation $0.7 < r < 0.89$ strong correlation, and $0.9 < r < 1$ very strong correlation [64].

Table 4. Potential of peaks and cumulative peak areas for skins and seeds of Merlot, Tannat, and Syrah during ripening.

		Ep,a1 (mV)	Ep,a2 (mV)	Q_{240mV} (μC/g DW)	Q_{520mV} (μC/g DW)	$Q_{520mV}-Q_{240mV}$ (μC/g DW)	Q_{800mV} (μC/g DW)	Q_{240mV}/Q_{800mV} (%)
Skins								
Merlot	Green stage	137 ± 3 [b]	391 ± 4 [a]	44 ± 6 [a]	153 ± 26 [a]	110 ± 19 [a]	262 ± 55 [a]	17 ± 1 [ab]
	Close to veraison	134 ± 2 [b]	383 ± 4 [a]	39 ± 3 [a]	126 ± 14 [a]	87 ± 11 [a]	166 ± 1 [b]	22 ± 3 [a]
	Veraison	159 ± 5 [a]	363 ± 2 [b]	15 ± 1 [b]	57 ± 2 [b]	42 ± 1 [b]	154 ± 4 [b]	13 ± 1 [b]
	Maturity	157 ± 3 [a]	370 ± 1 [b]	22 ± 1 [b]	75 ± 5 [b]	53 ± 4 [b]	118 ± 7 [b]	19 ± 1 [a]
Tannat	Green stage	139 ± 5 [b]	392 ± 5 [a]	65 ± 8 [a]	211 ± 20 [a]	145 ± 13 [a]	315 ± 36 [a]	21 ± 1 [a]
	Close to veraison	133 ± 1 [b]	383 ± 2 [b]	42 ± 10 [b]	134 ± 37 [b]	92 ± 27 [b]	215 ± 5 [b]	18 ± 6 [a]
	Veraison	130 ± 9 [b]	356 ± 3 [c]	21 ± 6 [c]	64 ± 18 [c]	43 ± 12 [c]	154 ± 24 [b]	16 ± 8 [a]
	Maturity	164 ± 2 [a]	362 ± 1 [c]	27 ± 5 [bc]	105 ± 16 [bc]	78 ± 11 [bc]	174 ± 3 [b]	18 ± 5 [a]
Syrah	Green stage	137 ± 1 [b]	383 ± 1 [a]	36 ± 5 [a]	119 ± 21 [a]	83 ± 16 [a]	172 ± 27 [a]	21 ± 1 [a]
	Close to veraison	126 ± 2 [c]	377 ± 3 [ab]	29 ± 5 [ab]	91 ± 18 [ab]	62 ± 13 [ab]	152 ± 11 [a]	18 ± 3 [ab]
	Veraison	160 ± 5 [a]	362 ± 3 [bc]	21 ± 1 [b]	77 ± 4 [ab]	56 ± 3 [ab]	141 ± 6 [a]	16 ± 1 [ab]
	Maturity	141 ± 3 [b]	359 ± 2 [c]	16 ± 3 [b]	59 ± 5 [b]	42 ± 3 [b]	129 ± 1 [a]	14 ± 2 [b]
Seeds								
Merlot	Green stage	129 ± 4 [a]	390 ± 8 [bc]	358 ± 36 [a]	905 ± 90 [a]	547 ± 54 [a]	1232 ± 152 [bc]	30 ± 3.64 [a]
	Close to veraison	133 ± 3 [a]	449 ± 4 [a]	393 ± 24 [a]	958 ± 53 [a]	565 ± 29 [a]	1407 ± 35 [ab]	28 ± 1 [ab]
	Veraison	132 ± 2 [a]	397 ± 1 [b]	379 ± 8 [a]	944 ± 23 [a]	564 ± 15 [a]	1471 ± 65 [a]	26 ± 0.63 [ab]
	Maturity	128 ± 1 [a]	380 ± 3 [c]	252 ± 19 [b]	639 ± 56 [b]	387 ± 39 [b]	1036 ± 94 [c]	24 ± 0.47 [b]
Tannat	Green stage	135 ± 3 [a]	377 ± 6 [b]	206 ± 29 [b]	555 ± 64 [b]	349 ± 35 [b]	808 ± 112 [b]	26 ± 1.63 [a]
	Close to veraison	128 ± 1 [a]	392 ± 6 [ab]	319 ± 22 [a]	827 ± 49 [a]	508 ± 28 [a]	1313 ± 52 [a]	24 ± 1.08 [a]
	Veraison	129 ± 3 [a]	418 ± 20 [a]	302 ± 16 [a]	746 ± 49 [a]	444 ± 33 [a]	1112 ± 162 [ab]	27 ± 2.45 [a]
	Maturity	129 ± 4 [a]	379 ± 2 [b]	216 ± 7 [b]	532 ± 20 [b]	316 ± 16 [b]	813 ± 61 [b]	27 ± 1.14 [a]
Syrah	Green stage	136 ± 3 [a]	397 ± 5 [c]	302 ± 18 [b]	724 ± 36 [b]	516 ± 179 [ab]	1165 ± 26 [ab]	26 ± 2.24 [a]
	Close to veraison	127 ± 2 [b]	438 ± 6 [a]	388 ± 24 [a]	937 ± 75 [a]	549 ± 50 [a]	1497 ± 15 [a]	23 ± 0.33 [a]
	Veraison	129 ± 1 [b]	409 ± 4 [b]	268 ± 20 [b]	691 ± 80 [b]	424 ± 30 [ab]	1082 ± 44 [ab]	25 ± 0.84 [a]
	Maturity	126 ± 4 [b]	391 ± 4 [c]	177 ± 33 [c]	463 ± 93 [c]	286 ± 60 [b]	818 ± 42 [b]	24 ± 2.6 [a]

Values represent means of triplicate determination ± SD. Different letters indicate the significant differences between stages according to Tukey's test, $p < 0.05$. DW: Dry weight.

Table 5. Pearson's correlation coefficients of antioxidant capacity using spectrophotometric tests, electrochemical parameters, flavanols, and anthocyanins.

					Skins					
	Folin	DPPH	ABTS	FRAP	Q_{240mV}	Q_{520mV}	$Q_{520mV}-Q_{240mV}$	Q_{800mV}	Flavanols	Anthocyanins
Folin	1									
DPPH	0.83	1								
ABTS	0.80	0.75	1							
FRAP	0.94	0.79	0.84	1						
Q_{240mV}	0.88	0.81	0.89	0.86	1					
Q_{520mV}	0.90	0.82	0.86	0.87	0.99	1				
$Q_{520mV}-Q_{240mV}$	0.90	0.81	0.85	0.87	0.98	1.00	1			
Q_{800mV}	0.84	0.69	0.69	0.75	0.84	0.85	0.85	1		
Flavanols	0.93	0.86	0.86	0.94	0.87	0.86	0.85	0.72	1	
Anthocyanins	−0.62	−0.55	−0.62	−0.68	−0.60	−0.53	−0.49	−0.50	−0.77	1

					Seeds				
	Folin	DPPH	ABTS	FRAP	Q_{240mV}	Q_{520mV}	$Q_{520mV}-Q_{240mV}$	Q_{800mV}	Flavanols
Folin	1								
DPPH	0.78	1							
ABTS	0.77	0.92	1						
FRAP	0.67	0.44	0.56	1					
Q_{240mV}	0.76	0.56	0.66	0.62	1				
Q_{520mV}	0.79	0.59	0.69	0.66	0.99	1			
$Q_{520mV}-Q_{240mV}$	0.66	0.56	0.62	0.41	0.89	0.90	1		
Q_{800mV}	0.60	0.41	0.49	0.51	0.88	0.88	0.79	1	
Flavanols	0.67	0.66	0.71	0.58	0.80	0.80	0.74	0.64	1

In skins, a strong correlation was found between TPC and electrochemical parameters ($r = 0.88$ vs. Q_{240mV}, $r = 0.90$ vs. Q_{520mV}, and $r = 0.84$ vs. Q_{800mV}). It was shown in the literature that TPC is significatively correlated with electrochemical responses [65], especially with cumulative response up to relatively high potentials [32]. In this study, TPC was better correlated with Q_{240mV} than Q_{800mV}. Colorimetric antioxidant assays (DPPH, ABTS, and FRAP) were strongly correlated with all electrochemical parameters. The best correlation was found with Q_{240mV} ($r = 0.81$ vs. DPPH, $r = 0.89$ vs. ABTS, and $r = 0.86$ vs. FRAP) than with Q_{800mV} ($r = 0.69$ vs. DPPH, $r = 0.69$ vs. ABTS, and $r = 0.75$ vs. FRAP). The methods used are well correlated because they are all based on electron transfer from antioxidant to oxidized compounds [32]. Flavanols content were well correlated with colorimetric assays ($r = 0.93$ vs. Folin-Ciocalteu, $r = 0.86$ vs. DPPH, $r = 0.86$ vs. ABTS, $r = 0.94$ vs. FRAP) as well as electrochemical parameters ($r = 0.87$ vs. Q_{240mV}, $r = 0.72$ vs. Q_{800mV}). The strong correlation between flavanols and Q_{240mV} compared with Q_{800mV} indicates that these compounds are the easiest antioxidant compounds that oxidized at a low potential (240 mV). A negative correlation between anthocyanins and the antioxidant tests have been shown, this result is an agreement with a previous study [59].

In seed grape extracts, the best correlation was found between flavanols and electrochemical parameters ($r = 0.80$ vs. Q_{240mV}, $r = 0.80$ vs. Q_{520mV}, and $r = 0.64$ vs. Q_{800mV}) than with spectrophotometric methods ($r = 0.67$ vs. Folin, $r = 0.66$ vs. DPPH, $r = 0.71$ vs. ABTS, and $r = 0.58$ vs. FRAP). A strong correlation was observed between Folin-Ciocalteu, DPPH, and ABTS ($r = 0.78$ vs. DPPH and $r = 0.77$ vs. ABTS) whereas a moderate correlation was found between Folin-Ciocalteu and FRAP ($r = 0.67$). Contrary to skin grape extracts, in seed grape extracts, FRAP have the lowest correlation with all assays compared with the other colorimetric methods. This result illustrates the specificity of each assay and the variability of phenolic composition between skin and seed grape extracts.

The antioxidant capacity was mainly related to the TPC of extracts in accordance with previous results [9,12–14,58,62,66,67] and especially to the flavanols content [14]. The antioxidant capacity of polyphenols is mainly linked to their structures, compounds that have more than one aromatic ring, more than one hydroxyl groups in different positions are able to have a highest antioxidant capacity. This may explain the variability of Pearson correlation between the different methods and between skins and seeds.

Principal Components Analysis (PCA)

Figure 3 shows the Biplot graphic that represents the association of the phenolic composition with the antioxidant assays on skin and seed grapes extracts during ripening. The first two principal components explained 94.2% of the total variability. The first axis accounted for 88.6% and the second axis only for 5.6%. From the Biplot, skin grape extracts are separated in the left side from seed grape extracts in the right side.

For skin grape extracts, the stages of maturity were well separated depending mainly on the content of anthocyanins, flavanols, as well as antioxidant capacity, down the stages before veraison (have the highest flavanols content and antioxidant capacity) and up the stages from veraison to maturity (beginning of synthesis and accumulation of anthocyanins, low antioxidant capacity, and flavanols content). For seed grape extracts, it is more difficult to separate the different stages of maturity because the variables are very close.

Flavanols were compounds with the highest positive contribution to the antioxidant capacity, while the anthocyanins were the highest negative contribution in the three varieties studied. As it can be seen in Figure 3, the content of flavanols and the antioxidant capacity were higher in seed than in skin grape extracts.

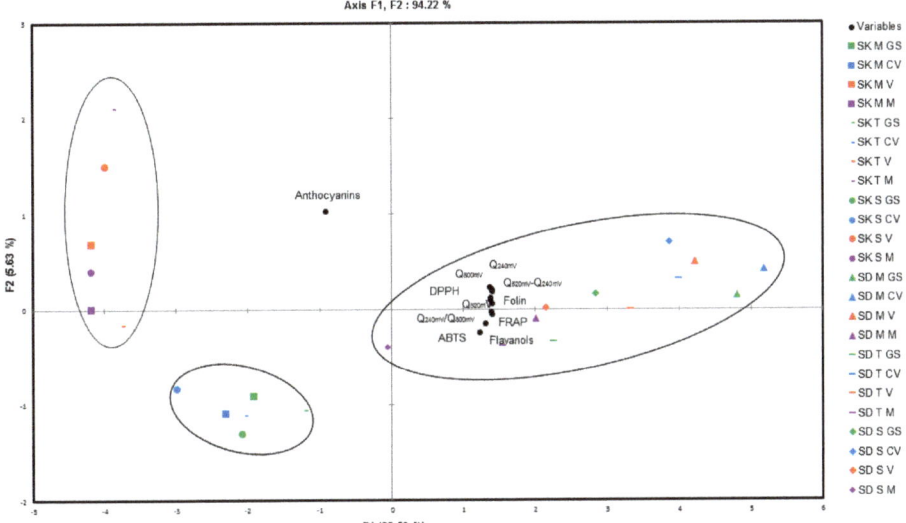

Figure 3. Biplot of the first PCs obtained from PCA for seeds (SD) and skins (SK) of three grape varieties Merlot (M), Tannat (T), and Syrah (S) at different stages of ripening (green stage (GS), close to veraison (CV), veraison (V), and maturity (M)).

4. Conclusions

Total phenolic content, antioxidant capacity, flavanol, and anthocyanin contents of grape skin and seed extracts of three red grape varieties were studied at different stages of ripening. At all stages of ripening, the total phenolic content was higher in seed than in skin grape extracts. The green stage had the highest total phenolic content in grape skin extracts, whereas in grape seed extracts, they were the close to veraison and the veraison that had the highest content.

To measure the antioxidant capacity of extracts, different colorimetric methods were used (DPPH, ABTS, and FRAP) in addition to cyclic voltammetry. In skin grape extracts, the total antioxidant capacity was higher at the green stage than at maturity, in seed grape extracts, they were the close to veraison and the veraison that had the highest content with all assays. Generally, stages that had the highest phenolic content presented also the highest antioxidant capacity.

The correlation between electrochemical results using disposable electrodes and the colorimetric assays indicates that electrochemical assays can be considered as an alternative to these routine tests in the determination and the characterization of the antioxidant capacity in a short time.

Supplementary Materials: The following are available online at http://www.mdpi.com/2076-3921/9/9/800/s1. Table S1: Dates corresponding to the different stages of ripening for the three varieties Merlot, Tannat, and Syrah; Figure S1: The experimental electrochemical set up using GCE (A) and SWCNT (B) electrodes.

Author Contributions: Conceptualization, N.B. and F.G.; methodology, N.B. and F.G.; formal analysis, N.B.; investigation, N.B. and F.G.; resources, N.B. and C.S.; data curation, N.B.; writing—original draft preparation, N.B. and F.G.; writing—review and editing, N.B., F.G., C.S., and T.R.; visualization, F.G. and C.S.; supervision, F.G., C.S., and T.R. All authors have read and agreed to the published version of the manuscript.

Funding: This work was supported in part by a PhD grant (N.B.) from the government of Algeria (Ministère algérien de l'Enseignement Supérieur et de la Recherche Scientifique).

Acknowledgments: The authors would like to thank the Algerian government for financing this thesis. Marie Zerbib is also thanked for her experimental work assistance.

Conflicts of Interest: The authors declare no conflict of interest.

References

1. Liang, Z.; Owens, C.L.; Zhong, G.-Y.; Cheng, L. Polyphenolic profiles detected in the ripe berries of *Vitis vinifera* germplasm. *Food Chem.* **2011**, *129*, 940–950. [CrossRef]
2. Cavaliere, C.; Foglia, P.; Gubbiotti, R.; Sacchetti, P.; Samperi, R.; Laganà, A. Rapid-resolution liquid chromatography/mass spectrometry for determination and quantitation of polyphenols in grape berries. *Rapid Commun. Mass Spectrom.* **2008**, *22*, 3089–3099. [CrossRef]
3. Yilmaz, Y.; Göksel, Z.; Erdoğan, S.S.; Öztürk, A.; Atak, A.; Özer, C. Antioxidant Activity and Phenolic Content of Seed, Skin and Pulp Parts of 22 Grape (*Vitis vinifera* L.) Cultivars (4 Common and 18 Registered or Candidate for Registration): Antioxidant Activity of Grapes. *J. Food Process. Preserv.* **2015**, *39*, 1682–1691. [CrossRef]
4. Nawaz, H.; Shi, J.; Mittal, G.S.; Kakuda, Y. Extraction of polyphenols from grape seeds and concentration by ultrafiltration. *Sep. Purif. Technol.* **2006**, *48*, 176–181. [CrossRef]
5. Obreque-Slier, E.; Peña-Neira, Á.; López-Solís, R.; Zamora-Marín, F.; Ricardo-da Silva, J.M.; Laureano, O. Comparative Study of the Phenolic Composition of Seeds and Skins from Carménère and Cabernet Sauvignon Grape Varieties (*Vitis vinifera* L.) during Ripening. *J. Agric. Food Chem.* **2010**, *58*, 3591–3599. [CrossRef]
6. Fanzone, M.; Zamora, F.; Jofré, V.; Assof, M.; Peña-Neira, Á. Phenolic Composition of Malbec Grape Skins and Seeds from Valle de Uco (Mendoza, Argentina) during Ripening. Effect of Cluster Thinning. *J. Agric. Food Chem.* **2011**, *59*, 6120–6136. [CrossRef]
7. Hubner, A.; Sobreira, F.; Vetore Neto, A.; Pinto, C.A.S.D.O.; Dario, M.F.; Díaz, I.E.C.; Lourenço, F.R.; Rosado, C.; Baby, A.R.; Bacchi, E.M. The Synergistic Behavior of Antioxidant Phenolic Compounds Obtained from Winemaking Waste's Valorization, Increased the Efficacy of a Sunscreen System. *Antioxidants* **2019**, *8*, 530. [CrossRef]
8. Gil-Muñoz, R.; Fernández-Fernández, J.I.; Crespo-Villegas, O.; Garde-Cerdán, T. Elicitors used as a tool to increase stilbenes in grapes and wines. *Food Res. Int.* **2017**, *98*, 34–39. [CrossRef]
9. Balík, J.; Kyseláková, M.; Vrchotová, N.; Tříska, J.; Kumšta, M.; Veverka, J.; Híc, P.; Totušek, J.; Lefnerová, D. Relations between polyphenols content and antioxidant activity in vine grapes and leaves. *Czech. J. Food Sci.* **2009**, *26*, S25–S32. [CrossRef]
10. Aguirre, M.J.; Chen, Y.Y.; Isaacs, M.; Matsuhiro, B.; Mendoza, L.; Torres, S. Electrochemical behaviour and antioxidant capacity of anthocyanins from Chilean red wine, grape and raspberry. *Food Chem.* **2010**, *121*, 44–48. [CrossRef]
11. Rockenbach, I.I.; Rodrigues, E.; Gonzaga, L.V.; Caliari, V.; Genovese, M.I.; Gonçalves, A.E.D.S.S.; Fett, R. Phenolic compounds content and antioxidant activity in pomace from selected red grapes (*Vitis vinifera* L. and *Vitis labrusca* L.) widely produced in Brazil. *Food Chem.* **2011**, *127*, 174–179. [CrossRef]
12. Bozan, B.; Tosun, G.; Özcan, D. Study of polyphenol content in the seeds of red grape (*Vitis vinifera* L.) varieties cultivated in Turkey and their antiradical activity. *Food Chem.* **2008**, *109*, 426–430. [CrossRef] [PubMed]
13. Coklar, H. Antioxidant capacity and phenolic profile of berry, seed, and skin of Ekşikara (*Vitis vinifera* L.) grape: Influence of harvest year and altitude. *Int. J. Food Prop.* **2017**, *20*, 2071–2087. [CrossRef]
14. Guendez, R. Determination of low molecular weight polyphenolic constituents in grape (*Vitis vinifera* sp.) seed extracts: Correlation with antiradical activity. *Food Chem.* **2005**, *89*, 1–9. [CrossRef]
15. Hosu, A.D.; Cimpoiu, C.; Miclaus, V.; Jantschi, L. Antioxidant Content of Three Different Varieties of Wine Grapes. *Biotechnol. Biotechnol. Equip.* **2011**, *25*, 2217–2221. [CrossRef]
16. Ky, I.; Teissedre, P.-L. Characterisation of Mediterranean Grape Pomace Seed and Skin Extracts: Polyphenolic Content and Antioxidant Activity. *Molecules* **2015**, *20*, 2190–2207. [CrossRef] [PubMed]
17. Lingua, M.S.; Fabani, M.P.; Wunderlin, D.A.; Baroni, M.V. From grape to wine: Changes in phenolic composition and its influence on antioxidant activity. *Food Chem.* **2016**, *208*, 228–238. [CrossRef]
18. Rababah, T.M.; Ereifej, K.I.; Al-Mahasneh, M.A.; Ismaeal, K.; Hidar, A.-G.; Yang, W. Total Phenolics, Antioxidant Activities, and Anthocyanins of Different Grape Seed Cultivars Grown in Jordan. *Int. J. Food Prop.* **2008**, *11*, 472–479. [CrossRef]
19. Kadouh, H.C.; Sun, S.; Zhu, W.; Zhou, K. α-Glucosidase inhibiting activity and bioactive compounds of six red wine grape pomace extracts. *J. Funct. Foods* **2016**, *26*, 577–584. [CrossRef]

20. Sales, P.M.; Souza, P.M.; Simeoni, L.A.; Magalhães, P.O.; Silveira, D. α-Amylase Inhibitors: A Review of Raw Material and Isolated Compounds from Plant Source. *J. Pharm. Pharm. Sci.* **2012**, *15*, 141. [CrossRef]
21. Lee, H.J.; Kwon, O.; Kim, J.Y. Supplementation of a polyphenol extract from Ecklonia cava reduces body fat, oxidative and inflammatory stress in overweight healthy subjects with abdominal obesity: A randomized, placebo-controlled, double-blind trial. *J. Funct. Foods* **2018**, *46*, 356–364. [CrossRef]
22. Jack, B.U.; Malherbe, C.J.; Mamushi, M.; Muller, C.J.F.; Joubert, E.; Louw, J.; Pheiffer, C. Adipose tissue as a possible therapeutic target for polyphenols: A case for Cyclopia extracts as anti-obesity nutraceuticals. *Biomed. Pharmacother.* **2019**, *120*, 109439. [CrossRef] [PubMed]
23. Callcott, E.T.; Santhakumar, A.B.; Luo, J.; Blanchard, C.L. Therapeutic potential of rice-derived polyphenols on obesity-related oxidative stress and inflammation. *J. Appl Biomed.* **2018**, *16*, 255–262. [CrossRef]
24. Khurana, S.; Piche, M.; Hollingsworth, A.; Venkataraman, K.; Tai, T.C. Oxidative stress and cardiovascular health: Therapeutic potential of polyphenols. *Can. J. Physiol. Pharmacol.* **2013**, *91*, 198–212. [CrossRef]
25. Amiot, M.-J.; Riollet, C.; Landrier, J.-F. Polyphénols et syndrome métabolique. *Médecine Mal. Métaboliques* **2009**, *3*, 476–482. [CrossRef]
26. Richard, T.; Temsamani, H.; Delaunay, J.-C.; Krisa, S.; Mérillon, J.-M. Stilbènes: De la chimie à la neuroprotection. *Cah. Nutr. Diététique* **2014**, *49*, 173–180. [CrossRef]
27. Lorrain, B.; Ky, I.; Pechamat, L.; Teissedre, P.-L. Evolution of Analysis of Polyhenols from Grapes, Wines, and Extracts. *Molecules* **2013**, *18*, 1076–1100. [CrossRef]
28. Hoyos-Arbeláez, J.; Vázquez, M.; Contreras-Calderón, J. Electrochemical methods as a tool for determining the antioxidant capacity of food and beverages: A review. *Food Chem.* **2017**, *221*, 1371–1381. [CrossRef]
29. Dai, Y.-Q.; Shiu, K.-K. Glucose Biosensor Based on Multi-Walled Carbon Nanotube Modified Glassy Carbon Electrode. *Electroanalysis* **2004**, *16*, 1697–1703. [CrossRef]
30. Chowdhry, A.; Kaur, J.; Khatri, M.; Puri, V.; Tuli, R.; Puri, S. Characterization of functionalized multiwalled carbon nanotubes and comparison of their cellular toxicity between HEK 293 cells and zebra fish in vivo. *Heliyon* **2019**, *5*, e02605. [CrossRef]
31. Liu, M.; Xiang, J.; Zhou, J.; Ding, H. A disposable amperometric sensor for rapid detection of serotonin in the blood and brain of the depressed mice based on Nafion membrane-coated colloidal gold screen-printed electrode. *J. Electroanal. Chem.* **2010**, *640*, 1–7. [CrossRef]
32. Giné Bordonaba, J.; Terry, L.A. Electrochemical behaviour of polyphenol rich fruit juices using disposable screen-printed carbon electrodes: Towards a rapid sensor for antioxidant capacity and individual antioxidants. *Talanta* **2012**, *90*, 38–45. [CrossRef] [PubMed]
33. Pasakon, P.; Mensing, J.P.; Phokaratkul, D.; Karuwan, C.; Lomas, T.; Wisitsoraat, A.; Tuantranont, A. A high-performance, disposable screen-printed carbon electrode modified with multi-walled carbon nanotubes/graphene for ultratrace level electrochemical sensors. *J. Appl. Electrochem.* **2019**, *49*, 217–227. [CrossRef]
34. Zerbib, M.; Mazauric, J.-P.; Meudec, E.; Le Guerneve, C.; Lepak, A.; Nidetzky, B.; Cheynier, V.; Terrier, N.; Saucier, C. New flavanol O-glycosides in grape and wine. *Food Chem.* **2018**, *266*, 441–448. [CrossRef]
35. Kennedy, J.A.; Jones, G.P. Analysis of Proanthocyanidin Cleavage Products Following Acid-Catalysis in the Presence of Excess Phloroglucinol. *J. Agric. Food Chem.* **2001**, *49*, 1740–1746. [CrossRef]
36. Pérez-Magariño, S.; González-San José, M.L. Evolution of Flavanols, Anthocyanins, and Their Derivatives during the Aging of Red Wines Elaborated from Grapes Harvested at Different Stages of Ripening. *J. Agric. Food Chem.* **2004**, *52*, 1181–1189. [CrossRef]
37. Ricci, A.; Olejar, K.J.; Parpinello, G.P.; Mattioli, A.U.; Teslić, N.; Kilmartin, P.A.; Versari, A. Antioxidant activity of commercial food grade tannins exemplified in a wine model. *Food Addit. Contam. Part A* **2016**, *33*, 1761–1774. [CrossRef]
38. Brand-Williams, W.; Cuvelier, M.E.; Berset, C. Use of a free radical method to evaluate antioxidant activity. *LWT Food Sci. Technol.* **1995**, *28*, 25–30. [CrossRef]
39. Re, R.; Pellegrini, N.; Proteggente, A.; Pannala, A.; Yang, M.; Rice-Evans, C. Antioxidant activity applying an improved ABTS radical cation decolorization assay. *Free Radic. Biol. Med.* **1999**, *26*, 1231–1237. [CrossRef]
40. Benzie, I.F.F.; Strain, J.J. The Ferric Reducing Ability of Plasma (FRAP) as a Measure of "Antioxidant Power": The FRAP Assay. *Anal. Biochem.* **1996**, *239*, 70–76. [CrossRef]

41. Torchio, F.; Cagnasso, E.; Gerbi, V.; Rolle, L. Mechanical properties, phenolic composition and extractability indices of Barbera grapes of different soluble solids contents from several growing areas. *Anal. Chim. Acta* **2010**, *660*, 183–189. [CrossRef] [PubMed]
42. Rolle, L.; Río Segade, S.; Torchio, F.; Giacosa, S.; Cagnasso, E.; Marengo, F.; Gerbi, V. Influence of Grape Density and Harvest Date on Changes in Phenolic Composition, Phenol Extractability Indices, and Instrumental Texture Properties during Ripening. *J. Agric. Food Chem.* **2011**, *59*, 8796–8805. [CrossRef] [PubMed]
43. Bindon, K.; Varela, C.; Kennedy, J.; Holt, H.; Herderich, M. Relationships between harvest time and wine composition in *Vitis vinifera* L. cv. Cabernet Sauvignon 1. Grape and wine chemistry. *Food Chem.* **2013**, *138*, 1696–1705. [CrossRef] [PubMed]
44. Kennedy, J.A.; Troup, G.J.; Pilbrow, J.R.; Hutton, D.R.; Hewitt, D.; Hunter, C.R.; Ristic, R.; Iland, P.G.; Jones, G.P. Development of seed polyphenols in berries from *Vitis vinifera* L. cv. Shiraz. *Aust. J. Grape Wine Res.* **2000**, *6*, 244–254. [CrossRef]
45. Pantelić, M.M.; Zagorac, D.Č.D.; Davidović, S.M.; Todić, S.R.; Bešlić, Z.S.; Gašić, U.M.; Tešić, Ž.L.; Natić, M.M. Identification and quantification of phenolic compounds in berry skin, pulp, and seeds in 13 grapevine varieties grown in Serbia. *Food Chem.* **2016**, *211*, 243–252. [CrossRef]
46. Mulero, J.; Pardo, F.; Zafrilla, P. Antioxidant activity and phenolic composition of organic and conventional grapes and wines. *J. Food Compos. Anal.* **2010**, *23*, 569–574. [CrossRef]
47. Delgado, R.; Martín, P.; del Álamo, M.; González, M.-R. Changes in the phenolic composition of grape berries during ripening in relation to vineyard nitrogen and potassium fertilisation rates. *J. Sci. Food Agric.* **2004**, *84*, 623–630. [CrossRef]
48. Niu, S.; Hao, F.; Mo, H.; Jiang, J.; Wang, H.; Liu, C.; Fan, X.; Zhang, Y. Phenol profiles and antioxidant properties of white skinned grapes and their coloured genotypes during growth. *Biotechnol. Biotechnol. Equip.* **2017**, *31*, 58–67. [CrossRef]
49. Ryan, J.-M.; Revilla, E. Anthocyanin Composition of Cabernet Sauvignon and Tempranillo Grapes at Different Stages of Ripening. *J. Agric. Food Chem.* **2003**, *51*, 3372–3378. [CrossRef]
50. Robinson, S.P.; Davies, C. Molecular biology of grape berry ripening. *Aust. J. Grape Wine Res.* **2000**, *6*, 175–188. [CrossRef]
51. Boido, E.; García-Marino, M.; Dellacassa, E.; Carrau, F.; Rivas-Gonzalo, J.C.; Escribano-Bailón, M.T. Characterisation and evolution of grape polyphenol profiles of *Vitis vinifera* L. cv. Tannat during ripening and vinification: Polyphenolic profiles of Tannat. *Aust. J. Grape Wine Res.* **2011**, *17*, 383–393. [CrossRef]
52. Haselgrove, L.; Botting, D.; Heeswijck, R.; Høj, P.B.; Dry, P.R.; Ford, C.; Land, P.G.I. Canopy microclimate and berry composition: The effect of bunch exposure on the phenolic composition of *Vitis vinifera* L. cv. Shiraz grape berries. *Aust. J. Grape Wine Res.* **2000**, *6*, 141–149. [CrossRef]
53. Kilmartin, P.A.; Zou, H.; Waterhouse, A.L. Correlation of Wine Phenolic Composition versus Cyclic Voltammetry Response. *Am. J. Enol. Vitic.* **2002**, *53*, 294–302.
54. Newair, E.F.; Kilmartin, P.A.; Garcia, F. Square wave voltammetric analysis of polyphenol content and antioxidant capacity of red wines using glassy carbon and disposable carbon nanotubes modified screen-printed electrodes. *Eur. Food Res. Technol.* **2018**, *244*, 1225–1237. [CrossRef]
55. Danilewicz, J.C. Folin-Ciocalteu, FRAP, and DPPH* Assays for Measuring Polyphenol Concentration in White Wine. *Am. J. Enol. Vitic.* **2015**, *66*, 463–471. [CrossRef]
56. Vilas-Boas, Â.; Valderrama, P.; Fontes, N.; Geraldo, D.; Bento, F. Evaluation of total polyphenol content of wines by means of voltammetric techniques: Cyclic voltammetry vs. differential pulse voltammetry. *Food Chem.* **2019**, *276*, 719–725. [CrossRef]
57. Kilmartin, P.A.; Zou, H.; Waterhouse, A.L. A Cyclic Voltammetry Method Suitable for Characterizing Antioxidant Properties of Wine and Wine Phenolics. *J. Agric. Food Chem.* **2001**, *49*, 1957–1965. [CrossRef]
58. Dudonné, S.; Vitrac, X.; Coutière, P.; Woillez, M.; Mérillon, J.-M. Comparative Study of Antioxidant Properties and Total Phenolic Content of 30 Plant Extracts of Industrial Interest Using DPPH, ABTS, FRAP, SOD, and ORAC Assays. *J. Agric. Food Chem.* **2009**, *57*, 1768–1774. [CrossRef]
59. Ky, I.; Lorrain, B.; Kolbas, N.; Crozier, A.; Teissedre, P.-L. Wine by-Products: Phenolic Characterization and Antioxidant Activity Evaluation of Grapes and Grape Pomaces from Six Different French Grape Varieties. *Molecules* **2014**, *19*, 482–506. [CrossRef]
60. El Rayess, Y.; Barbar, R.; Wilson, E.A.; Bouajila, J. *Analytical Methods for Wine Polyphenols Analysis and for Their Antioxidant Activity Evaluation*; Nova Science Publishers: New York, NY, USA, 2014.

61. Prior, R.L.; Wu, X.; Schaich, K. Standardized Methods for the Determination of Antioxidant Capacity and Phenolics in Foods and Dietary Supplements. *J. Agric. Food Chem.* **2005**, *53*, 4290–4302. [CrossRef]
62. Floegel, A.; Kim, D.-O.; Chung, S.-J.; Koo, S.I.; Chun, O.K. Comparison of ABTS/DPPH assays to measure antioxidant capacity in popular antioxidant-rich US foods. *J. Food Compos. Anal.* **2011**, *24*, 1043–1048. [CrossRef]
63. Tkacz, K.; Wojdyło, A.; Nowicka, P.; Turkiewicz, I.; Golis, T. Characterization in vitro potency of biological active fractions of seeds, skins and flesh from selected *Vitis vinifera* L. cultivars and interspecific hybrids. *J. Funct. Foods* **2019**, *56*, 353–363. [CrossRef]
64. Schober, P.; Boer, C.; Schwarte, L.A. Correlation Coefficients: Appropriate Use and Interpretation. *Anesth. Analg.* **2018**, *126*, 1763–1768. [CrossRef] [PubMed]
65. José Jara-Palacios, M.; Luisa Escudero-Gilete, M.; Miguel Hernández-Hierro, J.; Heredia, F.J.; Hernanz, D. Cyclic voltammetry to evaluate the antioxidant potential in winemaking by-products. *Talanta* **2017**, *165*, 211–215. [CrossRef]
66. Selcuk, A.R.; Demiray, E.; Yilmaz, Y. Antioxidant Activity of Grape Seeds Obtained from Molasses (Pekmez) and Winery Production. *Acad. Food J.* **2011**, *9*, 39–43.
67. Doshi, P.; Adsule, P.; Banerjee, K. Phenolic composition and antioxidant activity in grapevine parts and berries (*Vitis vinifera* L.) cv. Kishmish Chornyi (Sharad Seedless) during maturation. *Int. J. Food Sci. Technol.* **2006**, *41*, 1–9. [CrossRef]

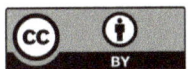

© 2020 by the authors. Licensee MDPI, Basel, Switzerland. This article is an open access article distributed under the terms and conditions of the Creative Commons Attribution (CC BY) license (http://creativecommons.org/licenses/by/4.0/).

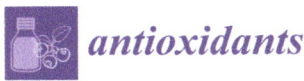

Article

Comparative Studies on Different *Citrus* Cultivars: A Revaluation of Waste Mandarin Components

Giulia Costanzo [1], Maria Rosaria Iesce [2], Daniele Naviglio [2], Martina Ciaravolo [2], Ermenegilda Vitale [1] and Carmen Arena [1,*]

[1] Dipartimento di Biologia, Università degli Studi di Napoli Federico II, Via Cinthia, 80126 Napoli, Italy; giul.costanzo@studenti.unina.it (G.C.); ermenegilda.vitale@unina.it (E.V.)
[2] Dipartimento di Scienze Chimiche, Università degli Studi di Napoli Federico II, Via Cinthia, 80126 Napoli, Italy; iesce@unina.it (M.R.I.); naviglio@unina.it (D.N.); martinaciaravolo@gmail.com (M.C.)
* Correspondence: c.arena@unina.it; Tel.: +39-081-679-173

Received: 17 May 2020; Accepted: 10 June 2020; Published: 12 June 2020

Abstract: Peel, pulp and seed extracts of three mandarin varieties, namely Phlegraean mandarin (*Citrus reticulata*), Kumquat (*Citrus japonica*), and Clementine (*Citrus clementina*) were compared and characterised in terms of photosynthetic pigment content, total polyphenols amount, antioxidant activity and vitamin C to assess the amount of functional compounds for each cultivar. The highest polyphenols content was found in the Phlegraean mandarin, especially in peel and seeds, whereas Kumquat exhibited the highest polyphenols amount in the pulp. The antioxidant activity was higher in the peel of Phlegraean mandarin and clementine compared to Kumquat, which showed the highest value in the pulp. The antioxidant activity peaked in the seeds of Phlegraean mandarin. The vitamin C in the Phlegraean mandarin was the highest in all parts of the fruit, especially in the seeds. Total chlorophyll content was comparable in the peel of different cultivars, in the pulp the highest amount was found in clementine, whereas kumquat seeds showed the greatest values. As regards total carotenoids, peel and pulp of clementine exhibited higher values than the other two cultivars, whereas the kumquat seeds were the richest in carotenoids. Among the analysed cultivars Phlegraean mandarin may be considered the most promising as a source of polyphenols and antioxidants, compared to the clementine and Kumquat, especially for the functional molecules found in the seeds. Moreover, regardless of cultivars this study also highlights important properties in the parts of the fruit generally considered wastes.

Keywords: ascorbic acid; antioxidant activity; chlorophyll and carotenoid content; phenolic compounds

1. Introduction

In recent years, clinical trials and epidemiological studies have established an inverse correlation between the intake of fruits and vegetables and the occurrence of chronic diseases, the most prevalent causes of death in the world [1,2]. This protective effect has been ascribed to the antioxidant properties of different compounds, which coordinate and balance the body system to protect tissues and fluids from damage by reactive oxygen species (ROS) or free radicals [1,3,4].

Besides health and nutritional benefits, antioxidants have an important role for the food industry. These compounds prevent the propagation reaction of free radicals during the oxidative process preserving food quality and shelf life during handling and storage [5–7].

In general, citrus fruits are considered as one of the natural sources of antioxidants. In fact, they contain an appreciable amount of ascorbic acid, flavonoids, and phenolic compounds [8–11] and even some essential minerals important for human nutrition [12–14].

Mandarin is a product with many desirable characteristics for consumers who are health aware [15]. Continuous improvements in transportation logistics have allowed its widespread distribution to consumers throughout the world. These reasons have increased the world demand for mandarin cultivation so that its products are in continuous growth [16].

In food manufacturing, citrus is mainly used for producing fresh juice or citrus-based drinks, so a large amount of citrus wastes such as peels and seeds must be discarded. The global volume of citrus processed every year is about 31.2 million tons [17], 50%–60% of which represents waste called "pastazzo" [18,19]. The management of a such amount of wastes represents a critical issue for the citrus industry due to the high costs involved for its disposal [18,20].

This encourages the implementation of recycling policies to promote potential new and innovative uses of citrus by-products. Currently, several technological innovations have been developed to valorise citrus wastes in order to convert possible environmental risks into a valuable resource, thus reducing the environmental impact [19]. Citrus by-products find utilisation in biogas production [21], ruminant feeding [22], and essential oil extraction [23].

Moreover, a very interesting perspective would be also to utilise citrus by-products as a source of bioactive compounds for human diet [24,25]. In fact, recent studies suggest that citrus waste could be used as natural sources of antioxidants [26,27]. However, it is well known that the chemical composition of fruits may be subjected to variations according to climate, cultivation practices, soil type, cultivar, fruit maturity, and even between parts of the same fruit [1]. In addition to the expected changes of fruit quality, variations in antioxidant properties during ripening have also been described [28,29]. For a revaluation of citrus by-products, it would be appropriate to focus the attention on varieties with very different provenance and traits, in order to have an indication about the potential associated to the wastes of diverse cultivars.

Starting from these considerations, the aim of this study was to determine the amount of specific functional compounds such as chlorophyll and carotenoid, total polyphenols, vitamin C as well as the antioxidant capacity in the pulp and more specifically in peel and seeds of three different cultivars of mandarin, namely Phlegraean mandarin (*Citrus reticulata* Blanco), Kumquat (*Citrus japonica*), and Clementine (*Citrus* × *clementina*). These cultivars have been selected for specific characteristics. In detail, clementine was chosen for its large demand and commercial consumption worldwide due mainly to ease of peeling and seedlessness, kumquat is very appreciated in food preparation but has a niche consumption, while the Phlegraean mandarin is specifically diffused only in a peculiar volcanic area of Southern Italy (Campi Flegrei, Naples, Italy). The mandarin cultivar from the Phlegraean fields, planted for the first time in Naples in the 19th Century, is considered a traditional product from Campania region. The mandarin and the liqueur derived from it, namely "mandarinetto", have been included by the Italian Ministry of Agriculture, Food and Forestry in the list of typical, traditional products of the Campania region (GU 168/2015). This citrus fruit variety has shown its maximum expression in the Phlegraean fields, a peculiar area surrounding the supervolcano, Vesuvius; the fertile soil, typical of a volcanic area as well as the proximity of the sea and the mild climate make the Phlegrean land unique and particularly favourable to the agriculture.

The outcomes of this study will be useful for a valorisation of mandarin waste products, encouraging their use and thus favouring the recycling practices and the bioeconomy strategies.

2. Materials and Methods

2.1. Plant Material and Sample Preparation

Three cultivars of mandarins (Phlegraean mandarin, *Citrus reticulata*; Kumquat, *Citrus japonica*; and Clementina, *Citrus clementina*) collected in the seasons 2019–2020 were used in this study. Fruits, used for the experiments, were homogeneously collected from five selected mandarin trees, for each cultivars. Phlegrean mandarin fruits were collected in the area of Bacoli, Phlegraean fields, (Naples, Southern Italy); mandarins from Clementine and Kumquat cultivars were sampled in private plantations at Sorrento peninsula (Naples, Southern Italy). Sampling was carried out during the harvest period typical for each cultivar, generally from November to January. The samples were placed in plastic bags and stored in dry ice, then they were transferred immediately to the laboratory and stored at −80 °C for subsequent analysis. Analyses were performed on each component of the fruit: peel, pulp and seeds for all the collected samples.

The fruits were washed with tap water, separated into the three components and homogenised, using mortar and pestle, by preventively powdering in liquid nitrogen. Powdered citrus tissues, obtained for each component of the fruit, were placed in test tubes and stored at −20 °C until analysis. At least three different trees for each mandarin cultivar were chosen to collect samples. For each mandarin cultivar a total of ten samples were analysed. Mandarins of two collections (seasons 2019 and 2020) for all cultivars were analysed in this study.

2.2. Photosynthetic Pigments Content Determination

Total chlorophylls and carotenoids contained in peel, pulp and seeds were determined according to Lichtenthaler (1987) [30]. Briefly, pigments were extracted from 0.25 g of powered sample in ice-cold 100% acetone and centrifuged (Labofuge GL, Heraeus Sepatech, Hanau, Germany) at 5000 rpm for 5 min. The absorbance was measured by spectrophotometer (Cary 100 UV-VIS, Agilent Technologies, Santa Clara, CA, USA) at wavelenghts of 470, 645 and 662 nm and pigment concentration expressed as mg g^{-1} fresh weight (FW).

2.3. Total Polyphenol Content

Total polyphenol content was measured according to the reported procedure [31]. Briefly, 0.25 g of powered sample was extracted with aqueous 80% methanol, at 4 °C (for 30 min) and then centrifuged at 11,000 rpm for 5 min. Extracts were combined with 1:1 (v/v) 10% Folin–Ciocalteu phenol reagent and water. After 3 min, 700 mM Na_2CO_3 solution was added to the resulting mixture in 5:1 (v/v). Samples were incubated for 2 h in darkness. Then, the absorbance at 765 nm was measured with a spectrophotometer (UV-VIS Cary 100, Agilent Technologies, Palo Alto, CA, USA). Gallic acid was used as a standard. Calibration curve was constructed analysing standard solutions in the interval of concentration 5–500 ppm. The total polyphenols concentration was calculated and expressed as gallic acid equivalents (mg GAE g^{-1} FW) from the calibration curve ($R^2 = 0.996$) using gallic acid.

2.4. Determination of Antioxidant Capacity and Ascorbic Acid

The antioxidant activity of the cultivars was evaluated by the Ferric Reducing Antioxidant Power (FRAP) assay, according to the reported method [32]. Briefly, 0.25 g of powered sample was mixed with 60:40 (v/v) methanol/water solution and centrifuged at 14,000 rpm for 15 min (4 °C). FRAP reagents (300 mM Acetate Buffer pH 3.6; 10 mM tripyridyltriazine (TPTZ), 40 mM HCl and 12 mM $FeCl_3$) were added to the extracts of each sample in 16.6:1.6:1.6 (v/v), respectively. After 1 h in darkness, the absorbance at 593 nm was measured with a spectrophotometer (UV-VIS Cary 100, Agilent Technologies, Palo Alto, CA, USA). Trolox (6-hydroxy-2,5,7,8-tetramethylchroman-2-carboxylic acid) was used as the standard and total antioxidant capacity was quantified and expressed as mmol Trolox equivalents (µmol Trolox Eq. mg^{-1} FW).

The ascorbic acid (AsA) content was determined using the Ascorbic Acid Assay Kit (MAK074, Sigma-Aldrich, St. Louis, MO, USA), following the reported procedure [33]. Briefly, 10 mg of sample was homogenized in 4 volumes of cold AsA buffer, and then centrifuged at 13,000 rpm for 10 min at 4 °C to remove insoluble material. The liquid fraction was mixed with AsA assay buffer to a final volume of 120 µL. The assay reaction was performed by adding the kit reagents to the samples.

In this assay, the AsA concentration was determined by a coupled enzyme reaction, which develops a colorimetric (570 nm) product, proportionate to the amount of ascorbic acid contained in the sample. The concentration of ascorbic acid in the samples was referred to a standard curve and expressed in mg L^{-1}.

2.5. Statistical Analysis

Statistical analysis was performed using Sigma Plot 12.0 (Jandel Scientific, San Rafael, CA, USA). Statistically significant differences among varieties were checked by one-way ANOVA followed by Holm Sidak test for multiple comparison tests, based on a significance level of $p < 0.05$. The normal distribution of data was verified by Shapiro–Wilk and Kolmogorov–Smirnov tests. Spearman correlation coefficient was used to test associations between variables. All data were expressed as means ± standard error (SE) ($n = 6$).

3. Results

3.1. Total Polyphenol Content

Total phenolic content of the peel, pulp and seeds extracts strongly varied among *Citrus* varieties and components of the fruit (Figure 1). Highest amounts ($p < 0.05$) of total polyphenols were found in *C. reticulata* peel (2.21 ± 0.19 mg GAE g^{-1} FW), followed by *C. japonica* (1.24 ± 0.013 mg GAE g^{-1} FW) and *C. clementina* (0.24 ± 0.011 mg GAE g^{-1} FW). No statistically significant difference was detected in the total polyphenol content for the pulp of all the examined Citrus varieties.

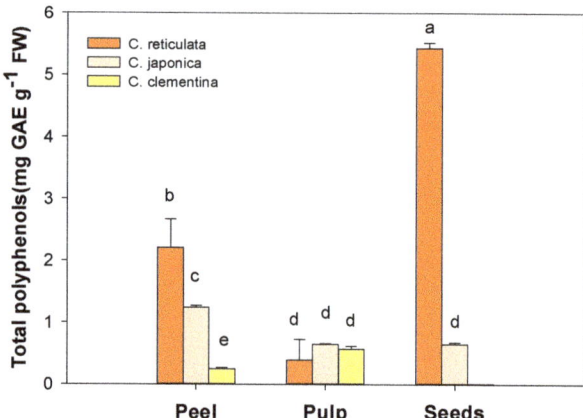

Figure 1. Total polyphenols in peel, pulp and seeds of the three different mandarin cultivars: *C. reticulata* (Phlegrean mandarin), *C. japonica* (Kumquat) and *C. clementina* (Clementine). Each bar represents the mean ± SE ($n = 6$). Different letters indicate statistically significant differences among mandarin varieties ($p < 0.05$). Results were analysed by one-way ANOVA followed by Holm–Sidak post hoc test for multiple comparisons. GAE: gallic acid equivalents; FW: fresh weight.

Among the fruit components, seeds of the *C. reticulata* cultivar exhibited the highest ($p < 0.001$) total polyphenol content (5.43 ± 0.04 mg GAE g^{-1} FW); this concentration was eight-fold higher than that measured in *C. japonica* seed extracts (0.65 ± 0.011 mg GAE g^{-1} FW).

3.2. Total Soluble Antioxidant Capacity

The total antioxidant capacity of the different cultivars is shown in Figure 2 for different parts of mandarin fruit: peel, seeds and pulp. The peel extracts of *C. reticulata* cultivar exhibited the highest ($p < 0.01$) total antioxidant capacity (14.69 ± 1.80 mmol eq Trolox mg^{-1} FW) compared to *C. clementina* (7.5 ± 1.0 mmol Trolox eq mg^{-1} FW) and *C. japonica*, which showed the lowest antioxidant capacity (2.1 ± 0.2 mmol Trolox eq mg^{-1} FW).

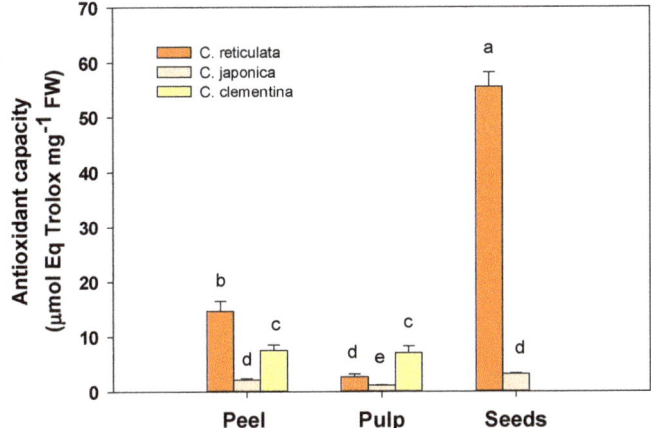

Figure 2. Total antioxidant capacity of peel, pulp and seeds in the three different mandarin cultivars: *C. reticulata* (Phlegrean mandarin), *C. japonica* (Kumquat) and *C. clementina* (Clementine). Each bar represents the mean ± SE ($n = 6$). Different letters indicate statistically significant differences among mandarin varieties ($p < 0.05$). Results were analysed by one-way ANOVA followed by Holm–Sidak post hoc test for multiple comparisons.

In the *C. clementina* pulp extracts, the total antioxidant capacity was found to be three-fold higher (7.1 ± 1.27 mmol Trolox eq mg^{-1} FW) ($p < 0.01$) than that measured in *C. reticulata* (2.6 ± 0.5 mmol Trolox eq mg^{-1} FW) and almost six-fold higher compared to *C. japonica* (1.2 ± 0.06 mmol Trolox eq mg^{-1} FW).

As observed for total polyphenols, among the different fruit parts, the seeds of *C. reticulata* showed the highest ($p < 0.001$) antioxidant capacity (55.6 ± 2.6 mmol Trolox eq mg^{-1} FW). This value was seventeen-fold more abundant compared to *C. japonica* (3.2 ± 0.15 mmol Trolox eq mg^{-1} FW).

3.3. Total Chlorophyll and Carotenoid Content

The concentration of pigments varied significantly among both cultivars and fruit components. Regarding peel, no difference in total chlorophyll content was detected among cultivars (Figure 3). Conversely, the total carotenoid content increased significantly ($p < 0.01$) in *C. clementina* peel (128.16 ± 3.03 mg g^{-1} FW) compared *C. reticulata* (70.99 ± 3.01 mg g^{-1} FW) and *C. japonica* (42.97 ± 1.72 mg g^{-1} FW) (Figure 3).

In the pulp of *C. clementina* cultivar the total chlorophyll content was very high ($p < 0.01$) (37.13 ± 0.67 mg g^{-1} FW) compared to values observed for *C. japonica* (2.93 ± 0.23 mg g^{-1} FW) and *C. reticulata* (0.73 ± 0.07 mg g^{-1} FW). The same trend was observed for carotenoid content in the pulp (Figure 3).

The total amount of chlorophyll increases significantly ($p < 0.001$) in *C. japonica* seeds (94.01 ± 7.92 mg g^{-1} FW), compared to *C. reticulata* (25.05 ± 1.78 mg g^{-1} FW). The highest concentration ($p < 0.01$) of carotenoids was detected in *C. japonica* seeds (Figure 3).

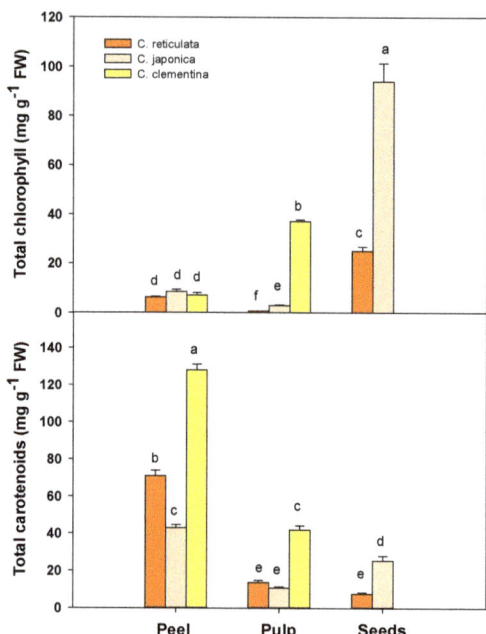

Figure 3. Total chlorophyll (a + b) and total carotenoid (x + c) content of peel, pulp and seeds in the three different mandarin cultivars: *C. reticulata* (Phlegrean mandarin), *C. japonica* (Kumquat) and *C. clementina* (Clementine). Each bar represents the mean ± SE ($n = 6$). Different letters indicate statistically significant differences among mandarin varieties ($p < 0.05$). Results were analysed by one-way ANOVA followed by Holm–Sidak post hoc test for multiple comparisons.

3.4. Ascorbic Acid

Ascorbic acid (AsA) content was very different among mandarin cultivars and fruit components. The highest values ($p < 0.01$) were found in peel, pulp and seed extracts of *C. reticulata* (Figure 4).

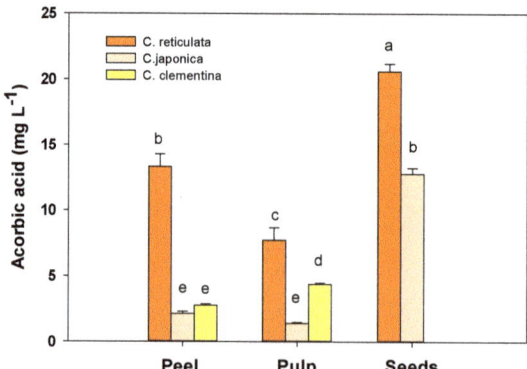

Figure 4. Total soluble antioxidant capacity expressed as ascorbic acid equivalents in peel, pulp and seeds in the three different tangerine cultivars: *C. reticulata* (Phlegrean mandarin), *C. japonica* (Kumquat) and *C. clementina* (Clementine). Each bar represents the mean ± SE ($n = 6$). Different letters indicate statistically significant differences among mandarin varieties ($p < 0.05$). Results were analysed by one-way ANOVA followed by Holm–Sidak post hoc test for multiple comparisons.

In particular, in the peel of *C. reticulata* the ascorbic acid concentration was higher ($p < 0.01$) (13.32 ± 0.96 mg L^{-1}) compared to that measured in *C. clementina* (2.75 ± 0.10 mg L^{-1}) and *C. japonica* (2.13 ± 0.16 mg L^{-1}). In pulp the trend was the same with the highest ($p < 0.01$) AsA concentration in extracts of *C. reticulata* (7.72 ± 0.97 mg L^{-1}) followed by *C. clementina* (4.37 ± 0.12 mg L^{-1}) and *C. japonica* (1.39 ± 0.07 mg L^{-1}) cultivars.

Finally, in the seeds of *C. reticulata*, the AsA amount was almost twice higher ($p < 0.01$) than that found in *C. japonica* (20.61 ± 0.57 mg L^{-1} and 12.78 ± 0.45 mg L^{-1}, respectively).

3.5. Relationship among Bioactive Compounds in the Seeds

The correlations among bioactive compounds in seeds are reported in Table 1. *C. reticulata* showed a significant positive correlation between antioxidant capacity and total chlorophyll, antioxidant capacity and carotenoids as well as between total chlorophylls and carotenoids. *C. japonica* exhibited a significant negative correlation between antioxidant capacity and ascorbic acid and a significant positive correlation between chlorophylls and carotenoids.

Table 1. Pearson correlations among bioactive compounds in the seeds (* $p < 0.05$; ** $p < 0.01$); total polyphenols—TP; antioxidant capacity—AC; total chlorophyll—Chl (a + b); total carotenoids—Car (x + c); ascorbic acid—AsA.

Cultivar	Variables	TP	AC	Chl (a + b)	Car (x + c)	AsA
	TP	1	0.373	0.094	0.096	−0.09
	AC		1	0.893 *	0.897 *	0.265
C. reticulata	Chl (a + b)			1	0.998 **	0.544
	Car (x + c)				1	0.548
	AsA					1
	TP	1	0.643	0.496	0.469	−0.414
	AC		1	−0.268	−0.239	−0.893 *
C. japonica	Chl (a + b)			1	0.837 *	0.546
	Car (x + c)				1	0.314
	AsA					1

4. Discussion

In this study, a comparison between different Citrus varieties was carried out to quantify the content of some bioactive compounds in the peel, pulp and seeds. Data collected allowed us to screen the most promising Citrus cultivar in terms of nutraceutical compounds and to valorise the parts of the fruit, such as peel and seeds, generally considered useless by-products of the production chain. Among cultivars, compelling experimental evidence emerges mainly from *C. reticulata* cultivar. The Phlegraean mandarin is a typical product of the volcanic Phlegraean area (Southern Italy, Naples), characterized by mild climate conditions and very fertile soils. This cultivar is not widespread outside the Campania region boundaries, obscured by the most famous Clementine and Kumquat varieties, with a broader national market.

From our data, it is evident that all fruit parts of the investigated citrus species showed strong antioxidant properties, especially peels and seeds, considered waste products, with limited or even without market value for the food industry [18,19].

Consistent with findings of other authors [34], the total pigment content was very high in the peel compared to the pulp in all tested varieties of mandarin, confirming the valuable antioxidant properties of this fruit part. Among cultivars, *C. clementina* showed the highest pigment content in both peel and pulp.

It is interesting to note that in seeds, *C. japonica* presented the highest content of carotenoids and chlorophylls compared to *C. reticulata*. This difference may be due to intrinsic characteristics of the species. It has been demonstrated that *Citrus* fruits are complex sources of pigments, especially carotenoids, with a broad diversity among the different species and cultivars in terms of types and amounts [35–37]. Therefore, most *Citrus* species show the same carotenoid profile, although some of them have higher concentrations [38].

Generally, the carotenoids are absent in seeds compared to peel and pulp, conversely to the concentration of chlorophylls. The presence of chlorophyll in the seeds of both *C. reticulata* and *C. japonica* cultivars is due to the chlorophyllous embryo. Especially in Kumquat, the cotyledon primordia were particularly evident under the outer seed integument (personal observation). The amount of chlorophyll in seeds is a valuable attribute because the chlorophyll presence ensures the activation of light capture mechanisms, as soon as germination begins [39]. Moreover, there are also some references about fruit photosynthesis: this process may be affected by light able to penetrate in fruit, temperature and ontogeny [40]. It is interesting to consider that the occurrence of a slight level of photosynthesis in mandarin fruit could determine the enrichment of the fruit biochemical profile.

Differently from chlorophylls, the presence of carotenoids in seeds and non-green tissues is common in many species such as maize, pumpkins, sunflowers [41].

The occurrence of carotenoids in plant tissues is associated with a protective function. They develop more abundantly in seedlings at a later time, to enlarge the sunlight harvesting and to defend the photosynthetic apparatus from damages due to excess of light. The carotenoids contribute, as antioxidants, to contrast the deterioration of the membranes induced by free radicals and ageing [42,43].

The function of carotenoids in the seed is less clear than in other plant tissues; however, previous researches have demonstrated that carotenoid presence in the grain is essential for the production of abscisic acid (ABA) and the induction of seed dormancy [44]. The dormancy is one of the mechanisms by which plants can delay germination when the environmental conditions are unfavourable to sprouting [45]. Generally, the number of plants with dormant seeds increases with increasing distance from the equator, in response to seasonality and habitat diversity [46]. It may be hypothesised that the higher content of carotenoids in the *C. japonica* seeds serves for higher production of ABA, in response to the plant's need to maintain seeds quiescent for a longer time compared to *C. reticulata*. On the other hand, *C. reticulata* does not require a quiescent strategy for seeds because it is particularly diffused in Mediterranean ecosystems where the mild climate favours germination conditions.

Furthermore, carotenoids in seeds also contribute to the antioxidant defence of embryonal tissues limiting the membrane deterioration due to free radical and ROS production during seed ageing [42,43]. The presence of carotenoids ensures healthy and long-lived mandarin seeds and together with chlorophylls contributes to improve the fruit value, as chlorophyll and carotenoids are important antioxidant compounds in the human diet [47].

The most relevant result of our study regards the antioxidant power found in mandarin by-products. Our data demonstrate that considerable amounts of polyphenols, water-soluble antioxidants and ascorbic acid were found in the peel and extremely high concentrations of these compounds were measured in seeds, especially in *C. reticulata* cultivar. The peels, and even more so the seeds, are considered wastes of the citrus industry and currently to our knowledge, they are not used for the human diet, but only for ruminant nutrition [22].

The peel is generally the tissue richer in polyphenols and antioxidant activity than other fruit parts [26], even if the antioxidant properties are strictly related to the species. Our results evidence an interesting exception for the *C. reticulata* cultivar, where the highest concentration of total polyphenols and the most elevated antioxidant capacity was found in the seeds. According to other authors [48], we assume the elevated content of compounds with antioxidant action, located in particular in peel and seeds, represents a defence mechanism of the fruit and the embryo against external agents. Indeed, it is well known that these compounds are involved in the protection of the fruit and the embryo against herbivores and fungal pathogen attacks [49].

For the highest cumulative capacity to scavenge free radicals compared to peel and pulp, the seeds of *C. reticulata* are worthy of particular attention. The concurrent increase in total polyphenol and ascorbic acid contents suggests that these molecules may, in part, contribute to the seed antioxidant power in this species. The *C. japonica* seeds exhibited different nutraceutical traits compared to *C. reticulata*, showing a lower antioxidant capacity and polyphenol and ascorbic acid content, but a higher amount of chlorophylls and carotenoids. *C. reticulata* seeds also showed a positive relationship among chlorophylls, carotenoids and antioxidant capacity, while *C. japonica* revealed a positive relationship between chlorophylls and carotenoids but a negative relationship between ascorbic acid and antioxidant capacity, indicating that ascorbic acid does not contribute so much to the antioxidant power.

The absence of relationships among ascorbic acid and antioxidant capacity in the peel and pulp of mandarin cultivars suggests that other compounds should be responsible for the antioxidant power of these fruit components [27].

Several studies report that various phenolic compounds, compared to ascorbic acid, mainly influence antioxidant activity [50,51]. However, according to the literature [6], it may be argued that the phenolic compounds in citrus fruits contribute less than vitamin C to the antioxidant activity. This evidence seems to be confirmed for the seeds of the *C. reticulata* cultivar, where we have found a very high content of vitamin C. However, it cannot be excluded that other antioxidant compounds, such as flavonoids may be present in seeds enhancing the antioxidant power. In addition, other factors may contribute to this distinctive trait in Phlegrean mandarin, such as the plant age or the stage of fruit ripeness [52]. It is noteworthy that antioxidant properties found in the different parts of mandarin fruit are strictly related to intrinsic species characteristics. In fact, conversely to Phlegrean mandarin, in other citrus fruits such as orange, lemon and grapefruit, the higher amount of phenolic compounds, flavonoids, vitamin C, and antioxidant activity, were found in the peels compared to the inner wasted parts (pulp and seeds) [26]. Starting from this evidence, the high antioxidant charge of Phlegrean mandarin seeds assumes a great commercial value for diverse purposes. Lyophilised or fresh seeds extracts might be used as food additives or included in pharmaceutical formulations as promising alternatives to the common preparations [53]. The current challenge is to improve the extraction techniques of bioactive compounds from vegetable wastes to preserve the properties of these molecules over time and obtain a full by-product valorisation.

5. Conclusions

The comparison among diverse mandarin cultivars and fruit components revealed some important insights about the nutraceutical value associated with species and fruit parts. For all tested cultivars the peel is more abundant in antioxidants compared to pulp and may be potentially used as a dietary supplement. However, the most significant result concerns the seeds of the Phlegraean mandarin, which have proved to be highly rich in polyphenols, ascorbic acid, and antioxidant activity, compared to the other parts of the fruit and other citrus varieties.

Seeds could be inexpensive and readily available resources of bioactive compounds (such as natural antioxidants) for use in the food and pharmaceutical industries. The seed consumption would also reduce the problem of large amounts of wastes derived annually from the agri-food industry.

A sustainable re-utilisation of seeds and peels for industrial and pharmacological applications could represent a strong boost toward circular economy initiatives in Southern Italy.

Further analyses are needed to improve this initial research, allowing a deepen characterisation of bioactive molecules responsible for the high antioxidant power of the seeds.

From the economic point of view, the evidence that the Phlegraean mandarin is richer in bioactive compounds than the most commercialised varieties (i.e., kumquat and clementine) promotes the valorisation of a potentially unexploited resource typical of the Campania region (Southern Italy), whose economy is mainly based on the tourism and agriculture.

Author Contributions: Conceptualization, C.A., M.R.I.; methodology, C.A., G.C.; investigation, C.A., G.C., E.V., M.C.; resources, M.R.I., D.N.; data curation, E.V.; writing—original draft preparation, C.A., G.C.; writing—review and editing, C.A., M.R.I, D.N.; supervision, C.A., M.R.I. All authors have read and agreed to the published version of the manuscript.

Funding: This research received no external funding.

Conflicts of Interest: The authors declare no conflict of interest.

References

1. De Moraes Barros, H.R.; Aparecida, T.; de Castro Ferreira, P.; Genovese, M.I. Antioxidant capacity and mineral content of pulp and peel from commercial cultivars of citrus from Brazil. *Food Chem.* **2012**, *134*, 1892–1898. [CrossRef] [PubMed]
2. Boeing, H.; Bechthold, A.; Bub, A.; Ellinger, S.; Haller, D.; Kroke, A.; Leschik-Bonnet, E.; Muller, M.J.; Oberritter, H.; Schulze, M.; et al. Critical review: Vegetables and fruit in the prevention of chronic diseases. *Eur. J. Nutr.* **2012**, *51*, 637–663. [CrossRef] [PubMed]
3. Huang, G.D.; Ou, B.; Prior, R.L. The chemistry behind antioxidant capacity assays. *J. Agric. Food Chem.* **2005**, *53*, 1841–1856. [CrossRef] [PubMed]
4. Patil, B.S.; Jayaprakasha, G.K.; Murthy, K.N.C.; Vikram, A. Bioactive compounds: Historical perspectives, opportunities, and challenges. *J. Agric. Food Chem.* **2009**, *57*, 8142–8160. [CrossRef]
5. Masuda, T.; Inaba, Y.; Takeda, Y. Antioxidant mechanism of carnosic acid: Structural identification of two oxidation products. *J. Agric. Food Chem.* **2001**, *49*, 5560–5565. [CrossRef]
6. Arena, E.; Fallico, B.; Maccarone, E. Evaluation of antioxidant capacity of blood orange juices as influenced by constituents, concentration process and storage. *Food Chem.* **2001**, *74*, 423–427. [CrossRef]
7. Saito, S.; Okamoto, Y.; Kawabata, J. Effects of alcoholic solvents on antiradical abilities of protocatechuic acid and its alkyl esters. *J. Biosci. Biotechnol. Biochem.* **2004**, *68*, 1221–1227. [CrossRef]
8. Al-Juhaimi, F.Y.; Ghafoor, K. Bioactive compounds, antioxidant and physico- chemical properties of juice from lemon, mandarin and orange fruits cultivated in Saudi Arabia. *Pak. J. Bot.* **2013**, *45*, 1193–1196.
9. Ebrahimzadeh, M.A.; Hosseinimehr, S.J.; Gayekhloo, M.R. Measuring and comparison of vitamin C content in citrus fruits: Introduction of native variety. *Indian J. Chem. B.* **2004**, *1*, 650–652.
10. Fernandez-Lopez, J.; Zhi, N.; Aleson-Carbonell, L.; Perez-Alvarez, J.A.; Kuri, V. Antioxidant and antibacterial activities of natural extracts: Application in beef meatballs. *Meat Sci.* **2005**, *69*, 371–380. [CrossRef]
11. Jayaprakasha, G.K.; Patil, B.S. In vitro evaluation of the antioxidant activities in fruit extracts from citron and blood orange. *Food Chem.* **2007**, *101*, 410–418. [CrossRef]
12. Barros, L.; Dueñas, M.; Dias, M.I.; Sousa, M.J.; Santos-Buelga, C.; Ferreira, I.C.F.R. Phenolic profiles of in vivo and in vitro grown *Coriandrum sativum* L. *Food Chem.* **2012**, *132*, 841–848. [CrossRef]
13. Gorinstein, S.; Belloso, O.M.; Park, Y.; Haruenkit, R.; Lojek, A.; Ciz, M.; Caspi, A.; Libman, I.; Trakhtenberg, S. Comparison of some biochemical characteristics of different citrus fruits. *Food Chem.* **2001**, *74*, 309–315. [CrossRef]
14. Topuz, A.; Topakci, M.; Canakci, M.; Akinci, I.; Ozdemir, F. Physical and nutritional properties of four orange varieties. *J. Food Eng.* **2005**, *66*, 519–523. [CrossRef]
15. Goldemberg, L.; Yaniv, Y.; Porat, R.; Carmi, N. Mandarin fruit quality: A review. *J. Sci. Food Agric.* **2018**, *98*, 18–26. [CrossRef]
16. Putnik, P.; Barba, F.J.; Lorenzo, J.M.; Gabric, D.; Shpigelman, A.; Cravotto, G.; Kovačević, D.B. An integrated approach to mandarin processing: Food safety and nutritional quality, consumer preference, and nutrient bioaccessibility. *Compr. Rev. Food Sci. Saf.* **2017**, *16*, 1345–1358. [CrossRef]
17. BP Statistical Review of World Energy. 2012. Available online: http://www.bp.com/assets/bp_internet/globalbp/globalbp_uk_english/reports_and_publications/statistical_energy_review_2011/STAGING/local_assets/pdf/statistical_review_of_world_energy_full_report_2012.pdf (accessed on 5 September 2012).
18. Sharma, K.; Mahato, N.; Cho, M.H.; Lee, Y.R. Converting citrus wastes into value-added products: Economic and environmentally friendly approaches. *Nutrition* **2017**, *34*, 29–46. [CrossRef]
19. Wikandari, R.; Nguyen, H.; Millati, R.; Niklasson, C.; Taherzadeh, M.J. Improvement of biogas production from orange peel waste by leaching of limonene. *BioMed Res. Int.* **2015**, *2015*, 494182. [CrossRef]
20. Ledesma-Escobar, C.A.; de Castro, M.D.L. Towards a comprehensive exploitation of citrus. *Trends Food Sci. Technol.* **2014**, *39*, 63–75. [CrossRef]
21. Lin, C.S.K.; Pfaltzgraff, L.A.; Herrero-Davila, L.; Mubofu, E.B.; Abderrahim, S.; Clark, J.H.; Koutinas, A.A.; Kopsahelis, N.; Stamatelatou, K.; Dickson, F.; et al. Food waste as a valuable resource for the production

of chemicals, materials and fuels. Current situation and global perspective. *Energy Environ. Sci.* **2013**, *6*, 426–464. [CrossRef]
22. Bampidis, V.A.; Robinson, P.H. Citrus by-products as ruminant feeds: A review. *Anim. Feed Sci. Technol.* **2006**, *128*, 175–217. [CrossRef]
23. Calabrò, P.S.; Pontoni, L.; Porqueddu, I.; Greco, R.; Pirozzi, F.; Malpei, F. Effect of the concentration of essential oil on orange peel waste biomethanization: Preliminary batch results. *Waste Manag.* **2016**, *48*, 440–447. [CrossRef] [PubMed]
24. Deng, G.F.; Shen, C.; Xu, X.R.; Kuang, R.D.; Guo, Y.J.; Zeng, L.S.; Gao, L.-L.; Lin, X.; Xie, J.-F.; Xia, E.; et al. Potential of fruit wastes as natural resources of bioactive compounds. *Int. J. Mol. Sci.* **2012**, *13*, 8308–8323. [CrossRef] [PubMed]
25. Manthey, J.A.; Grohmann, K. Phenols in citrus peel by products: Concentrations of hydroxycinnamates and polymethoxylated flavones in citrus peel molasses. *J. Agric. Food Chem.* **2001**, *49*, 3268–3273. [CrossRef]
26. Elkhatim, K.A.S.; Elagib, R.A.A.; Hassan, A.B. Content of phenolic compounds and vitamin C and antioxidant activity in wasted parts of Sudanese citrus fruits. *Food Sci. Nutr.* **2018**, *6*, 1214–1219. [CrossRef] [PubMed]
27. Bocco, A.; Cuvelier, M.; Richard, H.; Berset, C. Antioxidant activity and phenolic composition of citrus peel and seed extracts. *J. Agric. Food Chem.* **1998**, *46*, 2123–2129. [CrossRef]
28. Fattahi, J.; Hamidoghli, Y.; Ghazvini, R.F.; Ghasemnejad, M.; Bakhshi, D. Assessment of fruit quality and antioxidant activity of three citrus species during ripening. *South-West. J. Hortic. Biol. Environ.* **2011**, *2*, 113–128.
29. Moulehi, I.; Bourgou, S.; Ourghemmi, I.; Tounsi, M.S. Variety and ripening impact on phenolic composition and antioxidant activity of mandarin (*Citrus reticulate* Blanco) and bitter orange (*Citrus aurantium* L.) seeds extracts. *Ind. Crop. Prod.* **2012**, *39*, 74–80. [CrossRef]
30. Lichtenthaler, H.K. Chlorophylls and carotenoids: Pigments of photosynthetic biomembranes. *Methods Enzymol.* **1987**, *148*, 350–382.
31. Porzio, L.; Buia, M.C.; Lorenti, M.; Vitale, E.; Amitrano, C.; Arena, C. Ecophysiological response of *Jania rubens* (Corallinaceae) to ocean acidification. *Rend. Lincei-Sci. Fis.* **2018**, *29*, 543–546. [CrossRef]
32. George, B.; Kaur, C.; Khurdiya, D.S.; Kapoor, H.C. Antioxidants in tomato (*Lycopersium esculentum*) as a function of genotype. *Food Chem.* **2004**, *84*, 45–51. [CrossRef]
33. Arena, C.; Vitale, L.; Bianchi, A.R.; Mistretta, C.; Vitale, E.; Parisi, C.; Guerriero, G.; Magliulo, V.; De Maio, A. The ageing process affects the antioxidant defences and the poly (ADPribosyl)ation activity in *Cistus incanus* L. leaves. *Antioxidants* **2019**, *8*, 528. [CrossRef] [PubMed]
34. Agócs, A.; Nagy, V.; Szabó, Z.; Márk, L.; Ohmacht, R.; Deli, J. Comparative study on the carotenoid composition of the peel and the pulp of different citrus species. *Innov. Food Sci. Emerg. Technol.* **2007**, *8*, 390–394. [CrossRef]
35. Kato, M.; Ikoma, Y.; Matsumoto, H.; Sugiura, M.; Hyodo, H.; Yano, M. Accumulation of carotenoids and expression of carotenoid biosynthetic genes during maturation in citrus fruit. *Plant Physiol.* **2004**, *134*, 824–837. [CrossRef] [PubMed]
36. Fanciullino, A.L.; Dhuique-Mayer, C.; Luro, F.; Casanova, J.; Morillon, R.; Ollitrault, P. Carotenoid diversity in cultivated Citrus is highly influenced by genetic factors. *J. Agric. Food Chem.* **2006**, *54*, 4397–4406. [CrossRef]
37. Matsumoto, H.; Ikoma, Y.; Kato, M.; Kuniga, T.; Nakajima, N.; Yoshida, T. Quantification of carotenoids in citrus fruit by LC-MS and comparison of patterns of seasonal changes for carotenoids among citrus varieties. *J. Agric. Food Chem.* **2007**, *55*, 2356–2368. [CrossRef]
38. Conesa, A.; Manera, F.C.; Brotons, J.M.; Fernandez-Zapata, J.C.; Simón, I.; Simón-Grao, S.; Alfosea-Simón, M.; Nicolás, J.J.M.; Valverde, J.M.; Garcìa-Sanchez, F. Changes in the content of chlorophylls and carotenoids in the rind of Fino 49 lemons during maturation and their relationship with parameters from the CIELAB color space. *Sci. Hortic.* **2019**, *243*, 253–260. [CrossRef]
39. Casodoro, G.; Rascio, N. Cotyledonal chloroplasts in the hypogeal seeds of clementine. *Planta* **1987**, *170*, 300–307. [CrossRef]
40. Marcelis, L.F.M.; Hofman-Eijer, L.R.B. The contribution of fruit photosynthesis to the carbon requirement of cucumber fruits as affected by irradiance, temperature and ontogeny. *Physiol. Plant* **1995**, *93*, 476–483. [CrossRef]
41. Howitt, C.A.; Pogson, B.J. Carotenoid accumulation and function in seeds and non-green tissues. *Plant Cell Environ.* **2006**, *29*, 435–445. [CrossRef]

42. Pinzino, C.; Capocchi, A.; Galleschi, L.; Saviozzi, F.; Nanni, B.; Zandomeneghi, M. Aging, free radicals, and antioxidants in wheat seeds. *J. Agric. Food Chem.* **1999**, *47*, 1333–1339. [CrossRef] [PubMed]
43. Calucci, L.; Capocchi, A.; Galleschi, L.; Ghiringhelli, S.; Pinzino, C.; Saviozzi, F.; Zandomeneghi, M. Antioxidants, free radicals, storage proteins, puroindolines, and proteolytic activities in bread wheat (*Triticum aestivum*) seeds during accelerated aging. *J. Agric. Food Chem.* **2004**, *52*, 4274–4281. [CrossRef] [PubMed]
44. Maluf, M.P.; Saab, I.N.; Wurtzel, E.T.; Sachs, M.M. The viviparous 12 maize mutant is deficient in abscisic acid, carotenoids, and chlorophyll synthesis. *J. Exp. Bot.* **1997**, *48*, 1259–1268. [CrossRef]
45. Fenner, M.; Thompson, K. *The Ecology of Seeds*; Cambridge University Press: Cambridge, UK, 2005; p. 260. [CrossRef]
46. Bewley, J.D.; Bradford, K.; Hilhorst, H.; Nonogaki, H. *Seeds. Physiology of Development, Germination and Dormancy*, 3rd ed.; Springer: New York, NY, USA, 2013; p. 392.
47. Zakynthinos, G.; Varzakas, T. Carotenoids: From plants to food industry. *Curr. Res. Nutr. Food Sci.* **2016**, *4*, 38–51. [CrossRef]
48. Ortuno, A.; Baidez, A.; Gomez, P.; Arcas, M.C.; Porras, I.; Garcia-Lidon, A.; Del Rio, J.A. *Citrus paradisi* and *Citrus sinensis* flavonoids: Their influence in the defence mechanism against *Penicillium digitatum*. *Food Chem.* **2006**, *98*, 351–358. [CrossRef]
49. Jayaprakasha, G.K.; Murthy, K.N.C.; Patil, B.S. Antioxidant activities of polyphenol containing extracts from Citrus. *Funct. Food Health Dis.* **2008**, *24*, 264–276.
50. Manganaris, G.A.; Goulas, V.; Vicente, A.R.; Terry, L.A. Berry antioxidants: Small fruits providing large benefits. *J. Sci. Food Agric.* **2014**, *94*, 825–833. [CrossRef]
51. Silva, F.G.D.; O'Callaghan, Y.; O'Brien, N.M.; Netto, F.M. Antioxidant capacity of flaxseed products: The effect of in vitro digestion. *Plant Food Hum. Nutr.* **2013**, *68*, 24–30. [CrossRef]
52. Al-Juhaimi, F.A. Citrus fruits by-products ad sources of bioactive compounds with antioxidant potential. *Pak. J. Bot.* **2014**, *46*, 1459–1462.
53. Jimenez-Moreno, N.; Esparza, I.; Bimbela, F.; Gandìa, L.M.; Ancín-Azpilicueta, C. Valorization of selected fruit and vegetable wastes as bioactive compounds: Opportunities and challenges. *Crit. Rev. Environ. Sci. Technol.* **2019**, 1–48. [CrossRef]

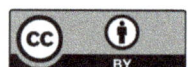

© 2020 by the authors. Licensee MDPI, Basel, Switzerland. This article is an open access article distributed under the terms and conditions of the Creative Commons Attribution (CC BY) license (http://creativecommons.org/licenses/by/4.0/).

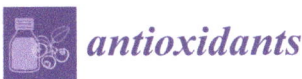

Article

Electroactive Phenolic Contributors and Antioxidant Capacity of Flesh and Peel of 11 Apple Cultivars Measured by Cyclic Voltammetry and HPLC–DAD–MS/MS

Danuta Zielińska * and Marcin Turemko

Department of Chemistry, University of Warmia and Mazury in Olsztyn, Plac Lodzki 4, 10-727 Olsztyn, Poland; marcin.turemko@uwm.edu.pl
* Correspondence: danuta.zielinska@uwm.edu.pl; Tel.: +48-89-523-39-35

Received: 29 August 2020; Accepted: 26 October 2020; Published: 28 October 2020

Abstract: In this study, 11 apple cultivars were characterized by their total phenolic content (TPC) and total flavonoid content (TFC) and antioxidant, reducing, and chelating capacity by 2,2-diphenyl-1-picrylhydrazyl (DPPH) test, cyclic voltammetry (CV), and ferric reducing antioxidant power (FRAP) assays; and ferrous ion chelating capacity. The phenolic compounds in flesh and peel were determined by liquid chromatography coupled to mass spectrometry and diode array detector (HPLC–DAD–MS/MS) and their electroactivity by CV. The results showed higher TPC, TFC, and antioxidant capacity by DPPH test in the peels of all apple cultivars as compared to the respective flesh. The peel extracts also showed two-fold higher FRAP values as compared to the flesh extracts. The reducing capacity of the peel and flesh determined by CV measurements confirmed the results achieved by spectrophotometric methods of evaluating antioxidant capacity. There was no significant difference in chelating capacity in the peel and flesh. The HPLC–DAD–MS/MS analysis showed the presence of 11 phenolic compounds in the peel and flesh which varied in antioxidant, reducing, and chelating activity. The order of the phenolic compound content in flesh and peel in Quinte cultivar, which showed the highest antioxidant capacity, was as follows: epicatechin > chlorogenic acid > quercetin 3-arabinoside > quercetin 3-glucoside > cyanidin 3-galactoside > quercetin 3-rhamnoside > catechin > phloridzin > rutin > phloretin = quercetin. CV results were highly correlated with those obtained by spectrophotometry and HPLC–DAD–MS/MS, providing evidence to support the use of cyclic voltammetry as a rapid method to determine the phenolic profile and reducing the power of apple flesh and peel. The association between antioxidant assays and phenolic compound content showed that the highest contribution to the antioxidant capacity of apple peel and flesh was provided by catechin, epicatechin, and cyadinin-3-galactoside, while phloretin, phloridzin, and chlorogenic acid were the main contributors to chelating activity. Results from this study clearly indicate that removing the peel from apples may induce a significant loss of antioxidants.

Keywords: apples; phenolic compounds; antioxidant; reducing and chelating capacity; cyclic voltammetry; HPLC–DAD–MS/MS

1. Introduction

Apple is a popularly consumed fruit, mostly because of the pleasant taste and the fact that it is cultivated worldwide. Apples are a significant part of the human diet and are ranked in the top five consumed fruits in the world [1]. The beneficial health effects of apples have been ascribed to the polyphenolic compounds, a group of secondary plant metabolites, of which several thousand structurally different compounds have been identified [2,3]. Phenolic compounds are generally recognized as the main determinants of the biological activities of apples, such as the prevention of cardiovascular diseases, asthma and other lung dysfunctions, diabetes, obesity, and cancer [4–7] as well as age-related neurodegeneration [8,9]. The potential health benefits of polyphenols have been reviewed by Scalbert et al. [10]. Moreover, the content and composition of polyphenols present in apples are important because of their contribution to the sensory quality of fresh fruit and processed apple products [11].

Apples contain a variety of phenolic compounds that can be classified into five major sub-classes, with procyanidins being the most abundant class (between 40% and 89%), followed by hydroxycinnamic acids, dihydrochalcones, flavonols, anthocyanins, and flavan-3-ols [12]. Anthocyanins that contribute to the red color of apple fruits are exclusively found in the peel and represent less than 8% of total phenolics [13–15].

The flavan-3-ols can be found in the form of monomers, oligomers, and polymers (procyanidins), and flavonols are often associated with sugar moieties. The main sugars involved in glycosylation are galactose, glucose, rhamnose, arabinose, and xylose, and rutinose, a disaccharide, has also been found in apple. Dihydrochalcones are mainly associated with glucose and xyloglucose [16]. Moreover, the distribution and profile of phenolic compounds vary considerably among different cultivars, genotypes, ripening stages, and environmental conditions, and also within different tissues [13,15,17–21].

The antioxidant activity of polyphenolics has been studied extensively [22–24]. These compounds usually have a high redox potential, which allows them to act as reducing agents, hydrogen donors, and singlet oxygen quenchers [22]. Therefore, several methods to measure the antioxidant activity of polyphenols have been proposed and were recently reviewed [23,24]. Among other methods, scavenging stable radicals such as 2,2-diphenyl-1-picrylhydrazyl (DPPH) and 2,2'-azinobis(3-ethylbenzothiazoline-6-sulfonic acid) (ABTS), oxygen radical absorbance capacity (ORAC), total radical trapping antioxidant parameter (TRAP), ferric reducing antioxidant power (FRAP), and cupric ion (Cu^{2+}) reducing power (CUPRAC) were employed in foods [23]. The determination of antioxidant activity by electrochemical methods is of increasing interest. Electrochemical methods used to determine antioxidant activity are still being developed. Among electrochemical techniques, the most widely used for this purpose is cyclic voltammetry (CV). In contrast to the aforementioned methods, electrochemical assays are low-cost and usually do not require time-consuming sample preparation. CV is based on an analysis of the anodic current (AC) waveform, which is a function of the reactive potential of a given compound in the sample. The CV tracing indicates the ability of a compound to donate electrons at the potential of the anodic wave. Therefore, in the past couple of years, CV has proven to be highly practical and efficient in determining the phenolic composition and reducing the power of complex matrices, including fruit extracts, honey, wine, tea, coffee, and kiwifruit [25–29]. Methods involving cyclic voltammetry (CV) have also been suggested as an instrument in evaluating the reducing activity of a wide spectrum of bioactive compounds and food extracts [25,30,31].

In many works, the content and antioxidant properties of polyphenols present in all parts of the apple fruit (skin, pulp, and seeds) were determined for various cultivars [32–35]. However, these You jumped the numbers in between.studies mainly focused on the relationship between antioxidant activity and total phenolic content, while a limited amount of data were available on phenolic profiles and their contribution to the antioxidant activity of apple extracts. Additionally, the correlation between the different antioxidant activity evaluation assays, chelating activity, and contents of individual apple polyphenols has not yet been fully investigated. However, the feasibility of electrochemical methods in determining the antioxidant activity in the phenolic compounds of apple and extracts from the peel and flesh samples is yet to be studied.

In this study, the antioxidant properties and major phenolic contributors present in the flesh and peel extracts of 11 apple cultivars from Poland were addressed. We attempted a novel approach by investigating the feasibility of applying cyclic voltammetry (CV) to determine the reducing activity of major phenolic compounds and predicting the antioxidant capacity of apple extract from peel and flesh. The aims of this study were as follows: (1) to determine the antioxidant capacity of apple flesh and peel by peel by cyclic voltammetry and spectrophotometric assays, (2) to determine the profiles of phenolic compounds in the flesh and peel of popular apple cultivars by sensitive liquid chromatography (HPLC) coupled to mass spectrometry (MS) using the electrospray ionization (ESI) and diode array detector (DAD) methodology, (3) to determine the antioxidant activity of the identified phenolic compounds by cyclic voltammetry (CV) and spectrophotometric assays, and (4) to show the relationship between the content of individual phenolic compounds and the antioxidant capacity of apple flesh and peel.

2. Materials and Methods

2.1. Chemicals and Reagents

Chlorogenic acid, gallic acid, rutin, quercetin, quercetin-3-O-glucoside, quercetin-3-O-rhamnoside, (-)-epicatechin, and cyanidin-3-O-galactoside were supplied by Extrasynthese (Genay, France). Quercetin-3-O-arabinoside, (+)-catechin, phloretin, phloridzin, and other compounds were obtained from Sigma-Aldrich (Munich, Germany); 2,2-diphenyl-1-picrylhydrazyl (DPPH), 2,4,6-tri(2-pyridyl)-s-triazine (TPTZ) and 6-hydroxy-2,5,7,8-tetramethylchroman-2-carboxylic acid (Trolox) were purchased from Sigma (Sigma Chemical Co., St. Louis, MO, USA). Folin–Ciocalteu's reagent and others of reagent-grade quality were from POCh (Gliwice, Poland). Ultrapure water was purified with a Millipore Direct-Q UV 3 System (Bedford, MA, USA). Flavonoids and solvents were HPLC-grade quality, and other reagents were at least reagent-grade quality.

2.2. Sample and Standard Preparations

The studied material consisted of 11 first-quality grade apple cultivars at their ripe period of growth. Early varieties of apples such as Antonówka, Delikates, Early Geneva, Papierówka, Paulared, Sunrise, and Quinte were harvested in August, while Gloster, Jonagored, Ligol, and Rubinola cultivars, which are late varieties, were harvested in September, both during the 2019 season. All fruits were purchased from the Experimental and Production Institute "Pozorty" Sp. z o.o. in Olsztyn (Poland). Fruit samples (10 apple fruits randomly selected) were washed with distilled water to remove foreign substances and manually peeled using a hand peeler (1–2 mm thickness), cored, and cut into small pieces. The weighed apple flesh and peels were pooled separately. Before freeze drying (FD), the apple flesh and peels were frozen overnight at −25 °C and dried in the FreeZone 2.5 freeze dryer (Labconco, CA, USA). During FD, pressure was reduced to 16 Pa. The temperature in the drying chamber was −55 °C, and the shelf temperature was 26 °C. Apple flesh and peels were kept in the drying chamber for 24 h. The lyophilized samples were ground in a laboratory mill and stored at −20 °C up to further analysis. The moisture content of the peel from all apple cultivars ranged from 93.44 to 94.83%, and that of flesh was in the range from 91.63 to 93.01%. About 100 mg (for spectrophotometric methods) and 250 mg (for the electrochemical method) of lyophilized flesh and peel were extracted with 1 mL of 80% methanol by 30 s sonication. Then, the mixture was vortexed for 30 s, again sonicated and vortexed, and centrifuged for 5 min (13,200 rpm). This step was repeated five times and supernatant was collected in a 5 mL flask. Finally, all extracts were kept in dark-glass vials at −20 °C for further analysis.

2.3. Spectrophotometric Determination of Total Phenolic and Flavonoid Content

Total phenolic content (TPC) was determined according to the Folin–Ciocalteu (FC) assay as described by Shahidi and Naczk [36] with a slight modification. A volume of 90 µL of sample extract (10 mg/ml), 90 µL of FC reagent (diluted 1:10, v/v), 180 µL of saturated solution of Na_2CO_3, and 1440 µL of H_2O were mixed and allowed to react for 25 min in a thermomixer (Comfort, Eppendorf) at room temperature. The absorbance was measured at 725 nm in a UV-1800 spectrophotometer (Shimadzu, Japan) with a temperature controller (TCC-Controller, Shimadzu, CA, USA). Catechin was used as a standard and the results were based on the standard curve equation of catechin (0.0625–1.0 mM) and expressed as a catechin equivalent (CAE) in µg/g of fresh weight. The measurements were made in triplicate.

Total flavonoid content (TFC) was determined based on the method by Jia et al. [37] with some modifications. A volume of 1230 µL of extract (10 mg/mL) was mixed with 62 µL of 5% $NaNO_2$ solution (m/v). After incubation in the thermomixer (Comfort, Eppendorf) at room temperature for 6 min, 123 µL of 10% $AlCl_3·6H_2O$ was added. Again, the mixture was incubated under the same conditions for 6 min, then 410 µL of 1M NaOH was added and the mixture was centrifuged for 5 min at 2000 rpm (Centrifuge 5424, Eppendorf). The absorbance of the reaction mixture was measured against the reagent blank at 510 nm with the UV-1800 spectrophotometer with a temperature controller (TCC-Controller, Shimadzu, city, State, country). Catechin was used as a standard and the results were based on standard curve equation of catechin (0.0625–0.5 mM) and expressed as catechin equivalent (CAE) in µg/g of fresh weight. The measurements were done in triplicate.

2.4. Analysis of Phenolic Compounds by HPLC–DAD–MS/MS

The identification of phenolic compounds was done by means of liquid chromatography (HPLC) coupled to mass spectrometry (MS) using the electrospray ionization interface (ESI). Quantification of phenolic compounds was carried out by using HPLC with diode array detector (DAD). The analysis of phenolic compounds was performed on a micro-HPLC system (LC200, Eksigent, Dublin, CA, USA) with pump, autosampler, column oven, and system controller. The micro-HPLC was connected in series to a QTRAP 5500 mass spectrometer (AB Sciex, Canada) equipped with a triple quadrupole, ion trap, and an ion source of electrospray ionization (ESI). The analytical column was a Halo C18 column (50 mm × 0.5 mm, 2.7 µm i.d.; Eksigent, Dublin, CA, USA). Eluent A was water/formic acid, 99.05/0.95 (v/v); eluent B was acetonitrile/formic acid, 99.05/0.95 (v/v). A gradient elution program was used: 5–5–90–90–5–5% B in 0–0.1–2–2.5–2.7–3 min. Before chromatographic analysis, apple extract was centrifuged (20 min, 13,000 g). Aliquot (2 µL) of sample solution was injected, with flow rate of 15 µL/min, at a column temperature of 45 °C. Phenolic compounds detected in the apple extracts were identified according to their MS/MS fragmentation spectrum (m/z values). Mass spectrometry data were obtained in positive- and negative-ion mode. The optimal identification of phenolic compounds was achieved under the following conditions: curtain gas: 25 L/min, collision gas: 9 L/min, ions pray voltage: 5400 V (for positive-ion mode) and −4500 V (for negative-ion mode), temperature: 350 °C, 1 ion source gas: 35 L/min and 2 ion source gas: 30 L/min; and entrance potential: 10 V (for positive-ion mode) and −10 V (for negative-ion mode). Phenolic compounds were quantified from the determined multiple reaction monitoring pairs (MRM) as shown in Table 1 and the calibration curves of external standards (range of 10–1000 nM).

Table 1. MS data of phenolic compounds from apple.

Identification	(M)− (m/z)	(M)+ (m/z)	MS/MS (m/z)
Cyanidin 3-O-galactoside		449.0	287.0
Phloretin	273.1		227.1/166.8/123.1
Phloridzin	435.2		273.1
Catechin	289.2		245.3/203.1/109.1
Epicatechin	289.2		245.3/203.1/109.1
Chlorogenic acid	353.2		191.1/179.1
Rutin	609.0		463.0/301.0
Quercetin 3-O-glucoside	463.0		301.0
Quercetin	301.0		179.0/151.0
Quercetin 3-O-arabinoside	433.0		301.0
Quercetin 3-O-rhamnoside	447.0		301.0

2.5. Ferric Reducing Antioxidant Power (FRAP) Assay

The FRAP assay was carried out with some modifications according to the method of Benzie and Strain [38]. Briefly, the FRAP-2,4,6-tri(2-pyridyl)-s-triazine (TPTZ) reagent was prepared from the sodium acetate buffer (300 mM, pH 3.6), 10 mM 2,4,6-tri(2-pyridyl)-s-triazine (TPTZ) solution (40 mM HCl as solvent), and 20 mM $FeCl_3·6H_2O$ in a volume ratio of 10:1:1. The FRAP reagent was freshly prepared on the day of the measurements. An aliquot of 75 µL of the extract was mixed with 225 µL of ultrapure water and 2250 µL of FRAP reagent (pre-incubated for 5 min at 25 °C). The absorbance of the reagent mixture was measured at 593 nm after 30 min incubation at 25 °C. Samples were measured in 3 replicates. The standard curve was prepared using Trolox solution (0.034–0.612 mM), and the results were expressed as µmol of Trolox equivalent per gram of apple fresh weight (µmol TE/g FW).

2.6. DPPH Assay

DPPH assay was based on the method of Brand-Williams et al. [39]. The samples were diluted to a proper concentration to make sure that the test results were readable between the absorbance values of 0.2–0.8. A volume of 100 µL of sample was mixed with 2 mL of methanol and then reacted with 250 µL of DPPH solution (10 mg DPPH in 25 mL of methanol) The reaction mixture was incubated in the dark at room temperature for 20 min, after which the absorbance at 517 nm was recorded. The test was performed in triplicate. The Trolox calibration curve (0.1–1.0 mM) was plotted as a function of the decrease in absorbance. The percentage of inhibition of DPPH radical by tested samples was calculated using the following equation, expressed as µmol TE/g FW:

Scavenging activity % = 100 − [(Abs. of sample − Abs. of blank) × 100/Abs. of control]

2.7. Cyclic Voltammetry (CV) Assay

Cyclic voltammograms were recorded using a Gamry G 750 potentiostat (Warminster, PA, USA). The working electrode was a 3 mm diameter glassy carbon disk electrode (BAS MF-2012). An Ag/AgCl reference electrode was used in conjunction with a platinum wire as a counter electrode. Given the effect of polyphenol adsorption on the voltammetric response, which was observed in our previous work [40], it was considered important to run the voltammograms in as consistent a manner as possible. The following electrode cleaning procedure was undertaken between each run. The electrode was thoroughly hand-polished with 0.05 µm alumina powder (BAS CF-1050) on the polishing cloth (BAS MF-1040) and rinsed thoroughly with Milli-Q grade water. Before taking the cyclic voltammogram of the test solution, a background cyclic voltammogram was run in the buffer solution in the potential range from −0.1 to 1.3 V at a scan rate of 0.1 V s^{-1}, and the electrode was rinsed with Milli-Q grade water and methanol and dried. Apple extracts were diluted with Britton-Robinson (B-R) buffer (0.1 M, pH 7.4) at a 1:1 ratio, and the final extract concentration was 25 mg/mL. Cyclic voltammograms were taken in the potential range from −0.1 to 1.3 V at scan rate of 0.1 V s^{-1}, with only the first scan being recorded. Background cyclic voltammograms were subtracted from those obtained for apple extracts to allow the oxidation and reduction processes to be more clearly revealed. For the purpose of testing, the total anodic peak wave area of the voltammograms was calculated within the range of 0 to 1.1 V. This method was based on the correlations between the total anodic peak wave area of a cyclic voltammogram and the antioxidant capacity of the sample and reference substance. For the reference, a solution of Trolox within the concentration range of 0.15–1.00 mM was used, and the results were expressed as µmol TE/g FW.

2.8. Chelating Activity on Ferrous Ions

The chelating activity of ferrous irons was measured by the inhibition of the formation of an Fe^{2+}-ferrozine complex after treating the apple extracts with Fe^{2+} according to Mladénka et al. [41]. Briefly, 0.4 mL of apple extract (0.5 mg/mL) and 0.2 mL of HEPES (pH 7.5, 0.12 mM) were added to a solution of 0.4 mM FeSO$_4$·7H$_2$O (0.2 mL) and mixed for 2 min. Then, a volume of 800 µL of ferrozine solution (0.5 mM) was added and the absorbance of the ferrous ion–ferrozine complex was immediately measured at 562 nm. Ferrous ion solution was prepared daily and purged by argon 5.5 grade quality (Linde, Germany). For the comparison of ferrous chelating activity, deferoxamine (DEF) was used as a standard iron chelator. The amount of remaining ferrous ion was calculated from the difference of absorbance between the apple extract sample (with ferrozine) and its control blank (without ferrozine) was divided by the difference of the control sample (known amount of ferrous ion without apple extract) and its corresponding blank. A standard curve of Fe^{2+} ions was prepared within the range of concentration of 5–60 µM. The ferrous chelation efficiency of tested apple extract was expressed in %. Measurements were done at least in triplicate.

2.9. Analysis of Antioxidant Activity of Phenolic Compounds Identified by HPLC–DAD–MS/MS

The antioxidant activity of the phenolic compounds identified by HPLC–DAD–MS/MS in apple peel and flesh was provided by cyclic voltammetry and by spectrophotometric assays (DPPH, FRAP, and chelating activity). Stock solutions of each standard compound were also dissolved in 80% methanol (v/v, pH 6.0) and stored at −80 °C. Results were expressed as mM of Trolox of 9 independent experiments ($n = 9$). The ferrous chelation efficiency of apple phenolics was expressed in % of 9 replicates ($n = 9$).

2.10. Statistical Analyses

The analyses were performed in triplicate, and the results were displayed as the mean ± standard deviation (SD). The differences in identified phenolic contents in the peel and flesh of 11 apple cultivars were determined by one-way analysis of variance (ANOVA) with Fisher's least significant difference test ($p < 0.05$). Correlations between the antioxidant capacity assays and polyphenol compounds were analyzed using the Pearson correlation coefficient test. All analyses were performed using Statistica software (v. 12; StatSoft, Tulsa, OK, USA). Statistical significance thresholds for correlations were set at p-value < 0.05 (*), $p < 0.01$ (**) and $p < 0.001$ (***).

3. Results and Discussion

3.1. Total Phenolic Content (TPC) and Total Flavonoid Content (TFC)

According to several authors, the phenolic and flavonoid contents vary among different cultivars of fruits and vegetables, and within different tissues [42,43]. With respect to this condition, for this study, the cultivars were selected in order to eliminate the impact of soil, fertilizing method, and climatic conditions on apples, because all fruits were grown exclusively in one orchard (Pozorty, Olsztyn). It can be supposed that the antioxidant activity of apples depends, to a large extent, on the cultivar. The 11 apple cultivars selected for this study were characterized by an over-color of the peel that ranged from green-yellow (Papierówka and Antonówka) to red (Paulared, Quinte, Gloster, and Rubinola). The distribution of polyphenol compounds between the peel and flesh of analyzed cultivars for total phenolic content (TPC) for total flavonoid content (TFC) is shown in Table 2.

For all the studied cultivars, both the TPC and TFC were higher in the apple peel extract than in the flesh extract. Furthermore, significant differences were found between the cultivars ($p < 0.05$) in TPC and TFC. TPC ranged between 1821.3 and 3278.6 µg CAE/g fresh peel (Table 2). Quinte had the highest TPC, followed closely by Early Geneva and Jonagored (3278.6, 3147, and 3123.1 µg CAE/g fresh peel, respectively), whereas Ligol and Antonówka had the lowest TPC (1821.3 and 2051.6 µg CAE/g fresh peel, respectively). The remaining cultivars were intermediate, with a TPC varying between 2194.7 and 2916.1 µg CAE/g fresh peel. However, the total phenolics were lower in flesh than in peel, ranging from 535.5 to 1740.3 µg CAE/g fresh flesh (Table 2). Ligol and Gloster presented low contents with less than 600 µg CAE/g fresh flesh, whereas Quinte showed a concentration level of 1740.3 µg CAE/g fresh flesh. TPC values for the flesh and peel extracts of the studied apple cultivars were comparable with those previously reported by Tsao et al. [13] and Carbone et al. [18]. Tsao et al. [13] reported, for the eight most popular apple cultivars grown in Ontario, that the TPC ranged from 1016.5 to 2350.4 µg GAE/g of FW in the peel and 177.4 to 933.6 µg GAE/g of FW in the flesh. These values were found to be in agreement with our TPC results obtained for the 11 tested apple cultivars (1821.3 to 3278.6 µg CAE/g FW and 535.5 to 1740.3 µg CAE/g FW for peel and flesh, respectively). In the present study, the flavonoid content (TFC) ranged from 25% to 44.7% of the TPC in the peel and from 28.9% to 61.0% in the flesh, and these results are in agreement with those reported by Carbone et al. [18].

Table 2. Total phenolic content (TPC), total flavonoid content (TFC), Fe^{2+} chelation activity, and antioxidant activity by ferric-reducing/antioxidant power assay (FRAP), 2,2-diphenyl-1-picrylhydrazyl (DPPH), and cyclic voltammetry (CV) of the peel and flesh of different apple cultivars.

Apple Cultivars	FRAP	DPPH	CV	Chelating Activity	TPC	TFC
Apple Peel						
Quinte	21.31 ± 0.06a	7.51 ± 0.02d	6.09 ± 0.26b, c	51.80 ± 0.43b	3278.6 ± 29.0a	970.6 ± 6.3b
Jonagored	20.89 ± 0.23b	8.65 ± 0.02a	6.37 ± 0.32a, b	30.00 ± 0.39g	3123.1 ± 30.6b	830.1 ± 3.5e
Early Gen.	20.20 ± 0.21c	7.14 ± 0.01f	5.75 ± 0.15^c	48.23 ± 0.58d	3147.0 ± 38.1b	835.2 ± 23.3e
Paulared	19.38 ± 0.20d	7.39 ± 0.03e	6.80 ± 0.33a	39.90 ± 0.58e	2916.1 ± 42.5c	1303.8 ± 14.2a
Sunrise	17.44 ± 0.11e	6.90 ± 0.02g	5.86 ± 0.39c	36.36 ± 0.31f	2716.3 ± 37.2d	905.8 ± 5.6c
Gloster	16.90 ± 0.10f	8.19 ± 0.00b	5.69 ± 0.16c	24.27 ± 0.18h	2517.2 ± 56.2e	696.7 ± 3.1h
Delikates	14.70 ± 0.16g	6.67 ± 0.03h	5.23 ± 0.15d	30.71 ± 0.28g	2333.7 ± 16.1f	628.2 ± 10.9i
Papierówka	14.30 ± 0.16h	5.62 ± 0.03i	5.13 ± 0.31d	49.98 ± 0.88c	2194.7 ± 9.4g	875.1 ± 6.5d
Rubinola	14.21 ± 0.11h	7.91 ± 0.01c	4.97 ± 0.25d	23.59 ± 0.27h	2296.9 ± 4.1f	714.6 ± 2.4g
Antonówka	12.73 ± 0.23i	5.27 ± 0.03j	4.35 ± 0.22e	53.54 ± 0.61a	2051.6 ± 21.9h	766.6 ± 8.0f
Ligol	12.40 ± 0.14j	6.87 ± 0.02g	4.46 ± 0.15e	19.30 ± 0.36i	1821.3 ± 20.7i	553.1 ± 3.2j
Apple Flesh						
Quinte	10.15 ± 0.12a	4.65 ± 0.01a	3.95 ± 0.17a	45.89 ± 0.33d	1740.3 ± 19.4a	737.6 ± 3.9c
Jonagored	4.88 ± 0.07f	3.01 ± 0.01g	1.91 ± 0.04d	21.89 ± 0.12i	734.9 ± 7.2g	217.1 ± 1.9h, i
Early Gen.	9.28 ± 0.09b	4.20 ± 0.04b	3.14 ± 0.17b	47.51 ± 0.19c	1578.5 ± 33.3b	612.2 ± 9.2e
Paulared	7.51 ± 0.04d	3.48 ± 0.02d	3.04 ± 0.37b, c	33.52 ± 0.86e	1217.5 ± 4.1e	765.5 ± 6.6b
Sunrise	5.09 ± 0.09e	2.47 ± 0.02h	1.96 ± 0.22d	29.85 ± 0.23f	811.1 ± 11.1f	311.5 ± 4.0f
Gloster	3.15 ± 0.10i	2.23 ± 0.01k	1.49 ± 0.01e	23.02 ± 0.31h	544.3 ± 1.8i	223.0 ± 2.3h
Delikates	4.51 ± 0.05g	2.42 ± 0.01i	1.84 ± 0.25d	25.06 ± 1.12g	711.2 ± 7.3h	206.0 ± 6.3i
Papierówka	8.39 ± 0.02c	3.85 ± 0.01c	3.35 ± 0.20b	49.46 ± 0.54b	1356.2 ± 7.1c	831.1 ± 15.9a
Rubinola	4.80 ± 0.08f	3.12 ± 0.04f	1.92 ± 0.13d	24.99 ± 0.24g	830.4 ± 4.9f	296.9 ± 4.0g
Antonówka	7.60 ± 0.10d	3.19 ± 0.02e	2.83 ± 0.07c	60.0 ± 0.1a	1246.4 ± 13.4d	656.3 ± 5.9d
Ligol	3.44 ± 0.11h	2.37 ± 0.02j	1.44 ± 0.07e	18.31 ± 0.67j	535.6 ± 4.9i	178.7 ± 1.9j

Values represent the mean (n = 3) ± SD. Different letters a–j in the same column for peel or flesh indicate significant differences by ANOVA test ($p < 0.05$). Results for ferric reducing antioxidant power (FRAP), DPPH, and CV are expressed in Trolox equivalent per gram of apple fresh weight (µmol TE/g FW), and for chelating activity in % of chelating of Fe(II). TPC and TFC results are expressed in µg catechin equivalent (CAE)/g FW.

Recent studies also have demonstrated the influence of the apple cultivar on the fruit's phytochemical content [13,18] as well as a possible relationship between the color of different cultivars and their nutritional values [44]. In West Himalayan apple varieties, it was confirmed that there is a significant difference in phenolic content among cultivars and locations [45]. It was also confirmed that the variety and maturity of apples have a significant impact on chemical composition, the concentration of polyphenols, and level of antioxidant activity [35]. In a study of 120 apple varieties, a large diversity in polyphenolic compound content was observed depending on the variety [35]. According to this research, the highest phenolic content was found in Ozark Gold (~2116.03 mg/kg), and the lowest concentration was for Ligol (~814.17 mg/kg). The quality and quantity of polyphenols in apples directly influences their antioxidant activity [46].

While a TPC assay can adequately differentiate between apple cultivars that are high and low in polyphenols, it was less useful as a forecaster of potential health benefits. This is because the TPC measurements include nonabsorbable polymeric polyphenols as well as smaller, potentially absorbable polyphenolic compounds, which are thought to be mainly responsible for the observed physiological effects. Although some degradation products of polymeric polyphenols are absorbed in the colon, it is still not fully explained whether they have beneficial physiological effects. Whether the magnitude of polyphenol content has any relevance to the health properties of apples must then be tested by measuring the individual small molecular weight polyphenols.

3.2. Antioxidant and Chelating Capacity of Apple Flesh and Peel Determined by Spectrophotometric Assays

The antioxidant capacity of food should be evaluated with a variety of methods that can address the different mechanisms [47,48]. In the present study, spectrophotometric methods such as DPPH radical-scavenging activity and ferric reducing antioxidant power (FRAP) were used to determine the antioxidant capacity of apple extracts. The DPPH assay is based on a mixed mechanism of free radical DPPH• stabilization: hydrogen atom transfer and electron transfer. This assay presents some critical analytical points [49], but it has the great advantage of being easy to use. The FRAP assay is based on the ability of antioxidants to reduce ferric(III) ions to ferrous(II) ions by the electron transfer mechanism. The antioxidant capacity of apple peel and flesh extracts, evaluated by DPPH and FRAP assays and expressed as Trolox equivalent (μmol TE/g FW), is shown in Table 2.

The results obtained in the DPPH assay showed that, in general, the flesh and peel have intermediate radical-scavenging activity, with peels being better scavengers than flesh. Apple peel extracts from Jonagored (8.65 μmol TE/g FW), Gloster (8.19 μmol TE/g FW), and Rubinola (7.91 μmol TE/g FW) had the highest and extracts from Papierówka (5.62 μmol TE/g FW) and Antonówka (5.27 μmol TE/g FW) showed the lowest free radical scavenging capacity among the tested apple cultivars. In the case of apple flesh extracts, the DPPH values ranged between 2.23 and 4.65 μmol TE/g FW for Gloster and Quinte cultivars, respectively. These results were consistent with those reported for different apple varieties by Carbone et al. [18]. A highly significant relationship was found between the DPPH antiradical activity of apple flesh extracts and the concentration of TPC ($r = 0.96$; $p < 0.001$) and TFC ($r = 0.82$; $p < 0.01$). Panzela et al. [50] also found a good correlation between the percentage of reduced DPPH and the concentration of total polyphenols ($r = 0.79$) and total flavan-3-ols ($r = 0.77$).

For all the tested apple cultivars, peel extracts had a much greater ferric-reducing antioxidant power than flesh extracts, with a two-fold difference (Table 2). Quinte and Jonagored peel extracts had the highest FRAP values (21.31 μmol TE/g FW and 20.89 μmol TE/g FW, respectively), and Antonówka and Ligol peel extracts had the lowest (12.73 μmol TE/g FW and 12.40 μmol TE/g FW, respectively). These results were consistent with the total polyphenol and total flavonoid concentration in Early Geneva, Quinte, and Jonagored and in Ligol. The FRAP activity of the extracts from different apple cultivars was positively correlated with both total phenolic and total flavonoid content ($r = 0.9972$ and 0.8229, respectively). These results were in agreement with the findings of Tsao et al. [13], who studied the total phenolic compounds of eight apple cultivars and also obtained a good correlation between the TPC and FRAP activity ($r = 0.95$).

The phenolic compounds of apple may act as reducing agents, hydrogen donors, free radical scavengers, and singlet oxygen quenchers, and may exhibit antioxidant activity via the chelation of metal ions [23]. In this study, ferrous ion chelating activity was measured by the inhibition of the formation of a Fe(II)–ferrozine complex after the treatment of peel and flesh extracts with Fe(II). The chelating capacity of apple peel ranged from 51.80 (Quinte cultivar) to 19.30% (Ligol cultivar), while in flesh it was within the range of 49.46 (Papierówka cultivar) to 18.31% (Ligol cultivar). The chelating activities of peels of individual apple cultivars were significantly different and the same observation was noted for apple flesh ($p < 0.05$).

3.3. Reducing Capacity of Apple Flesh and Peel Determined by Cyclic Voltammetry

In this study, we conducted a critical evaluation of the cyclic voltammetry method for the determination and rapid screening of the reducing capacity of peel and flesh of 11 apple cultivars compared with DPPH and FRAP assays. The representative cyclic voltammograms of peel and flesh extracts (25 mg/mL) were recorded from −0.1 to 1.3 mV at a scan rate of 100 mV/s (Figures 1 and 2).

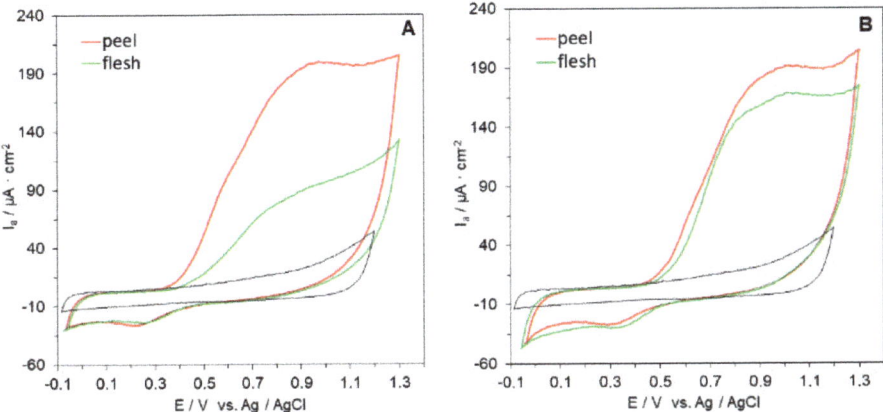

Figure 1. Cyclic voltammograms of peel and flesh extracts of selected apple cultivars: (**A**) Jonagored, (**B**) Antonówka. CV of electrolyte solution shown as dotted gray line. Operative conditions: extract concentration 25 mg/mL; pH 6.0; scan rate 0.1 V/s.

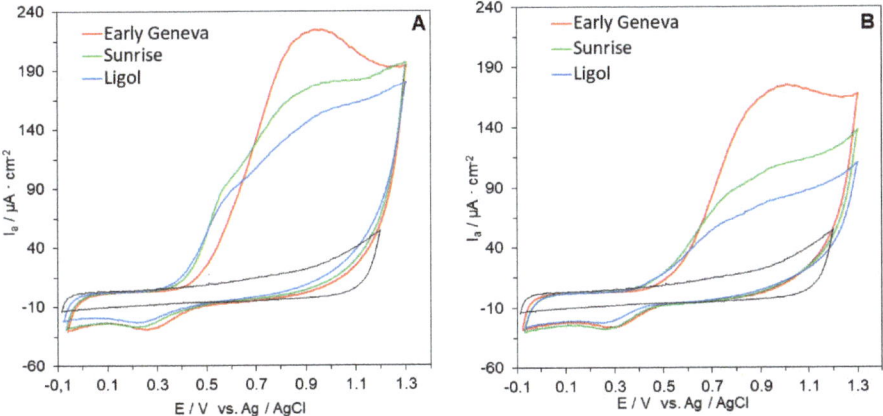

Figure 2. Cyclic voltammograms of selected apple cultivars: (**A**) extracts from peel; (**B**) extracts from flesh. CV of electrolyte solution shown as dotted gray line. Operative conditions: extract concentration 25 mg/mL; pH 6.0; scan rate 0.1 V/s.

The obtained voltammograms show that the apple extracts exhibited well defined oxidation and reduction voltammetric peaks. The area of each voltammetric peak was related to the concentration of antioxidants. A broad anodic peak between 0.4 and 1.0 V was observed. This peak was due to the response of several antioxidants with different oxidation potentials, mainly flavonoids and phenolic acids. The results show that the samples contained multiple reducing agents in the respective extracts. Therefore, the area under the anodic current waveform (area under the curve, AUC) was taken to reflect the reducing capacity of the samples compared to a set of Trolox solutions, as suggested by Chevion et al. [51], Martinez et al. [52], and Zielińska and Zieliński [40]. This provides a marked advantage in some cases, particularly when the AUC wave represents more than a single component. Higher AUC indicates a higher reducing capacity of the investigated extract.

The reducing capacity of peels as shown by CV ranged from 6.80 to 4.35 μmol TE/g FW (Table 2). The highest reducing capacity was noted for Paulared, Jonagored, and Quinte cultivars and the lowest for Rubinola, Antonówka, and Ligol. In contrast, the reducing capacity of apple flesh was noted to be at least twice as low (Table 2), ranging from 3.95 (Quinte) to 1.44 (Ligol) µmol TE/g FW. The reducing capacity of peels as shown by CV was positively correlated with both the total phenolic content ($r = 0.867$; $p < 0.01$) and total flavonoid content ($r = 0.752$, $p < 0.01$). The same trend in correlation efficient values was noted for apple flesh. This result was in agreement with other studies, in which CV was shown to be an efficient instrumental tool for evaluating the reducing capacity of plant, food, and biological samples. An advantage of electrochemical measurement compared to DPPH and FRAP is that it is fast. CV measurement is carried out in <10 min, so it is less tedious. Moreover, it is not necessary to use expensive reagents that include free radicals, thus lowering the cost. In addition, the use of a small amount of organic solvent reduces the amount of organic waste produced.

3.4. Profile and Content of Phenolic Compounds in Apple Flesh and Peel Measured by HPLC–DAD–ESI-MS/MS

Detailed knowledge of the polyphenol profile and content in apple cultivars is necessary in order to evaluate their antioxidant activity and potential beneficial health effects. A comprehensive qualitative analysis of the phenolic compounds of the studied apple peel and flesh samples was achieved by HPLC–DAD–MS/MS. The composition and concentrations of identified compounds in the peel and flesh are presented in Table 3. Eleven polyphenolic compounds belonging to five major groups were identified: chlorogenic acid (hydroxycinnamic acid), phloretin and phloridzin (dihydrochalcones), catechin and epicatechin (flavonols), and quercetin, and four derivatives (flavonols) and cyanidin 3-galactoside (anthocyanins). It was found that phenolic acids and flavonols were the two main groups of polyphenols identified in the studied apple cultivars, as previously reported [53]. Concentrations of individual phenolic compounds in peel and flesh identified by HPLC–DAD–MS/MS are shown in Table 3.

Among flavan-3-ols, epicatechin was the major compound of this group in apple peel and flesh. The highest concentration of epicatechin in peel was found for Quinte (297.77 µg/g FW) and Early Geneva (278.11 µg/g FW), while Delikates had the lowest content (94.79 µg/g FW). In the flesh, the Quinte cultivar was also found to possess the highest concentration of epicatechin (325.04 µg/g FW), followed by Early Geneva and Paulared (270.76 and 221.56 µg/g FW, respectively). These results are in accordance with those reported by Tsao et al. [13] for eight apple cultivars, in which epicatechin ranged from 17.9 to 591.6 µg/g FW in the peel and 16.0 to 142.3 µg/g FW in the flesh. Catechin was present in smaller amounts in peel extracts (3.83 to 92.16 µg/g FW) as well as flesh extracts (1.64 to 75.90 µg/g FW). These data are also in agreement with those obtained for eight traditional apple cultivars of Southern Italy [50], for which the concentration of catechin ranged from 0 to 76.7 µg/g FW).

Chlorogenic acid, which is the major compound of hydroxycinnamic acids, was mostly located in the apple flesh, except for Gloster, Jonagored, and Ligol cultivars, where the content of chlorogenic acid in peel was higher than in flesh. In the flesh, chlorogenic acid levels ranged between 18.21 and 451.53 µg/g FW, with the highest amounts being recorded in Papierówka, followed by Quinte, Antonówka, and Rubinola (Table 3). The lowest amounts were found in Delikates and Gloster (20.01 and 18.21 µg/g FW, respectively). The concentrations of chlorogenic acid obtained for some cultivars tested in this work, particularly Papierówka, were twice those found in the cultivars studied by Khanizadeh et al. [53] and Panzella et al. [50]. These observations indicate that the range of differences between the polyphenol profiles of apples are highly cultivar dependent.

Table 3. Concentrations of the individual phenolic compounds identified by the HPLC–DAD–MS/MS analysis in the apple peel and flesh in different cultivars.

	Quinte	Jonagored	Early Geneva	Paulared	Sunrise	Gloster	Delikates	Papierówka	Rubinola	Antonówka	Ligol
					Apple Peel						
Phloretin	0.96 ± 0.02d	0.91 ± 0.08d	0.85 ± 0.02e	0.64 ± 0.01g	1.38 ± 0.08b	1.32 ± 0.02b	b0.73 ± 0.03f	2.25 ± 0.05a	1.24 ± 0.05c	1.20 ± 0.01c	0.66 ± 0.04g
Phloridzin	23.91 ± 0.48d	24.65 ± 1.63d	24.45 ± 0.49d	16.43 ± 0.76e	48.08 ± 0.80b	43.45 ± 2.59c	18.30 ± 1.74e	84.10 ± 1.60a	42.90 ± 3.21c	23.37 ± 0.45d	16.51 ± 0.73e
Catechin	92.16 ± 1.99a	7.93 ± 0.07h, i	28.56 ± 0.62d	53.66 ± 0.46b	41.34 ± 0.29c	7.32 ± 0.53i	3.83 ± 0.31j	17.93 ± 1.21e	10.56 ± 0.80g	12.40 ± 0.12e	8.58 ± 0.29h
Epicatechin	297.77 ± 0.91a	103.17 ± 5.97h	278.11 ± 15.55b	161.68 ± 10.26e	198.36 ± 5.41c	142.23 ± 1.43f	94.79 ± 4.34h	165.57 ± 12.39e	182.86 ± 5.22d	127.72 ± 8.40g	101.28 ± 6.79h
Chlorogenic acid	188.59 ± 9.98c	57.00 ± 6.46g	57.41 ± 2.45g	68.97 ± 4.14f	87.27 ± 2.24e	61.67 ± 0.74g	8.05 ± 0.36h	259.58 ± 3.19a	206.97 ± 1.09b	137.17 ± 2.99d	58.62 ± 1.08g
Rutin	14.54 ± 0.60f	15.33 ± 0.47e, f	3.36 ± 0.07h	16.52 ± 0.49e	73.03 ± 0.94a	27.55 ± 2.38c	12.21 ± 0.67g	2.97 ± 0.08h	22.97 ± 0.74d	32.35 ± 0.72b	10.59 ± 3.31g
Quercetin 3-glucoside	131.46 ± 2.06b	120.55 ± 1.62c	33.80 ± 5.66h	76.04 ± 0.48e	265.76 ± 0.56a	125.36 ± 2.05c	95.13 ± 7.38d	52.41 ± 1.69g	68.01 ± 4.92f	49.20 ± 3.38g	70.20 ± 4.40f
Quercetin 3-arabinoside	0.98 ± 0.01a	0.73 ± 0.00d, e	0.65 ± 0.01g	0.77 ± 0.00c	0.81 ± 0.01b	0.69 ± 0.00f	0.73 ± 0.00d	0.71 ± 0.00e	0.80 ± 0.01b	0.61 ± 0.02h	0.76 ± 0.03c
Quercetin 3-rhamnoside	185.98 ± 0.69b	167.01 ± 1.68c	98.70 ± 2.20e	100.39 ± 2.96e	241.28 ± 8.75a	179.38 ± 14.91b	112.36 ± 0.94d	97.04 ± 0.98e	58.45 ± 0.88g	87.63 ± 5.37f	83.94 ± 3.32f
Quercetin	97.45 ± 14.86d	112.52 ± 1.94c	90.41 ± 2.41d	40.72 ± 1.12h	222.37 ± 1.80b	114.83 ± 3.98c	74.87 ± 0.97f	39.96 ± 1.51h	235.08 ± 0.43a	51.05 ± 1.08g	82.41 ± 4.61e
Cyanidin 3-galactoside	99.16 ± 2.16b	45.93 ± 0.48e	31.21 ± 1.32f	63.82 ± 4.79c	18.00 ± 1.52g	101.92 ± 0.31a	49.20 ± 0.95d	1.15 ± 0.00h	103.69 ± 2.17a	1.24 ± 0.00h	30.69 ± 1.00f
					Apple Flesh						
Phloretin	0.72 ± 0.03b	0.42 ± 0.01g	0.72 ± 0.01b	0.51 ± 0.02e	0.60 ± 0.03d	0.41 ± 0.00g	0.47 ± 0.01e, f	0.75 ± 0.03b	0.65 ± 0.03c	1.38 ± 0.08a	0.43 ± 0.01f, g
Phloridzin	18.89 ± 0.98d	7.17 ± 0.17h	20.63 ± 0.80c	10.37 ± 0.36f	14.68 ± 0.84e	5.86 ± 0.16i	9.14 ± 0.06g	23.46 ± 0.77b	18.09 ± 0.22d	45.05 ± 1.79a	6.61 ± 0.14h, i
Catechin	39.46 ± 0.20b	1.07 ± 0.01i	21.83 ± 0.61e	75.90 ± 1.44a	30.91 ± 0.49c	1.64 ± 0.57i	3.91 ± 0.22h	25.90 ± 0.33d	10.67 ± 0.39g	14.00 ± 0.29f	1.66 ± 0.06i
Epicatechin	325.04 ± 1.63a	18.64 ± 3.02g	270.76 ± 8.20b	221.56 ± 24.07c	68.76 ± 0.68f	4.99 ± 0.13h	68.27 ± 3.92f	154.17 ± 7.08d	100.67 ± 2.23e	78.23 ± 2.56f	13.81 ± 0.35g, h
Chlorogenic acid	307.17 ± 3.22b	43.56 ± 0.73g	154.91 ± 0.73e	265.59 ± 4.52d	85.07 ± 1.80f	18.21 ± 0.71h	20.01 ± 2.19h	451.53 ± 19.59a	264.47 ± 10.42d	293.56 ± 7.19c	26.74 ± 2.63h
Rutin	0.79 ± 0.00d	1.07 ± 0.05a	0.70 ± 0.01g	0.84 ± 0.00c	1.00 ± 0.00b	0.72 ± 0.01f	0.75 ± 0.00e	0.64 ± 0.00h	0.75 ± 0.01e	0.64 ± 0.00h	0.69 ± 0.03g
Quercetin 3-glucoside	2.12 ± 0.03a	1.58 ± 0.02c	1.27 ± 0.03e	1.97 ± 0.03b	1.96 ± 0.07b	1.06 ± 0.12g	1.34 ± 0.02d	1.06 ± 0.03g	1.03 ± 0.05g	0.81 ± 0.00h	1.18 ± 0.04f
Quercetin 3-arabinoside	n.d.	n.d.	n.d.	n.d.	n.d.	n.d.	n.d.	n.d.	n.d.	n.d.	n.d.
Quercetin 3-rhamnoside	6.89 ± 0.17a	5.69 ± 0.45b	4.10 ± 0.08d	4.84 ± 0.19c	4.60 ± 0.40c	2.33 ± 0.25f	1.47 ± 0.05g, h	2.84 ± 0.21e	1.76 ± 0.15g	1.21 ± 0.01h	2.76 ± 0.02e
Quercetin	1.63 ± 0.04g	15.39 ± 0.32a	1.12 ± 0.02i	1.38 ± 0.02h	10.55 ± 0.36h	3.01 ± 0.04f	1.72 ± 0.06g	3.68 ± 0.05e	4.67 ± 0.29d	1.15 ± 0.04h, i	6.22 ± 0.12c
Cyanidin 3-galactoside	1.29 ± 0.06a	0.68 ± 0.01e	1.10 ± 0.00b	0.83 ± 0.01c	0.70 ± 0.00d, e	0.59 ± 0.00g	0.72 ± 0.00d	0.54 ± 0.00h	0.65 ± 0.01f	0.55 ± 0.00h	0.61 ± 0.00g

Values represent the mean ($n = 4$) ± SD. Different letters a–j in the same row related to apple peel or flesh indicate significant differences by ANOVA test ($p < 0.05$). n.d., not detected. Results are expressed in µg/g FW.

Differences were also observed in the content of dihydrochalcones. Phloridzin (phloretin 2′-glucoside) was the predominant dihydrochalcone found and identified in all tested apple peel and flesh extracts. Phloretin and phloretin derivatives have occasionally been found in apple in trace amounts [13]. Phloridzin concentration was higher in apple peel, with a mean value of 33.28 μg/g FW compared to 16.38 μg/g FW in flesh (Table 3). Khanizadeh et al. [53] reported an average concentration of phloridzin in the peel and flesh of 10.4 and 55.4 μg/g FW, respectively. Among the tested apple cultivars, Papierówka in particular was characterized by the highest level of phloridzin (84.10 μg/g FW in peel), whose anti-diabetic properties have recently been reported by Masumoto et al. [54]. Even though dihydrochalcones exist in relatively low amounts due to the uniqueness of the apple and their different profiles among different cultivars, they have been used to distinguish apple from a number of other fruits and to identify apple cultivars [13].

Flavonols represent the second largest group in terms of concentration in apple peel. These polyphenols were constituted mainly by quercetin 3-arabinoside, followed by 3-rhamnoside and 3-glucoside, and slightly by quercetin and rutin. Depending on the cultivar, the total flavonols in the peel varied from 193.09 to 808.25 μg/g FW, with Sunrise showing the highest concentration (Table 3). These data are consistent with those reported by Tsao et al. [13]. On the other hand, in the flesh extracts of studied apple cultivars, only small amounts of quercetin 3-arabinoside, 3-rhamnoside, and 3-glucoside were detected (Table 3).

The major anthocyanins in apple are cyanidin glycosides, among which 3-galactoside is the predominant individual compound. Anthocyanins were found only in apples characterized by red and partially red skin (Quinte, Paulared, Gloster, and Rubinola), and only cyanidin 3-galactoside was identified in our study (Table 3). Cyanidin 3-galactoside content ranged from 1.15 to 103.69 μg/g FW and was the highest for Rubinola. This observation was consistent with that reported by Khanizadeh et al. [53].

According to Kschonsek et al. [43], the most abundant flavonoids that occur in apples (raw, with skin) are (-)-epicatechin, (+)-catechin, and cyanidin. The same flavonoids were found in apples without skin, but also a high amount of (-)-epigallocatechin. The main polyphenols that can be found in apples are quercetin, (-)-epicatechin, (+)-catechin, procyanidines, and anthocyanidines; dihydrochalcones; phloretin and phloridzin derivatives; and other phenolic compounds, such as chlorogenic acid. In addition, it was important that apples were shown to have the highest portion of free phenolics when compared to other fruits [4]. Apple's bound phenolics have lower bioavailability as compared to free phenolics since they need to be released from the food matrix after digestion [55].

3.5. Antioxidant, Reducing, and Chelating Activities of Phenolic Compounds in Apple Flesh and Peel

The antioxidant, reducing, and chelating activities of phenolic compounds identified in apple peel and flesh by HPLC–DAD–MS/MS are shown in Table 4. The antioxidant activity of phenolic compounds from apple flesh and peel, determined as free radical-scavenging activity against stable, nonbiological relevant DPPH radicals, is expressed as Trolox equivalent. As it was defined, antioxidant activity is equal to the millimolar concentration of a Trolox solution that has antioxidant capacity equivalent to a 1.0 mM solution of the substance under investigation.

Quercetin, cyanidin 3-galactoside, rutin, catechin, and chlorogenic acid (2.09–1.45 mM Trolox) showed the highest ability to scavenge DPPH radicals, followed by quercetin 3-glucoside, epicatechin, quercetin 3-rhamnoside, and quercetin 3-arabinoside (1.42–0.95 mM Trolox), while the ability to scavenge DPPH radicals by phloretin (0.19 mM Trolox) and phloridzin (0.06 mM Trolox) was the lowest.

The order of reducing activity as shown by the FRAP assay was as follows: cyanidin 3-galactoside > quercetin > chlorogenic acid > quercetin 3-glucoside > catechin > epicatechin > quercetin 3-rhamnoside > rutin > quercetin 3-arabinoside > phloretin > phloridzin (5.69–0.18 mM Trolox). This order was supported by a study on the structure–activity relationship (SAR) of flavonoids [56,57].

Table 4. Antioxidant, reducing, and chelating activities of phenolic compounds identified in apple peel and flesh by HPLC–DAD–MS/MS.

Compound/Assay	Antioxidant Activity (mM Trolox)	Reducing Activity (mM Trolox)		Chelating Activity (%)
	DPPH	FRAP	CV	FZ
Phloretin	0.19 ± 0.01	0.95 ± 0.02	0.46 ± 0.02	1.15 ± 0.06
Phloridzin	0.06 ± 0.01	0.18 ± 0.01	0.26 ± 0.03	5.68 ± 0.30
Catechin	1.55 ± 0.02	1.97 ± 0.01	0.39 ± 0.03	74.56 ± 3.65
Epicatechin	1.37 ± 0.01	1.95 ± 0.15	0.69 ± 0.03	70.14 ± 2.80
Chlorogenic acid	1.45 ± 0.01	3.71 ± 0.07	0.34 ± 0.02	88.47 ± 2.65
Rutin	1.69 ± 0.02	1.64 ± 0.06	0.46 ± 0.01	85.33 ± 2.56
Quercetin 3-glucoside	1.42 ± 0.03	2.08 ± 0.01	0.23 ± 0.03	70.25 ± 2.10
Quercetin	2.09 ± 0.03	3.68 ± 0.19	0.90 ± 0.04	76.84 ± 2.31
Quercetin 3-arabinoside	0.95 ± 0.03	1.52 ± 0.01	0.19 ± 0.20	69.74 ± 2.10
Quercetin 3-rhamnoside	1.27 ± 0.02	1.89 ± 0.03	0.24 ± 0.01	68.13 ± 2.38
Cyanidin 3-galactoside	2.07 ± 0.03	5.69 ± 0.02	0.65 ± 0.02	29.11 ± 1.02

Results were provided by DPPH radical scavenging activity assay. FRAP: ferric-reducing/antioxidant power assay; CV: cyclic voltammetry assay; FZ: ferrozine assay. Data expressed as the mean ± standard deviation ($n = 9$).

In this study, cyclic voltammograms of the phenolic compounds identified in apple flesh and peel were recorded in the range of −100 to +1300 mV at a scanning rate of 100 mV s^{-1}. Cyclic voltammograms of 0.25 mM solutions of examined compounds in 0.1 M Britton–Robinson (B–R) buffer (pH 6.0) in 80% methanol are shown in Figure 3.

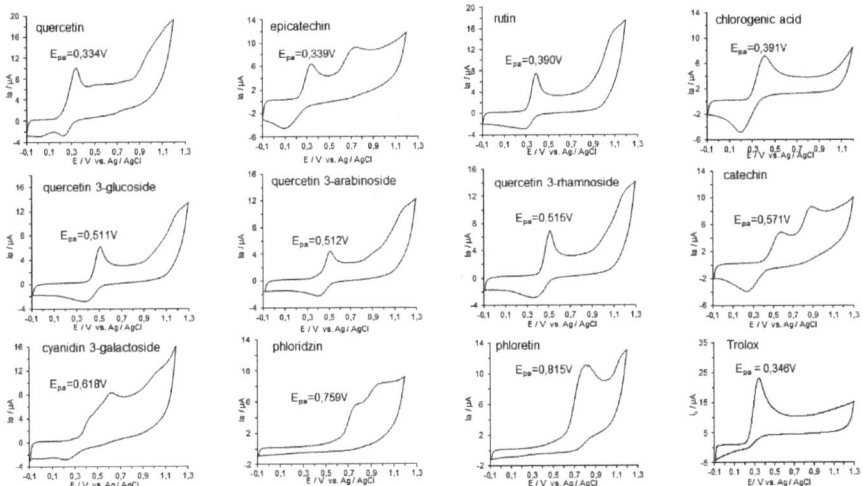

Figure 3. Cyclic voltammograms of 0.25 mM of standard solutions (final concentration) of phenolic compounds in apple cultivars identified by HPLC–DAD–MS/MS analysis in Britton–Robinson (B–R) buffer (0.1 M; pH 7.4) recorded from −100 to +1300 mV; scan rate 100 mV s^{-1}.

The cyclic voltammograms showed that all compounds had well defined reversible waves with the first oxidation peak potential. The first anodic peak potential (E_{pa}) of the investigated compounds varied according to the following gradation: phloretin (0.815 V) > phloridzin (0.759 V) > cyanidin 3-galactoside (0.618 V) > catechin (0.571 V) > quercetin 3-rhamnoside (0.515 V) > quercetin 3-arabinoside

(0.512 V) ≥ quercetin 3-glucoside (0.511 V) > chlorogenic acid (0.391 V) ≥ rutin (0.390 V) > epicatechin (0.339 V) ≥ quercetin (0.334 V) as compared to Trolox (0.346 V). Higher Ep_a values were associated with lower reducing activity of the tested compound. Therefore, taking into account the values of the first oxidation potential of the studied compounds, almost all phenolic compounds identified in apple flesh and peel can be described as having high (intermediate) antioxidant power (Ep < 0.8 V), while phloretin had low antioxidant power (0.8 V < Ep < 1.3 V). This conclusion was drawn based on the work by Blasco et al. [58], in which the differentiation of the antioxidant power of phenolic compounds was based on their oxidation potential. When the calculation of antioxidant activity was based on the area under the anodic current waveform within the range of 0 to 1100 mV for each compound and Trolox, then the order of antioxidant activity was as follows: quercetin > epicatechin > cyanidin 3-galactoside > rutin ≥ phloretin > catechin > chlorogenic acid > phloridzin ≥ quercetin 3-rhamnoside ≥ quercetin 3-glucoside > quercetin 3-arabinoside (0.90–0.19 mM Trolox). The gradation of samples for reducing activity as determined by CV mirrored that obtained with the FRAP assay.

The highest ferrous ion chelating activity was shown by chlorogenic acid (88.47%), followed by rutin, quercetin, catechin, epicatechin, quercetin 3-glucoside, quercetin 3-arabinoside, and quercetin 3-rhamnoside (68.13%); activity twice as low was noted for cyanidin 3-galactoside, and the lowest was for phloridzin and phloridzin (5.68 and 1.15%, respectively).

3.6. Phenolic Contribution to Antioxidant Activity

A correlation analysis was performed to assess the contribution of polyphenolic compounds to antioxidant capacity. Interestingly, the association between antioxidant assays and the content of bioactive compounds differed between apple peel and flesh (Table 5).

In apple peel, catechin and epicatechin content was positively correlated to FRAP assay, while cyadinin-3-galactoside was highly associated with DPPH. Moreover, a strong correlation was found between the total phenolic and flavonoid content and FRAP and CV (Table 5).

Table 5. Correlation coefficient between phenolic compounds and antioxidant capacity tests and linear correlation coefficient between different methods for antioxidant capacity assessment in apple peel and flesh.

	FRAP	DPPH	CV	Chelating Activity
Apple Peel				
Phloretin	−0.189	−0.388	−0.232	0.295
Phloridzin	−0.155	−0.258	−0.134	0.156
Catechin	0.628 *	0.079	0.541	0.526
Epicatechin	0.659 *	0.083	0.332	0.549
Chlorogenic acid	−0.110	−0.312	−0.232	0.420
Rutin	−0.093	−0.015	0.045	−0.090
Quercetin-3-glucoside	0.198	0.270	0.362	−0.174
Quercetin	0.299	0.353	0.365	−0.029
Quercetin-3-arabinose	0.460	0.330	0.509	0.027
Quercetin-3-rhamnoside	−0.045	0.439	0.015	−0.439
Cyadinin-3-galactoside	0.190	0.744 **	0.350	−0.393
Total polyphenol	0.980 ***	0.553	0.867 **	0.324
Total flavonoid	0.607 *	0.069	0.752 **	0.498
FRAP	1.000	–	–	–
DPPH	0.413	1.000	–	–
CV	0.824 **	0.600	1.000	–
Chelating activity	0.451	−0.562	0.104	1.000

Table 5. Cont.

	FRAP	DPPH	CV	Chelating Activity
		Apple Flesh		
Phloretin	0.551	0.372	0.491	0.862 **
Phloridzin	0.590	0.412	0.519	0.879 ***
Catechin	0.524	0.508	0.642 *	0.340
Epicatechin	0.874 ***	0.915 ***	0.897 ***	0.587
Chlorogenic acid	0.773 **	0.719 *	0.791 **	0.737 *
Rutin	−0.272	−0.174	−0.225	−0.444
Quercetin-3-glucoside	0.203	0.282	0.321	−0.122
Quercetin	−	−	−	−
Quercetin-3-arabinose	0.379	0.521	0.455	0.020
Quercetin-3-rhamnoside	−0.447	−0.360	−0.466	−0.508
Cyadinin-3-galactoside	0.604 *	0.720 *	0.626 *	0.267
Total polyphenol	0.988 ***	0.956 ***	0.978 ***	0.838 **
Total flavonoid	0.905 ***	0.820 **	0.939 ***	0.841 **
FRAP	1.000	−	−	−
DPPH	0.943 ***	1.000	−	−
CV	0.975 ***	0.939 ***	1.000	−
Chelating activity	0.866 **	0.694 *	0.816 **	1.000

*, **, *** Significant correlation at $p < 0.05$, $p < 0.01$, $p < 0.001$, respectively.

In the apple flesh, FRAP showed a very strong correlation with epicatechin, chlorogenic acid, and cyaniding-3-galactoside. Similarly, DPPH and CV were correlated with the same compounds, and CV was additionally correlated with catechin. The chelating activity assay showed the strongest correlation with phloretin, phloridzin, and chlorogenic acid (Table 5). Among the antioxidant capacity tests, the strongest correlation was observed between CV and FRAP in apple peel, and between all assays in apple flesh.

4. Conclusions

It needs to be noted that the ripe apples are a good source of phenolic compounds, being present in both peel and flesh. According to the available literature, the geographical origin and variety of apples influence the content of phenolic compounds and are highly related to their antioxidant activity fluctuation. In this study, the apple peel and flesh of early varieties such as Antonówka, Delikates, Early Geneva, Papierówka, Paulared, Sunrise, Quinte showed higher total phenolic and flavonoids content as compared to the late varieties such as Gloster, Jonagored, Ligol and Rubinola. The HPLC–DAD–MS/MS analysis showed that the dominant compounds were catechin, epicatechin, chlorogenic acid, quercetin 3-glucoside, quercetin 3-arabinoside, quercetin 3-rhamnoside, cyanidin 3-galactoside and phloridzin whereas phloretin, quercetin and rutin were present in low concentration. These phenolic compounds varied considerably among apple cultivars and their content was higher in peels than in flesh. Information about cultivar–typical apple polyphenol content and profile is important for bioactivity studies and, consequently, essential for the development of consumer-relevant products with particular nutritional functionalities. Therefore, it can be concluded that whole ripe apples should be used as a relevant source of phenolics in our diet since the removal of peel from apple may induce a significant loss of antioxidants. On the other hand, apple peels can be a good component to formulate functional foods after currently proposed "cold-pressing technology" as an effective method for peeling and deseeding apple fruits, with a positive effect on phenolic compounds retention in pomace. This study showed that the application of HPLC–DAD–MS/MS analysis of phenolic compounds with the spectrophotometric methods for the determination of their antioxidant, reducing and chelating capacity and their electroactivity provided by cyclic voltammetry was essential to show their contribution to the antioxidant capacity of apple peel and flesh. This study also provides evidence to support the application of cyclic voltammetry as a rapid method in determining the phenolic profile and reducing power of apple flesh and peel.

Author Contributions: Conceptualization, D.Z.; methodology, D.Z., M.T.; formal analysis, D.Z., M.T.; investigation, writing—original draft preparation, D.Z., M.T.; writing—review and editing, D.Z. All authors have read and agreed to the published version of the manuscript.

Funding: The project was financially supported by the Ministry of Science and Higher Education within the Regional Initiative of Excellence program for 2019–2022, project no. 010/RID/2018/19, amount of funding PLN 12,000,000.

Conflicts of Interest: The authors declare no conflict of interest.

References

1. Chodak, A.D.; Tarko, T.; Satora, P.; Sroka, P.; Tuszyński, T.T. The profile of polyphenols and antioxidant properties of selected apple cultivars grown in Poland. *J. Fruit. Ornam. Plant Res.* **2010**, *18*, 39–50.
2. Sies, H. Polyphenols and health: Update and perspectives. *Arch Biochem. Biophys.* **2010**, *501*, 2–5. [CrossRef]
3. Bizjak, B.K.; Vodopivec, B.M.; Eler, K.; Ogrinc, N.; Mulič, I.; Masuero, D.; Vrhovšek, U. Primary and secondary metabolites as a tool for differentiation of apple juice according to cultivar and geographical origin. *LWT-Food Sci. Technol.* **2018**, *90*, 238–245.
4. Boyer, J.; Liu, L.H. Apple phytochemicals and their health benefits. *Nutr. J.* **2004**, *3*, 1–15. [CrossRef]
5. Graziani, G.; D'Argenio, G.; Tuccillo, C.; Loguercio, C.; Ritieni, A.; Morisco, F. Apple polyphenol extracts prevent damage to human gastric epithelial cells in vitro and to rat gastric mucosa in vivo. *Gut* **2005**, *54*, 193–200. [CrossRef]
6. Leopoldini, M.; Russo, N.; Toscano, M. The molecular basis of working mechanism of natural polyphenolic antioxidants. *Food Chem.* **2010**, *125*, 288–306. [CrossRef]
7. Zielińska, D.; Laparra-Llopis, J.M.; Zieliński, H.; Szawara-Nowak, D.; Gimenez Bastida, J.A. Role of Apple Phytochemicals, Phloretin and Phloridzin, in Modulating Processes Related to Intestinal Inflammation. *Nutrients* **2019**, *11*, 1173. [CrossRef]
8. Spencer, J.P.E. The impact of fruit flavonoids on memory and cognition. *Br. J. Nutr.* **2010**, *104*, S40–S47. [CrossRef] [PubMed]
9. Giomaro, G.; Karioti, A.; Bilia, A.R.; Bucchini, A.; Giamperi, L.; Donata, R.D.; Fraternale, D. Polyphenols profile and antioxidant activity of skin and pulp of a rare apple from Marche region (Italy). *Chem. Cent. J.* **2014**, *8*, 45–55. [CrossRef]
10. Scalbert, A.; Manach, C.; Morand, C.; Remsey, C.; Jimenez, L. Dietary polyphenols and the prevention of diseases. *Crit. Rev. Food Sci. Nutr.* **2005**, *45*, 287–306. [CrossRef]
11. Sun, J.; Chu, Y.F.; Wu, X.; Liu, R.H. Antioxidant and antiproliferative activities of common fruits. *J. Agric. Food Chem.* **2002**, *50*, 7449–7454. [CrossRef]
12. Oleszek, W.; Lee, C.Y.; Jaworski, A.W.; Price, K.R. Identification of some phenolic compounds in apples. *J. Agric. Food Chem.* **1988**, *36*, 430–432. [CrossRef]
13. Tsao, R.; Yang, R.; Young, J.C.; Zhu, H. Polyphenolic profiles in eight apples cultivars using high-performance liquid chromatography (HPLC). *J. Agric. Food Chem.* **2003**, *51*, 6347–6353. [CrossRef]
14. Alonso-Salces, R.M.; Barranco, A.; Abad, B.; Berrueta, L.A.; Gallo, B.; Vicente, F. Polyphenolic profiles of basque cider apples cultivars and their technological properties. *J. Agric. Food Chem.* **2004**, *52*, 2938–2952. [CrossRef]
15. Awad, M.A.; De Jager, A.; van Westing, L.M. Flavonoid and chlorogenic acid levels in apple fruit: Characterization and variation. *Sci. Hortic.* **2000**, *83*, 249–263. [CrossRef]
16. Guyot, S.; Marnet, N.; Laraba, D.; Sanonerm, P.; Drilleau, J.F. Reversed-phase HPLC following thiolysis for quantitative estimation and characterization of the four main classes of phenolic compounds in different tissue zones of a French cider apple variety. *J. Agric. Food Chem.* **1998**, *46*, 1698–1705. [CrossRef]
17. McRae, K.B.; Lidster, P.D.; de Marco, A.C.; Dick, A.J. Comparison of the polyphenol profiles of the apple fruit cultivars by correspondence analysis. *J. Sci. Food Agric.* **1990**, *50*, 329–342. [CrossRef]
18. Carbone, K.; Giannini, B.; Picchi, V.; Lo Scalzo, R.; Cecchini, F. Phenolic composition and free radical scavenging activity of different apple cultivars in relation to the cultivar, tissue type and storage. *Food Chem.* **2011**, *127*, 493–500. [CrossRef]

19. Napolitano, A.; Cascone, A.; Graziani, G.; Ferracane, R.; Scalfi, L.; Di Vaio, C. Influence of variety and storage on the polyphenol composition of apple flesh. *J. Agric. Food Chem.* **2004**, *52*, 6526–6531. [CrossRef]
20. Scalzo, J.; Politi, A.; Pellegrini, N.; Mezzetti, B.; Battino, M. Plant genotype affects total antioxidant capacity and phenolic contents in fruits. *Nutrition* **2005**, *21*, 207–213. [CrossRef]
21. Volz, R.K.; McGhie, T.K. Genetic variability in apple fruit polyphenol composition in *Malus x domestica* and *Malus sieversil* germplasm grown in New Zealand. *J. Agric. Food Chem.* **2011**, *59*, 11509–11521.
22. Kahkonen, M.P.; Hopia, A.I.; Vuorela, H.J.; Rauha, J.P.; Pihlaja, K.; Kujala, T.S.; Heinonen, M. Antioxidant activity of plant extracts containing phenolic compounds. *J. Agric. Food Chem.* **1999**, *47*, 3954–3962.
23. Gulcin, I. Antioxidant activity of food constituents: An overview. *Arch Toxicol.* **2012**, *86*, 345–391. [PubMed]
24. Sanchez-Moreno, C. Review: Methods used to evaluate the free radical scavenging activity in foods and biological systems. *Food Sci. Technol. Int.* **2002**, *8*, 121–137. [CrossRef]
25. Arteaga, J.F.; Ruiz-Montoya, M.; Palma, A.; Alonso-Garrido, G.; Pintado, S.; Rodriguez-Mellad, J.M. Comparison of the simple cyclic voltammetry (CV) and DPPH assay for the determination of antioxidant capacity of active principles. *Molecules* **2012**, *17*, 5126–5138. [CrossRef] [PubMed]
26. Gomes, S.M.; Ghica, M.-E.; Rodrigues, I.A.; de Souza Gil, E.; Oliveira-Brett, A.M. Flavonoids electrochemical detection in fruit extracts and total antioxidant capacity evaluation. *Talanta* **2016**, *154*, 284–291. [CrossRef] [PubMed]
27. Lino, F.; de Sá, L.; Torres, I.; Rocha, M.; Dinis, T.; Ghedini, P. Voltammetric and spectrometric determination of antioxidant capacity of selected wines. *Electrochim. Acta* **2014**, *128*, 25–31. [CrossRef]
28. de Oliveira Neto, J.R.; Rezende, S.G.; Lobón, G.S.; Garcia, T.A.; Macedo, I.Y.L.; Garcia, L.F. Electroanalysis and laccase-based biosensor on the determination of phenolic content and antioxidant power of honey samples. *Food Chem.* **2017**, *237*, 1118–1123. [CrossRef]
29. Jiao, Y.; Kilmartin, P.A.; Fan, M.; Quek, S.Y. Assessment of phenolic contributors to antioxidant activity of new kiwifruit cultivars using cyclic voltammetry combined with HPLC. *Food Chem.* **2018**, *268*, 77–85. [CrossRef]
30. Lugonja, N.M.; Stankovic, D.M.; Spasic, S.D.; Roglic, G.M.; Manojlovic, D.D.; Vrvic, M.M. Comparative electrochemical determination of total antioxidant activity in infant formula with breast milk. *Food Anal. Methods* **2014**, *7*, 337–344. [CrossRef]
31. Gulaboski, R.; Mirceski, V.; Mitrev, S. Development of a rapid and simple voltammetric method to determine total antioxidative capacity of edible oils. *Food Chem.* **2013**, *138*, 116–121. [CrossRef] [PubMed]
32. Hossain, M.A.; Salehuddin, S.M.; Kabir, M.J.; Rahman, S.M.M.; Rupasinghe, H.P.V. Sinensetin, rutin, 3′-hydroxy-5,6,7,4′-teramethoxyflavone and rosmarinic acid contents and antioxidative effect of the skin of apple fruit. *Food Chem.* **2009**, *113*, 185–190. [CrossRef]
33. Kondo, S.; Tsuda, K.; Muto, N.; Ueda, J. Antioxidant activity of apple skin or flesh extracts associated with fruit development on selected apple cultivars. *Sci. Hortic.* **2002**, *96*, 177–185. [CrossRef]
34. Lu, Y.; Foo, L.Y. Antioxidant and radical scavenging activities of polyphenols from apple pomace. *Food Chem.* **2000**, *68*, 81–85. [CrossRef]
35. Oszmiański, J.; Wolniak, M.; Wojdyło, A.; Wawer, I. Influence of apple puree preparation and storage on polyphenol contents and antioxidant activity. *Food Chem.* **2008**, *107*, 1473–1484. [CrossRef]
36. Shahidi, F.; Naczk, M. Methods of analysis and quantification of phenolic compounds. In *Food Phenolic: Sources, Chemistry, Effects and Applications*; Shahidi, F., Naczk, M., Eds.; Technomic Publishing Company: Lancaster, UK, 1995; pp. 287–293.
37. Jia, Z.; Tang, M.; Wu, J. The determination of flavonoid contents in mulberry and their scavenging effects on superoxides radical. *Food Chem.* **1998**, *64*, 555–559.
38. Benzie, I.F.F.; Strain, J.J. Ferric reducing antioxidant power assay: Direct measure of total antioxidant activity of biological fluids and modified version for simultaneous measurement of total antioxidant power and ascorbic acid concentration. *Method. Enzymol.* **1999**, *299*, 15–27.
39. Brand-Williams, W.; Cuvelier, M.E.; Berset, C. Use of a free radical method to evaluate antioxidant activity. *LWT-Food Sci. Technol.* **1995**, *28*, 25–30. [CrossRef]
40. Zielińska, D.; Zieliński, H. Antioxidant activity of flavone C-glucosides determined by updated analytical strategies. *Food Chem.* **2011**, *124*, 672–678. [CrossRef]
41. Mladenka, P.; Zatloukalova, L.; Filipsky, T.; Hrdina, R. Cardiovascular effects of flavonoids are not caused only by direct antioxidant activity. *Free Radical Biol. Med.* **2010**, *49*, 963–975. [CrossRef]

42. Van der Sluis, A.A.; Dekker, M.; de Jager, A.; Wim Jongen, M.F. Activity and concentration of polyphenolic antioxidants in apple: Effect of cultivar, harvest year, and storage condition. *J. Agric. Food Chem.* **2001**, *49*, 3606–3613. [CrossRef]
43. Kschonsek, J.; Wolfram, T.; Stöckl, A.; Böhm, V. Polyphenolic compounds analysis of old and new apple cultivars and contribution of polyphenolic profile to the in vitro antioxidant capacity. *Antioxidants* **2018**, *7*, 20. [CrossRef]
44. Drogoudi, P.D.; Michailidis, Z.; Pantelidis, G. Peel and flesh antioxidant content and harvest quality characteristics of seven apple cultivars. *Sci. Hortic.* **2008**, *115*, 149–153. [CrossRef]
45. Bahukhandi, A.; Dhyani, P.; Bhatt, I.D.; Rawal, R.S. Variation in polyphenolics and antioxidant activity of traditional apple cultivars from West Himalaya, Uttarakhand. *Hortic. Plant J.* **2018**, *4*, 151–157. [CrossRef]
46. Wojdyło, A.; Oszmiański, J.; Laskowski, P. Phenolic composition and antioxidant activity of selected apple from Europe. *J. Clin. Biochem. Nutr.* **2018**, *43*, 548–553.
47. Huang, D.; Ou, B.; Prior, R.L. The chemistry behind antioxidant capacity assays. *J. Agric. Food Chem.* **2005**, *53*, 1841–1856. [CrossRef]
48. Perez-Jimenez, J.; Arranz, S.; Tabernero, M.; Diaz-Rubio, E.; Serrano, J.; Goni, I. Updated methodology to determine antioxidant capacity in plant foods, oils and beverages: Extraction, measurements and expression of results. *Food Res. Int.* **2008**, *41*, 274–285. [CrossRef]
49. Prior, R.L.; Wu, X.; Schaich, K. Standardized methods for the determination of antioxidant capacity and phenolics in foods and dietary supplements. *J. Agric. Food Chem.* **2005**, *53*, 4290–4302. [CrossRef]
50. Panzela, L.; Petriccone, M.; Rega, P.; Scortichini, M.; Napolitano, A. A reappraisal of traditional apple cultivars from Southern Italy as a rich source of phenols with superior antioxidant activity. *Food Chem.* **2013**, *140*, 672–679. [CrossRef]
51. Chevion, S.; Roberts, M.A.; Chevion, M. The use of cyclic voltammetry for the evaluation of antioxidant capacity. *Free Radic. Biol. Med.* **2000**, *28*, 860–870. [CrossRef]
52. Martinez, S.; Valek, L.; Resetic, J.; Rusic, D.F. Cyclic voltammetry study of plasma antioxidant capacity–comparison with the DPPH and TAS spectrophotometric methods. *J. Electroanal. Chem.* **2006**, *588*, 68–73. [CrossRef]
53. Khanizadeh, S.; Tsao, R.; Rekika, D.; Yang, R.; Charles, M.T.; Rupasinghe, H.P.V. Polyphenol composition and total antioxidant capacity of selected apple genotypes for processing. *J. Food Compost. Anal.* **2008**, *21*, 396–401. [CrossRef]
54. Masumoto, S.; Akimoto, Y.; Oike, H.; Kobori, M. Dietary phloridzin reduces blood glucose levels and reverses Sglt1 expression in the small intestine in streptozotocin-induced diabetic mice. *J. Agric. Food Chem.* **2009**, *57*, 4651–4656. [CrossRef]
55. Williamson, G.; Kay, C.D.; Crozier, A. The Bioavailability, Transport, and Bioactivity of Dietary Flavonoids: A Review from a Historical Perspective. *Compr. Rev. Food Sci. Food Saf.* **2018**, *17*, 1054–1112. [CrossRef]
56. Rice-Evans, C.A.; Miller, N.J.; Bolwell, P.G.; Bramley, P.M.; Pridham, J.B. The relative antioxidant activities of plant-derived polyphenols flavonoids. *Free Radic. Res.* **1995**, *22*, 375–383. [CrossRef]
57. Balasundram, N.; Sundram, K.; Samman, S. Phenolic compounds in plants and agri-industrial by-products: Antioxidant activity, occurrence, and potential uses. *Food Chem.* **2006**, *99*, 191–203. [CrossRef]
58. Blasco, A.J.; Rogerio, M.C.; Gonzalez, M.C.; Escarpa, A. "Electrochemical Index" as a screening method to determine "total polyphenolics" in foods: A proposal. *Anal. Chim. Acta* **2005**, *539*, 237–244. [CrossRef]

Publisher's Note: MDPI stays neutral with regard to jurisdictional claims in published maps and institutional affiliations.

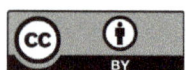

© 2020 by the authors. Licensee MDPI, Basel, Switzerland. This article is an open access article distributed under the terms and conditions of the Creative Commons Attribution (CC BY) license (http://creativecommons.org/licenses/by/4.0/).

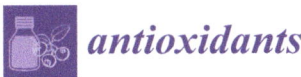 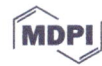

Article

Identification of a New Variety of Avocados (*Persea americana* Mill. CV. Bacon) with High Vitamin E and Impact of Cold Storage on Tocochromanols Composition

Celia Vincent [1,2], Tania Mesa [1,2] and Sergi Munne-Bosch [1,2,*]

1. Department of Evolutionary Biology, Ecology and Environmental Sciences, University of Barcelona, Faculty of Biology, Av. Diagonal 643, E-08028 Barcelona, Spain; cevisa96@gmail.com (C.V.); tmesapar7@alumnes.ub.edu (T.M.)
2. Research Institute of Nutrition and Food Safety (INSA), University of Barcelona, Faculty of Biology, Av. Diagonal 643, E-08028 Barcelona, Spain
* Correspondence: smunne@ub.edu; Tel.: +34-934-021-480

Received: 21 April 2020; Accepted: 6 May 2020; Published: 9 May 2020

Abstract: (1) Background: Tocochromanols are a group of fat-soluble compounds including vitamin E (tocopherols and tocotrienols) and plastochromanol-8, and just one avocado can contain up to 20% of the required vitamin E daily intake. (2) Methods: HPLC and LC-MS/MS analyses were performed in avocados of various varieties and origin for the identification and quantification of tocopherols, tocotrienols and plastochromanol-8. After selection of the variety with the highest vitamin E content, we evaluated to what extent short- (4 h) and long-term (10 d) cold storage influences the accumulation of tocochromanols. (3) Results: Analyses revealed that "Bacon" avocados (*Persea americana* Mill. cv. Bacon) were the richest in vitamin E compared to other avocado varieties (including the highly commercialized Hass variety), and they not only accumulated tocopherols (with 110 µg of α-tocopherol per g dry matter), but also tocotrienols (mostly in the form of γ-tocotrienol, with 3 µg per g dry matter) and plastochromanol-8 (4.5 µg per g dry matter). While short-term cold shock did not negatively influence α-tocopherol contents, it increased those of γ-tocopherol, γ-tocotrienol, and plastochromanol-8 and decreased those of δ-tocotrienol. Furthermore, storage of Bacon avocados for 10 d led to a 20% decrease in the contents of α-tocopherol, whereas the contents of other tocopherols, tocotrienols and plastochromanol-8 were not affected. (4) Conclusions: It is concluded that Bacon avocados (i) are very rich in α-tocopherol, (ii) not only contain tocopherols, but also tocotrienols and plastochromanol-8, and (iii) their nutritional vitamin E value is negatively influenced by long-term cold storage.

Keywords: avocados (*Persea americana* Mill.); low temperatures; plastochromanol-8; tocotrienols; tocopherols; tocochromanols

1. Introduction

Tocochromanols are a group of amphiphilic molecules that includes tocopherols, tocotrienols and plastochromanol-8 [1,2]. These are all composed by a polar chromanol head and a highly apolar polyprenyl side chain that provide them with the capacity to exert an antioxidant function in membranes, from cyanobacteria and plants where they are synthetized until a variety of tissues in animals and humans, which incorporate tocochromanols regularly from their daily dietary intake [1,2]. While tocopherols have a saturated phytyl-derived side chain, tocotrienols and plastochromanol-8 tails are more unsaturated since they derive from geranylgeranyl-diphospate and solanesyl-diphospate, respectively [3]. Both tocopherols and tocotrienols include various homologues according to the position and methylation degree in the chromanol head, thus identifying four different molecules for each group (α-, β-, γ- and δ-tocopherols and -tocotrienols). All tocochromanols exert an efficient antioxidant activity by inhibiting the propagation of lipid peroxidation through scavenging lipid peroxyl radicals and by preventing it through the (physical) quenching and (chemical) scavenging of singlet oxygen, not only in plant tissues where they are synthetized, but also in humans, although such a role is mainly generally attributed to α-tocopherol in the human body, since this is the major form transported by a specific protein [4].

While α-tocopherol is a universal molecule found in plants, animals and humans, tocotrienols have not been described in all photosynthetic tissues; rather, they accumulate in seeds and fruits of some plant species only [5,6]. Similarly, plastochromanol-8 is not present universally, despite being found in many plant tissues such as seeds, leaves, buds, flowers and fruits of several species [2,7,8]. Interestingly, in vitro studies in hydrophobic solvents show a higher antioxidant activity against singlet oxygen for tocotrienols and plastochromanol-8 than for tocopherols, which has been attributed to their more apolar structure of the side chain [2]. New nutraceutical functions have been recently attributed to tocotrienols. For instance, antiangiogenic properties against osteoporosis, atherosclerosis, inflammatory processes and many types of cancer (like colorectal, prostate, lung and pancreas cancer) have been reported, mainly for δ- and γ-tocotrienol forms [9]. Otherwise, despite not being considered a molecule belonging to the vitamin E family, the antioxidant activity of plastochromanol-8 is of great relevance in plants and it may also probably display beneficial properties in humans, although to our knowledge this has not been studied thus far in detail.

Cold storage of fruits is an effective means to prevent food deterioration, particularly in climacteric fruits such as avocados (*Persea americana* Mill), where low temperatures reduce ethylene production and therefore inhibit fruit over-ripening [10,11]. Indeed, introducing avocado fruits in cold chambers is a common technique implemented for preventing their early deterioration, thus increasing fruit marketability. However, the cellular redox balance in fruits may be threatened by the extent of low temperature exposure in storage chambers before fruits reach the consumers. Indeed, low temperature shocks or long-term cold exposure can cause a loss of cellular antioxidant defenses in fruits [12–14]. As a result, oxidative reactions may occur in an uncontrolled manner resulting in sustained oxidative stress and tissue damage [13]. To fight against oxidation reactions at low temperatures, tocopherols, mainly α-tocopherol, have been suggested to be essential for attaining acclimation in plants [3]. Additionally, some studies have reported that tocotrienols may be as effective as tocopherols in protecting leaves from photooxidation processes under low temperatures [1]. Although several studies have been performed in leaves of *Arabidopsis* and other model plant species to link tocopherol accumulation and low temperature acclimation [15–18], very few studies have investigated thus far the influence of cold temperature storage on the accumulation of tocochromanols in fruits; except for an increase in tocopherols upon 3 d of storage at cold temperatures in sweet cherries, which is a fruit with low concentrations of fatty acids and vitamin E [19] and a maintenance of constant α-tocopherol contents in oil of Fuerte avocados upon exposure to 5 °C for three weeks [20]. To our knowledge, the effects of low temperatures on the accumulation of tocochromanols in other avocado varieties, and of tocotrienols and plastochromanol-8 in fruits in general have not been investigated thus far.

Avocados (*Persea americana* Mill) are highly valuable fruits with increasing interest for consumers thanks to their nutraceutical properties due to antioxidant contents, such as ascorbate (vitamin C, 8.8 mg/100 g) and B-type vitamins (such as vitamin B_6, 0.29 mg/100 g), fiber (6.8 g/100 g), phytosterols (83.1 mg/100 g), monounsaturated fatty acids (9.8 g/100 g) and vitamin E (2.36 mg/100 g) [21]. These are originally from Mexico where tropical environmental conditions permitted hybridization techniques that have led to the wide number of varieties currently found worldwide [22]. Nevertheless, the main producing countries are still those with warm climates which export a huge percentage of their production to other continents [23]. Hass is the most widely produced and commercialized avocado variety worldwide, while Bacon, a hybrid variety originally cultivated in 1954 by James Bacon in California, occupies the third position (after Hass and Fuerte) in terms of agricultural production in

Spain, the main avocado producer in Europe [24]. Here, avocado fruits (*Persea americana* Mill) were investigated aiming to determine (i) the amounts and composition of tocochromanols in the edible part of various avocado varieties and (ii) how cold storage in the short and long term influences tocochromanol contents in Bacon avocados. This study shows to what extent cold storage implemented along the supply chain can negatively influence the nutritional quality of avocados in terms of vitamin E accumulation.

2. Material and Methods

2.1. Plant Material and Samplings

Avocados (*Persea americana* Mill.), either collected at commercial harvest maturity in the field or purchased from supermarkets in a non-ripe stage (depending on the experiments, see details below), were immediately brought to the laboratory at the University of Barcelona (Barcelona, NE Spain) and used for assays. In all cases, fruits were selected for homogeneity according to their size and lack of pathogen symptoms. Three independent experiments were performed.

For the identification of tocochromanols in various avocado varieties and origins (experiment 1), fruits were purchased in local supermarkets or markets, as follows. Non-ripe Hass avocados originated from Brazil, Perú and Spain, and identified as such in their label, were obtained from a supermarket in Barcelona (NE Spain) and immediately transported at room temperature by car to the laboratory. Non-ripe Hass and Fuerte avocados from Chile and Govín avocados from Cuba were obtained from local markets and transported by plane and car to the laboratory. Finally, Bacon avocados were obtained from a commercial orchard in Málaga (south Spain) at a mature stage and brought to the laboratory after 12 h of transportation at 8–10 °C. All fruits were then exposed to room temperature in the laboratory at the University of Barcelona and when firmness attained levels of 3N for all fruits from all varieties and origins, then the mesocarp tissue of four fruits per variety and origin was sampled and immediately frozen in liquid nitrogen and stored at −80 °C until analyses. With these samples, tocochromanols were quantified by high-performance liquid chromatography (HPLC) and identification of compounds confirmed by liquid chromatography coupled to electrospray ionization mass spectrometry in tandem (LC-ESI-MS/MS).

The influence of short-term, cold shock exposure on tocochromanol accumulation in Bacon avocados (experiment 2) was examined by performing samplings just before and after 4 h of cold shock of fruits at 4 °C in a cold storage chamber (Frimatic, S.A., Barcelona, Spain). Samples from 18 randomly selected fruits at each time point including 0 h and 4 h were immediately frozen in liquid nitrogen and stored at −80 °C until analyses. With these samples, tocochromanols were quantified by HPLC while the extent of lipid peroxidation and changes in photosynthetic pigments were estimated spectrophotometrically, as described below.

The influence of long-term exposure to low temperatures on tocochromanol accumulation in Bacon avocados (experiment 3) was examined by performing samplings just before and during exposure for a period of 10 d of cold storage of fruits at 4 °C using the same cold chamber (Frimatic, S.A.). Mesocarp samples from 18 randomly selected fruits at times including 0 d, 2 d, 5 d, 7 d and 10 d of low temperature exposure were immediately frozen in liquid nitrogen and stored at −80 °C until analyses. With these samples, tocochromanols were quantified by HPLC while the extent of lipid peroxidation and changes in photosynthetic pigments were estimated spectrophotometrically, as described below.

2.2. Tocochromanol Analyses

The quantification of the different tocochromanol forms, including tocopherols, tocotrienols and plastochromanol-8, was performed as described previously [25] with some modifications. One-hundred mg of avocado (mesocarp) sample was extracted with 1 mL of methanol containing 0.01% (*w/v*) butyl-hydroxytoluene (BHT) and 5 ppm (*w/v*) of tocol as an internal standard. Extraction was performed using 30 min of ultrasonication (Bransonic ultrasonic bath 2800, Emerson Industrial, Danbury, CT,

USA) just after vortexing for 20 s. Then, samples were centrifuged at 600 g during 10 min at 4 °C to subsequently recover supernatants with a hydrophobic PTFE filter 0.22 µm (Phenomenex, Torrance, CA, USA). Tocochromanols were separated by HPLC at room temperature using an Inertsil 100A column (5 µm, 30 × 250 mm, GL Sciences Inc., Tokyo, Japan). Quantification was performed using a Jasco fluorescence detector (FP-1520, Tokyo, Japan) and a calibration curve established with each of the tocochromanols analyzed and corrected with the tocol recovery, which was always above 97%.

The identification of tocochromanols was confirmed by using high-performance liquid chromatography coupled to electrospray ionization mass spectrometry in tandem (LC-ESI-MS/MS) as described previously [26]. Methanolic extracts were obtained as described before for the HPLC analyses and used here for the identification of tocochromanols by LC-ESI-MS/MS. Tocochromanol separation was performed with an Inertsil 100A column (5 µm, 30 × 250 mm, GL Sciences Inc. (Tokyo, Japan), and an isocratic flow of hexane:dioxane (95.5:4.5 v/v) mobile phase. The MS acquisition was performed using negative ionization between m/z 100 and 650, with the Turbo Ionspray source. In addition, quadrupole time-of-flight (QqToF) mass spectrometry was used to obtain product ion information. The MS parameters were: ion spray voltage, −4200; declustering potential (DP), −40; focusing potential (FP), −150; declustering potential two (DP2), −10; ion release delay (IRD), 6 V; ion release width (IRW), 5 ms; nebulizer gas, 50 (arbitrary units); curtain gas, 60 (arbitrary units), and auxiliary gas N_2, 6000 cm^3 min^{-1} heated at 500 °C.

2.3. Lipid Peroxidation Assays

To determine the extent of lipid peroxidation, primary (lipid hydroperoxide) and secondary (malondialdehyde, MDA) lipid peroxidation products were analyzed, as follows. For lipid hydroperoxides analyses, frozen samples (100 mg) were repeatedly (three times) extracted with 1 mL methanol + 0.01% BHT (w/v) at 4 °C using 30 min of ultrasonication (Bransonic ultrasonic bath 2800). After centrifugation, supernatants were collected, combined and used for analyses using the Fox-2 reagent (consisting in a solution of 90% methanol (v/v) containing 25 mM sulfuric acid, 4 mM butylhydroxyltoulene (BHT), 250 µM iron sulfate ammonium (II) and 10 µM xylenol orange) as described in Bou et al. [27]. Absorbances were measured at 560 nm and 800 nm. A calibration curve using hydrogen peroxide 37% (v/v) was used for quantification.

For estimation of the MDA content, the thiobarbituric acid-reactive substances (TBARS) assay, which considers the possible influence of interfering compounds, was used [28]. In short, 100 mg of sample was extracted with 3 mL of ethanol 80% (v/v) containing 0.01% (w/v) BHT, vortexed for 20 s and exposed to ultrasonication for 15 min (Bransonic ultrasonic bath 2800). After centrifuging at room temperature for 13 min at 600 g, the supernatant was recovered, and the pellet re-extracted twice using the same procedure. Then, two tubes were used: (a) − TBA, with 1 mL extract + 1 mL 20% trichloroacetic acid (w/v) with 0.01% BHT (w/v) and (b) + TBA, with 1 mL extract + 1 mL 20% trichloroacetic acid (w/v), 0.01% BHT (w/v) and 0.65% thiobarbutiric acid (w/v). Tubes were incubated for 25 min at 95 °C and then the reaction was stopped by maintaining them at 4 °C for 10 min. After centrifugation at 600 g at room temperature for 5 min, MDA content in samples were analyzed by spectrophotometry at 440, 532 and 600 nm and quantified using the equations developed by Hodges et al. [28].

2.4. Chlorophyll Content

To determine total chlorophyll content, samples (100 mg) were extracted in 1 mL of methanol + 0.01% BHT as explained before, using vortex and ultrasonication for 30 min at 4 °C. Supernatants were collected after centrifugation for 10 min at 600 g and 4 °C. Chlorophylls were measured spectrophotometrically reading absorbances at 653, 666 and 750 nm and measuring chlorophyll content as described [29].

2.5. Statistical Analyses

Statistical analyses were performed by one-way ANOVA and Tukey posthoc tests were used for multiple comparisons among time (IBS SPSS Statistics 19; SPSS Inc., Chicago, IL., USA). Differences were considered significant when p values were under the significance level $\alpha = 0.05$.

3. Results

3.1. Identification of Tocochromanols in Various Avocado Varieties

In order to determine the presence and amount of tocochromanols in the mesocarp (edible part of the fruit) of different avocado varieties, HPLC and LC-ESI MS/MS analyses were performed. Among the various varieties and origins tested, Bacon avocados from Spain showed the largest amount of vitamin E (Table 1A). Bacon avocados contained 2.4 mg α-tocopherol per 100 g of edible fruit, which coincided with a very low quantity of its precursor γ-tocopherol in the tissue (Table 1A). Bacon was the variety with the highest tocochromanol content among all studied varieties. By contrast, Govín from Cuba, Hass from Brazil and Hass from Perú were the avocados showing the lowest amounts of total tocochromanols.

Table 1. Contents of tocochromanols in different avocado varieties, including various origins.

	(A) Tocochromanol (µg/100 g FW)						
	α-T	β-T	γ-T	γ-TT	δ-TT	PC-8	Total TCs
Bacon Spain	2371 ± 148[c]	140.3 ± 22.7[d]	50.3 ± 11.2	42.2 ± 3.3	47.7 ± 5.7	191 ± 23[b]	2848 ± 181[c]
Fuerte Chile	2190 ± 52[bc]	79.8 ± 4.9[bcd]	29.9 ± 4.5	32.1 ± 5.0	ND	192 ± 17[b]	2524 ± 53[abc]
Hass Chile	2068 ± 48[bc]	88.4 ± 7.6[cd]	51.4 ± 5.1	27.4 ± 3.8	ND	300 ± 18[cd]	2535 ± 61[bc]
Govín Cuba	2004 ± 129[bc]	ND	25.5 ± 5.5	29.6 ± 1.8	ND	93 ± 4[a]	2152 ± 133[a]
Hass Spain	1997 ± 211[bc]	57.9 ± 8.2[abc]	50.5 ± 4.3	39.2 ± 3.7	ND	284 ± 21[c]	2434 ± 296[abc]
Hass Perú	1592 ± 225[b]	14.1 ± 8.2[a]	36.4 ± 3.4	32.1 ± 11.5	ND	378 ± 22[d]	2062 ± 224[ab]
Hass Brazil	816 ± 209[a]	18.0 ± 6.8[ab]	31.8 ± 4.7	42.9 ± 6.3	ND	226 ± 12[b]	1138 ± 217[ab]
	(B) Tocochromanol (µg/g DW)						
	α-T	β-T	γ-T	γ-TT	δ-TT	PC-8	Total TCs
Bacon Spain	127.3 ± 10.7[c]	7.5 ± 1.2[b]	2.7 ± 0.6[b]	2.2 ± 0.1[bc]	2.5 ± 0.3	10.3 ± 1.4[b]	153 ± 13[b]
Fuerte Chile	47.3 ± 4.8[ab]	1.7 ± 0.1[a]	0.6 ± 0.1[a]	0.7 ± 0.1[a]	ND	4.2 ± 0.7[a]	54 ± 5[a]
Hass Chile	60.4 ± 1.6[ab]	2.6 ± 0.3[a]	1.5 ± 0.2[ab]	0.8 ± 0.1[a]	ND	8.8 ± 0.6[ab]	74 ± 2[a]
Govín Cuba	174.2 ± 16.2[d]	ND	2.2 ± 0.4[a]	2.6 ± 0.2[c]	ND	8.1 ± 0.8[ab]	187 ± 17[a]
Hass Spain	62.3 ± 5.2[ab]	1.8 ± 0.2[a]	1.6 ± 0.05[a]	1.2 ± 0.09[ab]	ND	9.0 ± 1.0[ab]	76 ± 5[a]
Hass Perú	78.4 ± 9.8[b]	0.7 ± 0.4[a]	1.8 ± 0.08[a]	1.7 ± 0.6[abc]	ND	18.7 ± 0.6[c]	102 ± 10[a]
Hass Brazil	33.5 ± 8.4[a]	0.7 ± 0.3[a]	1.3 ± 0.2[a]	1.8 ± 0.4[abc]	ND	9.4 ± 0.5[b]	47 ± 8[a]

(**A**) Per 100 g fresh weight and (**B**) per g dry weight (DW). Data, which were obtained using the mesocarp of fruits in their optimum stage of ripening, show the mean of $n = 4$ fruits. Lower case letters (a–d) indicate differences between avocado varieties when $p < 0.05$. Trace amounts of δ-tocopherol and α-tocotrienol could not be properly quantified and are not shown here. T, tocopherol; TT, tocotrienol; PC-8, plastochromanol-8; ND, not detected.

A comparison of four origins of Hass avocados (Chile, Spain, Perú and Brazil) revealed that the origin had a very strong effect on tocochromanol contents, including α-tocopherol (Table 1). All avocado varieties behaved similarly to Bacon avocados from Spain in terms of accumulating most of the tocochromanols in the form of α-tocopherol but both Bacon from Spain and Govín from Cuba presented a larger amount of α-tocopherol than the highly commercialized Hass variety irrespective of its origin. Furthermore, although plastochromanol-8 was present in all avocado varieties, its contents were higher in Hass varieties (irrespective of the origin) than in Bacon and Govín (from Spain and Cuba, respectively). Notably, δ-tocotrienol seemed to be exclusively present in Bacon (Table 1A). Results differed slightly when comparing the vitamin E amounts per unit of dry weight in different varieties; Bacon occupied the second position in terms of vitamin E accumulation, just after Govín, as the contents of α-tocopherol were higher in these two varieties than in Hass or Fuerte (Table 1B). Moreover, total tocochromanol contents were also higher in Bacon when compared to the other highly commercialized varieties, except for Govín which occupied the first position just before Bacon variety (Table 1B).

The major tocochromanol present in the mesocarp (edible tissue) of Bacon avocados was α-tocopherol (with an 87.8%), as clearly observed in the HPLC chromatogram (Figure 1A), followed by plastochromanol-8, β- and γ-tocopherols, and δ- and γ-tocotrienols (Table 1A). HPLC identification by retention time was confirmed by LC-ESI MS/MS using the corresponding authentic standards, which showed exactly the same fragmentation patterns as the corresponding peaks in the samples (Figure 1). This tocochromanol profile in Bacon avocados, enriched in the α-tocopherol form and with the presence of δ-tocotrienol, is different from that found for the Hass variety (Table 1, see also [30,31]).

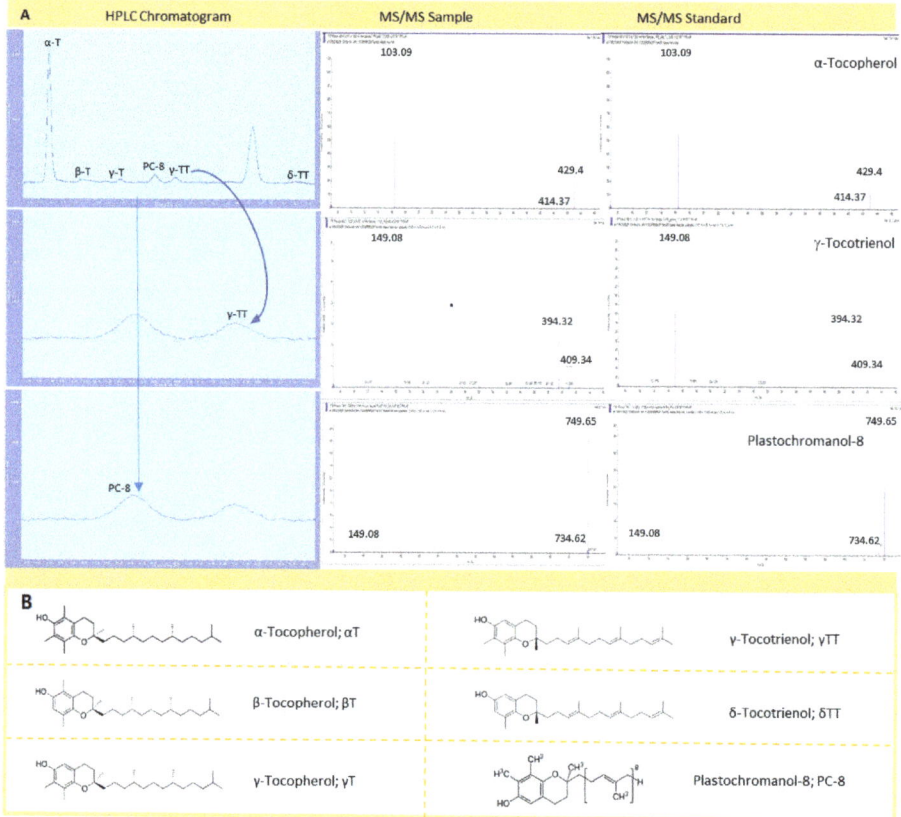

Figure 1. (**A**): Separation (by HPLC, *left*) and identification (by liquid chromatography coupled to electrospray ionization mass spectrometry in tandem [LC-ESI-MS/MS], *center* and *right*) of tocochromanols in Bacon avocados. (**B**): Chemical formula of tocochromanols identified in Bacon avocados.

3.2. Cold-induced Changes in Tocochromanol Composition in Bacon Avocados

After a low temperature shock for 4 h, the contents of the major tocochromanol present in the mesocarp of Bacon avocados, α-tocopherol, were not altered (Figure 2). The same was observed for β-tocopherol, but not for the other tocochromanols. While the contents of plastochromanol-8, γ-tocopherol and γ-tocotrienol increased, those of δ-tocotrienol decreased, with the latter showing a reduction by 60% under cold treatment (Figure 2). This cold-induced shift in the tocochromanol composition was accompanied by an increase in the extent of lipid peroxidation, as indicated by 60% increases in lipid hydroperoxides and malondialdehyde contents, while chlorophyll levels and the chlorophyll a/b ratio remained unaltered (Figure 3).

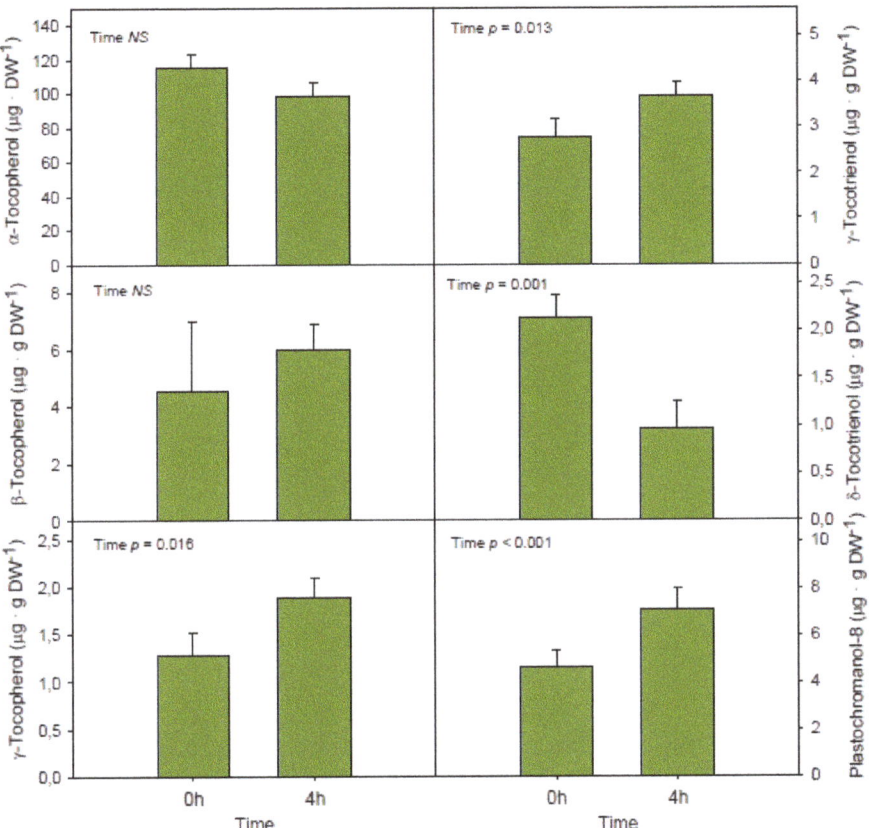

Figure 2. Influence of short-term (4 h) exposure of Bacon avocados to cold temperatures (4 °C) in the contents of tocochromanols. Data represent the mean ± SE of $n = 18$ fruits. Differences were considered significant when $p < 0.05$. DW, dry weight.

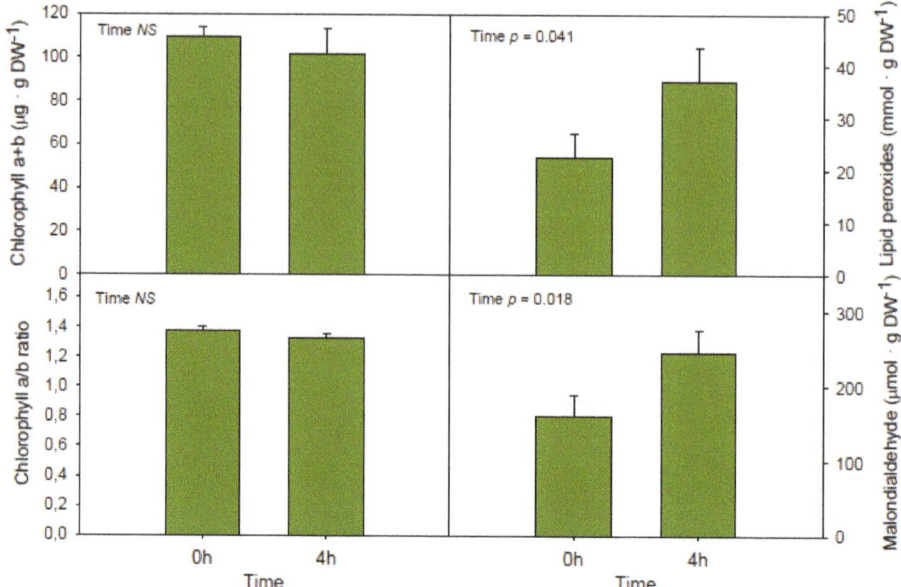

Figure 3. Influence of short-term (4 h) exposure of Bacon avocados to cold temperatures (4 °C) in the contents of chlorophylls, chlorophyll a/b ratio and the extent of lipid peroxidation (estimated as the contents of lipid hydroperoxides and malondialdehyde, as indicators of primary and secondary lipid peroxidation, respectively). Data represent the mean ± SE of n = 18 fruits. Differences were considered significant when $p < 0.05$. DW, dry weight.

Total tocochromanol contents showed a decrease by 16% after 10 d of storage at low temperatures, which was mostly due to a significant decrease in tocopherols but not tocotrienols (Figure 4). Part of this loss was related to the decrease in the major tocochromanol form in Bacon avocados, α-tocopherol, which decreased by 20% after 10 d of cold storage (Figure 4). When α-tocopherol contents were expressed on a fresh weight basis (either per 100 g FW, per fruit, half fruit or serving), a decrease in its contents was also observed, thus offering a lower amount (by 15%) of α-tocopherol per amount of fruit consumed (Figure 4). This reduction in vitamin E contents occurred progressively over time, as revealed by the time-course evolution of α-tocopherol contents (Figure S1), but most particularly between 5 d and 10 d of cold storage. In contrast to short-term exposure to cold temperature, the other tocochromanol forms were not clearly affected by long-term cold storage, although γ-tocopherol and δ-tocotrienol showed slight variations over time (Figure S1). Reductions of α-tocopherol during long-term storage at low temperatures was coincident with a 3.4-fold increase in malondialdehyde contents after 10 d of cold storage (Figure S2).

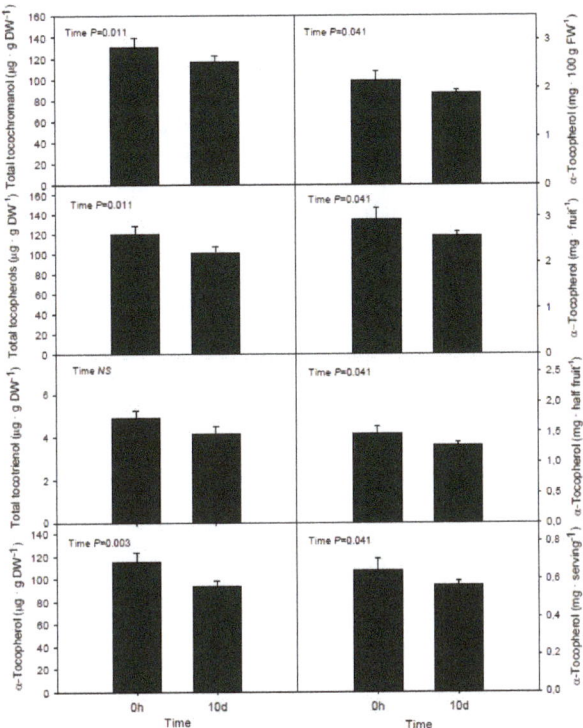

Figure 4. Influence of long-term (10 d) storage of Bacon avocados at cold temperatures (4 °C) in the contents of total tocochromanols, tocopherols, tocotrienols and α-tocoperol. Contents of α-tocopherol are also shown in mg per 100 g of mesocarp in fresh weight (FW), per one fruit (136 g FW), per a half (68 g FW) and per serving according to the Nutrition Labelling and Education Act (NLEA; corresponding to 30 g FW). Data represent the mean ± standard error of $n = 18$ fruits. Differences were considered significant when $p < 0.05$. DW, dry weight.

4. Discussion

4.1. Bacon is a Variety of Avocados with High Tocochromanol Contents

Among the avocado varieties examined in our study, Bacon from Spain was the one showing the highest vitamin E content. All varieties showed a similar tocochromanol composition, so that the major tocochromanol was α-tocopherol, except Bacon, which also accumulated some amounts of δ-tocotrienol. Hence, tocochromanols composition was in general enriched in α-tocopherol, with a diminished accumulation of other tocopherols and tocotrienols, with the overall most notable exception of γ-tocochromanols in all varieties and additionally of δ-tocotrienol in Bacon. Varietal differences might be associated not only with the geographical origin of the fruit, as shown in our results, but also with the highly heterozygous genetic origin of avocado races. *Persea americana* includes *P. americana* var. *drymifolia* (commonly known as Mexican race), var. *guatemalensis* (known as Guatemalan race) and var. *americana* (or West Indian race). While Bacon is obtained from the hybridization of Mexican × Guatemalan races, Hass variety is generally reported to have a pure Guatemalan origin [32]. However, breeding strategies, cross- and self-pollination techniques, different strategies of cultivation and the posterior selection according to farmer preferences, like high yield, fruit quality and long shelf life, usually give rise to quite heterogenic crops in the same variety, which might lead to the observed differences in the Hass avocados from different origins studied here that showed notable differences in the accumulation of tocochromanols.

Plastochromanol-8 accumulation in fruits may be of particular relevance since this is also a powerful antioxidant, even showing higher antioxidant activity than α-tocopherol in hydrophobic environments due to its more highly unsaturated prenyl chain [2]. Plastochromanol-8 was found in mesocarp tissue of avocado fruit at relatively low amounts compared to α-tocopherol, but some differences between cultivars were observed. In this case, Hass was the variety with the greatest amount of this compound compared to the other studied varieties, including Bacon. Furthermore, we reported here on the accumulation of tocotrienols in avocados, which contrasts with a recent report [8] showing the accumulation of plastochromanol-8 but not of tocotrienols in Hass avocado. Our study shows that tocotrienols may accumulate in avocado fruits, in particular in some varieties such as Bacon. Notably, δ-tocotrienol was only found in Bacon among all studied varieties. Beneficial properties for humans have recently been attributed to this compound, in particular to help in the prevention of the development of various cancers, including breast, colorectal, lung and many other types of cancer, apart from providing anticholesterolemic and antidiabetic benefits [33–35]. Although the contents of δ- and γ-tocotrienols were relatively low compared to that of α-tocopherol in Bacon avocados, these compounds might, to some extent, exert an additional beneficial response in the human body, an aspect that deserves further investigations.

4.2. Effects of Short and Long-Term Storage on Tocochromanol Contents

While a low temperature shock for 4 h did not alter α-tocopherol contents in the mesocarp of Bacon avocados, long-term storage for 10 d led to significant decreases in vitamin E contents. In contrast to unaltered contents of tocopherols after 4 h of low temperature exposure, the contents of plastochromanol-8, γ-tocopherol and γ-tocotrienol increased, and those of δ-tocotrienol decreased, the latter showing a reduction by 60% under cold treatment. Therefore, cold shock led to significant reductions in the levels of δ-tocotrienol and the cold-induced shift in the tocochromanol composition was accompanied by an increase in the extent of lipid peroxidation, as indicated by 60% increases in lipid hydroperoxides and malondialdehyde contents. Interestingly, chlorophyll contents were unaltered during the same period and Bacon avocados stored for 5d did not show alterations in the extent of lipid peroxidation, as indicated by the same measurements. This suggests that the cold-induced shift in tocochromanol composition was mainly due to metabolic alterations that resulted in transient lipid peroxidation, but this was not accompanied with a quality loss. In contrast, α-tocopherol contents decreased during long-term storage of Bacon avocado fruits at low temperatures, a decrease that was accompanied by an increase in the extent of lipid peroxidation, which was reflected by an increase in malondialdehyde. This result contrasts with a previous study [20] showing that α-tocopherol in oil obtained from Fuerte avocados keeps stable after 3 weeks of storage at 5 °C. This difference may be due to different reasons, including not only the study of a different variety (Fuerte in [20] and Bacon in our study), but also to a higher stability of α-tocopherol in oil at 5 °C [20] than in entire fruits at 4 °C in our study. Unfortunately, little research has been performed thus far to evaluate how cold storage temperature influences tocochromanol composition in vitamin E-rich fruits and further studies are required to better understand the causes of vitamin E instability in avocado fruits and oils.

4.3. Balance between Storage and Nutritional Value

According to the Nutritional Labelling and Education Act (NLEA) and the National Health and Nutrition Examination Survey (NHANES), the serving of avocado is recommended to be of 30 g or half of an avocado, respectively, which corresponds to an intake of 0.59 mg and 1.34 mg of α-tocopherol, respectively. Interestingly, when the nutritional value in terms of vitamin E was measured over time of cold storage, a decrease in tocochromanols occurred, which was mostly attributed to a progressive drop in α-tocopherol content, so that the daily vitamin E intake is significantly lower if avocados are stored for 10 d at 4 °C. In contrast, other tocochromanols were not affected. According to the results presented in our study, avocados stored for 10 d at low temperatures start to suffer oxidation processes, which might be related to the stress situation experienced by the mesocarp due to cold temperatures, which can lead to oxidative damage. Indeed, α-tocopherol levels dropped up to 20% after 10 d of cold storage, and this loss of α-tocopherol contents may slightly contribute to a lesser intake and absorption of vitamin E in the human diet under the levels of reference [36]. Furthermore, the loss in detoxifying oxygen radicals function by a loss of antioxidants such as vitamin E due to cold storage of fruits for long periods may contribute to a higher risk of suffering from cardiovascular diseases like atherosclerosis, cancer and cataracts, among other diseases related to degenerative processes [37–40].

5. Conclusions

In conclusion, Bacon has been shown to be the variety with very high tocochromanol contents relative to other studied varieties, presenting values greater than those of the highly commercialized Hass variety. Furthermore, Bacon variety marketing should be fostered not only because of the high amounts of vitamin E but also because it was the only variety showing δ-tocotrienol, a compound that might have additional beneficial effects. Moreover, according to procedures implemented along the supply chain which consist of introducing fruits into cold chambers, our study showed that 10 d might be the threshold where cold stress is starting to induce losses in vitamin E, hence decreasing nutritional value and fruit quality.

Supplementary Materials: The following are available online at http://www.mdpi.com/2076-3921/9/5/403/s1, Figure S1: Variations in the contents of tocochromanols during long-term (10 d) storage of "Bacon" avocados at cold temperatures (4 °C), Figure S2: Variations in the contents of chlorophylls, chlorophyll a/b ratio and the extent of lipid peroxidation (estimated as the contents of lipid hydroperoxides and malondialdehyde, as indicators of primary and secondary lipid peroxidation, respectively) during long-term (10 d) storage of "Bacon" avocados at cold temperatures (4 °C).

Author Contributions: Conceptualization, C.V. and S.M.-B.; methodology, C.V. and T.M.; software, C.V.; validation, C.V., T.M. and S.M.-B.; formal analysis, C.V.; investigation, C.V. and T.M.; resources, S.M.-B.; data curation, C.V.; writing—original draft preparation, C.V. and S.M.-B.; writing—review and editing, C.V., T.M. and S.M.-B.; visualization, C.V.; supervision, S.M.-B.; project administration, S.M.-B.; funding acquisition, S.M.-B. All authors have read and agreed to the published version of the manuscript.

Funding: This research was funded by Generalitat de Catalunya, grant number 2017 SGR 980.

Acknowledgments: We are very grateful to Paula Muñoz and Maren Müller for their help in the quantification and identification of tocochromanols, respectively, to Camila Ribalta for providing the avocados from Chile, and to Marina Pérez and Andrea Casadesús for their help in samplings.

Conflicts of Interest: The authors declare no conflict of interest.

References

1. Falk, J.; Munné-Bosch, S. Tocochromanol functions in plants: Antioxidation and beyond. *J. Exp. Bot.* **2010**, *61*, 1549–1566. [CrossRef]
2. Kruk, J.; Szymanska, R.; Cela, J.; Munné-Bosch, S. Plastochromanol-8: Fifty years of research. *Phytochemistry* **2014**, *108*, 9–16. [CrossRef]
3. Menné-Saffrané, L.; DellaPena, D. Biosynthesis, regulation and functions of tocochromanols in plants. *Plant Physiol. Biochem.* **2010**, *48*, 301–309. [CrossRef]
4. Kono, N.; Ohto, U.; Hiramatsu, T.; Urabe, M.; Uchida, Y.; Satow, Y.; Arai, H. Impaired a-TTP–PIPs interaction underlies familial vitamin E deficiency. *Science* **2013**, *340*, 1106–1110. [CrossRef] [PubMed]
5. Müller, M.; Cela, J.; Asensi-Fabado, M.; Munné-Bosch, S. Tocotrienols in plants: Occurrence, Biosynthesis and Functions. In *Tocotrienols: Vitamin E beyond Tocopherols*, 2nd ed.; Tan, B., Ed.; CRC Press Taylor & Francis Group: Boca Raton, FL, USA, 2013.
6. Chun, J.; Lee, J.; Ye, L.; Exler, J.; Eitenmiller, R.R. Tocopherol and tocotrienol contents of raw and processed fruits and vegetables in the United States diet. *J. Food Compost. Anal.* **2006**, *19*, 196–204. [CrossRef]
7. Georgiadou, E.C.; Goulas, V.; Ntourou, T.; Manganaris, G.A.; Kalaitzis, P.; Fotopoulos, V. Regulation of on-tree vitamin E biosynthesis in olive fruit during successive growing years: The impact of fruit development and enviornmental cues. *Front. Plant Sci.* **2016**, *7*, 1656. [CrossRef] [PubMed]

8. Trela, A.; Szymanska, R. Less widespread plant oils as a good source of vitamin E. *Food Chem.* **2019**, *296*, 160–166. [CrossRef] [PubMed]
9. Tan, B.; Watson, R.R.; Preedy, V.R. *Tocotrienols: Vitamin E Beyond Tocopherols*; CRC Press Taylor and Francis Group: Boca Raton, FL, USA, 2013.
10. Kassim, A.; Workneh, T.S.; Bezuidenhout, C.N. A review on postharvest handling of avocado fruit. *Afr. J. Agric. Res.* **2013**, *8*, 2385–2402. [CrossRef]
11. Arpaia, M.L.; Collin, S.; Sievert, J.; Obenland, D. 'Hass' avocado quality as influenced by temperature and ethylene prior to and during final ripening. *Postharvest Biol. Technol.* **2018**, *140*, 76–84. [CrossRef]
12. Blokhina, O.; Virolainen, E.; Fagerstedt, K.V. Antioxidants, oxidative damage and ocygen deprivation stress: A review. *Ann. Bot.* **2003**, *91*, 179–194. [CrossRef] [PubMed]
13. Foyer, C.H.; Noctor, G. Redox regulation in photosynthetic organisms: Signalling, acclimation, and practical implications. *Antiox. Redox Signal.* **2009**, *11*, 861–905. [CrossRef] [PubMed]
14. Das, K.; Roychoudhury, A. Reactive oxygen species (ROS) and response of antioxidants as ROS-scavengers during environmental stress in plants. *Front. Environ. Sci.* **2014**, *2*, 53. [CrossRef]
15. Leipner, J.; Fracheboud, Y.; Stamp, P. Effect of growing season on the photosynthetic apparatus and leaf antioxidative defenses in two maize genotypes of different chilling tolerance. *Environ. Exp. Bot.* **1999**, *42*, 129–139. [CrossRef]
16. Maeda, H.; Song, W.; Sage, T.L.; DellaPenna, L. Tocopherols play a crucial role in low-temperature adaptation and phloem leading in Arabidopsis. *Plant Cell* **2006**, *18*, 1710–1732. [CrossRef]
17. Gabruk, M.; Habina, I.; Kruk, J.; Dluzewska, J.; Szymanska, R. Natural variation in tocochromanols content in *Arabidopsis thaliana* accessions – the effect of temperature and light intensity. *Physiol. Plant.* **2016**, *157*, 147–160. [CrossRef]
18. Xiang, N.; Li, C.; Li, G.; Yu, Y.; Hu, J.; Guo, X. Comparative evaluation on vitamin E and carotenoid accumulation in sweet corn (*Zea mays* L.) seedlings under temperature stress. *J. Agric. Food Chem.* **2019**, *67*, 9772–9781. [CrossRef]
19. Tijero, V.; Teribia, N.; Muñoz, P.; Munné-Bosch, S. Implication of abscisic acid on ripening and quality in sweet cherries: Differential effects during pre- and post-harvest. *Front. Plant Sci.* **2016**, *7*, 602. [CrossRef]
20. Prabath Pathinara, U.A.; Sekozawa, Y.; Sugaya, S.; Gemma, H. Changes in lipid oxidation stability and antioxidant properties of avocado in response to 1-MCP and low oxygen treatment under low-temperature storage. *Int. Food Res. J.* **2013**, *20*, 1065–1075.
21. USDA (US Department of Agriculture). Avocado, almond, pistachio and walnut composition. In *Nutrient Data Laboratory. USDA National Nutrient Database for Standard Reference, Release 24*; US Department of Agriculture: Washington, DC, USA, 2011.
22. Yahia, E.M. Avocado. In *Crop Post-Harvest: Science and Technology*, 1st ed.; Rees, D., Ed.; Blackwell Publishing Ltd.: Oxford, UK, 2013.
23. FAO: Food and Agriculture Organization of the United Nations. Agriculture Database. 2014. Available online: http://www.fao.org/faostat/en/#data/QC (accessed on 20 February 2020).
24. Diaz-Robledo, J. An update of the spanish avocado industry. In *Proceedings of Second World Avocado Congress*; Lovatt, C.J., Ed.; University of California: Riverside, CA, USA, 1991; pp. 647–651.
25. Amaral, J.S.; Casal, S.; Torres, D.; Seabra, R.M.; Oliveira, B.P.P. Simultaneous determination of tocopherols and tocotrienols in hazelnuts by a normal phase liquid chromatographic method. *Anal. Sci.* **2005**, *21*, 1545–1548. [CrossRef]
26. Soba, D.; Müller, M.; Aranjuelo IMunné-Bosch, S. Vitamin E in legume nodules: Occurrence and antioxidant function. *Phytochemistry* **2020**, *172*, 112261. [CrossRef]
27. Bou, R.; Codony, R.; Tres, A.; Decker, E.A.; Guardiola, F. Determination of hydroperoxides in foods and biological samples by the ferrous oxidation-xylenol orange method: A review of the factors that influence the method's performance. *Anal. Biochem.* **2008**, *377*, 1–15. [CrossRef]
28. Hodges, D.M.; DeLong, J.M.; Forney, C.F.; Prange, R.K. Improving the thiobarbituric acid-reactive-substances assay for estimating lipid peroxidation in plant tissues containing anthocyanin and other interfering compounds. *Planta* **1999**, *207*, 604–611. [CrossRef]
29. Wang, W.; Bostic, T.R.; Gu, L. Antioxidant capacities, procyanidins and pigments in avocados of different strains and cultivars. *Food Chem.* **2010**, *122*, 1193–1198. [CrossRef]

30. Vinha, A.F.; Moreira, J.; Barreira, S. Physiochemical parameters, phytochemical composition and antioxidant activity of the algarvian avocado (*Persea americana* Mill.). *J. Agric. Sci.* **2013**, *5*, 100–109. [CrossRef]
31. Corral-Aguayo, R.D.; Yahia, E.M.; Carrillo-Lopez, A.; González-Aguilar, G. Correlation between some nutritional components and the total antioxidant capacity measured with six different assays in eight horticultural crops. *J. Agric. Food Chem.* **2008**, *56*, 10498–10504. [CrossRef]
32. Lahav, E.; Lavi, U. Avocado: Genetics and breeding. In *Breeding Plantation Tree Crops: Tropical Species*; Jain, S.M., Priyadarshan, P.M., Eds.; Springer: New York, NY, USA, 2009.
33. Guthrie, N.; Gapor, A.; Chambers, A.F.; Carroll, K.K. Inhibition of proliferation of estrogen receptor-negative MDA-MB-435 and -positive MCF-7 human breast cancer cells by palm oil tocotrienols and tamoxifen, alone and in combination. *J. Nutr.* **1997**, *127*, 544S–548S. [CrossRef]
34. Qureshi, A.A.; Mo, H.; Packer, L.; Peterson, D.M. Isolation and identification of novel tocotrienols from rice bran with hypocholesterolemic, antioxidant, and antitumor properties. *J. Agric. Food Chem.* **2000**, *48*, 3130–3140. [CrossRef]
35. Nakagawa, K.; Shibata, A.; Yamashita, S.; Tsuzuki, T.; Kariya, J.; Oikawa, S.; Miyazawa, T. In vivo angiogenesis is suppressed by unsaturated vitamin E, tocotrienol. *J. Nutr.* **2007**, *137*, 1938–1943. [CrossRef]
36. Dreher, M.L.; Davenport, A.J. Hass avocado composition and potential health effects. *Crit. Rev. Food Sci. Nutr.* **2013**, *53*, 738–750. [CrossRef]
37. Thorin, E. Vascular disease risk in patients with hypertriglyceridemia: Endothelial progenitor cells, oxidative stress, accelerated senescence and impaired vascular repair. *Can. J. Cardiol.* **2011**, *27*, 538–540. [CrossRef]
38. Reiner, Z. Hypertriglyceridaemia and risk of coronary arteria disease. *Nat. Rev. Cardiol.* **2017**, *14*, 401–411. [CrossRef] [PubMed]
39. Saha, S.K.; Lee, S.B.; Won, J.; Choi, H.Y.; Kim, K.; Yang, G.M.; Dayem, A.A.; Cho, S. Correlation between oxidative stress, nutrition and cancer initiation. *Int. J. Mol. Sci.* **2017**, *18*, 1544. [CrossRef] [PubMed]
40. Ames, B.N.; Shigenaga, M.K.; Hagen, T.M. Oxidants, antioxidants, and the degenerative diseases of aging. *Proc. Natl. Acad. Sci. USA* **1993**, *90*, 7915–7922. [CrossRef] [PubMed]

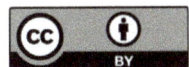

© 2020 by the authors. Licensee MDPI, Basel, Switzerland. This article is an open access article distributed under the terms and conditions of the Creative Commons Attribution (CC BY) license (http://creativecommons.org/licenses/by/4.0/).

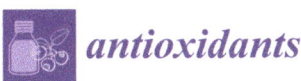

Article

Chemical Profile and Antioxidant Activity of the Kombucha Beverage Derived from White, Green, Black and Red Tea

Karolina Jakubczyk, Justyna Kałduńska, Joanna Kochman and Katarzyna Janda *

Department of Human Nutrition and Metabolomics, Pomeranian Medical University in Szczecin, 24 Broniewskiego Street, 71-460 Szczecin, Poland; jakubczyk.kar@gmail.com (K.J.); justynakaldunska@wp.pl (J.K.); kochmaan@gmail.com (J.K.)
* Correspondence: Katarzyna.Janda@pum.edu.pl; Tel.: +48-091-441-4818

Received: 27 April 2020; Accepted: 21 May 2020; Published: 22 May 2020

Abstract: Kombucha is a fermented tea beverage prepared as a result of the symbiotic nature of bacterial cultures and yeast, the so-called SCOBY (*Symbiotic Cultures of Bacteria and Yeasts*). Kombucha is characterised by rich chemical content and healthy properties. It includes organic acids, minerals and vitamins originating mainly from tea, amino acids, and biologically active compounds—polyphenols in particular. Kombucha is prepared mainly in the form of black tea, but other tea types are increasingly often used as well, which can significantly impact its content and health benefits. This work shows that the type of tea has a significant influence on the parameters associated with the antioxidant potential, pH, as well as the content of acetic acid, alcohol or sugar. Red tea and green tea on the 1st and 14th day of fermentation are a particularly prominent source of antioxidants, especially polyphenols, including flavonoids. Therefore, the choice of other tea types than the traditionally used black tea and the subjection of these tea types to fermentation seems to be beneficial in terms of the healthy properties of kombucha.

Keywords: kombucha; tea; fermentation; antioxidant; flavonoids; polyphenols

1. Introduction

Unhealthy lifestyle, intense physical exercising, stress, and environmental pollution are factors that influence the excessive synthesis of reactive oxygen species. The disturbance in homeostasis caused by free radicals leads to the formation of oxidative stress and damage to the structures of the human organism [1–4]. Illnesses that can be caused by free radical disorders include atherosclerosis, neurodegenerative diseases, such as Parkinson's or Alzheimer's disease, or even obesity. In order to maintain the balance between the production and removal of reactive oxygen species, it is important to search for easily accessible sources of antioxidants [1]. The main and the most widespread antioxidants are vitamins E, A and C, as well as polyphenolic compounds [1–3]. Phenolic compounds are an essential part of the human diet and are of considerable interest due to their health-promoting properties, including antioxidant effects. They are capable of capturing peroxide anions, lipid radicals, hydroxyl radicals and reactive oxygen species. Plant-derived polyphenols have a beneficial impact on slowing down the ageing process and reducing the risk of age-related neurodegenerative conditions, such as Alzheimer's disease, Parkinson's disease or ischaemic brain injury [5,6]. Antioxidant sources are mainly searched for in natural plant resources. Antioxidants are present in many easily available sources, such as tea, coffee, fruits, vegetables, spices and herbs. They complement everyday diet, contributing to good health.

Kombucha is a fermented tea drink created with the use of symbiotic cultures of bacteria and yeast, the so-called SCOBY (*Symbiotic Cultures of Bacteria and Yeasts*). Kombucha is prepared by combining tea with sugar (10%), sourdough from previous fermentation (10%) and SCOBY. SCOBY, when added to sugared tea, initiates fermentation, which results in the formation of various new bioactive compounds. The fermentation is conducted at room temperature for a period of 7–14 days. Various tea types can be used to produce kombucha, including green tea, as well as fermented, e.g., red, black or yellow tea. However, black tea and white sugar (saccharose) are considered the traditional and best ingredients that condition the proper content of the drink as well as its healthy properties. The taste of the drink is described as sour, slightly fruity and delicately sparkling, but after a few days of storage it becomes similar to the taste of wine vinegar [7].

Studies of kombucha proved its anti-bacterial, antioxidant, anti-diabetic properties, as well as its ability to reduce the concentration of cholesterol, to support the immune system and to stimulate the detoxification of the liver [8,9]. Kombucha drinks also feature minerals originating mainly from tea (potassium, manganese, fluoride ions), vitamins (E, K, B), amino acids (especially theanine, a derivative of glutamine), as well as other compounds that are formed as the result of numerous reactions occurring during the fermentation of the tea. During the oxidation of polyphenolic compounds, catechins, flavonoids and other compounds with health benefits for the organism are formed [8,10,11].

Various parameters influence the properties and content of kombucha, including the type of tea, fermentation time, the content of SCOBY colonies, and temperature. Despite the increase in the popularity of this drink's consumption, information regarding the influence of the many parameters or tea types on the properties and content is still not fully available. Hence, the aim of this research was to analyse the antioxidant properties and the content of the drink prepared from black, green, white and red teas at different time points of fermentation [10].

2. Material and Methods

2.1. Plant Material

The material consisted of four types of leaf tea (*Camellia sinensis*): black Ceylon originating in India, green Gunpowder, white tea and red tea (Pu-ERH) originating in China or India.

2.2. Preparation of Kombucha

The kombucha starter cultures, also known as SCOBY (which generally consists of *Acetobacter xylinum*, *Gluconobacter*, *S. cerevisiae*), were obtained from a commercial source from Poland. The starter culture used in the present article was stored in a refrigerator (4 °C) and consisted of sour broth and cellulosic layer (SCOBY floating on the liquid surface). One hundred grams of sugar (100.0 g/L, 10.0%), eight grams of tea (8.0 g/L, 0.8%) and 1 litre of hot, distilled water (90 °C) were mixed. The solution was infused for 10 min in a sterile conical flask. After cooling (30 °C), the tea decoction was filtered through nylon filters (0.45 µm, diam. 25 mm, Sigma-Aldrich, Poznań, Poland) into clean glass bottles.

2.3. Fermentation of Kombucha

Kombucha cultures were kept under aseptic conditions. Fermentation was carried out by incubating the kombucha culture at 28 ± 1 °C for 1, 7 and 14 days. Replicates were prepared so that each replicate was completely collected after its stipulated period of fermentation. The kombucha obtained was filtered and analysed.

2.4. Antioxidant Activity by the DPPH Methods

The antioxidant activity of samples was measured with the spectrophotometric method using synthetic radical DPPH (2.2-Diphenyl-1-Picrylhydrazyl, Sigma, Poznań, Poland) according to Brand-Williams et al. and Pekkarinen et al. [12,13]. The spectral absorbance was immediately measured at 518 nm (Agilent 8453UV). All assays were performed in triplicate. The results are shown in % of DPPH radical inhibition.

Antioxidant potential (antioxidant activity, inhibition) of tested solutions has been expressed by the percent of DPPH inhibition, using the following formula:

$$\% \text{ inhibition} = \frac{A0 - As}{A0} \times 100$$

where:
A0—absorbance of DPPH solution at 518 nm without tested sample
As—absorbance of DPPH solution at 518 nm with tested sample

2.5. The Determination of the Ferric Ion Reducing Antioxidant Power (FRAP) Method

The FRAP method, used to determine the total reduction potential, which also means the antioxidant properties of tested ingredient, is based on the ability of the test sample to reduce Fe^{3+} ions to Fe^{2+} ions. The FRAP unit determines the ability to reduce 1 micromole Fe^{3+} to Fe^{2+} according to Benzie and Strain [14,15]. Absorbance at 593 nm was measured (8453UV, AGILENT TECHNOLOGIES, Santa Clara, CA, USA). All assays were performed in triplicate. The ferric ion reducing antioxidant power was determined from the calibration curve using Fe(II)/L as the reference standard (0–5000 µM Fe(II)/L).

2.6. The Determination of the Total Polyphenols Content (TPC)

Determination of polyphenols was performed according to ISO 14502-1; Singleton and Rossi method using the Folin-Ciocalteu reagent [16]. Absorbance at 765 nm was measured (8453UV, AGILENT TECHNOLOGIES, Santa Clara, USA). All assays were performed in triplicate. The content of polyphenols was determined from the calibration curve using gallic acid as the reference standard (0–200 mg/L of gallic acid).

2.7. The Determination of the Total Flavonoids Content (TFC)

Determination of total flavonoids content was performed according to the Pękal and Pyrzynsk and Hu methods [17,18]. Different concentrations of flavonoids were used in the plotting of the standard calibration curve. The content of flavonoids was determined from the calibration curve using rutin equivalent as the reference standard (0–120 mg/L of rutin equivalent). Absorbance at 510 nm was measured (8453UV, AGILENT TECHNOLOGIES, Santa Clara, CA, USA). All assays were performed in triplicate.

2.8. The Determination of pH

The pH of both the fermented beverage and the unfermented control was determined by a pH meter (SCHOTT Instruments; SI Analytics Mainz, Mainz, Germany).

2.9. The Determination of Acetic Acid

Samples of tea and kombucha at 1, 7 and 14 days of fermentation were filtered through nylon filters (0.45 µm, diam. 25 mm, Sigma-Aldrich, Poznań, Poland). Acetic acid (AA) was analysed by high performance liquid chromatography (HPLC) using a 1200 series HPLC connected to a 1100 series RI detector (Agilent Technologies, Santa Clara, CA, USA) with a Rezex ROA-Organic Acid H^+ (8%) column (Phenomenex, Torrance, CA, USA). The column was eluted with a degassed mobile phase containing 5 mM H_2SO_4, pH 2.25 at 60 °C with a flow rate of 0.5 mL/min for 30 min per sample [19,20]. The results are shown in mg acetic acid/L.

2.10. The Determination of Alcohol

The alcohol content was measured using an alcoholometer (Browin, Łódź, Poland). The alcoholometer was immersed in the liquid and the result was read from the scale.

2.11. The Determination of Sugar Content

The total sugar content was measured with a laboratory refractometer RL3 (Polish Optical Works, Warsaw, Poland) from Brix scale.

2.12. Statistical Analysis

In all the experiments, three samples were analysed, and all the assays were carried out at least in triplicate. The statistical analysis was performed using Stat Soft Statistica 13.0 and Microsoft Excel 2017 (StatSoft Polska, Poland. The results are expressed as mean values and standard deviation (SD). To assess the differences between the examined parameters, the Tukey post hoc test was used. Differences were considered significant at $p \leq 0.05$. To control type I errors, the false discovery rate (FDR) approach was used. The calculations were performed using the p. adjust function of the stats package in R (R Foundation for Statistical Computing, Vienna, Austria).

3. Results

3.1. The Analysis of the Antioxidant Properties of Kombucha

The analysis of the antioxidant potential of the studied samples revealed that the content of antioxidant compounds was in the range between 70.62% and 94.61% DPPH inhibition (Table 1). The time of fermentation and the type of tea had an influence on the anti-radical properties of kombucha. In terms of the type of tea, kombucha prepared from green tea was characterised by the highest antioxidant potential, achieving the highest value on the first day of fermentation. In the case of each of the analysed kombucha drinks, the ability to deactivate free radicals decreased with the increase in the time of fermentation.

The highest content of reductive compounds labelled by the FRAP method was observed in all tea types before the fermentation process (5374.1–4486.7 µM Fe(II)/L). The addition of sourdough caused a rapid decrease in the reductive properties of kombucha (3626.3–2274.0 µM Fe(II)/L), but after 7 days of fermentation, the potential increased (4801.1–2725.9 µM Fe(II)/L), then it became lower on the 14th day of fermentation (3172.9–1573.9 µM Fe(II)/L). When analysing the type of the selected tea, kombucha made from green tea was characterised by the highest reductive potential (Table 1).

The analysis of the total content of polyphenols in kombucha, as well as the tea types used for its preparation, revealed that the content of compounds belonging to this group fluctuated in the range from 183.12 mg/L in black tea before the addition of sourdough and SCOBY to 320.12 mg/L in kombucha prepared from green tea on the 14th day of fermentation. In the case of kombucha from green, red and white teas, the highest polyphenol content was observed on the 14th day of fermentation. In kombucha made from green and white tea, the concentration of polyphenolic compounds increased proportionally with the increase in the duration of fermentation. The content of flavonoids, a compound from the group of polyphenols, was the highest for all tea types before starting the fermentation process (395.93 mg/L in red tea). The addition of sourdough significantly reduced flavonoid content in the analysed samples. The decrease in flavonoid content was progressing, achieving the lowest values on the 7th day of fermentation. During the next labelling (14th day of fermentation), there was another increase in the content of this compound (Table 1). In the case of most of the studied parameters, statistically significant differences were observed between tea types as well as the time of fermentation (Table 1).

Table 2 presents the statistically significant correlations between polyphenol content, flavonoids, antioxidant potential (DPPH, FRAP) and the duration of fermentation. Statistical analysis of the results showed significant correlations between the parameters characterising the kombucha antioxidant potential. It was shown that the correlations between the tested parameters are very different, depending on the type of tea (Table 2).

Table 1. Antioxidant potential: DPPH (2,2-Diphenyl-1-Picrylhydrazyl) free radical method, ferric ion reducing antioxidant power (FRAP)), the total polyphenols content (TPC) and total flavonoids content (TFC) in Kombucha tea.

Type of Beverage	Time Points (Day)	Total Flavonoids Content (TFC) [mg/L]	DPPH [%]	FRAP [µM Fe(II)/L]	Total Polyphenols Content (TPC) [mg/L]
Green Tea Kombucha—GK	tea	254.1 ± 8.6 *,2,3,4,5	80.33 ± 2.00 *,2,3,4	5374.1 ± 62.1 *,1,2,3,5,9,13	269.0 ± 0.9 *,3,4,5,9,13
	1	196.2 ± 2.6 *,1,3,4,10,14	94.61 ± 1.29 *,1,3,4,6,10,14	3626.3 ± 36.8 *,1,3,4,6,10,14	277.6 ± 0.4 *,3,4,6,10,14
	7	146.8 ± 3.4 *,1,2,4,7,11,15	91.40 ± 0.57 *,1,2,4,7,11,15	4801.1 ± 69.2 *,1,2,7,11,15	299.6 ± 3.1 *,1,2,4,7,11,15
	14	181.3 ± 4.8 *,1,2,3,8,12,16	88.23 ± 0.83 *,1,2,3,8,12,16	3172.9 ± 379.7 *,1,2,8,12,16	320.1 ± 3.5 *,1,2,3,8,12,16
Black Tea Kombucha—BK	tea	231.7 ± 11.0 *,1,6,7,8,9,13	70.40 ± 0.78 *,1,6,8,9,13	4486.7 ± 65.0 *,1,6,7,8,9,13	183.1 ± 2.3 *,6,7,8
	1	149.1 ± 0.6 *,2,5,7,8,10,14	78.62 ± 0.63 *,2,5,7,8,10,14	2274.0 ± 36.2 *,2,5,7,10,14	201.0 ± 5.7 *,5
	7	90.5 ± 0.7 *,5,6,8,11	70.63 ± 0.53 *,6,3,11,15	2725.9 ± 41.0 *,5,6,8,7,11,15	219.5 ± 2.1 *,5,3,7,15
	14	126.7 ± 5.2 *,5,6,7	61.04 ± 1.99 *,4,5,6,7,12,16	1573.9 ± 182.1 *,4,5,7,12,16	206.0 ± 1.2 *,5,4,6,12
White Tea Kombucha—WK	tea	209.3 ± 3.1 *,5,10,11,12	78.55 ± 0.35 *,10,12,1	4890.0 ± 8.90 *,1,5,10,11,12,13	184.6 ± 2.0 *,10,11,12
	1	132.6 ± 4.8 *,2,6,9,11,12,14	89.01 ± 0.99 *,9,11,12	2555.4 ± 26.2 *,2,6,9,11,12,14	200.8 ± 7.6 *,9,10,11
	7	83.8 ± 3.3 *,7,9,10,12	79.13 ± 0.93 *,9,10,12,3,7,15	3263.8 ± 46.3 *,3,7,9,10,12,15	205.6 ± 3.0 *,3,7,9,10,12,15
	14	111.6 ± 2.2 *,9,10,11	70.42 ± 1.38 *,9,10,11,16	2290.6 ± 171.0 *,4,8,9,10,11,16	228.1 ± 0.5 *,4,8,9,10,11,16
Red Tea Kombucha—RK	tea	395.9 ± 2.0 *,1,5,9,14,15,16	78.54 ± 0.06 *,5,14,16	5261.9 ± 26.5 *,1,5,9,14,15,16	229.5 ± 2.9 *,9,15,16,15,9
	1	292.5 ± 2.3 *,2,6,10,13,15,16	89.56 ± 0.08 *,13,15,16	2704.6 ± 7.3 *,2,6,10,13,15,16	219.8 ± 22.8 *,15,16
	7	198.1 ± 2.9 *,3,7,11,13,14,16	77.37 ± 0.80 *,3,7,11,14,16	4314.3 ± 53.5 *,3,7,11,13,14,16	270.5 ± 2.4 *,3,7,11,13,14
	14	242.5 ± 4.8 *,4,8,12,13,14,15	74.78 ± 2.11 *,12,13,14,15	2692.5 ± 202.8 *,4,8,12,13,14,15	271.9 ± 3.6 *,4,8,12,13,14

* FDR $p \leq 0.05$ between type of Kombucha (0, 1, 7, 14 days of fermentation), $p \leq 0.05$ between of particular subgroup: [1]—GK tea, [2]—GK 1, [3]—GK 7, [4]—GK 14, [5]—BK tea, [6]—BK 1, [7]—BK 7, [8]—BK 14, [9]—WK tea, [10]—WK 1, [11]—WK 7, [12]—WK 14, [13]—RK tea, [14]—RK 1, [15]—RK 7, [16]—RK.

Table 2. Statistically significant (at $p \leq 0.05$) correlation (r) between parameters for kombucha tea * p value ≤ 0.05.

Kombucha	Correlations (r) between Analysed Parameters			
	Green Tea	Black Tea	White Tea	Red Tea
Time vs	TPC (r = 0.92) * FRAP (r = 0.73) * DPPH (r = −0.94) *	TPC (r = 0.37) * DPPH (r = −0.96) *	TPC (r = 0.89) * FRAP (r = 0.86) * DPPH (r = −0.98) *	TPC (r = 0.69) * FRAP (r = 0.62) * DPPH (r = −0.84) *
Flavonoids vs	FRAP (r = −0.66) *	TPC (r = −0.37) * FRAP (r = −0.88) *	TPC (r = −0.43) * FRAP (r = −0.55) *	TPC (r = −0.66) * FRAP (r = −0.78) * DPPH (r = 0.56) *
TPC vs	Time (r = 0.92) * FRAP (r = 0.75) * DPPH (r = −0.85) *	Time (r = 0.36) * Flavonoids (r = −0.36) *	Time (r = 0.89) * Flavonoids (r = −0.43) * DPPH (r = −0.91) *	Time (r = 0.69) * Flavonoids (r = −0.66) * FRAP (r = 0.87) * DPPH (r = −0.80) *
FRAP vs	Time (r = 0.73) * Flavonoids (r = −0.65) * TPC (r = 0.75) * DPPH (r = −0.70) *	Flavonoids (r = −0.88) *	Time (r = 0.86) * Flavonoids (r = −0.55) * TPC (r = 0.93) * DPPH (r = −0.87) *	Time (r = 0.62) * Flavonoids (r = −0.78) * DPPH (r = −0.84) *
DPPH vs	Time (r = −0.94) * TPC (r = −0.85) * FRAP (r = −0.70) *	Time (r = −0.96) *	Time (r = −0.98) * TPC (r = −0.91) * FRAP (r = −0.87) *	Time (r = −0.84) * Flavonoids (r = 0.56) * TPC (r = −0.80) * FRAP (r = −0.84) *

3.2. The Analysis of pH, Content of Acetic Acid, Sugar and Alcohol in Kombucha

During the analysis of pH values, it was observed that the pH of all of the studied samples decreased with the increase in the duration of fermentation and the increase in the content of acetic acid. The rapid decrease in this parameter (1.8 unit in the case of kombucha prepared from black tea, up to 2.97 in the case of white kombucha) was caused by the addition of sourdough and SCOBY culture (1st day of fermentation). Further fermentation did not have a significant influence on the change in pH values. No significant differences were observed in terms of pH between drinks prepared from different tea types (Table 3).

With time, the acetic acid content of the fermentation increased, regardless of the type of tea used to prepare kombucha. On the 14th day of fermentation, acetic acid concentration was the highest for all tested beverages (9071.02–9147.40 mg/L) (Table 3).

The refractometric analysis of sugar content showed that all of the tea types were characterised by the highest concentration of saccharose before the beginning of the fermentation process. When it comes to kombucha prepared with the use of black or white tea, with progressing fermentation the content of saccharose decreased, achieving the lowest value on the 14th day of fermentation (7.5 and 9.5 °Bx, respectively). However, in the case of kombucha made from red and green tea types, the content of saccharose decreased directly after the addition of sourdough, increasing and approaching initial values at the moment of measurement on the 7th day of fermentation. The continuation of the process caused a slow decrease in the content of saccharose in these samples (Table 3).

The concentration of alcohol increased with time, achieving maximum value on the 7th day of fermentation—from 3.0% to 3.5% depending on the tea type. Subsequently, a decrease in alcohol content was observed in all types of kombucha drink (14th day of fermentation).

In the case of most of the studied parameters, statistically significant differences were observed between the time of fermentation. The smallest statistically significant differences were observed between kombucha drinks prepared from various tea types using the same fermentation time (Table 3). Statistical analysis of the results showed significant correlations between the parameters characterising the basic chemical composition of kombucha (Table 4).

Table 3. The content of alcohol, sugar, pH and acidity in Kombucha tea. * FDR $p \leq 0.05$ between type of Kombucha (0, 1, 7, 14 days of fermentation), $p \leq 0.05$ between particular subgroups: [1]—GK 0, [2]—GK 1, [3]—GK 7, [4]—GK 14, [5]—BK 0, [6]—BK 1, [7]—BK 7, [8]—BK 14, [9]—WK 0, [10]—WK 1, [11]—WK 7, [12]—WK 14, [13]—RK 0, [14]—RK 1, [15]—RK 7, [16]—RK 14.

Type of Beverage	Time Points (Day)	Alcohol [%]	pH	Saccharose [° Brix-g/100mL]	Acidity [mg acetic acid /L]
Green Tea Kombucha—GK	0	0.0 ± 0.00 *,2,4	5.54 ± 0.01 *,2,3,4,5	10.75 ± 0.00 *,3,4	20.12 ± 0.01 *,2,3,4
	1	0.2 ± 0.00 *,1,3	3.50 ± 0.04 *,1,3,4	9.75 ± 0.35 *,3,4,6	610.34 ± 0.02 *,1,3,4
	7	3.0 ± 0.00 *,2,4	2.61 ± 0.03 *,1,2,7	10.0 ± 0.00 *,1,2,4,7,11	7039.21 ± 0.12 *,1,2,7,11,15
	14	2.75 ± 0.50 *,1,3	2.49 ± 0.04 *,1,2	8.75 ± 0.00 *,1,3,4	9147.40 ± 0.31 *,1,2,12,16
Black Tea Kombucha—BK	0	0.0 ± 0.00	5.34 ± 0.03 *,1,6,7,8,9,13	11.0 ± 0.00 *,6,7	23.50 ± 0.01 *,6
	1	0.3 ± 0.00	3.54 ± 0.04 *,5,7,8	10.88 ± 0.18 *,5,7,8,2	501.02 ± 0.11 *,5
	7	3.25 ± 0.50 *,6,8,3,11,15	2.62 ± 0.03 *,3,5,6,8,15	9.5 ± 0.00 *,5,6,8,3	7039.08 ± 0.23 *,6,3,11,15,
	14	2.0 ± 0.00 *,5,7,12,16	2.53 ± 0.03 *,5,6,7,12,16	7.5 ± 0.00 *,6,7	9083.03 ± 0.36 *,5,6,712,16
White Tea Kombucha—WK	0	0.0 ± 0.00	6.53 ± 0.05 *,5,10,11,12	10.75 ± 0.00	21.09 ± 0.01 *,10,11,12
	1	0.4 ± 0.00	3.56 ± 0.06 *,9,11,12	10.13 ± 0.18	620.13 ± 0.09 *,9,11,12
	7	3.5 ± 0.50 *,3,7	2.53 ± 0.05 *,9,10,12	10.13 ± 0.00 *,3	7048.06 ± 0.17 *,9,10,12,3,7
	14	3.0 ± 0.00 *,4,8	2.37 ± 0.05 *,8,9,10,11	9.5 ± 0.00	9132.20 ± 0.43 *,9,10,11,8,16
Red Tea Kombucha—RK	0	0.0 ± 0.00	5.58 ± 0.07 *,5,14,15,16	10.75 ± 0.00 *,14,15,16	20.42 ± 0.03 *,14,15,16
	1	0.4 ± 0.50	3.62 ± 0.01 *,13,15,16	10.25 ± 0.35 *,13,15,16	600.09 ± 0.26 *,13,15,16
	7	3.5 ± 0.50 *,3,7	2.38 ± 0.04 *,7,13,14	10.75 ± 0.00 *,13,14,16	7059.47 ± 0.75 *,7,13,14,16
	14	3.0 ± 0.00 *,4,8	2.32 ± 0.02 *,8,13,14	9.5 ± 0.00 *,14,15	9071.02 ± 0.62 *,4,8,13,14,15

Table 4. Statistically significant (at $p \leq 0.05$) correlation (r) between parameters for kombucha tea. * p value ≤ 0.05.

Kombucha	Green Tea	Black Tea	White Tea	Red Tea
Time vs	Acidity ($r = 0.85$) * pH ($r = 0.81$) *	Acidity ($r = 0.93$) * pH ($r = 0.96$) *	Acidity ($r = 0.99$) * Alcohol ($r = -0.88$) * pH ($r = 0.99$) *	Acidity ($r = 0.99$) * Alcohol ($r = -0.88$) * pH ($r = 0.86$) *
Acidity vs	Time ($r = 0.85$) * Alcohol ($r = -0.61$) * Saccharose ($r = -0.75$) * pH ($r = 0.73$) *	Time ($r = 0.93$) * Saccharose ($r = -0.52$) * pH ($r = 0.88$) *	Time ($r = 0.99$) * Alcohol ($r = -0.93$) * pH ($r = 0.99$) *	Time ($r = 0.99$) * Alcohol ($r = -0.90$) * pH ($r = 0.82$) *
Alcohol vs	Acidity ($r = -0.61$) * Saccharose ($r = 0.65$) *	Saccharose ($r = -0.56$) *	Time ($r = -0.88$) * Acidity ($r = -0.93$) * Saccharose ($r = -0.52$) * pH ($r = -0.91$) *	Time ($r = -0.88$) * Acidity ($r = -0.91$) * pH ($r = -0.65$) *
Saccharose vs	Acidity ($r = -0.75$) * Alcohol ($r = -0.65$) *	Acidity ($r = -0.52$) *, Alcohol ($r = -0.56$) *	Acidity ($r = -0.52$) * pH ($r = -0.47$) *	Alcohol ($r = -0.72$) *
pH vs	Time ($r = 0.81$) * Acidity ($r = 0.73$) *	Time ($r = 0.96$) * Acidity ($r = 0.88$) *	Time ($r = 0.99$) * Acidity ($r = 0.99$) * Alcohol ($r = -0.91$) *	Time ($r = 0.86$) * Alcohol ($r = -0.65$) *

4. Discussion

The popularity of fermented drinks is increasing as consumers perceive fermentation as a mild method for the preservation of food and value the products themselves for their health benefits. Kombucha, as a fermented tea drink, is consumed not only in Asia, where it originally comes from, but also increasingly often in Europe. It is mainly formed from black tea, but other forms of kombucha made from different tea variants, such as green, white or red tea, are becoming increasingly available on the market. Despite the fact that kombucha has been researched in detail in terms of its microbiological content and antibacterial properties, there are not enough studies regarding the various tea types and their health benefits. This is why our study includes different, most frequently consumed tea types (black, green, white and red) and this is why we analysed the content, antioxidant potential depending on the time of fermentation and the type of tea selected for the preparation of kombucha.

This study has demonstrated that the health benefits as well as the chemical content depend both on the type of tea as well as fermentation time. Kombucha is characterised by high antioxidant potential. Green tea was characterised by the most significant antioxidant properties, slightly lower potential was observed for red and white tea types, whereas black tea featured the lowest values. The same tendency was observed for kombucha prepared from a given tea type. In the case of DPPH, the fermentation process had an influence on the increase in antioxidant properties in reference to tea, and with subsequent days of fermentation the potential decreased regardless of the tea type. A reverse situation was observed in the case of the reductive potential (FRAP). Fermentation had an influence on the decrease in reductive properties with reference to tea. The highest reductive potential was observed for kombucha on the 7th day. Therefore, a strong positive correlation was observed between the time of fermentation and the reductive potential (FRAP) as well as polyphenol content. On the other hand, a negative correlation was observed between the time and the antioxidant potential (DPPH). The differences in the antioxidant potential measured by FRAP and DPPH methods are due to different mechanisms of both methods. In the latter method, the DPPH radical uses the free electron transfer reaction, and the FRAP method utilizes metal ions for oxidation. Additionally, the DPPH method does not allow for the determination of hydrophilic antioxidant activity. FRAP was primarily used to determine the absolute reduction in body fluid. Recently, it has also been adapted for plant-based antioxidant research. In our study, both methods showed high reproducibility. However, the DPPH method has been shown to be more stable [21].

These results are similar to those achieved by Gaggia et al. in a study where the highest antioxidant potential (DPPH) was observed in relation to green tea, slightly lower for white tea, and the lowest for red tea. However, in this case, the 7th day of fermentation had the most positive influence on this parameter. It should be highlighted that the authors did not study kombucha on day one. In all cases, the fermentation process increase the antioxidant properties of the drink [19]. An increase in the antioxidant potential of kombucha in comparison to tea was also observed in the study by Chakravorty et al. [22]. The DPPH and ABTS (2,2'-Azino-bis-3-ethylbenzthiazoline-6-sulphonic acid) radicals' scavenging activity increased by 39.7% and 38.36%, respectively, after 21 days [22]. It was also observed that the microbiological content is the most diverse on the 7th day of fermentation. This might indicate that the increase in the diversity of microorganisms plays a significant role in the increase in the antioxidant properties of kombucha tea. Moreover, the change of the domination of yeast to lactic acid bacteria on the 7th day is also responsible for the increased antioxidant activity [22].

Tea, which is also the main ingredient of the drink, is rich in catechins-theaflavin and tearubigin. Polyphenols present in tea are responsible for the antioxidant activity of kombucha. A positive correlation was observed between the content of polyphenols and reductive potential. This study confirms the observations carried out by Chakravorty et al., in which an increase in polyphenols was observed during fermentation [22]. During fermentation, there is an increase in polyphenols, including flavonoids, whereas tearubigin is transformed into theaflavin, resulting in the change in kombucha's colour from dark to light with the progressing time of fermentation [22]. On the basis of our studies, it can be concluded that the general content of polyphenols depended on the type of tea. The highest concentration was observed for green tea, slightly lower for red and white tea types, the lowest for black tea. Fermentation time had an influence on the increase in the content of these compounds. Furthermore, an increase in the content of polyphenols in kombucha in comparison to tea alone has also been observed. For kombucha prepared from green and black tea types, the content of polyphenolic compounds increased with the time of fermentation, achieving the highest concentration on the 14th day. Our studies confirm those of other authors. The highest antioxidant potential was also observed in green tea, but on the 7th day of fermentation (100.33 mg/g). Kombucha prepared from red tea included the smallest amount of polyphenols, but they were stable and their concentration did not change during the fermentation process. This kombucha included a lot of flavonoids [19]. The increase in the content of polyphenolic compounds can be associated with numerous reactions occurring during the fermentation of tea, e.g., the oxidation of polyphenolic compounds by some enzymes leads to the formation of catechins, flavonoids and other compounds with healthy properties, including antioxidant properties, which is the result of a microbial hydrolysis reaction [10]. Moreover, microorganisms such as *Candida tropicalis* are able to degrade various polyphenols [23]. Catechins included in the tea can be broken down through the activity of bacteria and yeast into simpler particles, increasing antioxidant strength [10,24]. In addition, fermentation induces the structural breakdown of plant cell walls, leading to the liberation or synthesis of various antioxidant compounds. These antioxidant compounds can act as free radical terminators, metal chelators, singlet oxygen quenchers or hydrogen donors. The production of protease, α-amylase and some other enzymes might be influenced by fermentation possessing metal ion chelation activity [25].

Our study provides an extensive body of evidence that red tea and kombucha are good sources of polyphenols, among them flavonoids with undisputed antioxidant effects Additionally, they helps seal blood vessels, have anti-inflammatory properties and support immune system function [26]. Flavonoids, present in large quantities in red tea, can significantly contribute to its antioxidant properties. A good source of flavonoids also seems to be green tea and kombucha prepared from this variant. However, fermentation contributes to the degradation of this compound. Its highest concentration in red tea subjected to fermentation was observed on day 1 and day 14: 292.54 and 242.5 mg/L, respectively. The value for tea alone was 395.9 mg/L. In comparison, buckwheat—considered as one of the best sources of flavonoids—contains 62.30 mg/100 g of fresh weight of the resource. The tea drink available on the market included only 1.968 mg/L of the resource. Out of 14 of the studied infusions from various tea types, green tea included the highest content of flavonoids—37.13 mg/L [27].

Lactic fermentation is responsible for the breakdown of glucose, which results from the activity of bacteria of lactic fermentation. Another fermentation type is alcoholic fermentation. Yeast, a constituent of the drink's microflora, is responsible for the breakdown of glucose into ethyl alcohol with the appearance of carbon dioxide. Yeast consists of *Schizosaccharomyces pombe*, as well as *Candida krusei* and *Issatchenkia orientalis* [8]. In our study, on day 7, the highest concentration of alcohol was achieved with as much as 3.5% for kombucha prepared from white and red tea types, 3.25% for green tea and 3.0% for black tea. On the 14th day the content of alcohol slightly decreased in the case of all of the studied variants to the level of 2–3%. In a study by Gaggia et al., the content of alcohol on day 14 was higher— at the level of 5.83% for white tea, 4.18% for green tea and only 1.14% for black tea, but this depends on the fermentation conditions, such as temperature or microbiological composition [19]. In the next phase, *Acetobacter* bacteria [8] use ethyl alcohol as a substrate to create acetic acid. The dominating bacteria included in kombucha are the bacteria of acetic acid AAB: *Acetobacter xylinoides, Acetobacter aceti, Acetobacter pasteurianus, Bacterium gluconicum* and *Gluconobacter oxydans*. This is why on the 14th day of the fermentation process, the content of alcohol decreased, and there was an increase in acidity as well as the production of organic acids, including acetic acid. Acetic acid, which is the dominating acid present in a fermented solution, contributes to the decrease in pH from 5 to as low as 3 [10,28].

An important parameter that undergoes change during fermentation is pH and acidity, and thus the content of organic acids. The microorganisms present in SCOBY process the substances included in tea and sugar, producing various metabolites. This is why these parameters change with fermentation time. In this study, the pH of teas was from 5.34 to 6.53. In the case of kombucha, there was a significant decrease in this parameter: from 2.31 to 2.53 on the 14th day of fermentation. There was also a small decrease in pH between the 7th and 14th day of fermentation, which indicates that the reactions responsible for the decrease in this parameter were inhibited. Our results are similar to the findings of other authors [29–31]. Chakravorty et al. observed that the initial pH before fermentation was about 5.03 and decreased abruptly to 2.28 after 7 days of fermentation [22]. It has to be remembered that consuming drinks with a very low pH may negatively influence the digestive system [32]. This is why the fermentation time of kombucha is important, as well as the amount of the consumed drink.

The organic acids present in kombucha include acetic, glucuronic, gluconic, tartaric, malic, citric, lactic, succinic and malonic acids [8,10]. The biochemical content of the drink may slightly differ due to the change of parameters, such as: the amount of sugar, the type and quantity of tea, temperature, pH and the time of fermentation. In this study, for all kombucha types, there was a significant increase in the content of acids during fermentation. The sudden production of organic acids occurred after the 7th day of fermentation. The content of acetic acid on the 14th day of fermentation was the highest for green tea (9147.40 mg/L) and white tea (9132.20 mg/L), the lowest for red tea (9071.02 mg/L) and black tea (9083.03 mg/L). These results correspond to those present in other studies. The research showed differences in metabolite content between the drinks prepared from black tea, green tea and rooibos on different days of fermentation [19]. The content of acetic acid on the 7th day of fermentation present in a study by Gaggìa et al. was the highest in white tea (9.18 mg/mL) and green tea (7.65 mg/mL), while the lowest in rooibos (4.89 mg/mL) [19]. Shahbazi et al. determined that acetic acid was the main acid present in kombucha, and its content significantly decreased during fermentation [29]. Chen and Liu (2000) observed that the concentration of acetic acid increased to 8000 mg/L at the end of the storage period Jayabalan et al. (2007) studied the changes in organic acids of kombucha tea during fermentation [10,33]. They observed that green tea was characterised by the highest content of acetic acid (9500 mg/L) on the 15th day of fermentation [10]. The concentration of lactic acid significantly increased during fermentation. Its concentration was at the level of 145.71 mg/L on the 16th day of fermentation [29]. Malbaša, Lončar and Djurić (2008) used molasses as a source of sugar for the fermentation of kombucha. The content of lactic acid was from 0.16 to 0.4 g/L [34]. It is also worth highlighting that the pH of the solution and the presence of some organic acids determines the growth of microorganisms, and so also the chemical content of the drink [19]. Low pH and high acidity enable the growth of only those microbes that are able to colonise such a niche, so those that can provide a certain kind of protection against unwanted microorganisms [35].

Sugar content in kombucha also changes in time and depends on fermentation. The initial increase in reducing sugar content can be attributed to the hydrolysis of saccharose into glucose and fructose by yeast. With the progressing fermentation, yeast uses sugar in an oxygen-free way to produce ethanol [10]. In our study, the content of sugar decreased with the time of fermentation. The highest decrease (32%) was observed for black tea vs. kombucha on the 14th day of fermentation. Gaggìa et al. checked the content of glucose, fructose and saccharose in kombucha prepared from black, green and red tea types on the 7th and 14th day of fermentation. The content of complex carbohydrates, i.e., saccharose, decreased during fermentation, while the content of simple carbohydrates–glucose–increased. The concentration of fructose increased during fermentation. The highest content of sugars on the 14th day of fermentation was observed in kombucha prepared from red tea [19].

In this study, a strong positive correlation was observed between time, acetic acid and pH, whereas a negative correlation was observed between acetic acid and the content of alcohol and sugar. The observed correlations confirm the changes occurring in kombucha during the process of fermentation. The increase in acidity and pH with the time of fermentation, as well as the decrease in alcohol and sugar content are associated with the production of organic acids and the use of substrates for their production.

Kombucha has many health-promoting properties, including antioxidant ones. Therefore, to support one's antioxidative response, a regular diet should include kombucha, especially in cases of increased exposure to mental and physical stress. Considering the antioxidant properties of kombucha, the most valuable one is derived from red and green tea. However, longer fermentation leads to a decrease in the pH of the drink, which is why consumption of kombucha should be avoided by people suffering from ulcers or gastrointestinal reflux. Of note, kombucha may contain lead from an inadequate vessel, which may be another health hazard [36,37].

5. Conclusions

Kombucha, the fermented tea, has strong antioxidant properties associated with high polyphenol content, particularly flavonoids. Therefore, it should be consumed by people particularly exposed to oxidative stress. The antioxidant activity of kombucha is diverse and depends on the type and composition of the tea infusion before fermentation and on the content of SCOBY, which determines the character of the forming metabolites and conditions the type of the forming products of polyphenol compound transformation. A particularly rich source of antioxidants, especially flavonoids, are red and green tea types on the 1st and 14th day of fermentation. Therefore, the selection of tea other than black tea, and the subsequent subjection to fermentation, are beneficial to human health.

Author Contributions: Conceptualization, K.J. (Karolina Jakubczyk) and K.J. (Katarzyna Janda); Data curation, J.K. (Joanna Kochman); Funding acquisition, K.J. (Karolina Jakubczyk) and K.J. (Katarzyna Janda); Investigation, K.J. (Karolina Jakubczyk) and J.K. (Justyna Kałduńska); Methodology, K.J. (Karolina Jakubczyk) and J.K. (Justyna Kałduńska); Project administration, K.J. (Karolina Jakubczyk) and K.J. (Katarzyna Janda); Resources, J.K. (Joanna Kochman); Supervision, K.J. (Karolina Jakubczyk) and K.J. (Katarzyna Janda); Writing—original draft, K.J. (Karolina Jakubczyk); Writing—review & editing, K.J. (Karolina Jakubczyk) and J.K. (Joanna Kochman). All authors have read and agreed to the published version of the manuscript.

Funding: The project is financed from the program of the Minister of Science and Higher Education under the name "Regional Initiative of Excellence" in 2019-2022 project number 002/RID/2018/19 amount of financing 12 000 000 PLN.

Acknowledgments: The authors are thankful to company Naturalnie naturalni (https://naturalnienaturalni.com/) for providing the materials (Kombucha SCOBY) for this research.

Conflicts of Interest: The authors declare no conflict of interest.

References

1. Blokhina, O.; Virolainen, E.; Fagerstedt, K.V. Antioxidants, Oxidative Damage and Oxygen Deprivation Stress: A Review. *Ann. Bot.* **2003**, *91*, 179–194. [CrossRef] [PubMed]
2. Jakubczyk, K.J.P.; Piotrowska, G.; Janda, K. Characteristics and biochemical composition of kombucha–fermented tea. *Med. Ogólna Nauki Zdrowiu* **2020**. [CrossRef]
3. Chandrakala, S.K.; Lobo, R.O.; Dias, F.O. 16—Kombucha (Bio-Tea): An Elixir for Life? In *Nutrients in Beverages*; Grumezescu, A.M., Holban, A.M., Eds.; Academic Press: Cambridge, MA, USA, 2019; pp. 591–616.
4. Kim, J.; Adhikari, K. Current Trends in Kombucha: Marketing Perspectives and the Need for Improved Sensory Research. *Beverages* **2020**, *6*, 15. [CrossRef]
5. Shahidi, F.; Ambigaipalan, P. Phenolics and polyphenolics in foods, beverages and spices: Antioxidant activity and health effects—A review. *J. Funct. Foods* **2015**, *18*, 820–897. [CrossRef]
6. Jakubczyk, K.; Kałduńska, J.; Dec, K.; Kawczuga, D.; Janda, K. Antioxidant properties of small-molecule non-enzymatic compounds. *Pol. Merkur. Lekarski* **2020**, *48*, 128–132.
7. Blanc, P.J. Characterization of the tea fungus metabolites. *Biotechnol. Lett.* **1996**, *18*, 139–142. [CrossRef]
8. Villarreal-Soto, S.A.; Beaufort, S.; Bouajila, J.; Souchard, J.-P.; Taillandier, P. Understanding Kombucha Tea Fermentation: A Review. *J. Food Sci.* **2018**, *83*, 580–588. [CrossRef]
9. Kapp, J.M.; Sumner, W. Kombucha: A systematic review of the empirical evidence of human health benefit. *Ann. Epidemiol.* **2019**, *30*, 66–70. [CrossRef]
10. Jayabalan, R.; Malini, K.; Sathishkumar, M.; Swaminathan, K.; Yun, S.-E. Biochemical characteristics of tea fungus produced during kombucha fermentation. *Food Sci. Biotechnol.* **2010**, *19*, 843–847. [CrossRef]
11. Ivanišová, E.; Meňhartová, K.; Terentjeva, M.; Harangozo, Ľ.; Kántor, A.; Kačániová, M. The evaluation of chemical, antioxidant, antimicrobial and sensory properties of kombucha tea beverage. *J. Food Sci. Technol.* **2020**, *57*, 1840–1846. [CrossRef]

12. Brand-Williams, W.; Cuvelier, M.E.; Berset, C. Use of a free radical method to evaluate antioxidant activity. *LWT Food Sci. Technol.* **1995**, *28*, 25–30. [CrossRef]
13. Pekkarinen, S.S.; Stöckmann, H.; Schwarz, K.; Heinonen, I.M.; Hopia, A.I. Antioxidant activity and partitioning of phenolic acids in bulk and emulsified methyl linoleate. *J. Agric. Food Chem.* **1999**, *47*, 3036–3043. [CrossRef] [PubMed]
14. Benzie, I.F.; Strain, J.J. The ferric reducing ability of plasma (FRAP) as a measure of "antioxidant power": The FRAP assay. *Anal. Biochem.* **1996**, *239*, 70–76. [CrossRef] [PubMed]
15. Benzie, I.F.; Strain, J.J. Ferric reducing/antioxidant power assay: Direct measure of total antioxidant activity of biological fluids and modified version for simultaneous measurement of total antioxidant power and ascorbic acid concentration. *Methods Enzymol.* **1999**, *299*, 15–27. [PubMed]
16. Singleton, V.L.; Rossi, J.A. Colorimetry of Total Phenolics with Phosphomolybdic-Phosphotungstic Acid Reagents. *Am. J. Enol. Vitic.* **1965**, *16*, 144–158.
17. Hu, S.; Yuan, C.; Zhang, C.H.; Wang, P.; Li, Q.; Wan, J.; Chang, H.; Ye, J.; Guo, X. Comparative Study of Total Flavonoid Contents from the Different Tissues and Varieties of Abelmoschus Esculentus. *Int. J. Med. Sci. Biotechnol.* **2013**, *1*, 26–30.
18. Pękal, A.; Pyrzynska, K. Evaluation of Aluminium Complexation Reaction for Flavonoid Content Assay. *Food Anal. Methods* **2014**, *7*, 1776–1782. [CrossRef]
19. Gaggìa, F.; Baffoni, L.; Galiano, M.; Nielsen, D.S.; Jakobsen, R.R.; Castro-Mejía, J.L.; Bosi, S.; Truzzi, F.; Musumeci, F.; Dinelli, G.; et al. Kombucha Beverage from Green, Black and Rooibos Teas: A Comparative Study Looking at Microbiology, Chemistry and Antioxidant Activity. *Nutrients* **2018**, *11*, 1. [CrossRef]
20. Crafack, M.; Mikkelsen, M.B.; Saerens, S.; Knudsen, M.; Blennow, A.; Lowor, S.; Takrama, J.; Swiegers, J.H.; Petersen, G.B.; Heimdal, H.; et al. Influencing cocoa flavour using Pichia kluyveri and Kluyveromyces marxianus in a defined mixed starter culture for cocoa fermentation. *Int. J. Food Microbiol.* **2013**, *167*, 103–116. [CrossRef]
21. Schlesier, K.; Harwat, M.; Böhm, V.; Bitsch, R. Assessment of Antioxidant Activity by Using Different In Vitro Methods. *Free Radic. Res.* **2002**, *36*, 177–187. [CrossRef]
22. Chakravorty, S.; Bhattacharya, S.; Chatzinotas, A.; Chakraborty, W.; Bhattacharya, D.; Gachhui, R. Kombucha tea fermentation: Microbial and biochemical dynamics. *Int. J. Food Microbiol.* **2016**, *220*, 63–72. [CrossRef] [PubMed]
23. Ettayebi, K.; Errachidi, F.; Jamai, L.; Tahri-Jouti, M.A.; Sendide, K.; Ettayebi, M. Biodegradation of polyphenols with immobilized Candida tropicalis under metabolic induction. *FEMS Microbiol. Lett.* **2003**, *223*, 215–219. [CrossRef]
24. Tanaka, T.; Matsuo, Y.; Kouno, I. Chemistry of Secondary Polyphenols Produced during Processing of Tea and Selected Foods. *Int. J. Mol. Sci.* **2009**, *11*, 14–40. [CrossRef] [PubMed]
25. Hur, S.J.; Lee, S.Y.; Kim, Y.-C.; Choi, I.; Kim, G.-B. Effect of fermentation on the antioxidant activity in plant-based foods. *Food Chem.* **2014**, *160*, 346–356. [CrossRef] [PubMed]
26. Hosseinzadeh, H.; Nassiri-Asl, M. Review of the protective effects of rutin on the metabolic function as an important dietary flavonoid. *J. Endocrinol. Investig.* **2014**, *37*, 783–788. [CrossRef] [PubMed]
27. Price, K.R.; Rhodes, M.J.C.; Barnes, K.A. Flavonol Glycoside Content and Composition of Tea Infusions Made from Commercially Available Teas and Tea Products. *J. Agric. Food Chem.* **1998**, *46*, 2517–2522. [CrossRef]
28. ZhenJun, Z.; YuCheng, S.; HuaWei, W.; CaiBi, Z.; XianChun, H.; Jian, Z. Flavour chemical dynamics during fermentation of kombucha tea. *Emir. J. Food Agric.* **2018**, *30*, 732–741.
29. Shahbazi, H.; Hashemi Gahruie, H.; Golmakani, M.; Eskandari, M.H.; Movahedi, M. Effect of medicinal plant type and concentration on physicochemical, antioxidant, antimicrobial, and sensorial properties of kombucha. *Food Sci. Nutr.* **2018**, *6*, 2568–2577. [CrossRef]
30. Changes in Major Components of Tea Fungus Metabolites during Prolonged Fermentation—Chen—2000—Journal of Applied Microbiology—Wiley Online Library. Available online: https://onlinelibrary.wiley.com/doi/full/10.1046/j.1365-2672.2000.01188.x (accessed on 18 June 2019).
31. Sreeramulu, G.; Zhu, Y.; Knol, W. Kombucha Fermentation and Its Antimicrobial Activity. *J. Agric. Food Chem.* **2000**, *48*, 2589–2594. [CrossRef]
32. Malbaša, R.V.; Lončar, E.S.; Vitas, J.S.; Čanadanović-Brunet, J.M. Influence of starter cultures on the antioxidant activity of kombucha beverage. *Food Chem.* **2011**, *127*, 1727–1731. [CrossRef]

33. Chen, C.; Liu, B.Y. Changes in major components of tea fungus metabolites during prolonged fermentation. *J. Appl. Microbiol.* **2000**, *89*, 834–839. [CrossRef] [PubMed]
34. Malbaša, R.V.; Lončar, E.S.; Djurić, M. Comparison of the products of Kombucha fermentation on Sucrose and molasses. *Food Chem.* **2008**, *106*, 1039–1045. [CrossRef]
35. Greenwalt, C.J.; Steinkraus, K.H.; Ledford, R.A. Kombucha, the Fermented Tea: Microbiology, Composition, and Claimed Health Effects. *J. Food Prot.* **2000**, *63*, 976–981. [CrossRef] [PubMed]
36. Jayabalan, R.; Malbaša, R.V.; Lončar, E.S.; Vitas, J.S.; Sathishkumar, M. A Review on Kombucha Tea—Microbiology, Composition, Fermentation, Beneficial Effects, Toxicity, and Tea Fungus. *Compr. Rev. Food Sci. Food Saf.* **2014**, *13*, 538–550. [CrossRef]
37. Srinivasan, R.; Smolinske, S.; Pharm, D.; Greenbaum, D. Probable Gastrointestinal Toxicity of Kombucha Tea. *J. Gen. Intern. Med.* **1997**, *12*, 643–645. [CrossRef] [PubMed]

 © 2020 by the authors. Licensee MDPI, Basel, Switzerland. This article is an open access article distributed under the terms and conditions of the Creative Commons Attribution (CC BY) license (http://creativecommons.org/licenses/by/4.0/).

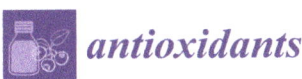

Article

Antioxidant Metabolism and Chlorophyll Fluorescence during the Acclimatisation to Ex Vitro Conditions of Micropropagated *Stevia rebaudiana* Bertoni Plants

José Ramón Acosta-Motos [1,2,†], Laura Noguera-Vera [1,†], Gregorio Barba-Espín [1], Abel Piqueras [1] and José A. Hernández [1,*]

1. Group of Fruit Tree Biotechnology, CEBAS-CSIC, 30100 Murcia, Spain; jacosta@cebas.csic.es (J.R.A.-M.); lauranoguera.ln@gmail.com (L.N.-V.); gbespin@cebas.csic.es (G.B.-E.); piqueras@cebas.csic.es (A.P.)
2. Cátedra Emprendimiento en el Ámbito Agroalimentario, Universidad Católica San Antonio de Murcia (UCAM) Campus de los Jerónimos, no. 135 Guadalupe, 30107 Murcia, Spain
* Correspondence: jahernan@cebas.csic.es
† These authors contributed equally to this work.

Received: 19 November 2019; Accepted: 30 November 2019; Published: 3 December 2019

Abstract: In this study, the functioning of antioxidant metabolism and photosynthesis efficiency during the acclimatisation of *Stevia rebaudiana* plants to ex vitro conditions was determined. A high percentage of acclimatised plants (93.3%) was obtained after four weeks. According to the extent of lipid peroxidation, an oxidative stress occurred during the first hours of acclimatisation. A lower activity of monodehydroascorbate reductase (MDHAR) than dehydroascorbate reductase (DHAR) was observed after 2 days of acclimatisation. However, after 7 days of acclimatisation, stevia plants activated the MDHAR route to recycle ascorbate, which is much more efficient energetically than the DHAR route. Superoxide dismutase and catalase activities showed a peak of activity after 7 days of acclimatisation, suggesting a protection against reactive oxygen species. Peroxidase activity increased about 2-fold after 2 days of acclimatisation and remained high until day 14, probably linked to the cell wall stiffening and the lignification processes. In addition, a progressive increase in the photochemical quenching parameters and the electronic transport rate was observed, coupled with a decrease in the non-photochemical quenching parameters, which indicate a progressive photosynthetic efficiency during this process. Taken together, antioxidant enzymes, lipid peroxidation, and chlorophyll fluorescence are proven as suitable tools for the physiological state evaluation of micropropagated plants during acclimatisation to ex vitro conditions.

Keywords: acclimatisation; antioxidant defences; chlorophyll fluorescence; in vitro culture; peroxidase; stevia plants

1. Introduction

The application of in vitro culture techniques is a powerful vegetative proliferation tool for many plant species [1]. However, this process can be limited due to significant losses during acclimatisation to ex vitro conditions. For this raison, a better knowledge of the physiology and biochemistry of in vitro cultured plants that subsequently will be adapted to ex vitro conditions are of major interest. Light availability, and therefore the process of photosynthesis, is a key factor for ex vitro acclimatisation. Improvement of the photosynthetic activity is a critical step to reach a high survival rate during acclimatisation of in vitro plantlets [2]. In other words, proper photosynthesis activation is the key point to change the way to acquire carbon from heterotrophic or mixotrophic (in vitro conditions) to autotrophic (ex vitro conditions) sources. In grapevine, net photosynthesis and biomass are dependent on the increase in light intensity [2]. However, a distinct response was found in chestnut under the same conditions, where symptoms of photoinhibition were found during the acclimatisation process [2]. The transition from in vitro to ex vitro conditions has not been studied extensively, and an appropriate research model is still missing. Some of them have used the chlorophyll fluorescence technique as a non-destructive indicator to follow the acclimatisation process [1–3].

Micropropagated plants are very susceptible to environmental challenges after transferring to ex vitro conditions. For example, ex vitro plants are normally subjected to higher photosynthetic photon flux density (PPFD) than plants grown under in vitro conditions. In addition, the relative humidity (RH) is also lower under ex vitro conditions, thus plants are prone to suffer desiccation. Both phenomena, which contribute to photoinhibition damage and water stress, can induce the overproduction of reactive oxygen species (ROS). However, plants are provided with an efficient antioxidant defence mechanism to defend against the harmful effects of ROS. These defences include the ascorbate-glutathione (ASC-GSH) cycle enzymes (ascorbate peroxidase (APX), monodehydroascorbate reductase (MDHAR), dehydroascorbate reductase (DHAR) and glutathione reductase (GR)) and ROS-scavenging enzymes (superoxide dismutases (SODs), peroxidases (POX) and catalase (CAT)). The knowledge about the behaviour of the antioxidant machinery during ex vitro acclimatisation is very scarce, and only a few researchers have studied the changes on the enzymatic and non-enzymatic antioxidants during this process [1,3–5].

Stevia (*Stevia rebaudiana* Bertoni) is a perennial shrub belonging to the Asteraceae family. The leaves of *S. rebaudiana* contain a high concentration of steviol glycosides, stevioside and rebaudioside A being the prevalent forms, and used as natural sweeteners as a substitute for saccharose [6]. However, stevia seeds have little viability and the plant requires specific humidity, light, and nutrient conditions. The accumulation of steviol glycosides within *S. rebaudiana* is very variable due to significant genetic variability. The total steviol glycoside content changed not only between plants of the same cultivar, but also among similar plants in the same developmental stage [7]. In addition, a high antioxidant capacity of *S. rebaudiana* leaf extracts, related to their function as ROS-scavengers, has been reported [7–9]. These positive roles have been primarily associated with the presence of phenolic compounds [7]. Moreover, health-related effects of stevioside against type-II diabetes, hypertension, metabolic syndrome, and atherosclerosis have been reported [7]. Therefore, the production of in vitro clonal plants with a similar stevioside profile can be of commercial interest.

Accordingly, this work has focused on the acclimatisation to ex vitro conditions of stevia clones, originated from the micropropagation of plants previously characterised as high accumulators of steviol glycosides [10]. During the process of acclimatisation, the evolution of different parameters, including antioxidant metabolism, lipid peroxidation as an oxidative stress parameter, and chlorophyll fluorescence, were monitored to determine the oxidative stress that stevia plants might be suffering during the aforementioned process.

2. Material and Methods

2.1. Plant Material and Experimental Design

The plants were obtained from micropropagated stevia shoot cultures [10] (solid Murashige and Skoog (MS) medium supplemented with 60 mg L^{-1} phloroglucinol, 30 mg L^{-1} sequestrene, 0.8 mg L^{-1} meta-topolin, 6 mg L^{-1} adenine sulphate, 0.040 mg L^{-1} indole butyric acid, 3% sucrose, and a pH of 5.8). For elongation and rooting, shoots with three internodes were transferred to 1/2 MS medium without growth regulators, containing 40 mg L^{-1} sequestrene, 80 mg L^{-1} phloroglucinol, 250 mg L^{-1} MES buffer, 0.7% Agar, and a pH of 5.8. Under these conditions, the shoots elongated and rooted in 6 weeks. All cultures were maintained at 25 ± 2 °C in a growth chamber with a 16 h photoperiod (80 μmol m^{-2} s^{-1} photosynthetically active radiation, PAR). When the plantlets reached ca. 8–9 cm shoot length, the acclimatisation stage was initiated. For this, the rooted shoots were washed with distilled water to remove the agar and grown in an acclimatisation chamber (UBBINK propagator,

(Northampton, UK)), consisting of a plastic tray and a transparent plastic cover, containing 2 vents for the control of the RH* in a mixture of perlite and peat (1:2, *v:v*). The substrate was moistened with distilled water and a systemic fungicide–bactericide (Beltanol-L, Probelte, Murcia, Spain) at 0.1% (*v/v*), which was also applied to the plantlets. These plantlets were kept in a culture chamber with a 16 h photoperiod and 25 °C, firstly at 150 µmoles cm^{-2} s^{-1} PAR for a period of ten days, followed by 18 days at 350 µmoles cm^{-2} s^{-1} PAR to complete the acclimatisation to ex vitro conditions. During this period, the respirators were gradually open to decrease the humidity progressively. For the different analysis, samples were taken from in vitro plantlets, and from plants at 2, 7, 14, 21, and 28 days of acclimatisation.

2.2. Measurement of Chlorophyll Fluorescence

Chlorophyll fluorescence was measured with a chlorophyll fluorimeter (IMAGIM-PAM M-series, Heinz Walz, Effeltrich, Germany) during the acclimatisation period of stevia plants to ex vitro conditions, at 2, 7, 14, 21, and 28 days of the initiation of the acclimatisation period. After a dark incubation period (20 min), the minimum and the maximal fluorescence yields of the stevia leaves were monitored. Kinetic analyses were carried out with actinic light (81 µmol quanta m^{-2} s^{-1} PAR) and repeated pulses of saturating light at 2700 µmol quanta m^{-2} s^{-1} PAR for 0.8 s, and at intervals of 20 s [11,12]. The following parameters were also analysed: effective PSII quantum yield (Y(II)); the quantum yield of regulated energy dissipation (Y(NPQ)); the non-photochemical quenching (NPQ); the maximal PSII quantum yield (Fv/Fm); the coefficients of non-photochemical quenching (qN); the photochemical quenching (qP); and quantum yields of non-regulated energy dissipation Y(NO) [13].

2.3. Lipid Peroxidation

Stevia leaves were snap-frozen in liquid nitrogen and stored at −80 °C until use. The extent of lipid peroxidation was estimated by determining the concentration of thiobarbituric acid-reactive substances (TBARS) using a UV/Vis V-630 Bio spectrophotometer (Jasco, Tokyo, Japan). Leaf samples (0.2 g) were ground in liquid nitrogen into a fine powder and extracted in 1 M perchloric acid solution (1/10, w/v). Homogenates were centrifuged at 12,000× g for 10 min and 0.5 mL of the supernatant obtained was added to 1.5 mL 0.5% TBA in 1 M perchloric acid. The mixture was incubated at 90 °C in a shaking water bath for 20 min, and the reaction was stopped by placing the reaction tubes in an ice water bath. Then, the samples were centrifuged at 10,000× g for 5 min, and the absorbance of the supernatant was read at 532 nm. The value for non-specific absorption at 600 nm was subtracted. The amount of TBARS (red pigment) was calculated from the extinction coefficient 155 mM^{-1} cm^{-1} [10]. The lipid peroxidation was measured in plantlets under in vitro conditions as well as during the acclimatisation period of stevia plants to ex vitro conditions at 2, 7, 14, 21, and 28 days after the initiation of the acclimatisation process.

2.4. Enzyme Extraction and Analysis

Leaf samples were homogenized in liquid nitrogen and an extraction medium (1/5, *w/v*) containing 50 mM Tris-acetate buffer (pH 6.0); 0.1 mM EDTA; 2 mm cysteine; and 0.2 % (*v/v*) Triton X-100. For the ascorbate peroxidase (APX) activity, 20 mM sodium ascorbate was added to the extraction buffer. The extracts were centrifuged at 10,000× g for 20 min. The supernatant fraction was filtered on Sephadex NAP-10 columns (GE Healthcare, Chicago, IL, USA) equilibrated with the same buffer used for homogenisation and used for the enzymatic determinations. For the APX activity, 2 mM of sodium ascorbate was added to the equilibration buffer.

The enzymatic analyses were measured in plantlets under in vitro conditions as well as during the acclimatisation period of stevia plants to ex vitro conditions at 2, 7, 14, 21, and 28 days of the initiation of the acclimatisation process. The antioxidant enzyme determinations were carried according to protocols set up in our laboratory using a UV/Vis V-630 Bio spectrophotometer (Jasco) [11,14,15]. Specifically, APX (EC 1.11.1.11) was determined following the decrease at 290 nm due to the ascorbate oxidation by H_2O_2. MDHAR (EC 1.6.5.4) was determined following the decrease at 340 nm due to the NADH oxidation. DHAR (EC1.8.5.1) was determined by following the increase at 265 nm due to ascorbate formation. The reaction rate was corrected for the nonenzymatic reduction of DHA by reduced glutathione (GSH). GR (EC 1.6.4.2) was assayed by the decrease at 340 nm due to the NADPH oxidation. The reaction rate was corrected for the non-enzymatic oxidation of NADPH by oxidized glutathione (GSSH). SOD (EC 1.15.1.1) was assayed by the ferricytochrome c method using xanthine/xanthine oxidase as the source of superoxide radicals. CAT (EC 1.11.1.6) was measured following the decrease at 240 nm due to H_2O_2 consumption [14,15]. POX activity (EC. 1.11.1.7) was analysed following the oxidation of 4-methoxy-a-naphtol at 593 nm [15].

Protein contents were analysed according to [16] using a plate reader (Epoch2, BioTek, Winooski, VT, USA) and bovine serum albumin as standard.

2.5. Statistical Analysis

The data were analysed by one-way ANOVA followed by Tukey's Multiple Range Test ($p \leq 0.05$) to separate treatment means, using the SPSS 20.0 software (SPSS Inc., 2002, Chicago, IL, USA). Multivariate analysis using the StatGraphics Centurion XV software (StatPoint Technologies, Warrenton, VA, USA) were conducted by Principal Component Analysis (PCA), followed by a partial least squares discriminant analysis to assign the principal components displaying eigenvalues greater than or equal to 1.0.

3. Results

In the present work, the acclimatisation of in vitro *Stevia rebaudiana* Bertoni plants to ex vitro conditions was achieved with a high success rate, since 93.3% of the plants survived.

3.1. Chlorophyll Fluorescence Measurement

During the acclimatisation process, the evolution of the fluorescence parameters was monitored. At Day 2, the plants displayed higher values of the non-photochemical quenching parameters (Y(NPQ), Y(NO), NPQ and qN) and low values of the photochemical quenching parameters (Y(II), qP) (Table 1, Figure 1), as well as of the electron transport rate (ETR) (Figure 2). During the acclimatisation process, a progressive decrease in the non-photochemical quenching parameters and a constant increase in the photochemical-quenching parameters were observed. In that regard, Y(NPQ) continuously decreased, reducing its values by 40% and 50% after 21 and 28 days of the acclimatisation, respectively (Table 1, Figure 1). Concomitantly, Y(NO) declined during the acclimatisation assay, reaching a decrease near 40% and 30% after 21 and 28 days of acclimatisation, respectively (Table 1, Figure 1). NPQ displayed increases and decreases during the acclimatisation process. At first, after 7 days of acclimatisation this parameter increased by 22%. Then, the NPQ value increased by 63% after 14 days of acclimatization in relation to the precedent value (Day 7). One week later (day 21), again the NPQ value raised by 29% in comparison to the value observed in the second week (14 days). Finally, after 28 days of acclimatisation, a 30% decrease in the NPQ parameter was observed in relation to the value observed after 21 days (Table 1, Figure 1). However, although the qN values decreased during the acclimatisation process, the changes produced were not statistically significant (Table 1, Figure 1). Regarding the photochemical quenching parameters (Y(II) and qP), a progressive increase occurred during the acclimatisation. In both cases, the values increased near 3-fold after 7 and 14 days of acclimatisation, and about 5-fold after 21 and 28 days of the process (Table 1, Figure 1). Fv/Fm showed the lowest values after 2 days of acclimatisation. This parameter increased after 7 and 14 days, and then slightly decreased after 21 and 28 days of acclimatisation, but their values remaining statistically higher than the initial values (Table 1). The changes observed in Y(II) and qP correlated with the evolution of the ETR values, reaching an increase of near 6-fold at the end (28 days) of the acclimatisation process (Figure 2).

Table 1. Evolution of photochemical (Y(II), qP, Fv/Fm) Fv/Fm and non-photochemical quenching parameters (Y(NPQ), Y(NO), NPQ, qN) during the process of acclimatization to ex vitro conditions of *Stevia rebaudiana* Bertoni plants. [a] F: values from one-way ANOVA for the different chlorophyll fluorescence parameters at 99.9% level of significance (*).

Days	Y(II)	qP	Fv/Fm	Y(NPQ)	Y(NO)	NPQ	qN
2	0.090 ± 0.009c	0.160 ± 0.020c	0.747 ± 0.004c	0.544 ± 0.009a	0.393 ± 0.007a	0.354 ± 0.008b	0.719 ± 0.007a
7	0.256 ± 0.022b	0.445 ± 0.033b	0.782 ± 0.006ab	0.479 ± 0.020b	0.279 ± 0.008c	0.433 ± 0.017a	0.749 ± 0.012a
14	0.319 ± 0.048b	0.488 ± 0.038b	0.791 ± 0.005a	0.353 ± 0.023c	0.327 ± 0.012b	0.274 ± 0.019c	0.618 ± 0.022a
21	0.453 ± 0.014a	0.787 ± 0.013a	0.767 ± 0.002b	0.320 ± 0.016cd	0.226 ± 0.004d	0.355 ± 0.023b	0.706 ± 0.017a
28	0.446 ± 0.009a	0.710 ± 0.018a	0.772 ± 0.003b	0.272 ± 0.006d	0.282 ± 0.011c	0.248 ± 0.012c	0.605 ± 0.014a
[a] F	70.82*	88.59*	14.89*	62.85*	40.08*	25.81*	21.73*

Different letters in the same column indicate significant differences according to Tukey's Multiple Range Test ($p \leq 0.05$).

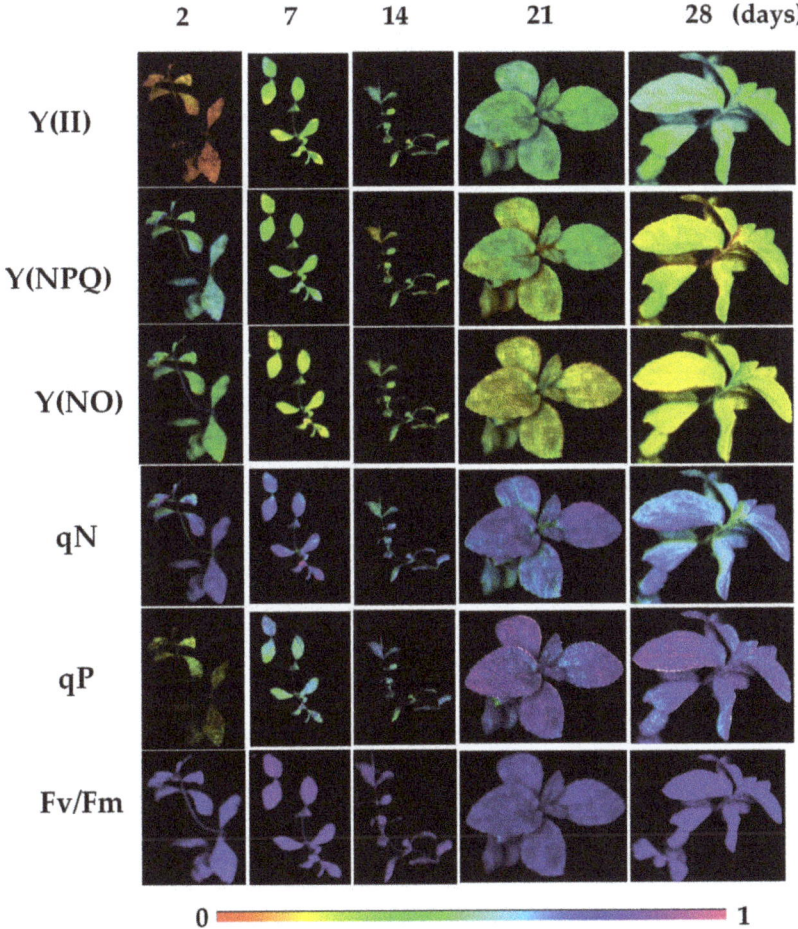

Figure 1. Evolution of the chlorophyll fluorescence parameters during the acclimatisation process of *S. rebaudiana* Bertoni plants to ex vitro conditions.

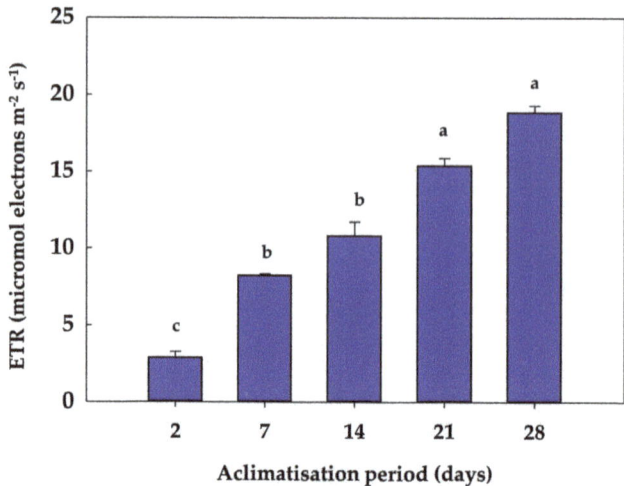

Figure 2. Evolution of the electron transport rate (ETR) during the acclimatization process of *S. rebaudiana* Bertoni plants to ex vitro conditions. Different letters in the same column indicate significant differences according to Tukey's Multiple Range Test ($p \leq 0.05$).

Complementarily, PCA was utilized as a mathematical tool to determine associations among the different chlorophyll fluorescence parameters, ETR, and the acclimatisation evolution (Figure 3). The first component (PC1), which explains 63% of the variability of the experiment (Table S1, Table S2 and Figure S1), indicated the greater relevance of the photosynthetic efficiency mechanisms to adapt to ex vitro conditions, as reflected by the positive values that show all the measured parameters related to the photochemical quenching parameters, such as Y(II), qP and Fv/Fm, and ETR. On the contrary, the contribution of the non-photochemical quenching parameters, related to heat dissipation in a regulated or unregulated way, was negative in the PC1. This was the case for qN, the NPQ, and Y (NPQ) in the first case (regulated dissipation), and Y (NO) in the second case (unregulated dissipation). Regarding the second component (PC2), which explained 24% of the variability of the experiment (Table S1, Table S2 and Figure S1), it indicated that in a second level of importance for the acclimatisation to ex vitro conditions the excess of light energy was also relevant, being not destined to perform photosynthesis, but dissipated safely as heat by regulated mechanisms as observed in the high positive values that show all the related measured parameters (qN, NPQ and Y(NPQ)). Again, as in PC1, any unregulated heat dissipation mechanism played a harmful role in the plant as reflected in the negative values of Y(NO).

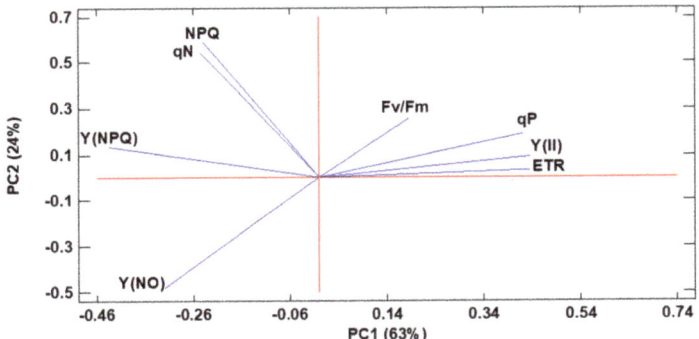

Figure 3. A principal component analysis applied to the fluorescence chlorophyll and electron transport rate (ETR) parameters. Two principal components (PC1 and PC2) resulted in a model that explained 87% of the total variance. The arrows denote eigen vectors characterised by the direction and the strength of the variable relative to PC1 and PC2.

3.2. Antioxidant Metabolism

3.2.1. Lipid Peroxidation Assay

During the first hours of the acclimatisation process, stevia plants seemed to experience stress due to the modification on the culture conditions, as observed by the increase in the lipid peroxidation levels, measured as TBARS. In that regard, a peak after 2 days was detected, increasing by 86% with respect to values in the plantlet (Figure 4). Thereafter, and as the acclimatisation process to ex-vitro conditions progressed, the lipid peroxidation values progressively decreased reaching initial values (Figure 4).

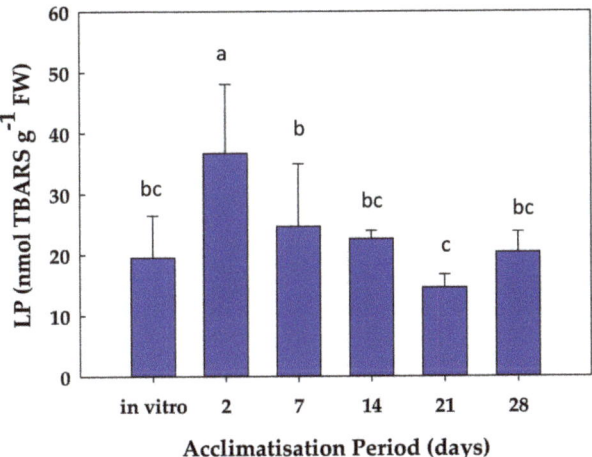

Figure 4. Levels of lipid peroxidation (LP) during the acclimatization process of *S. rebaudiana* Bertoni plants to ex vitro conditions. Different letters (a,b,c) in the same column indicate significant differences according to Tukey's Multiple Range Test ($p \leq 0.05$).

3.2.2. Antioxidant Enzymes

During the acclimatisation process of stevia plants to ex vitro conditions, the levels of some antioxidant enzymes, including the ASC-GSH cycle enzymes, superoxide dismutase (SOD), peroxidase (POX), and catalase (CAT), were analysed.

Regarding the ASC-GSH cycle enzymes, ascorbate peroxidase (APX) activity showed its highest activity in in vitro plants after 2 days of the acclimatisation process. The lowest APX activities were observed after 14 and 28 days, representing a decrease of ca. 35% with respect to the other time points (Figure 5). The monodehydroascorbate reductase (MDHAR) activity displayed its lower values at the beginning of the process of acclimatisation, i.e., under in vitro conditions and after 2 days of the acclimatisation process. Then, MDHAR activity progressively increased, especially after 21 and 28 days of acclimatisation, showing a 2.7- and 3.6-fold increase, respectively, with respect to values after 2 days (Figure 5). Regarding dehydroascorbate reductase (DHAR) activity, it behaved contrary to MDHAR activity. In that sense, DHAR showed its higher values after 2 days of the acclimatisation process, with a 40% increase in relation to the values observed in in vitro plants (Figure 5). Subsequently, DHAR activity progressively declined, with decreases ranging from 34% to 64% depending on the acclimatisation period, and a minimum DHAR activity observed after 14 days of acclimatisation (Figure 5). The GR activity behaved similarly to MDHAR activity. In that regard, GR increased as the plant acclimatisation process progressed, reaching their maximum values after 21 and 28 days of acclimatisation (4.2- and 3.2-fold increases, respectively) (Figure 5).

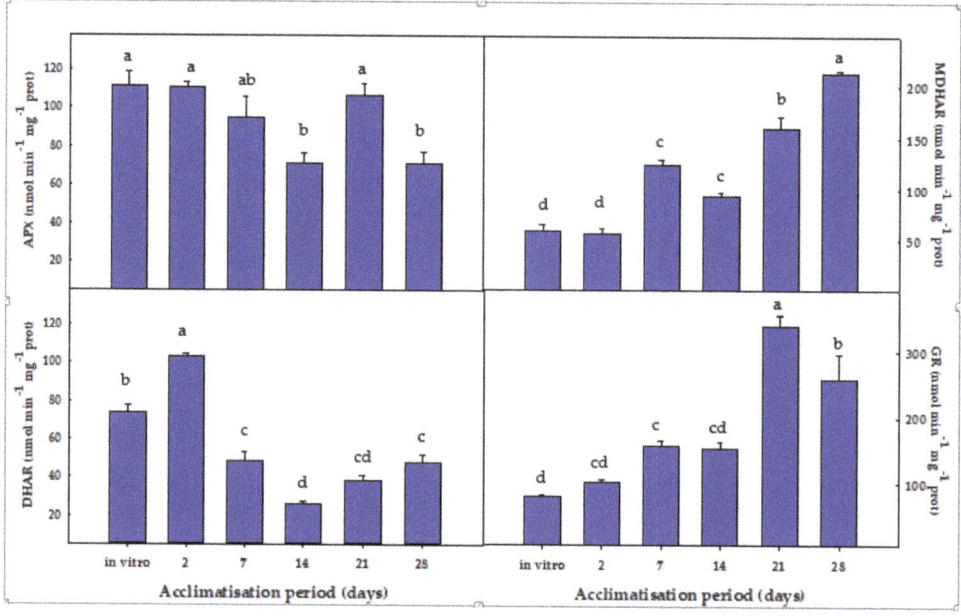

Figure 5. Evolution of the activity of the ASC-GSH cycle enzymes during the process of acclimatisation to ex vitro conditions of *S. rebaudiana* Bertoni plants. Different letters (a,b,c,d) in the same column indicate significant differences according to Tukey's Multiple Range Test ($p \leq 0.05$).

The activity SOD remained statistically invariable at all times except after 7 days of acclimatisation, where a 3.5-fold increase in relation to the initial values was observed (Figure 6). A similar response was observed for the CAT activity: a 1.7-fold increase occurred after 7 days of acclimatisation, whereas in the rest of the period the CAT activity displayed no significant differences in relation to the initial values (Figure 5). POX activity increased remarkably after 2 days, maintaining the value after 7 days

(2.4-fold increase with respect to in vitro plants). Thereafter, POX activity progressively declined until reaching a 4.2-fold decrease with respect to the values after 7 days (Figure 6).

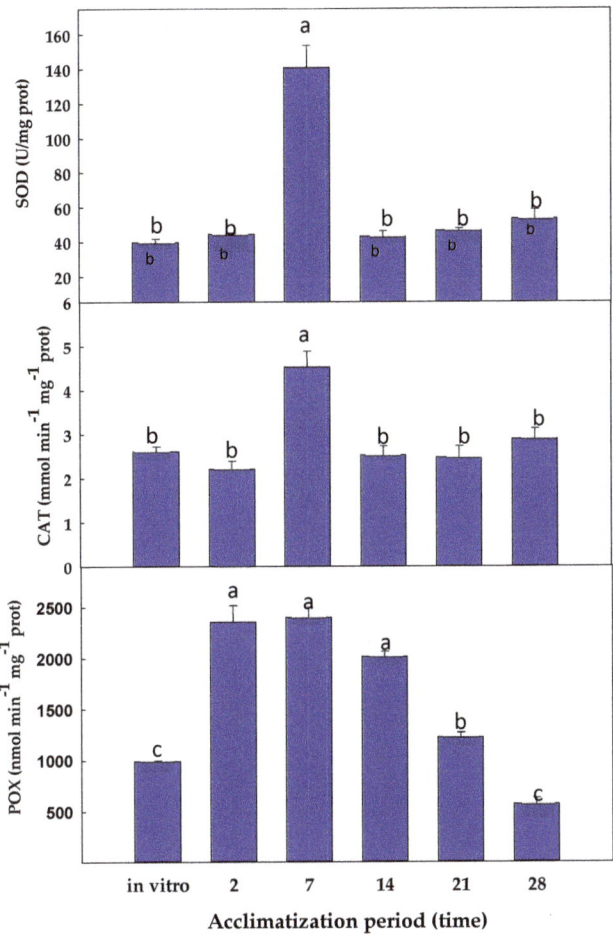

Figure 6. Evolution of the activity of SOD, CAT, and POX during the process of acclimatisation to ex vitro conditions of *S. rebaudiana* Bertoni plants. Different letters (a,b,c) in the same column indicate significant differences according to Tukey's Multiple Range Test ($p \leq 0.05$).

Complementarily, a PCA study was carried out to analyse the associations between the different antioxidant enzymes monitored, as well as lipid peroxidation during the evolution of acclimatisation to ex vitro conditions (Figure 7). The resulting model with two components explained 63% of the total variance. The first component (PC1), which explained 37% of the variability within the dataset (Table S3, Table S4 and Figure S2), indicates the importance of the defence mechanisms to protect from the cellular damage associated with lipid peroxidation (LP), allowing a faster acclimatisation to ex vitro conditions. The efficient antioxidant mechanisms are reflected by the positive values observed in the ROS-eliminating enzymes (SOD, POX and CAT), as well as MDHAR and GR, which guarantees redox homeostasis of the plant. However, the contribution of DHAR and APX was less important, as denoted by their negative values. With respect to the second component (PC2), explaining 26% of the variability of the experiment (Tables S3 and S4), the loadings for LP, DHAR, CAT, and POX appeared as the dominant variables, and were opposite to the positive contribution of APX. Moreover, the loadings for DHAR and LP clustered together, which may relate to the parallel evolution of both variables during the acclimatisation period.

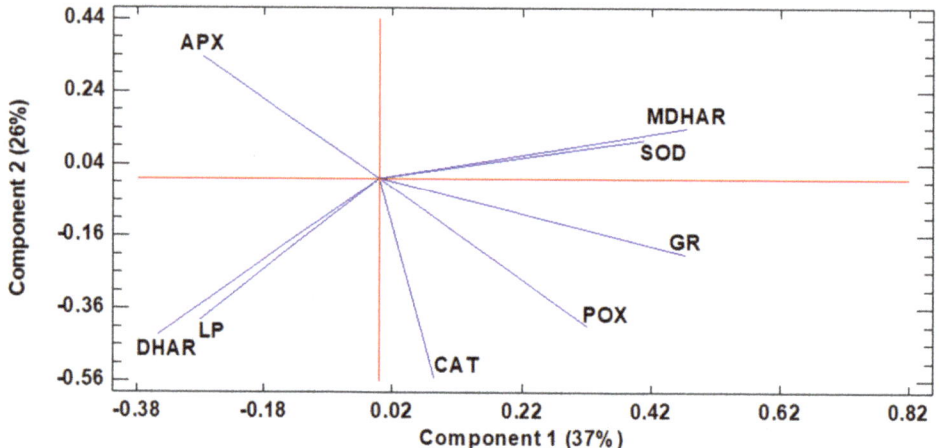

Figure 7. A principal component analysis applied to the antioxidant enzymes and lipid peroxidation variables. Two principal components (PC1 and PC2) resulted in a model that explained 63% of the total variance. The arrows denote eigen vectors characterised by the direction and the strength of the variable relative to PC1 and PC2.

4. Discussion

The acclimatisation to ex vitro conditions is a critical step for the survival of micropropagated in vitro plants. Light availability is an important factor for a successful process of acclimatisation, involving a proper activation of the photosynthesis process [2]. The transition from in vitro to ex vitro conditions has been achieved in numerous plant species, both herbaceous and woody plants [2,4,8,10,17–20].

The micropropagation and acclimatisation of stevia plants can be an excellent tool to ensure the production of clonal, uniform, and true-to-type plant material. This may be used as a by-pass to the problems associated to the low germination rate and the great variation in the profile of steviol glycosides of S. rebaudiana. As a consequence, the production of uniform S. rebaudiana plants with the same steviol glycosides profile is of important commercial interest. This is particularly interesting for rebaudioside A, which provides a superior flavour to food products compared to other steviosides [6]. In a previous work, carried out in our laboratory, we reported that the main steviol glycoside detected in stevia plants after 10 week of acclimatisation was stevioside, whereas after 12 weeks, the main steviol glycoside was rebaudioside A, whose levels were not affected by the presence of NaCl [10]

4.1. Chlorophyll Fluorescence

The use of the chlorophyll fluorescence technique has been used for different researchers to evaluate the acclimatisation process [1–3,21,22]. These authors found that acclimatised plants to ex vitro conditions increased the photosynthesis rate, which correlated with higher chlorophyll contents as well as Fv/Fm and Y(II) fluorescence parameters. In other studies, the authors used the photosynthesis rate or the chlorophyll a fluorescence technique, as well as the measurement of the antioxidant defences as indicators of the evolution of the acclimatisation process [1–4,17,19]. Accordingly, the monitoring of some physiological, biochemical, and molecular parameters can be useful tools to determine the success of ex vitro acclimatisation of in vitro plantlets.

Light intensity is another relevant abiotic factor influencing the acclimatization process. This was the case of grapevine and *Dieffenbachia* plantlets. In both cases, the increase in biomass or net photosynthesis was depending on the light intensity [2,5]. In grapevine, the photochemical quenching parameters, Y(II) and qP, showed higher values in the presence of 300 µmol m^{-2} s^{-1} of photons than in lower light intensities (100 µmol m^{-2} s^{-1}), indicating a better photosynthetic efficiency at higher intensities. However, during the acclimatisation of *Dieffenbachia* plantlets, the Fv/Fm decreased with the increase in light intensity, demonstrating that photoinhibition occurred after transplanting micropropagated plants [5]. In grapevine, immediately after transferring to ex vitro conditions, a reversible photoinhibition occurred, as denoted by an initial decrease in Fv/Fm and F'q/F'm parameters followed by a progressive increased until Day 7 [3]. The mentioned responses could be due to the presence of poorly developed chloroplasts in the in vitro established leaves, resulting in a low resistance against photoinhibition [23].

In this work, a decrease in the non-photochemical quenching parameters and an increase in the photochemical-quenching parameters were observed during acclimatisation to ex vitro conditions. This response was correlated with a progressive increase in ETR values, indicating a gain of chloroplast efficiency during the process. In this sense, Y(II) represents the proportion of the light absorbed by chlorophyll associated with PSII that is used for photochemistry, whereas qP gives an indication of the proportion of the PSII reaction centres that are open [13].

In contrast, the high values observed in the non-photochemical quenching parameters in the first steps of the acclimatisation process would indicate that part of the light captured by the chloroplasts may dissipate as heat, protecting the chloroplast against the excess of radiation and avoiding the formation of ROS, especially singlet oxygen. Different authors have previously described the increase in non-photochemical parameters as an efficient mechanism for dissipating excess light energy and thus minimizing ROS generation [13]. In addition, it has been demonstrated that NPQ and Y(NPQ) are parameters very sensitive in the early detection of stress conditions by using fluorescence images [24]. Both NPQ and Y(NPQ) are related to the energy dissipated as heat by regulated mechanism (i.e., the xanthophyll cycle) [25]. In contrast, Y(NO) reflects the fraction of energy passively dissipated as heat and fluorescence, mainly due to closed PSII reaction centres. Therefore, high values of Y(NO) are related to the inability of plants to protects itself from excess light. In that regard, after 2 days of acclimatisation, stevia plants showed the highest values of Y(NO), which progressively decreased during the acclimatisation process, reflecting a better regulation [26]. On the other hand, high values of the non-photochemical parameters indicated that plants are suffering a stress. However, as the plant adapts to the new ex vitro conditions, these parameters decreased.

4.2. Antioxidant Response

Several authors used biochemical parameters, including antioxidant enzymes and lipid peroxidation, to follow the acclimation of in vitro plantlets. In the ornamental African violet, SOD, CAT, and glutathione-peroxidase (GSH-POX) increased after 28 days of acclimatisation, concomitantly with the increase in the light irradiance, suggesting that plants were suffering an abiotic stress [4]. However, the lipid peroxidation extent, measured as malondialdehyde contents, was 2-fold higher under low irradiance (35 µmol m^{-2} s^{-1}) than in the presence of higher light intensities (70–100 µmol m^{-2} s^{-1}), indicating the presence of an oxidative stress. This response was associated with a lower activity of the antioxidants enzymes as well as a low reduced glutathione (GSH) content. In fact, GSH not only acts as an antioxidant substrate in the ASC-GSH cycle but also as an antioxidant to minimize oxidative stress [27]. In a recent work, [5] analysed the activity of some antioxidant enzymes (SOD, CAT, and GSH-POX) during the acclimatisation of different *Dieffenbachia* cultivars grown at different light intensities. SOD and GSH-POX activity were much higher in the presence of the higher photosynthetic photon flux density (PPFD). However, the effect of PPFD on CAT activity was less evident, although the activity was higher in the presence of 100 PPFD (µmol m^{-2} s^{-1}) than with lower light intensities (35 and 75 PPDF) [5]. According to these authors, this response of the antioxidant defences could be due to the higher ROS production induced by light stress.

In the present work, during the first days of ex vitro acclimatisation, an oxidative stress also occurred, as indicated by the lipid peroxidation levels. This variable is considered as an oxidative stress marker [12]; consequently, a damage to membrane lipids occurred, probably due to the change on the culture conditions. However, once this change on the culture conditions took place, the plants became progressively adapted to the new conditions, as reflected by the decrease in lipid peroxidation. A similar response has been described by [3] during the acclimatisation to ex vitro conditions of grapevine plantlets. These authors monitored the H_2O_2 levels, another oxidative stress marker, observing a 50% increase in H_2O_2 contents after 24 h of the acclimatisation process. Thereafter, H_2O_2 levels declined to the initial values and even lower [3]. In the same work, the increase in H_2O_2 after transfer to ex vitro conditions was followed by an increase in the expression of some antioxidant enzymes, including *APX1*, *GR1*, *SOD1*, and *SOD2* [3]. This response was partially similar to the observed in acclimatized stevia plants. In the present work, both MDHAR and GR activities increased during the acclimatisation process to ex vitro conditions, and other antioxidant enzymes as SOD, CAT, and POX peaked after 7 days of acclimatisation. In accordance with this, under in vitro conditions and after 2 days of acclimatisation, stevia plantlets displayed the highest DHAR activity, with values superior to MDHAR activity—the other ASC-recycling enzyme of the ASC-GSH cycle—at the same time. In that regard, after 2 days of acclimatisation the ratio DHAR/MDHAR was nearly 2. This suggests that, at that stage, DHAR activity is predominant in recycling ascorbate in stevia plants, using GSH as the electron donor. Subsequently, DHAR decreased and MDHAR progressively increased, reaching a DHAR/MDHAR ratio of 0.22 after 28 days of acclimatisation, where MDHAR activity was near 5-times higher than DHAR activity. Therefore, after 2 days of acclimatisation, stevia plants used the MDHAR way, spending NADH as a reducing power. It is necessary to clarify that the utilization of NADH to recycle the ASC is more efficient energetically than the use of GSH. Thus, different possibilities can be speculated to explain the higher DHAR activity under in vitro conditions and after 2 days of acclimatisation. The first is that under in vitro conditions, the culture media contained sucrose, so the plants had enough carbon source to generate energy through the glycolysis and respiration pathways, and thus they can afford the use GSH to recycle ASC (the inefficient way). The second possibility is that after 2 days of the acclimatisation process, the plants suffered an oxidative stress, as monitored by the lipid peroxidation data. Given that overexpression of *DHAR* has been associated with environmental stress tolerance [28], the higher DHAR activity observed at this stage could have a role coping with the stress resulting of the acclimatisation conditions. The third explanation is linked to the role of DHAR in plant growth and development [29]. Probably, after 2 days of acclimatisation the increased DHAR could have a function in plant growth and development processes. We also observed that MDHAR activity was enhanced after 7 days of acclimatisation. At this stage, photosynthesis seemed to work properly, as observed by the chlorophyll fluorescence and ETR values. Therefore, from that moment on, the plants produced their own sugars and energy to support plant growth. Probably, for this reason, plants changed the manner to recycle the ascorbate to an efficient way—via NADH.

On the other hand, it is known that DHAR and GR work together in the ASC-GSH cycle. We observed that under in vitro conditions and after 2 days of acclimatisation the ratio DHAR/GR was ca. 1, supporting the function of DHAR activity in the ascorbate recycling by using GSH as reducing power. However, from that moment on, the GR activity progressively increased, whereas DHAR significantly declined. This response supports the idea that most of the GSH produced in the GR reaction is used for other purposes, including the maintenance of redox homeostasis in stevia plants.

The peroxidase (POX) activity increased more than 2-fold after 2 days of acclimatisation and remained high until day 14, probably linked to the cell wall stiffening and the lignification processes that lead to hardening of the cell wall, as part of the plant differentiation process [30–32]. The overexpression of horseradish *POX* stimulated the growth of tobacco and hybrid aspen plants [33]. In pea seedlings and plants, a correlation between POX activity increase and growth was observed [34,35]. Thus, the observed increases in POX activity during the acclimatisation period can be linked to the plant growth and differentiation processes. However, a role of the POX eliminating H_2O_2 during the acclimatisation process cannot be ruled out. In fact, SOD, POX, and CAT displayed their maximum activities after 7 days of acclimatisation, indicating that these enzymes could work sequentially to eliminate $O_2\bullet^-$ and H_2O_2 at that time, since SOD generates H_2O_2, which is eliminated by the action of the H_2O_2-scavenging enzymes, such as POX, CAT, or even APX, which maintained its activity after 7 days of acclimatisation.

The results obtained by PCA confirmed the importance of the antioxidant mechanisms and the photosynthesis in the acclimatization of stevia plants. In general, greater efficiency in acclimatization to ex vitro conditions was more evident after 7 days of acclimatization and in the last two weeks (24 and 28 days), with increases in the antioxidant enzymes CAT, GR MDHAR, POX, and SOD, and also accompanied by decreases in lipid peroxidation (LP) in these same time periods.

5. Conclusions

Taken together, the data suggested that antioxidant enzymes, lipid peroxidation, and chlorophyll fluorescence parameters can be suitable tools for the evaluation of the physiological state of micropropagated plants during the acclimatisation to ex vitro conditions of stevia plants, providing very useful information to monitor the stress state of the plants during the process of acclimatisation. This work has practical implications, since clonal plants of stevia with a known and stable profile of steviol glycosides are a suitable source of edulcorates and natural antioxidants to a diet.

Supplementary Materials: The following are available online at http://www.mdpi.com/2076-3921/8/12/615/s1, Figure S1: Sedimentation graph where two PCA with eigenvalues greater than or equal to 1.0 were obtained to determine associations among the different chlorophyll fluorescence parameters, ETR and the acclimatisation evolution, Figure S2: Sedimentation graph where two PCA with eigenvalues greater than or equal to 1.0 were obtained to analyse the associations between the different antioxidant enzymes monitored, as well as lipid peroxidation during the evolution of acclimatisation to ex vitro conditions, Table S1: Weight of the Components for the fluorescence chlorophyll parameters and ETR, Table S2: Eigenvalues and percentage of variance of components for the fluorescence chlorophyll parameters and ETR, Table S3: Weight of the Components for the antioxidant enzymes and lipid peroxidation data (LP), Table S4: Eigenvalues and percentage of variance of components for the antioxidant enzymes and lipid peroxidation data.

Author Contributions: Conceptualization, J.A.H and A.P.; methodology, J.A.H, L.N.-V. and A.P.; formal analysis, J.A.H. and J.R.A.-M.; investigation J.A.H, L.N.-V. and A.P.; data curation J.A.H., J.R.A-M and G.B.-E.; writing—original draft preparation, J.A.H.; writing—review and editing, J.A.H, J.R.A.-M. and G.B.-E.

Funding: G.B.E. thanks the "Fundación Séneca" of the Agency of Science and Technology of the Region of Murcia for his research contract.

Conflicts of Interest: The authors declare no conflict of interest.

References

1. Van-Huylenbroeck, J.M.; Piqueras, A.; Debergh, P.C. The evolution of photosynthetic capacity and the antioxidant enzymatic system during acclimatization of micropropagated *Calathea* plants. *Plant Sci.* **2000**, *155*, 59–66. [CrossRef]
2. Carvalho, L.C.; Osorio, M.L.; Chaves, M.M.; Amâncio, S. Chlorophyll fluorescence as an indicator of photosynthetic functioning of in vitro grapevine and chestnut plantlets under ex vitro acclimatization. *Plant Cell Tissue Organ Cult.* **2001**, *67*, 271–280. [CrossRef]
3. Carvalho, L.C.; Vilela, B.J.; Vidigal, P.; Mullineaux, P.M.; Amâncio, S. Activation of the ascorbate-glutathione cycle is an early response of micropropagated *Vitis vinifera* L. explants transferred to ex Vitro. *Int. J. Plant Sci.* **2006**, *167*, 759–770. [CrossRef]
4. Dewir, Y.H.; El-Mahrouk, M.E.; Al-Shmgani, H.S.; Rihan, H.Z.; Teixeira da Silva, J.A.; Fuller, M.P. Photosynthetic and biochemical characterization of in vitro-derived African violet (*Saintpaulia ionantha* H. Wendl) plants to ex vitro conditions. *J. Plant Interact.* **2015**, *10*, 101–108. [CrossRef]

5. El-Mahrouk, M.E.; Dewir, Y.H.; Murthy, H.N.; Rihan, H.Z.; Al-Shmgani, H.S.; Fuller, M.P. Effect of photosynthetic photon flux density on growth, photosynthetic competence and antioxidant enzymes activity during ex vitro acclimatization of *Dieffenbachia* cultivars. *Plant Growth Regul.* **2016**, *79*, 29–37. [CrossRef]
6. Zeng, J.; Cheng, A.; Lim, D.; Yi, B.; Wu, W. Effects of salt stress on the growth, physiological responses, and glycoside contents of *Stevia rebaudiana* Bertoni. *J. Agric. Food Chem.* **2013**, *61*, 5720–5726. [CrossRef]
7. Ceunen, S.; Geuns, J.M.C. Steviol Glycosides: Chemical Diversity, Metabolism, and Function. *J. Nat. Prod.* **2013**, *76*, 1201–1228. [CrossRef]
8. Ghanta, S.; Banerjee, A.; Poddar, A.; Chattopadhyay, S. Oxidative DNA Damage Preventive Activity and Antioxidant Potential of *Stevia rebaudiana* (Bertoni) Bertoni, a Natural Sweetener. *J. Agric. Food Chem.* **2007**, *55*, 10962–10967. [CrossRef]
9. Jahan, I.A.; Mostafa, M.; Hossain, H.; Nimmi, I.; Sattar, A.; Alim, A.; Moeiz, S.M.I. Antioxidant activity of *Stevia rebaudiana* Bert. leaves from Bangladesh. *Bangladesh Pharm. J.* **2010**, *13*, 67–75.
10. Cantabella, D.; Piqueras, A.; Acosta-Motos, J.R.; Bernal-Vicente, A.; Hernandez, J.A.; Diaz-Vivancos, P. Salt-tolerance mechanisms induced in *Stevia rebaudiana* Bertoni: Effects on mineral nutrition, antioxidative metabolism and steviol glycoside content. *Plant Physiol. Biochem.* **2017**, *115*, 484–496. [CrossRef]
11. Acosta-Motos, J.R.; Díaz-Vivancos, P.; Álvarez, S.; Fernández-García, N.; Sánchez-Blanco, M.J.; Hernández, J.A. Physiological and biochemical mechanisms of the ornamental *Eugenia myrtifolia* L. plants for coping with NaCl stress and recovery. *Planta* **2015**, *242*, 829–846. [CrossRef] [PubMed]
12. Acosta-Motos, J.R.; Díaz-Vivancos, P.; Álvarez, S.; Fernández-García, N.; Sánchez-Blanco, M.J.; Hernández, J.A. NaCl-induced physiological and biochemical adaptative mechanisms in the ornamental *Myrtus communis* L. plants. *J. Plant Physiol.* **2015**, *183*, 41–51. [CrossRef] [PubMed]
13. Maxwell, K.; Johnson, G.N. Chlorophyll fluorescence: A practical guide. *J. Exp. Bot.* **2000**, *51*, 659–668. [CrossRef] [PubMed]
14. Ros Barceló, A.; Gómez-Ros, L.V.; Ferrer, M.A.; Hernández, J.A. The apoplastic antioxidant enzymatic system in the wood-forming tissues of trees. *Trees* **2006**, *20*, 145–156. [CrossRef]
15. Barba-Espín, G.; Clemente-Moreno, M.J.; Álvarez, S.; García-Legaz, M.F.; Hernández, J.A.; Díaz-Vivancos, P. Salicylic acid negatively affects the response to salt stress in pea plants: Effects on *PR1b* and *MAPK* expression. *Plant Biol.* **2011**, *13*, 909–917. [CrossRef]
16. Bradford, M.M. A rapid and sensitive method for the quantitation of microgram quantities of protein utilizing the principle of protein-dye binding. *Anal. Biochem.* **1976**, *72*, 248–254. [CrossRef]
17. Ďurkovič, J.; Čaňová, I.; Pichler, V. Water loss and chlorophyll fluorescence during ex vitro acclimatization in micropropagated black mulberry (*Morus nigra* L.). *Propag. Ornam. Plants* **2009**, *9*, 107–112.
18. Clemente-Moreno, M.J.; Piqueras, A.; Hernández, J.A. Implication of peroxidase activity in development of healthy and PPV-infected micropropagated GF305 peach plants. *Plant Growth Regul.* **2011**, *65*, 359–367. [CrossRef]
19. Chaari-Rkhis, A.; Maalej, M.; Chelli-Chaabouni, A.; Fki, L.; Drira, N. Photosynthesis parameters during acclimatization of in vitro-grown olive plantlets. *Photosynthetica* **2015**, *53*, 613–616. [CrossRef]
20. Diaz-Vivancos, P.; Faize, L.; Nicolas, E.; Clemente-Moreno, M.J.; Bru-Martinez, R.; Burgos, L.; Hernández, J.A. Transformation of plum plants with a cytosolic ascorbate peroxidase transgene leads to enhanced water stress tolerance. *Ann. Bot.* **2016**, *117*, 1121–1131. [CrossRef]
21. Pospisilova, J.; Ticha, I.; Kadlecek, P.; Haisel, D.; Plazakova, S. Acclimatization of micropropagated plants to ex vitro conditions. *Biol. Plant.* **1999**, *42*, 481–497. [CrossRef]
22. Van-Huylenbroeck, J.M.; Piqueras, A.; Debergh, P.C. Photosynthesis and carbon metabolism in leaves formed prior and during ex vitro acclimatization of micropropagated plants. *Plant Sci.* **1998**, *134*, 21–30. [CrossRef]
23. Lee, N.; Wetzstein, H.Y.; Sommer, H.E. Effects of quantum flux density on photosynthesis and chloroplast ultrastrucutre in tissue-cultured plantlets and seedling of *Liquidambar styraciflua* L. towards improved acclimatization and filed survival. *Plant Physiol.* **1985**, *78*, 637–664. [CrossRef] [PubMed]
24. Pérez-Bueno, M.L.; Ciscato, M.; vandeVen, M.; García-Luque, I.; Barón, M.; Valcke, R. Imaging viral infection: Studies on *Nicotiana benthamiana* plants infected with the pepper mild mottle virus. *Photosynth. Res.* **2006**, *90*, 111–123. [CrossRef] [PubMed]
25. Zhang, Q.Y.; Wang, L.Y.; Kong, F.Y.; Deng, Y.S.; Li, B.; Meng, Q.W. Constitutive accumulation of zeaxanthin in tomato alleviates salt stress-induced photoinhibition and photooxidation. *Physiol. Plant.* **2012**, *146*, 363–373. [CrossRef] [PubMed]

26. Klughammer, C.; Schreiber, U. Complementary PSII quantum yields calculated from simple fluorescence parameters measured by PAM fluorometry and the saturation pulse method. *PAM Appl. Notes (PAN)* **2008**, *1*, 27–35.
27. Alscher, R.G.; Donahue, J.L.; Cramer, C.L. Reactive oxygen species and antioxidant: Relationship in green cells. *Physiol. Plant.* **1997**, *100*, 224–233. [CrossRef]
28. Eltayeb, A.E.; Kawano, N.; Badawi, G.H.; Kaminaka, H.; Sanekata, T.; Morishima, I.; Shibahara, T.; Inanaga, S.; Tanaka, K. Enhanced tolerance to ozone and drought stresses in transgenic tobacco overexpressing dehydroascorbate reductase in cytosol. *Physiol. Plant.* **2006**, *127*, 57–65. [CrossRef]
29. Potters, G.; Horemans, N.; Caubergs, R.J.; Asard, H. Ascorbate and dehydroascorbate influence cell cycle progression in a tobacco cell suspension. *Plant Physiol.* **2012**, *124*, 17–20. [CrossRef]
30. Pomar, F.; Caballero, N.; Pedreño, M.A.; Ros Barceló, A. H_2O_2 generation during the auto-oxidation of coniferyl alcohol drives the oxidase activity of a highly conserved class III peroxidase involved in lignin biosynthesis. *FEBS Lett.* **2002**, *529*, 198–202. [CrossRef]
31. Sato, Y.; Demura, T.; Yamawaki, K.; Inoue, Y.; Sato, S.; Sugiyama, M.; Fukuda, H. Isolation and characterization of a novel peroxidase gene ZPO-C whose expression and function are closely associated with lignification during tracheary element differentiation. *Plant Cell Physiol.* **2006**, *47*, 493–503. [CrossRef] [PubMed]
32. Boerjan, W.; Ralph, J.; Baucher, M. Lignin biosynthesis. *Annu. Rev. Plant Biol.* **2003**, *54*, 519–546. [CrossRef] [PubMed]
33. Kawaoka, A.; Matsunaga, E.; Endo, S.; Kondo, S.; Yoshida, K.; Shinmyo, A.; Ebinuma, H. Ectopic expression of a horseradish peroxidase enhances growth rate and increases oxidative stress resistance in hybrid aspen. *Plant Physiol.* **2003**, *132*, 1177–1185. [CrossRef]
34. Diaz-Vivancos, P.; Barba-Espín, G.; Clemente-Moreno, M.J.; Hernandez, J.A. Characterization of the antioxidant system during the vegetative development of pea plants. *Biol. Plant.* **2010**, *54*, 76–82. [CrossRef]
35. Barba-Espín, G.; Diaz-Vivancos, P.; Clemente-Moreno, M.J.; Albacete, A.; Faize, L.; Faize, M.; Perez-Alfocea, F.; Hernandez, J.A. Interaction between hydrogen peroxide and plant hormones during germination and the early growth of pea seedlings. *Plant Cell Environ.* **2010**, *33*, 981–994. [CrossRef] [PubMed]

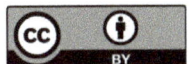

© 2019 by the authors. Licensee MDPI, Basel, Switzerland. This article is an open access article distributed under the terms and conditions of the Creative Commons Attribution (CC BY) license (http://creativecommons.org/licenses/by/4.0/).

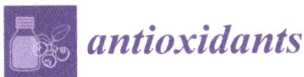

Article

Domestic Sautéing with EVOO: Change in the Phenolic Profile

Julián Lozano-Castellón [1,2], Anna Vallverdú-Queralt [1,2], José Fernando Rinaldi de Alvarenga [3], Montserrat Illán [1], Xavier Torrado-Prat [1] and Rosa Maria Lamuela-Raventós [1,2,*]

1. Nutrition, Food Science and Gastronomy Department, XaRTA, Institute of Nutrition and Food Safety (INSA-UB), School of Pharmacy and Food Sciences, University of Barcelona, 08028 Barcelona, Spain; julian.lozano@ub.edu (J.L.-C.); avallverdu@ub.edu (A.V.-Q.); millan@ub.edu (M.I.); xaviertorrado@ub.edu (X.T.-P.)
2. CIBER Physiopathology of Obesity and Nutrition (CIBEROBN), Institute of Health Carlos III, 28029 Madrid, Spain
3. Department of Food Science and Experimental Nutrition, School of Pharmaceutical Sciences, Food Research Center (FoRC), University of São Paulo, 05508-060 São Paulo, Brazil; zehfernando@gmail.com
* Correspondence: lamuela@ub.edu; Tel.: +34-934034843

Received: 11 December 2019; Accepted: 13 January 2020; Published: 16 January 2020

Abstract: (1) Background: The health benefits of extra-virgin olive oil (EVOO), a key component of the Mediterranean diet, are attributed to its polyphenol profile. EVOO is often consumed cooked, and this process may degrade and transform polyphenols. (2) Methods: In this work, we determined how temperature, time, and the interaction between them affects the EVOO polyphenolic profile during a domestic pan-frying process, simulating the cooking conditions of a home kitchen, without the control of light or oxygen. Applying a 2^2 full factorial design experiment, "Hojiblanca" EVOO was processed at two temperatures (120 °C and 170 °C) either for a short time or a long time, mimicking a domestic process, and polyphenol content was analyzed by UPLC-ESI-QqQ-MS/MS. (3) Results: Temperature degraded the polyphenols of EVOO during the sauté cooking process, whereas time had an effect on some individual phenols, such as hydroxytyrosol, but not on the total phenol content. The polyphenol content decreased by 40% at 120 °C and 75% at 170 °C compared to raw EVOO. (4) Conclusions: Cooked EVOO still meets the parameters of the EU's health claim.

Keywords: home-cooking; extra virgin olive oil; UPLC-ESI-QqQ-MS/MS; healthy cooking; Mediterranean diet

1. Introduction

Extra virgin olive oil (EVOO), the main source of fat in a Mediterranean diet, displays a singular fatty acid composition with a higher content of phenolic compounds and other antioxidants than other edible oils. Its health benefits are mainly attributed to these minor components, above all to simple phenols and polyphenols (both referred to henceforth as polyphenols) [1]. Its consumption has shown to play a protective role against a wide range of diseases [1,2], such as cancer [3], cardiovascular diseases [4], neurodegeneration [5], and diabetes [6]. EVOO phenolic concentration can be improved by changing agronomic and technical factors, such as the simple minimization of bruising by a selection of the variety [7].

The problem is that the Mediterranean consumption of EVOO is not only carried out by using it as a final seasoning; EVOO is also used in Mediterranean cuisine for roasting, sautéing (pan-frying), stir-frying, and deep-frying. All of these culinary techniques are thermal processes that could diminish the minor components of EVOO, such as polyphenols, by substances leaching (especially of more polar compounds) into the medium or by the degradation and transformation of its polyphenol content [8,9]. In addition to the loss of antioxidants, pro-oxidants formation can occur, especially when cooking at high temperatures, notably as a consequence of the lipid oxidation [10,11]. Nevertheless, EVOO polyphenols have been shown to reduce the heat-induced formation of undesired compounds, such as the cancerogenic heterocyclic amines [12], and the formation of acrolein and hexanal [13]. Finally, the polyphenols can act as lipid-derived carbonyl scavengers [14].

Most of the studies on cooking-induced changes in the polyphenol composition of EVOO have been carried out in laboratory conditions [15,16], applying non-conventional Mediterranean cooking techniques, like microwaving [17], or exploring the addition of a phenolic extract rather than EVOO [18]. Their results may not match those produced in a domestic setting because of the differences in oxygen and light availability or because polyphenol degradation in EVOO may be influenced by its content of other minor compounds [19].

On the other hand, previous studies carried out under more true-to-life conditions have focused on comparing the polyphenol content between raw and cooked foods [20] and between foods prepared with different cooking techniques [9]. However, they were not focused on evaluating EVOO polyphenol degradation or how this is affected by cooking factors, like temperature or time. When cooking factors, such as time, were explored, oil was heated for a longer time than the real cooking time, i.e., for 25 or even 36 h [21,22]. Furthermore, some works explored the degradation of total polyphenols measured by the Folin-Ciocalteau method, which is not selective and measures all antioxidant compounds [23]. Consequently, more research is required to determine the extent to which the loss of polyphenols during cooking is counteracted by the beneficial effects of EVOO, or how the phenolic profiles are altered during domestic cooking.

In this context, the aim of the present study was to determine changes in the EVOO polyphenolic profile during a domestic sautéing process commonly used in the Mediterranean diet [24], using a 2^2 full factorial design to assess the effect of time, temperature, and the interactions between these two factors, mimicking real conditions (without oxygen or light control). The polyphenolic profile was measured using ultra-high performance liquid chromatography coupled to a tandem mass spectrometer detector (UPLC-ESI-QqQ-MS/MS), providing information on how the polyphenolic profile changed and how individual polyphenols degraded at different rates.

2. Materials and Methods

2.1. Chemicals and Standards

Acetonitrile, methanol, formic acid, and acetic acid were purchased from AppliChem, Panreac Quimica SA (Barcelona, Spain). Hexane, *p*-coumaric acid, ferulic acid, luteolin, oleuropein, oleocanthal, and pinoresinol were purchased from Sigma-Aldrich (St. Louis, MO, USA). Hydroxytyrosol was acquired from Extrasynthese (Genay, France) and apigenin from Fluka (St. Louis, MO, USA). Ultrapure water was obtained using a Milli-Q purification system (Millipore, Bedford, MA, USA).

2.2. Samples

Polyphenol degradation was assessed in the common Spanish "Hojiblanca" variety of EVOO, which has a medium concentration of polyphenols [25]. It was provided by the Fundación Patrimonio Comunal Olivarero and was produced from olives milled in December 2016 in Spain.

2.3. Domestic Sauté Process

To simulate the home-cooking process of sauté, EVOO was heated in a pan (20 cm diameter, 0.8 mm thickness, stainless steel 18/10, Excalibur, Pujadas, Girona, Spain), and the influence of the cooking process on polyphenol degradation was monitored at two different temperatures: moderate (120 °C) and high (170 °C). In order to assess the influence of time, short and long cooking times were determined for each temperature, corresponding to the time needed to obtain "al dente" and well-cooked textures, respectively. For determining these times, 200 g of potatoes and 100 g of chicken (an average portion) were pan-fried at both temperatures, and the selected times for 120 °C were 30 and 60 min and the times for 170 °C were 15 and 30 min, time being a qualitative factor. A full-factorial design was performed (2^2) with three replicates per point to assess the effect of the temperature and time of cooking and the possible interaction between these two factors. The levels and the processing conditions are shown in Table 1.

Table 1. Levels and conditions of the full factorial design.

Experiment	Temperature (Level)	Time (Level)	Temperature	Time
1	−1	−1	120 °C	30
2	1	−1	170 °C	15
3	−1	1	120 °C	60
4	1	1	170 °C	30

The domestic sautéing was performed at the Food Torribera Campus, University of Barcelona (Santa Coloma de Gramenet, Spain). The pan was heated on an electrical cooking plate (180 mm diameter, 1500 W, model Encimera EM/30 2P, Teka®, Madrid, Spain) until the required temperature was reached. The temperature was monitored with a laser thermometer (error: ±1 °C, ScanTemp 410, TFA Dostmann GmbH & Co. KG, Wertheim, Germany) and maintained by turning the heat up or down as necessary. When the target temperature was achieved, 20 g of EVOO were added to the pan and heated for the chosen time. The pan was then removed from the heat and after a short cooling period, the oil was stored in a vacuum bag at −20 °C until extraction. The oxygen or light were not controlled to mimic the process carried out in a normal kitchen.

2.4. Polyphenol Extraction and Analysis

2.4.1. Polyphenol Extraction

The liquid-liquid extraction of phenolic compounds was performed following the method proposed by Kalogeropoulos et al. (2007) with minor modifications [26]. All of the extraction process was carried out over an ice bed. Briefly, 0.5 g of EVOO was suspended with 5 mL of methanol in a 10 mL centrifuge tube and stirred for 30 s. It was centrifuged for 3 min at 3000 rpm and 4 °C. The methanolic fraction was then transferred into a flask and the extraction was repeated. Both methanolic fractions were combined and evaporated under a reduced pressure. The residue was reconstituted with 2 mL of acetonitrile and washed twice with 2 mL of hexane. The acetonitrile was evaporated under a reduced pressure and the residue was reconstituted with 800 µL of MeOH:H$_2$O (4:1 v/v), filtered with Polytetrafluoroethylene syringe filters (0.2 µm), and was transferred to an amber glass vial and stored at −80 °C until analysis.

2.4.2. Polyphenol Analysis by UPLC-ESI-QqQ-MS/MS

The identification and quantification of phenolic compounds, except oleocanthal, oleacein and oleuropein and ligstroside aglycones, was performed following the method proposed by Suárez et al. (2008) with minor modifications [27], using an AcquityTM UPLC (Waters; Milford, MA, USA) coupled to an API 3000 triple-quadruple mass spectrometer (PE Sciex, Framingham, MA, USA) with a turbo ion spray source. The separation of compounds was achieved using an Acquity UPLC® BEH C18 Column (2.1 × 50 mm, i.d., 1.7 µm particle size) (Waters Corporation®, Wexford, Ireland) and an Acquity UPLC® BEH C18 Pre-Column (2.1 × 5 mm, i.d., 1.7 µm particle size) (Waters Corporation®, Wexford, Ireland). The exact chromatographic conditions were as detailed elsewhere [28].

The quantification of oleocanthal, oleacein, oleuropein aglycone, and ligstroside aglycone was performed using a methodology proposed by Sánchez de Medina et al. (2017) with some modifications [29]. Separation was achieved using an Acquity UPLC® BEH C18 Column (2.1 × 50 mm, i.d., 1.7 µm particle size) (Waters Corporation®, Wexford, Ireland) and Acquity UPLC® BEH C18

Pre-Column (2.1 × 5 mm, i.d., 1.7 μm particle size) (Waters Corporation®, Wexford, Ireland). The exact chromatographic conditions were as detailed elsewhere [28].

Ionization was performed using an electrospray (ESI) interface operating in the negative mode [M − H], and all of the compounds were monitored in the multiple reaction monitoring mode (MRM). The exact ionization and spectrometric conditions are detailed in the previous study [28], and the energies and retention times for each analyzed compound are shown in Tables S1 and S2. The system was controlled by Analyst version 1.4.2 software supplied by Applied Biosystems (Waltham, MA, USA).

Quantification was performed by an external standard calibration method, standards showed linearity in the concentration range 1–20 mg/L. Quantification was performed using oleuropein for hydroxydecarboxymethyl oleuropein aglycone (HDCM-OA), hydroxyoleuropein aglycone (HOA), elenolic acid, and hydroxyelenolic acid; hydroxytyrosol for hydroxytyrosol and hydroxytirsol acetate; the respective standards for ferulic acid, *p*-coumaric acid, pinoresinol, apigenin and luteolin were used; and oleocanthal was used for oleocanthal, ligstroside aglycone, oleacein, and oleuropein aglycone.

2.5. Statistical Analysis

The statistical differences between samples of EVOO taken in different cooking conditions were analyzed by Statistica version 10.0.228.8 (StatSoft Inc., Tulsa, OK, USA) using the factorial ANOVA test. The assumption of normalization was graphically checked. To assess the importance of the contributing factors, multiple linear regressions were calculated. The form of the regression is as follows:

$$\text{Concentration} = \beta_0 + \beta_1 \cdot T + \beta_2 \cdot t + \beta_3 \cdot Tt \quad (1)$$

where T stands for temperature, t stands for time, and each β is the contribution of these factors. If its *p*-value is lower than 0.05, then β is significantly different from 0. The statistic R^2 is adjusted to the size of the model and can decrease if insignificant factors are added [30]. This parameter measures the proportion of the total variability explained by the model [31,32]. Even if the factors were not statistically significant, they were added to the model as confusing variables, and it was assessed if the model was more accurate with or without them. The model with the largest adjusted R^2 was selected. In order to build the model, the low temperature was the point −1 and the high temperature point was +1, and the same was applied for the short (−1) and long (+1) cooking time. Then, the value of β multiplied per 2 is the difference between the two levels of a factor.

3. Results and Discussion

3.1. Total Polyphenols

The concentrations of different polyphenols and of the groups found in raw and cooked EVOO samples are presented in Table 2.

When EVOO was heated in a pan, the sumatory of polyphenolic content decreased by around 40% at the low temperature (120 °C) and 75% at the high temperature (170 °C). Casal et al. (2010) reported a decrease of 50% in the total phenolic content, measured by the Folin-Ciocalteu method, after heating olive oil in a domestic deep-fat fryer at 170 °C for 3 h. [23]. However, in this study, the oil was deep fried so the samples were less exposed to oxygen and light, which may explain why the results are different to those presented here. Moreover, Folin-Ciocalteau methods are not selective, so this variation is not measuring only the phenol content, but also other reducing compounds. For this reason, it is also difficult to compare the results with those showed by one recent study, in which the degradation of the total phenolic content during a sautéing process was evaluated. The authors showed a decrease of approximately 50% of the antioxidant capacity measured by the Folin-Ciocalteau method after sautéing typical Mediterranean vegetables (potato, eggplant, tomato, and pumkin) for 10 min at 100 °C [33].

Table 2. Polyphenolic concentration of raw and processed extra-virgin olive oil (EVOO) expressed in mg/kg of EVOO.

Group/Compound	Raw	↓T ↓t	↓T ↑t	↑T ↓t	↑T ↑t
Sum of phenols	860 ± 22	487 ± 29	498 ± 32	240 ± 19	218 ± 12
Secoiridoids	835 ± 22	466 ± 30	481 ± 31	231 ± 20	213 ± 12
Ligstroside aglycone	368 ± 7	190 ± 13	193 ± 11	94 ± 21	97 ± 7
Oleocanthal	81 ± 4	51 ± 3	53 ± 5	41 ± 3	41 ± 3
Oleuropein aglycone	79 ± 2	45 ± 3	47 ± 3	15 ± 2	12 ± 1
Oleacein	252 ± 9	134 ± 13	139 ± 15	46 ± 6	32 ± 4
HDCM-OA	23.6 ± 0.9	21 ± 2	22 ± 3	16 ± 2	9 ± 1
HOA	3.2 ± 0.2	2.3 ± 0.3	3.3 ± 0.5	2.3 ± 0.3	0.7 ± 0.1
Elenolic acid	25.1 ± 0.2	16 ± 2	16 ± 1	10 ± 1	10.9 ± 0.6
Hydroxyelenolic acid	1.9 ± 0.1	8 ± 1	8 ± 1	6.7 ± 0.8	9.1 ± 0.9
Phenolic alcohols	19.6 ± 0.5	18 ± 1	14 ± 1	5.9 ± 0.6	2.8 ± 0.2
Hydroxytyrosol acetate	4.5 ± 0.2	3.9 ± 0.3	4.0 ± 0.2	1.8 ± 0.2	1.4 ± 0.1
Hydroxytyrosol	15.2 ± 0.7	14 ± 1	10.0 ± 0.9	4.1 ± 0.5	1.5 ± 0.2
Flavonoids	1.8 ± 0.2	1.3 ± 0.4	1.3 ± 0.4	0.79 ± 0.08	0.86 ± 0.05
Apigenin	0.61 ± 0.04	0.7 ± 0.4	0.7 ± 0.4	0.48 ± 0.05	0.54 ± 0.03
Luteolin	1.16 ± 0.15	0.54 ± 0.08	0.61 ± 0.06	0.31 ± 0.04	0.32 ± 0.02
Phenolic acids	3.7 ± 0.3	1.4 ± 0.7	1.2 ± 0.4	1.2 ± 0.3	0.8 ± 0.2
Ferulic acid	3.3 ± 0.3	0.9 ± 0.7	0.7 ± 0.4	0.7 ± 0.3	0.4 ± 0.2
p-Coumaric acid	0.45 ± 0.01	0.49 ± 0.06	0.47 ± 0.04	0.47 ± 0.04	0.40 ± 0.02
Lignans	0.44 ± 0.05	0.48 ± 0.07	0.49 ± 0.05	0.60 ± 0.06	0.64 ± 0.07
Pinoresinol	0.44 ± 0.05	0.48 ± 0.07	0.49 ± 0.05	0.60 ± 0.06	0.64 ± 0.07

HDCM-OA: Hydroxydecarboxymethyloleuropein Aglycone; HOA: Hydroxyoleuropein Aglycone; T: temperature; t: time; ↑ high level of the factor; ↓ low level of the factor.

For the ANOVA and multiple regression models, the normality of residuals was verified. To check this assumption, normal probability plots of the residuals were plotted for each compound. The graph for the sum of polyphenols is shown in Figure 1. The results of the ANOVA test and the linear regression models are shown in Table 3. The temperature was mainly responsible for the polyphenols depletion and there were no significant effects from time or the interaction. These results are in accordance with those reported by Goulas et al. (2015), who showed that heating the oil at 180 °C for 1 h or for 5 h made no difference in polyphenol content decrease [8].

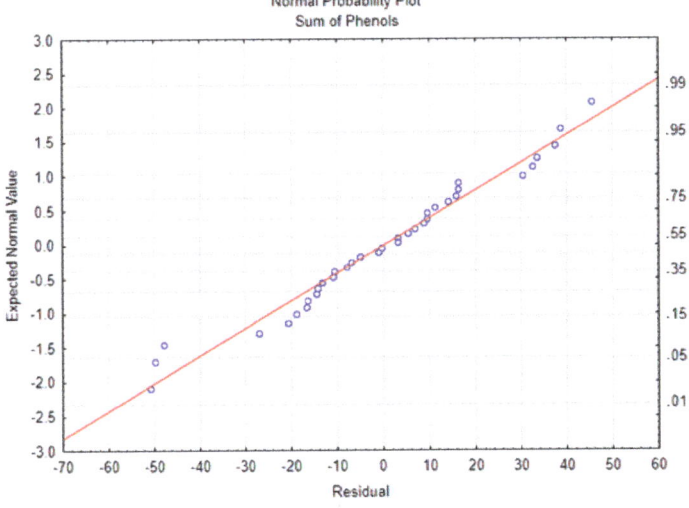

Figure 1. Normal probability plot of the sum of phenols.

Table 3. Statistical results of the ANOVA and the lineal models.

Group/Compound	R^2	β_0	Temperature F-Value	β_1	Time F-Value	β_2	Interaction F-Value	β_3
Sum of phenols	0.968	360.8 *	1038.8 *	−131.9 *	0.458	-	3.87	−8.05
Secoiridoids	0.965	347.9 *	946.9 *	−125.8 *	0.057	-	4.04	−8.22 *
Ligstroside aglycone	0.927	143.2 *	427.4 *	−47.8 *	0.443	-	0.0018	-
Oleocanthal	0.703	46.5 *	81.0 *	−5.31 *	0.603	-	0.232	-
Oleuropein aglycone	0.973	29.7 *	1276.1 *	−16.2 *	0.402	−0.287	8.96 *	−1.35 *
Oleacein	0.955	87.9 *	736.9 *	−48.6 *	1.59	−2.26	6.83 *	−4.68 *
HDCM-OA	0.845	17.2 *	144.3 *	−4.34 *	15.5 *	−1.42 *	33.7 *	−2.10 *
HOA	0.888	2.18 *	369.9 *	−0.660 *	0.718	−0.147 *	142.7 *	−0.645 *
Elenolic acid	0.824	13.2 *	159.8 *	−2.99 *	4.26 *	0.488 *	0.678	-
Hydroxyelenolic acid	0.444	7.92 *	0.002	-	17.1 *	0.654 *	11.9 *	0.546 *
Phenolic alcohols	0.978	10.1 *	1427.7 *	−5.78 *	124.6 *	−1.71 *	1.36	0.178
Hydroxytyrosol acetate	0.964	2.77 *	916.5 *	−1.18 *	3.28	−0.0705	12.6 *	−0.138 *
Hydroxytyrosol	0.971	7.37 *	1026.5 *	−4.60 *	129.9 *	−1.64 *	4.86 *	0.316 *
Flavonoids	0.396	1.06 *	23.1 *	−0.236 *	0.723	-	0.0038	-
Apigenin	0.121	0.615 *	5.54 *	−0.105 *	0.265	-	0.0648	-
Luteolin	0.855	0.446 *	202.4 *	−0.131 *	4.17 *	0.0187 *	2.44	−0.0144
Phenolic acids	0.090	1.15 *	3.35	−0.147	3.08	−0.141	0.0288	−0.0136
Ferulic acid	0.085	0.682 *	3.27	−0.133	2.97	−0.127	0.0158	−0.00927
p-Coumaric acid	0.111	0.463 *	3.43	−0.013	3.60	−0.0138	0.354	−0.00433
Lignans	0.520	0.553 *	39.2 *	0.068 *	1.16	0.0116	0.583	0.00827
Pinoresinol	0.526	0.553 *	39.2 *	0.068 *	1.16	0.0116	0.583	-

* Statistically significant difference (p-value < 0.05) for ANOVA (F-value) and for the linear regression analyses (β).

The model for the sum of polyphenols was great fitted, with a R^2 of 0.97, in which 97% of the variance is explained by the model. The slope for temperature was significantly different from 0, suggesting that a longer cooking period does not change the polyphenolic fraction when the EVOO is processed only once. As the low level is −1 and the high level is +1, and the β of the temperature is −131, then cooking using a high temperature decreased the polyphenol content 232 mg/kg more than applying a moderate temperature, which represents 27% of the raw EVOO concentration.

3.2. Secoiridoids

Secoiridoids are the largest group of EVOO polyphenols. Secoiridoids include oleuropein, ligstrosides, and their derivatives. Some of them have been reported to have important benefits to health, such as oleocanthal or oleacein [34]. Oleocanthal has demonstrated anti-inflammatory effects [35] and a protective role against some diseases, such as Alzheimer disease [34], and oleacein has proven to protect against cardiovascular diseases, reducing hypertension [36] and inhibiting neutrophils adhesion [37].

During the cooking process, secoiridoids decreased 45% at the low temperature and 70% at the high temperature. Among this group, a different behavior was observed in hydroxyelenolic acid, which is not a polyphenol but a related compound produced by the ester breakdown of ligstroside, oleuropein, and their aglycones [38]. Thus, the formation of hydroxyelenolic acid was enhanced by processing at a moderate temperature. However, a longer cooking period and a higher temperature promoted its degradation, giving a lower concentration.

According to ANOVA analysis, the factor responsible for the depletion of secoiridoids was temperature. However, different results were found for each secoiridoid, in which oleacein and oleuropein aglycone were also affected by the interaction of time and temperature, and hydroxydecarboxymethyl oleuropein aglycone and hydroxyoleuropein aglycon were affected by all of the evaluated factors. These results are in accordance with those reported by Attya et al. (2010), in which heating at 90 °C was shown to cause almost no degradation of oleocanthal and oleacein in EVOO, but at 170 °C the concentration of both compounds was reduced by half, reflecting the major role played by temperature in polyphenol degradation [16].

The models were properly fitted for most of the secoiridoids analyzed, however, oleocanthal showed a R^2 of 0.7 because of its high reactivity, which also prompted the development of a new method for its specific analysis [29]. Oleocanthal presents keto-enolic tautomerism, which impeded its proper analysis, as it reacts with the solvent during the chromatographic separation. Oleocanthal may have reacted more in some samples than others, but even with only a 70% model fit, the result indicates that the cooking time did not change the oleocanthal concentration. In contrast, it decreased by 100 mg/kg of oil after cooking at a high temperature compared to the moderate temperature.

In the case of the sum of secoiridoids, the ANOVA results showed that the interaction factor was not significant, although in the multiple regression model the β for the interaction was different to 0, indicating that there was an effect. This difference occurred because the test used for ANOVA and the test used for the regression model were different: ANOVA applies a F-test, and, for the regression models, a t-test is used. Despite the ANOVA result giving a p-value of over 0.05, it showed a trend that this factor had an effect on secoiridoid degradation (p-value = 0.052).

According to the slopes of the models, the temperature was mainly responsible for the depletion of seicoiridoids during a domestic sautéing process. Slopes were analyzed as a percentage of the initial concentration (in raw EVOO), as the initial concentration for each polyphenol differed substantially, making it difficult to compare the models between the different polyphenols. The results are shown in Table 3. The slopes represent the values ranging from 12% (ligstroside aglycone) to 20% (oleuropein aglycone) of their original concentrations. The most different one was oleocanthal, which showed just a 6.5% depletion and withstands better the temperature than oleuropein aglycone. The compounds with a o-diphenol group were the most reactive, with a slope representing between 18% (hydroxydecarboxymethyl oleuropein aglycone) an 20% (oleacein) of their initial concentration. On the other hand, oleocanthal and ligstroside aglycone (compounds with just one hydroxyl group) showed less reactivity. *ortho*-Diphenols are the most reactive, as they can be converted easily to *ortho*-quinones through a radical reaction [39–41]. Also, the intermediates of the reaction are radicals too, so they stabilized by the hydroxyl in the ortho position [40]. This rapid conversion may be responsible for the higher degradation compared to single phenols. This difference in the reactivity is also reflected in the activation energy, in which oleocanthal presents lower than oleacein because a higher temperature change is needed to degrade oleocanthal at the same rate as oleacein [16].

As mentioned above, hydroxyelenolic acid was an exception, its concentration was affected by the cooking time and the interaction between time and temperature, but not the temperature alone. For this compound and for elenolic acid, the time factor had a positive effect as the slopes were positive, indicating that frying with EVOO for longer periods may increase their concentration. Although the hydroxyelenolic acid model was not well fitted, the elenolic acid model showed an 82% fitness result. Like hydroxyelenolic acid, elenolic acid is not a phenol, but a derivative of oleuropein and ligstroside aglycones. Thus, despite a long cooking process degrading some of the polyphenols, it can enhance some related and new compounds.

3.3. Phenolic Alcohols and Others

Phenolic alcohols, mainly hydroxytyrosol and hydroxytyrosol acetate, are derivates from oleuropein, like the secoiridoids, but as their chemical behaviors are different, they are classified in a different group [27,28].

When frying at a low temperature for a short time, only 9% of phenolic alcohols decreased, although a depletion of 85% (90% in the case of hydroxytyrosol), when applying a high temperature and a long cooking time, was observed. At a low or moderate temperature, the hydroxytyrosol degradation, formed by the ester breakdown of oleuropein and its aglycones (Figure 2), may be counteracted by the rate of its generation. However, at a high temperature, its degradation is more likely to occur, resulting in a substantial reduction. Similar results are observed by Ramírez-Anaya et al. (2019), who showed that after sautéing typical Mediterranean vegetables at 100 °C, the hydroxytyrosol content only decreased between 25% and 50% [33]. Furthermore, a similar behavior was found by Krichene et al. (2015), who showed an increase in hytroxytyrosol concentration during the first months of storage due to the transformation of oleuropein and derivates in the compound, but after some months there was a high decrease in its concentration [42].

The concentration of phenolic alcohols was affected by temperature and time and hydroxytyrosol was also affected by their interaction, however, the β value for the temperature factor was higher, indicating that it is mainly responsible for their degradation.

Hydroxytyrosol was the most degraded compound by temperature, its slope represents 30% of its initial concentration. Thus, the amount of hydroxytyrosol diminished greatly—about 60% of the hydroxytyrosol concentration in the raw EVOO cooked at a high temperature compared to the EVOO cooked at a low temperature. So, cooking at low temperature should be recommended due to the fact that, according to the European Food and Safe Authority, it protects low-density lipoproteins (LDL) from oxidative damage [43] that have proven health effects.

The minor groups of polyphenols in EVOO are phenolic acids, lignans, and flavones. There was no possibility to build a model for those groups because of their low concentration. The only model properly fitted (>80%) for flavones was luteolin that was mainly affected by temperature. In the case of lignans, the only compound present in quantifiable amounts was pinoresinol, which increased during cooking probably because of the transformation of 1-acetoxypinoresinol and because of its high temperature stability [44].

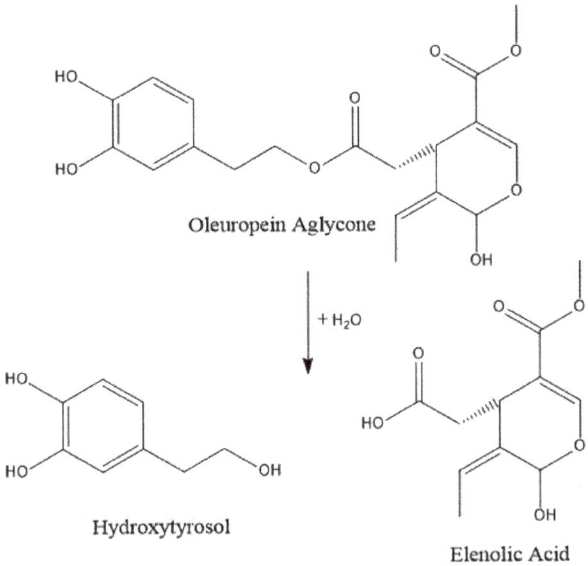

Figure 2. Normal probability plot of the sum of polyphenols.

4. Conclusions

In this work, we determined changes in the EVOO polyphenolic profile during a domestic sautéing process commonly used in the Mediterranean diet, simulating the cooking conditions of a home kitchen, without the control of light or oxygen. The cooking temperature was the most important factor in the degradation of EVOO polyphenols. In the case of time, it was only a significant factor for some polyphenolic compounds and was not a significant factor for the sum of the polyphenols. Sautéing at a low temperature changes the polyphenolic profile of EVOO by increasing the concentration of hydroxyelenolic acid and depleting other compounds. Besides, this oil would still have the amount of polyphenols, with values higher than 250 mg/kg of hydroxytyrosol, tyrosol, or the derivates necessary to inhibit LDL oxidation [43]. Furthermore, research is needed to determine if there are differences in EVOO polyphenol degradation when proteins or complex sugars are present and whether the presence of these phenolics for their antioxidant properties could avoid the formation of secondary undesirable compounds that originated from the cooking and food processing.

Supplementary Materials: The following are available online at http://www.mdpi.com/2076-3921/9/1/77/s1, Table S1: Ionization conditions for compounds analyzed with the method 1, Table S2: Ionization conditions for compounds analyzed with the method 2.

Author Contributions: Conceptualization, J.F.R.d.A. and R.M.L.-R.; Formal analysis, J.L.-C. and J.F.R.d.A.; Investigation, J.L.-C., A.V.-Q., M.I. and X.T.-P.; Methodology, J.L.-C. and J.F.R.d.A.; Supervision A.V.-Q. and R.M.L.-R.; Writing—original draft preparation, J.L.-C.; Writing—review and editing, A.V.-Q., J.F.R.d.A. and R.M.L.-R. All authors have read and agreed to the published version of the manuscript.

Funding: This research was funded by CICYT [AGL2016- 75329-R]. Julián Lozano-Castellón thanks the Ministry of Science Innovation and Universities for the FPI contract [BES-2017-080017]. Anna Vallverdú-Queralt thanks the Ministry of Science Innovation and Universities for the Ramon y Cajal contract (RYC-2016-19355). José Fernando Rinaldi de Alvarenga thanks the Fundação de Amparo a Pesquisa do Estado de São Paulo (FAPESP) for the post-doc grant [2019/11324-8].

Acknowledgments: The authors wish to thank the CCiT-UB for the mass spectrometry equipment. The authors also wish to thank the Fundación Patrimonio Comunal Olivarero for the EVOO.

Conflicts of Interest: Lamuela-Raventós reports receiving lecture fees from Cerveceros de España and receiving lecture fees and travel support from Adventia. The other authors declare no conflict of interest. The funders had no role in the design of the study; in the collection, analyses, or interpretation of data; in the writing of the manuscript, or in the decision to publish the results.

References

1. Cicerale, S.; Lucas, L.; Keast, R. Biological activities of phenolic compounds present in virgin olive oil. *Int. J. Mol. Sci.* **2010**, *11*, 458–479. [CrossRef]
2. Estruch, R.; Ros, E.; Salas-Salvadó, J.; Covas, M.-I.; Corella, D.; Arós, F.; Gómez-Gracia, E.; Ruiz-Gutiérrez, V.; Fiol, M.; Lapetra, J.; et al. Primary Prevention of Cardiovascular Disease with a Mediterranean Diet. *N. Engl. J. Med.* **2013**, *368*, 1279–1290. [CrossRef]
3. Gotsis, E.; Anagnostis, P.; Mariolis, A.; Vlachou, A.; Katsiki, N.; Karagiannis, A. Health benefits of the mediterranean diet: An update of research over the last 5 years. *Angiology* **2015**, *66*, 304–318. [CrossRef]
4. Nocella, C.; Cammisotto, V.; Fianchini, L.; D'Amico, A.; Novo, M.; Castellani, V.; Stefanini, L.; Violi, F.; Carnevale, R. Extra Virgin Olive Oil and Cardiovascular Diseases: Benefits for Human Health. *Endocr. Metab. Immune Disord. Drug Targets* **2017**, *18*, 4–13. [CrossRef]
5. Martínez-Lapiscina, E.H.; Clavero, P.; Toledo, E.; Estruch, R.; Salas-Salvadó, J.; San Julián, B.; Sanchez-Tainta, A.; Ros, E.; Valls-Pedret, C.; Martinez-Gonzalez, M.Á. Mediterranean diet improves cognition: The PREDIMED-NAVARRA randomised trial. *J. Neurol. Neurosurg. Psychiatry* **2013**, *84*, 1318–1325. [CrossRef] [PubMed]
6. Martínez-González, M.A.; Corella, D.; Salas-Salvadó, J.; Estruch, R.; Ros, E. Prevention of Diabetes with Mediterranean Diets. *Ann. Intern. Med.* **2014**, *161*, 157. [CrossRef] [PubMed]
7. Hussein, Z.; Fawole, O.A.; Opara, U.L. Preharvest factors influencing bruise damage of fresh fruits—A review. *Sci. Hortic.* **2018**, *229*, 45–58. [CrossRef]
8. Goulas, V.; Orphanides, A.; Pelava, E.; Gekas, V. Impact of Thermal Processing Methods on Polyphenols and Antioxidant Activity of Olive Oil Polar Fraction. *J. Food Process. Preserv.* **2015**, *39*, 1919–1924. [CrossRef]
9. Ramírez-Anaya, J.D.P.; Samaniego-Sánchez, C.; Castañeda-Saucedo, M.C.; Villalón-Mir, M.; De La Serrana, H.L.G. Phenols and the antioxidant capacity of Mediterranean vegetables prepared with extra virgin olive oil using different domestic cooking techniques. *Food Chem.* **2015**, *188*, 430–438. [CrossRef]
10. Engelsen, S.B. Explorative Spectrometric Evaluations of Frying Oil Deterioration. *JAOCS J. Am. Oil Chem. Soc.* **1997**, *74*, 1495–1508. [CrossRef]
11. Rannou, C.; Laroque, D.; Renault, E.; Prost, C.; Sérot, T. Mitigation strategies of acrylamide, furans, heterocyclic amines and browning during the Maillard reaction in foods. *Food Res. Int.* **2016**, *90*, 154–176. [CrossRef]
12. Persson, E.; Graziani, G.; Ferracane, R.; Fogliano, V.; Skog, K. Influence of antioxidants in virgin olive oil on the formation of heterocyclic amines in fried beefburgers. *Food Chem. Toxicol.* **2003**, *41*, 1587–1597. [CrossRef]
13. Sordini, B.; Veneziani, G.; Servili, M.; Esposto, S.; Selvaggini, R.; Lorefice, A.; Taticchi, A. A quanti-qualitative study of a phenolic extract as a natural antioxidant in the frying processes. *Food Chem.* **2019**, *279*, 426–434. [CrossRef]
14. Zamora, R.; Hidalgo, F.J. Carbonyl-Phenol Adducts: An Alternative Sink for Reactive and Potentially Toxic Lipid Oxidation Products. *J. Agric. Food Chem.* **2018**, *66*, 1320–1324. [CrossRef]
15. Esposto, S.; Taticchi, A.; Di Maio, I.; Urbani, S.; Veneziani, G.; Selvaggini, R.; Sordini, B.; Servili, M. Effect of an olive phenolic extract on the quality of vegetable oils during frying. *Food Chem.* **2015**, *176*, 184–192. [CrossRef]
16. Attya, M.; Benabdelkamel, H.; Perri, E.; Russo, A.; Sindona, G. Effects of conventional heating on the stability of major olive oil phenolic compounds by tandem mass spectrometry and isotope dilution assay. *Molecules* **2010**, *15*, 8734–8746. [CrossRef]
17. Cerretani, L.; Bendini, A.; Rodriguez-Estrada, M.T.; Vittadini, E.; Chiavaro, E. Microwave heating of different commercial categories of olive oil: Part I. Effect on chemical oxidative stability indices and phenolic compounds. *Food Chem.* **2009**, *115*, 1381–1388. [CrossRef]
18. Taticchi, A.; Esposto, S.; Urbani, S.; Veneziani, G.; Selvaggini, R.; Sordini, B.; Servili, M. Effect of an olive phenolic extract added to the oily phase of a tomato sauce, on the preservation of phenols and carotenoids during domestic cooking. *LWT Food Sci. Technol.* **2017**, *84*, 572–578. [CrossRef]

19. Bendini, A.; Cerretani, L.; Salvador, M.D.; Fregapane, G.; Lercker, G. Stability of the sensory quality of virgin olive oil during storage: An overview. *Ital. J. Food Sci.* **2009**, *21*, 389–406.
20. Kalogeropoulos, N.; Mylona, A.; Chiou, A.; Ioannou, M.S.; Andrikopoulos, N.K. Retention and distribution of natural antioxidants (α-tocopherol, polyphenols and terpenic acids) after shallow frying of vegetables in virgin olive oil. *LWT Food Sci. Technol.* **2007**, *40*, 1008–1017. [CrossRef]
21. Brenes, M.; García, A.; Dobarganes, M.C.; Velasco, J.; Romero, C. Influence of thermal treatments simulating cooking processes on the polyphenol content in virgin olive oil. *J. Agric. Food Chem.* **2002**, *50*, 5962–5967. [CrossRef]
22. Allouche, Y.; Jiménez, A.; Gaforio, J.J.; Uceda, M.; Beltrán, G. How Heating Affects Extra Virgin Olive Oil Quality Indexes and Chemical Composition. *J. Agric. Food Chem.* **2007**, *55*, 9646–9654. [CrossRef]
23. Casal, S.; Malheiro, R.; Sendas, A.; Oliveira, B.P.P.; Pereira, J.A. Olive oil stability under deep-frying conditions. *Food Chem. Toxicol.* **2010**, *48*, 2972–2979. [CrossRef]
24. Aubaile-Sallenave, F. La Méditerranée, une cuisine, des cuisines. In *Anthropologie de L'Alimentation*; SAGE: London, UK; Thousand Oaks, CA, USA; New Delhi, India, 1996; pp. 139–194.
25. García, A.; Brenes, M.; García, P.; Romero, C.; Garrido, A. Phenolic content of commercial olive oils. *Eur. Food Res. Technol.* **2003**, *216*, 520–525. [CrossRef]
26. Kalogeropoulos, N.; Chiou, A.; Mylona, A.; Ioannou, M.S.; Andrikopoulos, N.K. Recovery and distribution of natural antioxidants (α-tocopherol, polyphenols and terpenic acids) after pan-frying of Mediterranean finfish in virgin olive oil. *Food Chem.* **2007**, *100*, 509–517. [CrossRef]
27. Suárez, M.; Macià, A.; Romero, M.-P.; Motilva, M.-J. Improved liquid chromatography tandem mass spectrometry method for the determination of phenolic compounds in virgin olive oil. *J. Chromatogr. A* **2008**, *1214*, 90–99. [CrossRef]
28. López-Yerena, A.; Lozano-Castellón, J.; Olmo-Cunillera, A.; Tresserra-Rimbau, A.; Quifer-Rada, P.; Jiménez, B.; Pérez, M.; Vallverdú-Queralt, A. Effects of organic and conventional growing systems on the phenolic profile of extra-virgin olive oil. *Molecules* **2019**, *24*, 1986. [CrossRef]
29. Sánchez de Medina, V.; Miho, H.; Melliou, E.; Magiatis, P.; Priego-Capote, F.; Luque de Castro, M.D. Quantitative method for determination of oleocanthal and oleacein in virgin olive oils by liquid chromatography–tandem mass spectrometry. *Talanta* **2017**, *162*, 24–31. [CrossRef]
30. Douglas, C. *Montgomery: Design and Analysis of Experiments*; John Willy Sons: Hoboken, NJ, USA, 2000; p. 734.
31. Mariod, A.A.; Ibrahim, R.M.; Ismail, M.; Ismail, N. Antioxidant activity of the phenolic leaf extracts from monechma ciliatum in stabilization of corn oil. *JAOCS J. Am. Oil Chem. Soc.* **2010**, *87*, 35–43. [CrossRef]
32. Xiangli, F.; Wei, W.; Chen, Y.; Jin, W.; Xu, N. Optimization of preparation conditions for polydimethylsiloxane (PDMS)/ceramic composite pervaporation membranes using response surface methodology. *J. Membr. Sci.* **2008**, *311*, 23–33. [CrossRef]
33. Ramírez-Anaya, J.; Castañeda-Saucedo, M.C.; Olalla-Herrera, M.; Villalón-Mir, M.; De la Serrana, H.L.G.; Samaniego-Sánchez, C. Changes in the antioxidant properties of extra virgin olive oil after cooking typical mediterranean vegetables. *Antioxidants* **2019**, *8*, 246.
34. Lozano-Castellón, J.; López-Yerena, A.; Rinaldi de Alvarenga, J.F.; Romero del Castillo-alba, J.; Vallverdú-queralt, A.; Escribano-ferrer, E.; Lamuela-raventós, R.M. Health-promoting properties of oleocanthal and oleacein: Two secoiridoids from extra-virgin olive oil. *Crit. Rev. Food Sci. Nutr.* **2019**, 1–17. [CrossRef]
35. Beauchamp, G.K.; Keast, R.S.J.; Morel, D.; Lin, J.; Pika, J.; Han, Q.; Lee, C.H.; Smith, A.B.; Breslin, P.A.S. Ibuprofen-like activity in extra-virgin olive oil. *Nature* **2005**, *437*, 45–46. [CrossRef]
36. Hansen, K.; Adsersen, A.; Christensen, S.B.; Jensen, S.R.; Nyman, U.; Smitt, U.W. Isolation of an angiotensin converting enzyme (ACE) inhibitor from Olea europaea and Olea lancea. *Phytomedicine* **2011**, *2*, 319–325. [CrossRef]
37. Czerwińska, M.E.; Kiss, A.K.; Naruszewicz, M. Inhibition of human neutrophils NEP activity, CD11b/CD18 expression and elastase release by 3,4-dihydroxyphenylethanol-elenolic acid dialdehyde, oleacein. *Food Chem.* **2014**, *153*, 1–8. [CrossRef]
38. Obied, H.K.; Prenzler, P.D.; Ryan, D.; Servili, M.; Taticchi, A.; Esposto, S.; Robards, K. Biosynthesis and biotransformations of phenol-conjugated oleosidic secoiridoids from *Olea europaea* L. *Nat. Prod. Rep.* **2008**, *25*, 1167. [CrossRef]

39. Singleton, V.L. Oxygen with phenols and related reactions in musts, wines, and model systems: Observations and practical implications. *Am. J. Enol. Vitic.* **1987**, *38*, 69–77.
40. Hvattum, E.; Ekeberg, D. Study of the collision-induced radical cleavage of flavonoid glycosides using negative electrospray ionization tandem quadrupole mass spectrometry. *J. Mass Spectrom.* **2003**, *38*, 43–49. [CrossRef]
41. Vallverdu-Queralt, A.; Regueiro, J.; Rinaldi de Alvarenga, J.; Torrado, X.; Lamuela-Ravento, R.M. Home Cooking and Phenolics: Effect of Thermal Treatment and Addition of Extra Virgin Olive Oil on the Phenolic Profile of Tomato Sauces. *J. Agric. Food Chem.* **2014**, *62*, 3314–3320. [CrossRef]
42. Krichene, D.; Salvador, M.D.; Fregapane, G. Stability of Virgin Olive Oil Phenolic Compounds during Long-Term Storage (18 Months) at Temperatures of 5–50 °C. *J. Agric. Food Chem.* **2015**, *63*, 6779–6786. [CrossRef]
43. European Commission. European Commission Regulation EC No. 432/2012 establishing a list of permitted health claims made on foods, other than those referring to the reduction of disease risk and to children's development and health. *Off. J. Eur. Union L* **2012**, *136*, 1–40.
44. Daskalaki, D.; Kefi, G.; Kotsiou, K.; Tasioula-Margari, M. Evaluation of phenolic compounds degradation in virgin olive oil during storage and heating. *J. Food Nutr. Res.* **2009**, *48*, 31–41.

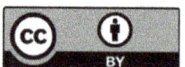 © 2020 by the authors. Licensee MDPI, Basel, Switzerland. This article is an open access article distributed under the terms and conditions of the Creative Commons Attribution (CC BY) license (http://creativecommons.org/licenses/by/4.0/).

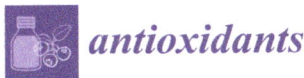

Review

Phenolic Compounds and Bioaccessibility Thereof in Functional Pasta

Valentina Melini *, Francesca Melini and Rita Acquistucci

CREA Research Centre for Food and Nutrition, Via Ardeatina 546, I-00178 Roma, Italy; francesca.melini@crea.gov.it (F.M.); rita.acquistucci@crea.gov.it (R.A.)
* Correspondence: valentina.melini@crea.gov.it

Received: 6 April 2020; Accepted: 20 April 2020; Published: 22 April 2020

Abstract: Consumption of food products rich in phenolic compounds has been associated to reduced risk of chronic disease onset. Daily consumed cereal-based products, such as bread and pasta, are not carriers of phenolic compounds, since they are produced with refined flour or semolina. Novel formulations of pasta have been thus proposed, in order to obtain functional products contributing to the increase in phenolic compound dietary intake. This paper aims to review the strategies used so far to formulate functional pasta, both gluten-containing and gluten-free, and compare their effect on phenolic compound content, and bioaccessibility and bioavailability thereof. It emerged that whole grain, legume and composite flours are the main substituents of durum wheat semolina in the formulation of functional pasta. Plant by-products from industrial food wastes have been also used as functional ingredients. In addition, pre-processing technologies on raw materials such as sprouting, or the modulation of extrusion/extrusion-cooking conditions, are valuable approaches to increase phenolic content in pasta. Few studies on phenolic compound bioaccessibility and bioavailability in pasta have been performed so far; however, they contribute to evaluating the usefulness of strategies used in the formulation of functional pasta.

Keywords: phenolic compounds; bioactive compounds; functional pasta; gluten-free pasta; bioaccessibility; bioavailability; whole grain; composite flour; legumes; food by-products

1. Introduction

Phenolic compounds are secondary plant metabolites with strong antioxidant activity [1]. The consumption of food products rich in phenolic compounds has been associated with a reduced risk of chronic disease onset and ageing [2,3]. Currently, Phenol-Explorer, the first comprehensive database on polyphenol content in foods, reports the content for 500 phenolic compounds in 400 foods, for a total of 35,000 values. Fruit and vegetables are the main source of these secondary plant-metabolites.

Cereal grains contain significant amounts of phenolic compounds, as well [4,5]. Nevertheless, daily consumed cereal-based products, such as bread and pasta, are not a carrier of phenolic compounds, since they are produced with refined flour or semolina. Most bioactive compounds are concentrated in the outer layers of cereal grains which are discarded as bran, while flour and semolina are obtained from the starchy endosperm layer [6]. Hence, phenolic compounds are commonly lost during milling.

Pasta is one of the staple foods of the Mediterranean diet. It composes the base of the food pyramid and a daily consumption is recommended [7]. Pasta is a good source of carbohydrates and energy. One serving of 100 g of pasta (cooked, unenriched, without added salt) contains about 31 g of carbohydrates, 26.01 g starch, 1.8 g total dietary fibre, 5.8 g protein, and 0.93 g lipid (fat), and provides about 158 kcal [8]. When pasta is cooked al dente, it also has a low glycemic index, ranging around 32–40, depending on the pasta type [9]. Pasta glycemic index is far lower than that of bread. Additionally, pasta can possibly slow digestion rates and may contribute to longer satiety [10–13]. Pasta has also additional unquestionable advantages, such as ease of preparation, long shelf-life, low price and global consumption. It is consumed by people of all ages and from all walks of life. Hence, it may be an optimal carrier of phenolic compounds.

Currently, the focus of nutritional science has shifted toward the concept of optimal nutrition, which aims at optimizing the daily diet in terms of nutrients and non-nutrients. Hence, the demand for functional food products with a well-balanced nutritional composition and contributing to maintaining wellbeing and health, has grown.

In this framework, novel formulations of functional pasta have been proposed and innovation in pasta-making has been prompted. The aim of this paper is to identify which formulations of functional pasta contribute to a higher intake of phenolic compounds, and greater bioaccessibility and bioavailability thereof. The consumption of food products with a high number of bioactive compounds does not necessarily imply beneficial effects on human health. Bioaccessibility studies are, thus, mandatory, to evaluate the bioactivity of a functional product. To this aim, the strategies used so far in formulation of functional pasta rich in phenolic compounds, both gluten-containing and gluten-free, will be reviewed. In addition, studies on phenolic compound bioaccessibility and bioavailability in pasta will be discussed, in order to evaluate the usefulness of these strategies and provide a basis for further investigations.

2. Dietary Phenolic Compounds

2.1. Structure

Phenolic compounds are a heterogeneous group of bioactive compounds produced in plants, via either the shikimate or the acetate pathway [14]. They include a variety of chemical structures having one or more phenolic groups as a common structural feature.

Based on the number of phenol rings and the structural elements that bind rings one to another, they can be classified into: (i) simple phenols; (ii) phenolic acids; (iii) flavonoids; (iv) xanthones; (v) stilbenes; and (vi) lignans [15], while a broader classification divides phenolic compounds into flavonoids and non-flavonoids [16]. Flavonoids show a distinctive benzo-γ-pyrone skeleton and occur as aglycones, glycosides and methylated derivatives. They comprise flavonols, flavan-3-ols, flavones, isoflavones, flavanones, anthocyanidins and dihydrochalcones. Non-flavonoids include diverse classes of polyphenols, such as phenolic acids and stilbenes [16]. Among non-flavonoids of dietary significance, phenolic acids play a pivotal role and are a major class in grains. They include hydroxybenzoic acids (C6–C1), such as gallic, *p*-hydroxybenzoic, vanillic, syringic, protocatechuic and ellagic acids, as well as hydroxycinnamic acids (C6–C3), namely *p*-coumaric, caffeic, ferulic, sinapic and chlorogenic acids (Table 1).

Phenolic compounds may occur in free, soluble conjugated, and bound form, depending on whether they are bound to other constituents, or otherwise. Hence, they can be classified as free phenolic compounds (FPCs), soluble conjugated phenolic compounds (EPCs) and insoluble bound phenolic compounds (BPCs) [17]. EPCs are esterified to other molecules such as fatty acids, while BPCs are covalently bound to cell wall constituents, such as pectin, cellulose, arabinoxylans and structural proteins. BPCs are the main fraction of phenolic compounds in wheat grains [18,19].

Table 1. Major classes of dietary phenolic compounds, skeleton structure thereof and common representatives.

Class	Subclass	Skeleton Structure	Common Representatives
Flavonoids	Flavonols		Kaempferol, quercetin
	Flavan-3-ols		Catechin, gallocatechin, epicatechin
	Flavones		Luteolin, apingenin
	Isoflavones		Genistein, daidzein
	Flavanones		Naringenin, hesperetin
	Anthocyanidins		Cyanidin, malvidin, delphinidin
	Dihydrochalcones		Phloretin

Table 1. Cont.

Class	Subclass	Skeleton Structure	Common Representatives
Non-Flavonoids	Phenolic acids—Hydroxybenzoic acids	(benzoic acid with R1, R2, R3 substituents; R1, R2, R3: –H or –OH)	Gallic acid, p-hydroxybenzoic acid, vanillic acid, syringic acid, protocatechuic acid, ellagic acid
	Phenolic acids—Hydroxycinnamic acids	(cinnamic acid skeleton with HO–, R1, R2 substituents; R1, R2, R3: –H or –OH)	p-coumaric acid, caffeic acid, ferulic acid, sinapic acid, chlorogenic acid
	Stilbenes	(stilbene skeleton)	Resveratrol

2.2. Bioaccessibility, Biotransformation and Bioavailability

The concept of bioavailability in nutrition has been borrowed from pharmacology. In this discipline, the term "bioavailability" refers to the fraction of the administered dose of drug that enters systemic circulation, so as to access the site of action [20]. In nutrition, bioavailability refers to the amount of a nutrient or bioactive compound which becomes available for normal physiological functions or storage, after absorption by the gut [21].

The first step, necessary for a food component to become bioavailable, is the release from the food matrix. The extent at which a nutrient or bioactive molecule is released from the food matrix into the gastrointestinal tract and is in the right form to be absorbed, is referred to as bioaccessibility [22].

The bioaccessibility and bioavailability of phenolic compounds are affected by factors related to phenolics, food matrix and host (Figure 1).

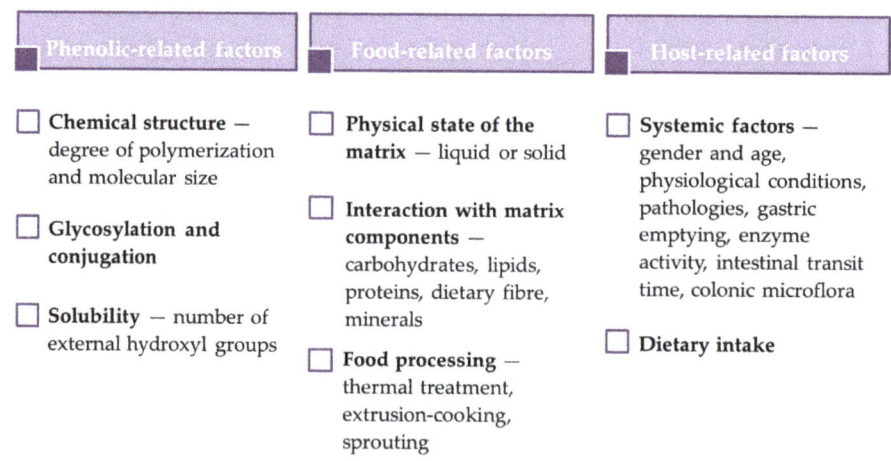

Figure 1. Factors affecting bioaccessibility and bioavailability of phenolic compounds.

As regards the relationship between phenolic characteristics and bioavailability, it has been observed that chemical structure (degree of polymerization and molecular size), glycosylation and conjugation with other phenolics, and solubility are critical factors [23]. For example, phenolic acids, isoflavones, catechins and quercetin glucosides are easily absorbed, while large polyphenols are poorly absorbed.

Generally, phenolic compounds in liquid foods are more bioaccessible than those in solid foods. However, differences in phenolic bioavailability among liquid matrices have been observed. The occurrence of alcohol, dietary fibre or other nutrients, such as carbohydrates, lipids and proteins, may in fact influence phenolic compound bioavailability because of the interactions between phenolics and matrix constituents. Food processing may positively or negatively affect phenolic compound bioaccesibility and bioavailability, as well. Lafarga et al. observed that cooking increased the bioaccessibility of phenolic compounds in pulses [24]. Zeng et al. found that the content of bioaccessible phenolics in brown rice and oat significantly decreased (by 31.09% and 30.95%, respectively) after improved extrusion-cooking treatment, while in wheat they were almost unchanged, possibly because of differences in the cereal matrix [25]. It should be also considered that processing can cause a loss of phenolic compounds while promoting their bioaccessibility. Hence, bioavailability is a compromise between the compounds lost during processing and those absorbed into the organism [26].

Host-related factors—such as physiological conditions, disorders or pathologies, gastric emptying, enzyme activity, intestinal transit time and colonic microflora—may influence bioaccessibility and bioavailability of phenolic compounds, as well.

The bioavailability of a phenolic compound implies: (i) its release from the food matrix; (ii) gastric and small-intestinal digestion (likely change of phenolic compound structure due to hydrolysis of glycosides and phase I/II metabolism); (iii) cellular uptake of aglycons and some conjugated phenolics by enterocytes; (iv) microbiological fermentation of non-absorbed polyphenols or phenolics re-excreted via bile or the pancreas, to produce additional metabolites; (v) modifications by phase I/II enzymes, upon uptake in the small intestine or in the colon; (vi) transport into the blood stream and redistribution to tissues; (vii) excretion via the kidney or re-excretion into the gut via bile and pancreatic juices (Figure 2).

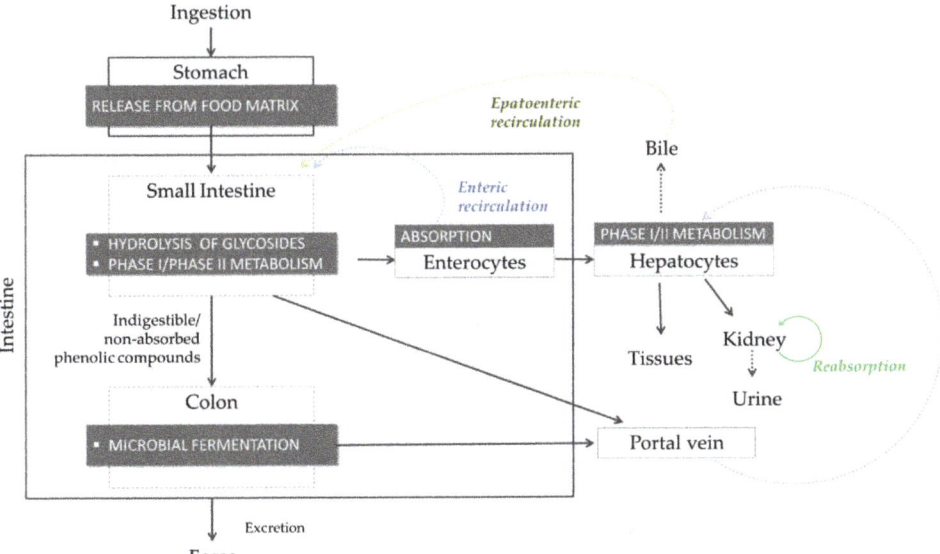

Figure 2. Representation of digestion, absorption and excretion of phenolic compounds and metabolites thereof.

Generally, after the absorption step, phenolics undergo phase I and II metabolic transformation, and metabolites with improved bioactivity or completely inactive can be obtained. As an example, protocatechuic acid, phloroglucinaldehyde, vanillic acid, and ferulic acid are bioactive metabolites obtained by the catabolism of cyanidine-3-O-glucoside in the gastrointestinal tract that contribute to maintaining intestinal integrity and function [27]. Hence, the evaluation of polyphenol bioavailability should include not only the determination of native compounds, but also of metabolites thereof.

Methods to Evaluate Phenolic Compound Bioaccessibility and Bioavailability

Several approaches have been proposed to evaluate phenolic compound bioaccessibility and bioavailability. They include the use of in vitro methods and in vivo models [23]. In vitro methods comprise simulated gastrointestinal (GI) digestion, artificial membranes, Caco-2 cell cultures and ussing chambers. As regards in vitro digestion models, they can be either static or dynamic [28]. Static models consist of multiple phases, including oral digestion (OD), gastric digestion (GD), intestinal digestion (ID) and dialysate (DIA). Each phase can vary slightly among studies. They can differ in the incubation time and characteristics of the digestive juices, and can also be adjusted for pH on the basis of the specific gut compartment [29]. However, they operate in static mode across the whole process, with prefixed conditions and parameters in terms of concentrations and volumes of digested materials, enzymes and salts, among others. The INFOGEST digestion method is an example of standardised static model [28,30].

Dynamic models include physical and mechanical processes and consider the changes that occur during the digestive process, as well as different physiological conditions. They were developed because static methods do not provide an accurate simulation of the complex dynamic physiological processes occurring under in vivo conditions. A common and very sophisticated gut model is the TIM system, a multi-compartmental dynamic computer-controlled model, used to simulate the human digestive system and to study the bioaccessibility of many compounds, such as vitamins, minerals, as well as phenolics [31].

In addition to the aforementioned methods, gastrointestinal organs in laboratory conditions (ex-vivo models) and intestinal perfusion in animals (in situ model) can be also applied in bioaccessibility/bioavailability determination [23]. In-vivo approaches are based on animal or human studies.

3. Strategies to Modulate Phenolic Compound Content in Pasta

According to tradition, pasta is seemingly a very simple food, produced with one ingredient, i.e., semolina of durum wheat (*Triticum turgidum* L. var. *durum*), and one "reactant", i.e., water. Pasta final configuration, made of starch granules dispersed within the protein network, is hence obtained upon the biochemical modification of the two main constituents of durum wheat semolina (that is, proteins and starch) prompted by water addition, and mechanical and thermal energy.

Pasta by itself is a healthy food. It is a good source of carbohydrates and energy. However, in recent years, scientists and producers have been striving to develop new formulas, so that pasta can not only provide nutrients and energy, but also beneficially modulate one or more targeted functions in the body, by enhancing a certain physiological response and/or reducing the risk of disease [32]. These new formulations are known as functional pasta products.

The use of functional ingredients, such as whole grain and composite flours, as well as the addition of extracts from plant foods and food wastes, has been increasingly explored as a strategy to improve phenolic content in pasta and gluten-free pasta. In addition, processing technologies have been specifically applied to raw materials or to the pasta-making process in order to increase the content of bioactive components and their bioavailability (Table 2).

Table 2. Modulation of phenolic compound content in pasta.

Strategy	Sub-Strategy	Pasta Products	Effect on Phenolic Compound Content/Profile	Reference
Use of functional ingredients in pasta-making	Whole Grain Flours	Whole grain wheat and whole grain spelt pasta (precooked)	↑ content of protocatechuic, 4-hydroxybenzoic, vanillic, syringic, trans-p-coumaric, cis-p-coumaric, trans-ferulic and cis-ferulic acids.	Wójtowicz et al. [33]
		Whole grain wheat products	TPAs: 226.7 µg/g	Chen et al. [34]
		Whole grain spaghetti	TPC (whole wheat spaghetti): 1263–1423 µg FAE/g dm TPC (regular spaghetti): 718–927 µg FAE/g dm	Hirawan et al. [35]
	Composite Flours	Pasta formulated with wheat semolina and 35% faba bean (Vicia faba L.) flour	TPC (functional pasta): 185.3 mg GAE/100 g dm TPC (control pasta): 63.8 mg GAE/100 g dm	Turco et al. [36]
		Pasta with varying proportions of wheat (T. durum L.) semolina (0–100%), chickpea flour (0–90%), and chia flour (0–10%)	TPC (pasta with 10:90 chia:chickpea flour): 16 mg GAE/g dm TPC (control pasta): 2 mg GAE/g	Cota-Gastélum et al. [37]
		Pasta prepared with carob flour (1–5%)	TPC (pasta with 1% of carob flour): 5.27 mg GAE/g dm TPC (pasta with 5% carob flour): 12.12 mg GAE/g dm TPC (control pasta): 3.51 mg GAE/g dm	Sęczyk et al. [38]
		Pasta prepared with amaranth seed flours and dried amaranth leaves (35%, 50%, 55% and 70%)	TPC (amaranth-added pasta): 1.54 to 3.37 mg FAE/g dm TPC (control pasta, 100% semolina): 0.98 mg FAE/g dm The highest value was observed in pasta with a semolina:amaranth flour/leaves ratio of 65:35.	Cárdenas-Hernández et al. [39]
		GF pasta (unripe plantain and chickpea flour) added with blue maize (Zea mays L.) at 25%, 50% and 75%	Samples containing 75% of blue maize presented the highest TPC retention after extrusion and cooking (approx. 70% and 80%, respectively). In the control pasta, the phenolic retention after extrusion and cooking was approx. 52% and 60%, respectively.	Camelo-Méndez et al. [40]
		GF pasta (with rice, maize and soy flour) added with white and brown sorghum	TPC (pasta with white sorghum): 2.41 g GAE/kg TPC (pasta with brown sorghum): 2.88 g GAE/kg TPC (rice pasta): 0.37 g GAE/kg TPC (soy pasta): 1.37 g GAE/kg TPC (corn pasta): 0.52 g GAE/kg	Palavecino et al. [41]

Table 2. Cont.

Strategy	Sub-Strategy	Pasta Products	Effect on Phenolic Compound Content/Profile	Reference
Use of functional ingredients in pasta-making	Powders and extracts from plant foods and food by-products	Pasta from wheat semolina and pearl-millet added with carrot powder (10%), mango peel powder (5%), moringa leaves powder (3%) and defatted soy flour (15%)	TFC (control pasta): 6.30 mg/100 g dm TFC (carrot-added pasta): 7.63 mg/100 g dm TFC (mango peel-added pasta): 16.53 mg/100 g dm TFC (moringa leaves-added pasta): 17.98 mg/100 g dm TFC (defatted soy flour-added pasta): 8.03 mg/100 g dm	Jalgaonkar et al. [42]
		Pasta added with mushroom (white button, shiitake and porcini) powder, at 5%, 10% and 15% semolina substitution levels	TPC values in mushroom pasta were significantly higher than in control pasta, except for 5% and 10% shiitake mushroom pasta. The greatest values were found in porcini mushroom pasta samples (approximately 4–5 mg GAE/g dm).	Lu et al. [43]
		Pasta added with onion powder, at 0%, 2.5%, 5% and 7.5% semolina substitution level	TPC (cooked pasta added with onion skin): approx. from 1.4 to 3 mg GAE/g dm TFC (cooked pasta added with onion skin): approx. from 0.7 to 3.8 mg QE/g dm TPC (cooked control pasta): approx. 0.5 mg GAE/g dm TFC (cooked control pasta): approx. 0.1 mg QE/g dm Cooked pasta showed TPC not significantly different from the corresponding raw sample, whichever addition level of onion skin powder.	Michalak-Majewska et al. [44]
		Durum spaghetti added with olive paste powder (10%)	TPC (enriched spaghetti): 245.08 µg/g dm TPC (control pasta): 82.39 µg/g dm Control and functional pasta differed also in the phenolic profile. Increased level of flavonoids (i.e., quercetin and luteolin) in functional pasta.	Padalino et al. [45]
		Spaghetti added with extracts from grape marc (grape skins, seeds, and stalks)	TPC (functional spaghetti): approx. 700 mg GAE/100g dm	Marinelli et al. [46]
		Pasta prepared from semolina and bran aqueous extract	TPC (functional spaghetti): 127 mg FAE/100 g fw TPC (control pasta): 97 mg FAE/100 g fw	Pasqualone et al. [47]

Table 2. Cont.

Strategy	Sub-Strategy	Pasta Products	Effect on Phenolic Compound Content/Profile	Reference
Use of functional ingredients in pasta-making	Powders and extracts from plant foods and food by-products	GF pasta added with chia (Salvia hispanica L.) milled seeds (5% and 10% substitution levels)	In raw samples— TPA (functional GF pasta—10% sub.): 164.3 µg/g TPA (durum wheat pasta): 149.08 µg/g TPA (functional GF pasta—5% sub.): 98.40 µg/g TPA (pasta produced with commercial GF flour): 10.30 µg/g In cooked samples— ↑TPAs in all pasta samples. TPA (functional GF pasta—10% sub.): 186.80 µg/g TPA (durum wheat pasta): 156.99 µg/g TPA (functional GF pasta—5% sub.): 123.53 µg/g TPA (pasta produced with commercial GF flour): 11.83 µg/g Control and functional pasta also differed in the phenolic profile.	Menga et al. [48]
		GF pasta (from a blend of rice and field bean flour) added with pear prickly fruit (Opuntia ficus indica (L.) Mill.) in different amounts (2.5%, 5%, 7.5%, 10%, 12.5% and 15%)	Pasta samples enriched with pear prickly fruit were rich in several phenolic acids, namely protocatechuic, caffeic, syryngic, 4-OH-benzoic, vanilic, gentisic, trans-sinapic, cis-sinapic, p-coumaric, ferulic, isoferulic, m-coumaric, 3,4-dimetoxycinnamic, and salicylic acids. The higher was the addition of pear prickly fruit, the higher was the content of phenolic acids. The dominant acid was isoferulic.	Oniszczuk et al. [49]
		GF pasta (from a blend of rice and field bean flour) added with chestnut fruit (Castanea sativa Mill.) in different amounts (10%, 20%, 30%, 40%, and 50%)	TPA content (10%): 38.93 µg/g dm TPA content (20%): 46.98 µg/g dm TPA content (30%): 51.47 µg/g dm TPA content (40%): 56.59 µg/g dm TPA content (50%): 65.01 µg/g dm The content of each phenolic acid also increased at the higher addition of chestnut fruit, with the exception of 4-hydroxy-benzoic and salicylic acids.	Oniszczuk et al. [50]

Table 2. Cont.

Strategy	Sub-Strategy	Pasta Products	Effect on Phenolic Compound Content/Profile	Reference
Raw material processing, pasta-making and pasta cooking	Debranning	Pasta enriched with a debranning fraction from purple wheat (25%)	Phenolic compounds in wheat flour and semolina were negligible compared to the debranning fraction from purple wheat. In pasta samples TPC was lower than it was expected. This was possibly due to the degradation of phenolics during the pasta-making process.	Abbasi et al. [51]
		Pasta enriched with the first and the second debranning fraction from purple wheat	Anthocyanin content (pasta enriched with the 1st debranning fraction): 67.9 µg/g dm Anthocyanin content (pasta added with the 2nd debranning fraction): 60 µg/g dm Anthocyanin content (control pasta with bran addition): 28 µg/g dm	Zanoletti et al. [52]
		Spaghetti enriched (30%) with debranning fractions of durum wheat	In raw samples— Free PAs were higher in the control pasta than in functional pasta. Conjugated PAs (functional pasta): 59.4 mg/kg dm Conjugated PAs (control pasta): 21.6 mg/kg dm Bound PAs (functional pasta): 650.0 mg/kg dm Bound PAs (control pasta): 27.2 mg/kg dm Conjugated TPC (functional pasta): 110.7 mg/kg dm Conjugated TPC (control pasta): 31.4 mg/kg dm Bound TPC (functional pasta): 1308.4 mg/kg dm Bound TPC (control pasta): 156.9 mg/kg dm In cooked samples— ↑ level of PAs, whichever form was considered ↓ free and conjugated TPC ↑ level of bound phenolic compound	Ciccoritti et al. [53]

Table 2. *Cont.*

Strategy	Sub-Strategy	Pasta Products	Effect on Phenolic Compound Content/Profile	Reference
Raw material processing, pasta-making and pasta cooking	Micronization	Pasta added with micronized fractions	In raw functional pasta— Conjugated PAs: 36.8 mg/kg dm Bound PAs: 357.3 mg/kg dm Conjugated TPs: 75.8 mg/kg dm Bound TPs: 113.3 mg/kg dm In cooked functional pasta (with respect to raw samples)— ↑ free PAs and conjugated PAs ↓ bound PAs ↓ conjugated TPs ↑ bound TPs	Ciccoritti et al. [53]
	Micronization	Pasta added with micronized fractions	Micronization preserved the content of phenolic acids, while conventional milling determined 89% decrease from seeds to cooked durum wheat pasta	Martini et al. [54]
	Cereal germination	Spaghetti formulated by using 30% dry tartary buckwheat sprouts	In raw samples— TPC (raw tartary buckwheat spaghetti): 3.7 mg GAE/g TPC (100% semolina spaghetti): 0.3 mg GAE/g In cooked samples— TPC (raw tartary buckwheat spaghetti): 2.2 mg GAE/g TPC (100% semolina spaghetti): 0.2 mg GAE/g	Merendino et al. [55]
	Legume germination	Pasta prepared with sprouted chickpea flour	TPC (sprouted chickpea pasta): 8.4 mg GAE/g TPC (non-sprouted chickpea pasta): 7.3 mg GAE/g	Bruno et al. [56]

Table 2. Cont.

Strategy	Sub-Strategy	Pasta Products	Effect on Phenolic Compound Content/Profile	Reference
Raw material processing, pasta-making and pasta cooking	Extrusion and Extrusion-cooking	GF precooked rice-yellow pea pasta	↑ TPC at higher screw speed (80 rpm)	Bouasla et al. [57]
		GF precooked pasta from roasted buckwheat (*Fagopyrum esculentum* Moench and *F. tataricum* Gaertner) flour	Highest level of benzoic acid derivatives (i.e., gallic, protocatechuic, gentisic, 4-hydroxybenzoic and salicylic acids) at 100 rpm extruder screw speed and 32% flour moisture content. Highest content in cinnamic acid derivatives (i.e., *trans*-caffeic, *trans*-*p*-coumaric, *cis*-*p*-coumaric and *cis*-ferulic acids) at 60 rpm extruder screw speed and 30% of flour moisture	Oniszczuk et al. [58]
		Barley pasta	↓ TPC after extrusion	De Paula et al. [59]
	Cooking	Barley pasta	TPAs were not greatly affected by cooking	De Paula et al. [59]
		Whole wheat	↑ free TPC	Podio et al. [60]
		GF pasta (i.e., pasta enriched with black rice, chickpea, red lentil, sorghum, amaranth and quinoa)	In raw GF pasta— Bound TPC > Free TPC Bound TPC (sorghum GF pasta): 7.58 mg GAE/100 g Bound TPC (quinoa GF pasta): 32.68 mg GAE/100 g In cooked GF pasta— Free TPC > Bound TPC Free TPC (black rice pasta): 27.27 mg GAE/100 g Free TPC (quinoa pasta): 19.27 mg GAE/100 g	Rocchetti et al. [61]

↓: decrease; ↑: increase; dm: dry matter; FAE: Ferulic Acid Equivalents; fw: fresh weight; GAE: Gallic Acid Equivalents; GF: Gluten-free; PAs: Phenolic Acids; QE: Quercetin Equivalents; TFC: Total Flavonoid Content; TPA(s): Total Phenolic Acid(s); TPC: Total Phenolic Content; TPs: Total Phenolics.

3.1. Use of Functional Ingredients in Pasta-Making

3.1.1. Whole Grain Flours

According to the HEALTHGRAIN Consortium, whole grains (WGs) shall consist of "the intact, ground, cracked or flaked kernel after the removal of inedible parts such as the hull and husk. The principal anatomical components—the starchy endosperm, germ and bran—are present in the same relative proportions as they exist in the intact kernel" [62]. While agreement on the definition of "whole grain" has been reached, there is a lack of consensus on the definition of whole-grain foods, including "whole grain pasta" [63].

In Germany and Italy, "whole grain pasta" is pasta where 100% of the grain component in the final product is whole grain; in Denmark, pasta containing a percentage of whole grain equal or higher than 60% on a dry matter basis, can be classified as "whole grain pasta"; in France and the Netherlands, there are no regulations nor guidelines for whole grain pasta definition [63].

Two main factors explain these different levels of whole grains admitted in whole grain products. On the one hand, foods with high whole grain content are not universally appreciated by consumers, hence manufacturers need to use whole grain ingredients in a level enabling to obtain products with good sensory qualities. On the other hand, the content of whole grain ingredients used for product preparation, must be adequate to guarantee nutritional benefits to consumers.

Cereals included in the whole grain definition are wheat (including spelt, emmer, faro, einkorn, khorasan wheat, durums), rice (including pigmented varieties), barley (including hull-less or naked barley but not pearled), corn, rye, oats (including hull-less or naked oats), millets, sorghum, teff, triticale, Canary seed, Job's tears, fonio, black fonio and Asian millet. Pseudocereals included in the whole grain definition are amaranth, buckwheat and tartar buckwheat, quinoa, and wild rice [62].

In whole grain flours, the outer multi-layered skin (bran) and the germ are retained together with the starchy main part of the grain. The bran is a major source of phenolic acids, dietary fibre (DF) and minerals, while the germ contains vitamins, minerals, fats and some proteins [64]. Phenolic acids, together with DF, are components responsible for many of the health effects associated with whole grain consumption [25]. They have shown to act synergistically and modulate favourably appetite, glucose metabolism, insulin sensitivity, and gut microbiota composition [65], and to have a role in the prevention and treatment of cardiovascular diseases [66,67]. Several studies have evidenced a lower risk from all causes and disease-specific mortality associated with a high intake of WGs [68].

The content of phenolic compounds in whole grain pasta has been, however, poorly investigated. Wójtowicz et al. determined the qualitative and quantitative profile of phenolic compounds in precooked pasta prepared from whole grain wheat and whole grain spelt [33]. Protocatechuic, 4-hydroxybenzoic, vanillic, syringic, *trans-p*-coumaric, *cis-p*-coumaric, *trans*-ferulic and *cis*-ferulic acids were identified in samples under investigation. *Cis*-ferulic acid was the main phenolic acid in both whole grain wheat and spelt pasta. In whole grain wheat pasta, vanillic acid was the second more abundant phenolic compound, while in whole grain spelt pasta, syringic and vanillic acids were identified as the main phenolics, after *cis*-ferulic acid. Compared to refined flours, the use of whole flours enabled to double the intake of phenolic acids. These data are in keeping with Chen et al. who found ferulic acid as the dominant phenolic compound in six whole grain wheat products, with values ranging between 99.9 and 316.0 µg/g [34]. In whole wheat pasta (41.4% fortification), Total Phenolic Acid (TPA) content was 226.7 µg/g dm.

Hirawan et al. determined the total phenolic content (TPC) in regular and whole grain spaghetti, and found that the former had a TPC level 2-fold lower than the latter [35]. TPC values in whole wheat spaghetti ranged between 1263 and 1423 µg/g Ferulic Acid Equivalents (FAE)/g dm, while in regular spaghetti TPC ranged between 718 and 927 µg/g FAE/g dm. It was also observed that all whole wheat spaghetti samples contained ferulic acid, while this compound was detected only in two out of regular spaghetti samples. However, TPC significantly decreased after cooking (about 40%), both in regular and whole wheat spaghetti. Despite the differences in the TPC, regular and whole grain spaghetti exhibited the same antioxidant capacity, possibly due to the antioxidant components, such as the Maillard reaction products, formed during pasta drying.

3.1.2. Composite Flours

Composite flours are blends of wheat and varying proportion of legumes, tubers or other cereals, including minor cereals, and pseudocereals. Cassava, maize, rice, sorghum, millets, potato, barley, sweet potato and yam are common ingredients of composite flours [69].

The concept of using composite flours in bread and pasta-making was first elaborated to tackle a low availability of wheat in areas whose climatic conditions are not suitable for wheat production, and to encourage the use of autochthonous crops with economic advantages for local producers and consumers [69]. The concept thus first had an economic value. However, partial or total wheat substitution with composite flours affects also the nutritional profile of the final product. Wheat is, in fact, deficient in essential amino acids, such as lysine and threonine, and, during milling, bioactive compounds and minerals are commonly lost. Hence, the use of composite flours contributes to counteracting these deficiencies. More recently, the concept of "composite flours" has been thus extended to blends of wheat flour/semolina and other flours richer in essential amino acids, minerals, vitamins and phenolic compounds.

Blends of cereal flours with pulse flours have been by far explored in pasta-making. Pulses are an important source of nutrients [69]. They have a low glycemic index and are rich in complex carbohydrates, DF, plant proteins, and micronutrients. They also have high levels of polyphenols with good antioxidant properties, and other plant secondary metabolites and components (i.e., isoflavones, phytosterols, bioactive carbohydrates, alkaloids, and saponins), that are being increasingly recognized for their bioavailability and potential benefits for human health. Among phenolic compounds, phenolic acids, flavonoids and condensed tannins are the most abundant [70].

The use of pulses in pasta-making and their contribution to the content of phenolic compounds have been recently investigated by Turco et al. [36]. They found that, in pasta formulated by wheat semolina and 35% faba bean (*Vicia faba* L.) flour, TPC increased from 63.8 mg Gallic Acid Equivalents (GAE)/100 g dry matter (dm) to 185.3 mg GAE/100 g dm. Cota-Gastélum et al. prepared functional pasta with varying proportions of wheat (*T. durum* L.) semolina (0–100%), chickpea flour (0–90%), and chia flour (0–10%) [37]. In raw samples, the highest phenolic content (approximately 16 mg GAE/g) was observed when durum semolina was totally replaced and a blend of 10% chia flour and 90% chickpea flour was used. This value was approximately 8-fold higher than in durum wheat pasta (2 mg GAE/g) [37]. Carob flour, which is obtained from carob seeds, has been also used in substitution of semolina in pasta-making. Sęczyk et al. produced pasta by using varying percentages of carob flour (1–5%) [38]. They found that the phenolic content in the produced functional pasta was higher than in the control pasta (3.51 mg GAE/g dm). In pasta with 1% of carob flour, TPC was 5.27 mg GAE/g dm, and it increased to 12.12 mg GAE/g dm in pasta with 5% carob flour [38].

Pseudocereal flours were also used to partially or totally replace semolina in pasta-making, in order to enhance pasta nutritional profile. Pseudocereals are, in fact, characterized by a high nutritional composition, in terms of high content in DF, high-quality protein, essential minerals, vitamins (e.g., folic acid), essential amino acids and unsaturated fatty acids [71,72]. They are also a valuable source of phenolic compounds [73]. Varying levels of amaranth seed flours and dried amaranth leaves (35%, 50%, 55% and 70%) were used as semolina substituents in the preparation of elbow-type pasta [39]. Both grains and leaves are, in fact, rich in bioactive compounds. Grains also show high levels of proteins (15 g/100 g) and are a source of vitamins, such as thiamine, niacin, riboflavin and folate, and minerals, namely iron, calcium, zinc, magnesium, phosphorus, copper, and manganese [74,75]. The study by Cárdenas-Hernández et al. showed that, whichever the substitution levels, amaranth pasta had a TPC higher than 100% semolina pasta (0.98 mg of FAE/g dm), with values ranging from 1.54 to 3.37 mg FAE/g dm [39]. The highest value was observed in pasta with a semolina:amaranth flour/leaves ratio of

65:35. A significant decrease in phenolic content (15–27%) was observed in all amaranth pasta samples, after cooking [39].

Composite flours have been also used to improve the nutritional value of gluten-free (GF) pasta. As a matter of fact, GF pasta is mainly produced with GF flours, such as rice and corn, which are low in micronutrients and bioactive compounds [76]. The use of blue maize in GF pasta-making has been recently explored. Blue maize (*Zea mays* L.), like the red and purple varieties, is rich in anthocyanidins (up to 325 mg/100 g dm), including cyanidin derivatives (75–90%), peonidin derivatives (15–20%) and pelargonidin derivatives (5–10%) [77]. Different percentages of blue maize (25%, 50% and 75%) were added to pasta dough produced with equal amounts of unripe plantain and chickpea flour [40]. It was observed that pasta samples containing 75% of blue maize presented the highest TPC retention after extrusion and cooking. Upon extrusion, TPC in pasta decreased between 20% and 30%, while an additional 10% loss occurred upon cooking. The phenolic compounds, retained after extrusion, were likely bound phenolics, whereas free phenolic species (e.g., free phenolic acids and anthocyanins), not physically trapped in the protein network, were leached into the cooking water.

The fortification of traditional GF flours with sorghum (*Sorghum bicolor* (L.) Moench) flour in pasta-making has been also studied. Sorghum has, in fact, high levels of a diverse array of beneficial bioactive components (e.g., polyphenols, especially flavonoids), and bioactive lipids (such as policosanols and phytosterols) [78–80]. Palavecino et al. produced GF pasta with white and brown sorghum [41]. They compared the two sorghum-based formulations to GF pasta produced with rice, maize and soy flour. Total phenolic compound content was higher in the two sorghum-based pasta samples than in the controls, with a value of 2.41 g GAE kg^{-1} and 2.88 g GAE kg^{-1} for white and brown sorghum, respectively. Sorghum pasta, after cooking, also showed higher radical scavenging activity and ferric reducing ability than the control samples, without significant differences between sorghum varieties.

3.1.3. Powders and Extracts from Plant Foods and Food By-Products

The use of powders and extracts from plant foods and food by-products in pasta-making is among the strategies recently explored to obtain functional pasta, both gluten-containing and gluten-free.

Functional pasta was prepared by incorporating carrot powder (10%), mango peel powder (5%), moringa leaves powder (3%) and defatted soy flour (15%) in a blend of wheat semolina and pearl-millet [42]. Total flavonoid content (TFC) was determined in order to evaluate the contribution of these ingredients to the phenolic content in pasta. It emerged that, in the control pasta, TFC was 6.30 mg/100 g. The addition of mango peel powder and moringa leaves powder provided the highest values (16.53 and 17.98 mg/100 g, respectively), while carrot powder and defatted soy flour contributed at a lower extent, with values of 7.63 and 8.03 mg/100 g, respectively.

Mushrooms can also contribute to the phenolic dietary intake. The study by Lu et al. investigated the contribution of mushroom powder addition to the phenolic content of spaghetti [43]. Three different powders were used: from white button, from shiitake and from porcini mushrooms. Three different semolina substitution levels were tested: 5 g, 10 g and 15 g/100 g (w/w). It emerged that all mushroom-powder-supplemented pasta samples showed TPC values significantly higher than semolina pasta, except for 5% and 10% shiitake mushroom pasta. The greatest values were found in porcini mushroom pasta samples (approximately 4–5 mg GAE/g dm), followed by the second button mushroom samples (approximately 2 mg GAE/g dm), and shiitake mushroom pasta.

Plant food industrial processing produces huge amounts of by-products that are a serious disposal issue. However, some by-products have shown to be an abundant source of valuable compounds [81]. Hence, in the domain of circular economy, they have been increasingly turned into functional ingredients. Vegetable wastes, such as peelings, trimmings, stems, seeds, shells, and bran are some by-products from which phenolic compounds can be extracted [82]. Ultrasound-assisted extraction, microwave-assisted extraction, supercritical fluid extraction, pressurized fluid extraction, pulsed electric field extraction and enzyme-assisted extraction are green technologies commonly used in the recovery of phenolic compounds from food wastes [82–84]. The choice of the extraction technique is related to factors including the functional ingredient to extract and the characteristics of the food matrix.

Onion dry skin powder has been used as a functional ingredient to modulate phenolic compound content in pasta [44]. Onion dry skins are by-products generated during industrial peeling and contain bioavailable compounds such as DF, fructo-oligosaccharides and quercetin aglycones. In the study by Michalak-Majewska et al., semolina was replaced by varying amounts of onion powder: 0%, 2.5%, 5% and 7.5%. TPC and TFC were determined both in raw and cooked samples. It was observed that pasta added with onion skin powder showed TPC and TFC higher than the control (100% semolina pasta). The highest TPC was found in pasta with 7.5% substitution level. Moreover, cooked pasta showed TPC not significantly different from the corresponding raw sample, whichever addition level of onion skin powder. Conversely, in the control pasta, TPC decreased after cooking. Hence, the functional pasta ensured a higher intake of phenolic compounds, compared to 100% semolina pasta. As regards TFC, the addition of onion skin powder enabled to obtain pasta with higher level of flavonoids, and after cooking a significant increase was observed.

Durum spaghetti were formulated by the addition of olive paste powder [45]. Olive paste is an industrial by-product of olive oil production, rich in phenolic compounds [45]. Two levels of olive paste powder were added to semolina: 10% and 15%. Phenolic content was determined on spaghetti with 10% addition of olive paste powder, since they showed the best sensory properties. TPC was 82.39 µg/g dm in the control pasta and 245.08 µg/g dm in the enriched spaghetti. In 100% semolina pasta, vanillic acid was the most abundant phenolic compound in free form (0.56 µg/g dm), while ferulic acid was the main bound phenolic compound (67.70 µg/g dm). In spaghetti enriched with olive paste powder, vanillic acid was the main phenolic acid in free form as in the control pasta; however, its content was higher (7.28 µg/g dm) than in the control. HPLC analysis also showed that the addition of olive paste powder increased the content of flavonoids, such as quercetin and luteolin.

Functional spaghetti were also produced by addition of extracts from grape marc, made up of skins, seeds, and stalks [46]. TPC was determined on fresh extruded spaghetti, pasteurized extruded spaghetti and dry spaghetti. It was found that, compared to the control, the addition of grape marc extract increased TPC in all enriched spaghetti samples (approximately 700 mg GAE/100g dm). The pasteurization and drying process did not significantly affect the TPC. Interestingly, after cooking an increase in TPC was observed, with respect to the raw samples.

Bran is the main by-product of cereal milling and is a great source of phenolic compounds and minerals. Despite its functionality, its use in pasta-making is challenging, since it has adverse effects on the quality of the final products, such as an increase of cooking loss, swelling index, and water absorption in pasta [85]. Recently, bran aqueous extract was used in the production of spaghetti [47]. The extract was obtained by ultrasound assisted-extraction at 20 °C for 25 min. The ratio between water and bran was 10 L/kg. The bran aqueous extract completely substituted processing water in pasta-making. A significant increase in phenolic compounds was observed in pasta samples due to the bran extract. In detail, TPC was 127 mg FAE/100 g fresh weight (fw) in functional spaghetti and 97 mg FAE/100 g fw in the control pasta.

As regards the formulation of functional GF pasta, different percentages (5% and 10%) of chia (*Salvia hispanica* L.) milled seeds were incorporated into rice flour dough [48]. Chia seed addition allowed increasing phenolic acid content, besides the slowly digestible starch fraction of rice, and protein and DF content. The highest content of TPAs was observed in raw samples of pasta produced with 10% milled chia seeds (164.3 µg/g). TPA content in functional GF pasta did not significantly differ from durum wheat pasta (164.3 vs 149.08 µg/g), but it was by far higher than in pasta produced with commercial GF flour (10.30 µg/g) [48].

After cooking, TPA content was higher in all pasta samples, with an increase of 5.3% in durum wheat pasta, 14.8% in commercial GF pasta, 25.5% in pasta with 5% of milled chia seeds and 13.7% in pasta with 10% of milled chia seeds. The highest content in TPAs was observed in pasta with a 10%

milled chia seeds (186.80 µg/g). The increase in TPA content in cooked samples was possibly due to the increased bioaccessibility of bound phenolic acids after boiling [48]. Samples also differed for the content of specific phenolic acids. Addition of milled chia seeds allowed obtaining pasta samples containing chlorogenic acid, which is otherwise absent in commercial GF and durum wheat pasta. Chia seed pasta was also rich in caffeic and vanillic acids, in contrast to durum wheat pasta. The higher was milled chia seed addition, the higher was the content of chlorogenic, caffeic, and vanillic acids.

Oniszczuk et al. investigated the phenolic profile of GF pasta prepared with a blend of rice and field bean flour, enriched with different amounts (2.5%, 5%, 7.5%, 10%, 12.5% and 15%) of pear prickly fruit (*Opuntia ficus indica* (L.) Mill.) [49]. The latter is a source of phenolic compounds and also provides vitamins (C, B1, B2, A, and E), minerals (calcium, potassium, magnesium, iron, and phosphorus), and other bioactive compounds, such as carotenoids and betalains. High-performance liquid chromatography/electrospray ionization tandem mass spectrometry (HPLC-ESI-MS/MS) showed that pasta samples enriched with the different amounts of pear prickly fruit were rich in several phenolic acids: protocatechuic, caffeic, syryngic, 4-OH-benzoic, vanilic, gentisic, *trans*-sinapic, *cis*-sinapic, *p*-coumaric, ferulic, isoferulic, *m*-coumaric, 3,4-dimetoxycinnamic, and salicylic acids. The dominant acid was isoferulic. The higher was the addition of pear prickly fruit, the higher was the content of phenolic acids. Antioxidant activity was also positively correlated with the addition of fruit.

The effect of chestnut fruit (*Castanea sativa* Mill.) addition (10%, 20%, 30%, 40%, and 50%) to the aforesaid blend of rice and field bean flour on pasta phenolic content, was also investigated [50]. Chestnut fruit is rich in phenolic compounds, as well as in proteins, unsaturated fatty acids, DF, vitamins and micronutrients. As regards the content of phenolic compounds, it was observed that the total content of free phenolic acids increased along with the chestnut addition. TPA content was 38.93, 46.98, 51.47, 56.59, and 65.01 µg/g dm in samples with 10%, 20%, 30%, 40% and 50% of chestnut flour, respectively [50]. The content of each phenolic acid also increased at a higher addition of chestnut fruit, with the exception of 4-hydroxy-benzoic and salicylic acids whose level decreased at the increase of chestnut flour addition. This trend might be explained by a content of these two acids higher in the rice and field bean flour blend than in chestnut fruit powder.

3.2. Raw Material Processing, Pasta-Making and Pasta Cooking

In addition to the use of raw materials naturally rich in phenolic compounds, such as whole grain flour, composite flours, and plant powders and extracts, raw material processing and modulation of pasta-making and pasta cooking parameters have been explored to increase the content of phenolic compounds in pasta.

Debranning, also known as pearling, is a technology based on the gradual removal of the outer bran layers prior to milling process. While in conventional milling the aleurone layer remains attached to the bran, in debranning it remains attached to the endosperm. As a consequence, semolina and flour obtained by debranning are richer in components commonly found in the grain aleurone. The technology also enables to isolate aleurone-rich fractions, which can be used as functional ingredients [86]. Abbasi et al. have recently formulated pasta enriched with a debranning fraction from purple wheat [51]. The debranning fraction (25%) was added to flour and to semolina by dry mixing, and macaroni pasta samples were prepared. Experimental analyses on raw materials showed that phenolic compounds in wheat flour and semolina were negligible compared to the debranning fraction. Despite the debranning technology enabled to obtain raw materials rich in phenolic compounds, pasta samples showed TPC lower than it was expected. This was possibly due to the degradation of phenolics during the pasta-making process, especially in the drying step.

One more study on the formulation of pasta products by using debranning fractions was reported by Zanoletti et al. [52]. Two functional pasta products enriched with a fraction obtained from either the first or the second debranning step of purple wheat were produced. The first fraction corresponded to a debranning level of 3.7% of whole grain, while the second fraction corresponded to 6% of the debranned grain after the first step. The content of anthocyanins, a subclass of phenolic compounds typical of many fruits, vegetables, and cereal grains with red, violet, and blue colour, was determined. The analysis of cooked samples showed that anthocyanin content was 67.9 µg/g dm in pasta enriched with the first debranning fraction and 60.0 µg/g dm in pasta added with the second debranning fraction. These two values were not significantly different. Moreover, anthocyanin content in functional pasta was higher than in pasta added with bran (28 µg/g dm) and used as control sample. In addition, both functional pasta products exhibited an antioxidant activity higher than the control.

Ciccoritti et al. prepared spaghetti enriched with debranning fractions of durum wheat cv Normanno. The addition level of debranning fraction was 30% w/w [53]. Phenolic acids (PAs) and TPC were determined in raw and cooked samples, in free, esterified and bound forms. It emerged that in raw samples, free PAs content was higher in the control pasta than in functional pasta. As far as conjugated and bound PAs are concerned, values were higher in enriched samples. Conjugated PAs were 59.4 mg/kg dm and bound PAs were 650.0 mg/kg dm in functional pasta, while in control pasta they were 21.6 and 27.2 mg/kg dm, respectively. A similar trend was observed for conjugated and bound TPC. The former was 110.7 mg/kg dm in functional pasta and 31.4 mg/kg dm in control pasta, while the latter was 1308.4 and 156.9 mg/kg dm, respectively. After cooking, it was observed a higher level of PAs, whichever form was considered. Conversely, free and conjugated TPC decreased, and bound TPC increased.

Ciccoritti et al. also explored the use of micronized fractions in pasta-making [53]. Micronization is a mechanical treatment consisting in reducing kernels into a fine powder. For this reason it is also known as ultrafine grinding. It differs from conventional milling because it produces wholegrain flour, without producing by-products such as bran. The treatment damages the fibre matrix, hence the phenolic compounds linked or embedded into the matrix are more bioaccessible. The content of PAs and total phenolics in experimental pasta was determined. Raw pasta prepared from debranned and micronized durum wheat had a higher level of PAs (conjugated and bound) and total phenolics (TPs) than the control. Conjugated PAs were 36.8 mg/kg dm and bound PAs were 357.3 mg/kg dm. The content of conjugated TPs was 75.8 mg/kg dm and bound TPs were 113.3 mg/kg dm. After cooking, the level of free PAs and conjugated PAs increased, while bound PAs decreased. As regards TPs, the content of free forms did not significantly differ from raw samples, while the content of conjugated TPs decreased and the level of bound TPs increased significantly. Data are in keeping with Martini et al. who observed that micronization preserved the content of phenolic acids, while conventional milling determined 89% decrease from seeds to cooked durum wheat pasta [54].

In addition to mechanical treatments, biological processes, such as germination and fermentation, are strategies enabling to increase the phenolic compound content in pasta products.

As regards germination, both cereal grains and pulses can be sprouted. Cereal seed germination may impact on nutritional properties of cereals [87] and possibly cereal-based products. An increase in phenolic compound content ranging from 1.2 to 3.6 folds was reported in wheat, barley, sorghum, rye, oat and brown rice, after germination [87–94]. During sprouting, cell wall-degrading enzymes, such as cellulases, endoxylanases and esterases, are biosynthesized. They can hydrolyze phenolic compounds bound to cell wall constituents, so as to increase the content of free phenolic compounds. Moreover, thanks to the effect of enzymes, bound phenolic compounds are more soluble in extraction solvents and more bioaccessible. Merendino et al. explored the use of sprouted cereals in pasta-making [55]. Spaghetti were formulated by replacing wheat semolina with 30% dry tartary buckwheat sprouts belonging to the Slovenian landrace Ljse. TPC in raw tartary buckwheat spaghetti was 3.7 mg GAE/g, while it was 0.3 mg GAE/g in 100% semolina spaghetti. After cooking, TPC was 2.2 and 0.2 mg GAE/g in tartary buckwheat and in control spaghetti, respectively. Flours from sprouted legumes have been also used in pasta-making, since sprouting increases phenolic compound content in legumes [95]. In detail, Bruno et al. investigated the contribution of sprouting to increasing phenolic content in chickpea pasta [56]. Pasta prepared with sprouted chickpea flour had phenolic content 15% higher than non-sprouted chickpea pasta.

Sourdough-fermented ingredients have been recently proposed to enhance the nutritional and functional properties of pasta [96]. However, to our knowledge, no study investigating the phenolic profile of pasta produced with sourdough-fermented flours has been so far published. Fermentation is indeed one more pre-processing technique that can increase the content of phenolic compounds in pasta ingredients, such as pulses and pseudocereals, and bran. Microorganisms responsible for the fermenting process, produce enzymes which boost the release of insoluble bound phenolic compounds from the food matrix, thus increasing their solubility and bioaccessibility. Rashid et al. reported a content of extractable phenolic compounds, in rice bran fermented by *Aspergillus oryzae*, 3.8-fold higher than in unfermented bran [97]. It was also observed that rice bran solid-state fermentation with *A. oryzae* affected the profile of phenolic acids. In unfermented bran, protocatechuic, coumaric and ferulic acids were found, while in fermented rice bran *p*-coumaric, protocatechuic, ferulic, caffeic and sinapic acids were detected. Moreover, the level of coumaric, ferulic and protocatechuic acids in the fermented bran increased by up to 3.2-fold, 52-fold and 3.2-fold, respectively, compared to its unfermented counterpart. Dey et al. studied the effect of solid state fermentation of wheat by *Rhizopus oryzae* RCK2012 on phenolic content and they found that TPC increased from 5.15 mg GAE/g to 24.55 mg GAE/g [98]. Călinoiu et al. explored the use of solid-state fermentation to improve phenolic content in wheat and oat bran [99]. A 112% increase in TPC was observed on day 3 fermentation in wheat bran and 83% increase on day 4 of fermentation in oat bran, with values reaching 0.84 mg GAE/g and 0.45 mg GAE/g, respectively. Based on these results, it can thus be speculated that fermentation of raw materials may contribute to increasing phenolic content in pasta; however, additional studies on the effect of pasta-making upon TPC are required.

The pasta-making process can also influence the content of phenolic compounds; process parameters and conditions may be thus set in order to limit/avoid phenolic compound degradation and/or increase their bioaccessibility.

Generally speaking, conventional pasta is produced by forcing flour/semolina dough through a die to obtain the required shape, and then drying it. Low shear and heat values (30–40 °C) are applied. Gluten-free and precooked pasta are prepared by extrusion-cooking, which is a high-temperature short-time process consisting in a short-term heating of dough, at a high temperature, under high pressure. During extrusion-cooking, raw materials are forced to flow through a die and thermal and shear energies cause structural, chemical, and nutritional transformations, including gelatinization and degradation of starch, denaturalization of proteins, oxidation of lipids, degradation of vitamins and bioactive compounds, and changes in bioavailability of minerals and solubility of dietary fibre [100]. The combination of high temperature, high pressure, and high shearing conditions during extrusion-cooking may affect the content in phenolic compounds. Heat can cause the decomposition of heat-labile phenolics and polymerization of some phenolic compounds, thus decreasing their content. At the same time, heat disrupts cell wall matrices which hinder phenolic molecules to gastrointestinal enzymes, thus promoting their accessibility [101]. Hence, the effect of extrusion-cooking on phenolic content and bioaccessibility depends on which effect prevails.

As regards the effect of extrusion-cooking parameters on phenolic content in pasta, Bouasla et al. observed that the application of higher screw speed (80 rpm) enabled to obtain higher phenolic content in GF precooked rice-yellow pea pasta [57]. As a matter of fact, in cereal grains phenolic acids are mainly found in the bound form and such complexes are difficult to break down at lower screw speeds [57]. Oniszczuk et al. studied the effect of extruder screw speed on free phenolic acid content of GF precooked pasta obtained from roasted buckwheat (*Fagopyrum esculentum* Moench and *F. tataricum* Gaertner) flour [58]. The qualitative and quantitative analysis of FAs in extruded pasta by high-performance liquid chromatography electrospray ionization tandem mass spectrometry (HPLC-ESI-MS/MS) showed that gallic, protocatechuic, gentisic, 4-hydroxybenzoic, vanilic, *trans*-caffeic, *cis*-caffeic, *trans*-*p*-coumaric, *cis*-*p*-coumaric, syryngic, *trans*-ferulic, *cis*-ferulic, salicylic, *trans*-sinapic and *cis*-sinapic acids were present in all pasta samples, regardless of moisture content (30%, 32% and 34%) and screw speed (60, 80, 100 and 120 rpm). However, in pasta samples produced at 100 rpm extruder screw speed and 32%

flour moisture content, benzoic acid derivatives (i.e., gallic, protocatechuic, gentisic, 4-hydroxybenzoic and salicylic acids) were present with the highest amounts. The highest content in cinnamic acid derivatives (i.e., *trans*-caffeic, *trans-p*-coumaric, *cis-p*-coumaric and *cis*-ferulic) was observed in samples of GF buckwheat pasta produced at 60 rpm extruder screw speed and 30% of flour moisture [58]. Conversely, De Paula et al. reported a significant reduction in total phenolic acid content after pasta extrusion, possibly due to oxidising reactions promoted by water, oxygen and heat [59].

Cooking is a necessary step for pasta consumption, and it may influence the content of phenolic compounds and/or change the ratio between free and bound form of phenolics. De Paula et al. investigated the effect of cooking on phenolic content in barley pasta and observed that TPAs were not greatly affected by this treatment, and both free and bound phenolic compounds were preserved [59]. Conversely, Podio et al. found that cooking promotes the release of bound phenolic compounds, thus increasing the content of the free forms. In addition, pasta-making and cooking produced a change in the phenolic profile with respect to the starting flour [60]. Results are in keeping with Rocchetti et al. who observed that cooking by boiling lowered the bound-to-free ratio of phenolics in GF pasta [61]. They studied six commercially available GF pasta samples (i.e., pasta enriched with black rice, chickpea, red lentil, sorghum, amaranth and quinoa) and observed that in raw GF pasta samples, bound TPC was higher than free TPC, with values ranging from 7.58 mg GAE/100 g (sorghum GF pasta) to 32.68 mg GAE/100 g (quinoa GF pasta). After cooking, the highest free TPC was observed in black rice and quinoa samples, with 27.27 and 19.27 mg GAE 100 g^{-1}, respectively ($p < 0.01$). In conclusion, from a nutritional point of view, understanding the effect of processing on phenolic content and on the ratio between free and bound forms is pivotal. As a matter of fact, the activity of phenolic acids is strictly dependent on the form they reach the gastrointestinal tract. The intake of free forms or soluble conjugated forms has systemic beneficial effects, such as inhibition of LDL cholesterol and liposome oxidation, since they are rapidly absorbed in the stomach and small intestine. Conversely, insoluble bound phenolic compounds reach the colon nearly intact where they are hydrolysed by the esterases and xylanase of colon microorganisms, thus having local activity and protecting against colon cancer [102]. However, the effects of phenolic compounds on human health depend on both the amount consumed and the bioavailability thereof.

4. Bioaccessibility of Phenolic Compounds in Pasta

As discussed above, several strategies have been explored in order to increase the phenolic content in pasta. Thanks to its low cost and long shelf life, pasta is consumed by people of all ages and all walks of life, hence it is appropriate to be used as a carrier of phenolic compounds, in order to promote health and wellbeing. However, a high dietary phenolic compound intake does not necessarily imply an appropriate bioactivity. As a matter of fact, bioactivity strictly depends on phenolic compound bioaccessibility and bioavailability. Several studies have been published and reviewed on the bioaccessibility of phenolic compounds in bread [29], while bioaccessibility of phenolic compounds in pasta products has been poorly investigated.

Phenolic compound bioaccessibility has been studied in pasta products formulated with whole-wheat flour or composite flours and in pasta samples produced with powders from plant materials or food by-products. Polyphenol bioaccessibility in GF pasta has been investigated, as well (Table 3). Static digestion models have been mainly used.

Table 3. Bioaccessibility studies on phenolic compounds in pasta.

Pasta Formulation	Phenolic Compounds Analysed	In Vitro Methods	Main Findings	Reference
Pasta produced with two varieties of whole wheat flour (*Triticum aestivum* L.)	TPC, 6G8AA, 8G6AA, cFA, ChDP, DFA (Isomers 1–12), FAD, HBADG, HBAG, HGPBA, pCoA, pCoFP, tFA, TFA	OD: human saliva, homogenization, pH adjustment to 2. GD: addition of pepsin solution (pepsin + 0.1 M HCl) to the homogenate; incubation with shaking for 2 h at 37 °C. ID and DIA: addition of a pancreatin/porcine bile solution and dialysis for 3 h at 37 °C.	After OD: release of 4.5–11% of TPC found in cooked supplemented pasta (depending on the variety). After GD: ↑ (344–370%) of TPC found in cooked supplemented pasta. After ID: ↑ (340–360%) of TPC found in cooked supplemented pasta. After DIA: ↑ (~140%) of TPC found in cooked supplemented pasta. Hydroxybenzoic acid diglucoside, hydroxybenzoic acid glucoside and *trans*-ferulic acid were the main compounds quantified in DIA samples.	Podio et al. [60]
Pasta from wheat flour fortified with partially-deoiled chia flour	QA, SA I/H, CTA, FTA, Try, CAH, CA, SA E/B/L, SF, RA, SA C, MeRA, MeQ	OD: human saliva; homogenization; pH adjustment to 2. GD: pepsin solution (pepsin + 0.1 M HCl) added to the homogenate; incubation with shaking for 2 h at 37 °C. ID and DIA: addition of a pancreatin/porcine bile solution and dialysis for 3 h at 37 °C.	After OD: release of 50% of the TPC found in cooked supplemented pasta. After GD and ID: ↑ (300–500%) of TPC found in cooked supplemented pasta. After DIA: ↑ (~50%) of TPC found in cooked supplemented pasta.	Pigni et al. [103]
Pasta produced with durum wheat semolina, red grape marc (RGM) and transglutaminase (TG)	TPC	GD: porcine pepsin; pH = 2.2–2.4; incubation with shaking for 1 h at 37 °C. ID: addition of porcine bile acid, pancreatin, α-amylase; pH = 7.2–7.6; treatment with nitrogen gas and shaking at 37 °C in a water bath for 2 h.	Bioaccessible TP in RGM/TG pasta vs control: 5.53 ± 0.61 vs. 4.16 ± 0.50 mg GAE/g dm	Marinelli et al. [104]
Pasta enriched with fruits from *Rubus* and *Ribes* genus	TPC	Based on the static method proposed by INFOGEST's scientists [30]	↑ (260%) of TPC (raspberry- and boysenberry-enriched pasta). ↑ (360%) of TPC (red- and blackcurrant enriched pasta).	Bustos et al. [105]

Table 3. Cont.

Pasta Formulation	Phenolic Compounds Analysed	In Vitro Methods	Main Findings	Reference
GF pasta formulated with blue maize, chickpea and unripe plantain flours	FPCs and TPC	OD: food was chewed for 15 s; each person rinsed his/her mouth with 5 mL of phosphate buffer. GD: HCl-KCl buffer; pH = 1.25; pepsin solution; incubation at 40 °C in a water bath for 60 min. ID: addition of a mixture of enzymes, incubated for 1 h at 37 °C in a water bath with constant agitation. DIA: dialysis tubing; pancreatic α-amylase solution; incubation at 37 °C.	After OD: release of FPCs. After GD: ↑ TPC release at the increase of blue maize flour percentage. After ID: release of 40% TPC.	Camelo-Méndez et al. [106]
GF pasta produced with white and brown sorghum	TPC	OD: simulated salivary fluid as reported in [108], sample disrupted in a Teflon pestle, incubated for 2 min at 37 °C. GD: simulated stomach fluid as reported in [108]; pH adjusted to 3; incubation for 2 h at 37°C. ID: simulated duodenal fluid as reported in [108]; pH adjusted to 7; incubation for 3 h at 37°C.	Phenolic compound bioaccessibility of white and brown sorghum GF pasta was 2.9- and 2.4-fold higher than in cooked pasta, respectively.	Palavecino et al. [41]
GF pasta produced with black rice, chickpea, red lentil, sorghum, amaranth and quinoa	TPC Flavonoids Lignans Stilbenes	Pre-incubation step with digestive enzymes. In vitro large intestine fermentation process.	After the large intestine fermentation process: - Flavonoid bioaccessibility: <1% - Hydroxycinnamic acid bioaccessibility: 0.6% to 8.6% (at 0 h), 0.6% to 1.6% (at 8 h) and 0.7% to 5.5% (at 24 h) - Lignan bioaccessibility: furofurans (very low); dibenzylbutyrolactones (2.7–12.2%); tyrosols and alkylresorcinols (the most bioaccessible).	Rocchetti et al. [107]

↑: increase; 6G8AA: 6-C-glucosyl-8-C-arabinosyl-apigenin; 8G6AA: 8-C-Glucosyl-6-C-arabinosyl-apigenin; CA: Caffeic acid; CAH: Caffeic acid hexoside; ChDP: Chrysoeriol-6,8-di-C-pentoside; cFA: cis-ferulic acid; CTA: Caftaric acid; DFA (Isomers 1, 2, 3, 4, 5, 6, 7, 8, 9, 10, 11, 12): Diferulic acid; DIA: dialysate; FAD: Ferulic acid derivative; FPCs: Free Phenolic Compounds; FTA: Fertaric acid; GD: gastric digestion; HBADG: Hydroxybenzoic acid diglucoside; HBAG: Hydroxybenzoic acid glucoside; HGPBA: 2-Hydroxy-3-O-β-D-glucopyranosylbenzoic acid; ID: intestinal digestion; MeQ: Methylquercetin; MeRA: Methylrosmarinate; OD: oral digestion; pCoA: p-coumaric acid; pCoFP: p-Coumaroyl-feruloylputrescine; QA: Quinic acid; RA: Rosmarinic acid; SA C: Salvianolic acid C; SA E/B/L: Salvianolic acid E/B/L; SA I/H: Salvianolic acid I/H; SF: Salviaflaside; tFA: trans-ferulic acid; TFA: Triferulic acid; TPC: Total Polyphenol Content; Try: Tryptophan.

Podio et al. investigated phenolic compound bioaccessibility in whole-wheat pasta by using an experimental model, simulating human gastrointestinal digestion and subsequent absorption [60]. They observed that the conditions found in the intestinal medium (e.g., alkaline pH, pancreatin and bile actions, etc.) are not favourable for the stability of some phenolic compounds, which are changed, among others, by enzymatic, oxidative and other transformations, and by aggregation with food matrix. Generally speaking, they observed that TPC significantly increased after gastric digestion (GD) and intestinal digestion (ID), but in the dialysate (DIA) it was significantly lower than in the GD and ID. As to the polyphenol profile, only 8 out of the 25 compounds identified and quantified in cooked pasta were detected in the four stages of the in vitro digestion. In particular, the analysis of dialysated samples showed that hydroxybenzoic acid diglucoside, hydroxybenzoic acid glucoside, tryptophan and *trans*-ferulic acid content increased with respect to the corresponding intestinal digestion. This is of paramount importance as these compounds represent the bioaccessible and dialyzable fraction of polyphenols, which pass into the blood stream to reach organs or tissues where they would exert their antioxidant action. The authors hypothesized that the alkaline conditions and the action of pancreatin/porcine bile acting during the intestinal phase boosted the release of these phenolic compounds from dietary fibre.

Pigni et al. performed a simulated in vitro gastrointestinal digestion of cooked samples of wheat pasta fortified with 10% of partially-deoiled chia flour (PDCF), to assess the absorption of individual polyphenols through the different stages [103]. Upon oral digestion (OD), a total of 50% of the TPC found in the cooked supplemented pasta was released. Gastric digestion and intestinal digestion determined a higher increase (i.e., 300–500%) indicating that the action of enzymes (pepsin, pancreatin) and pH enables an effective release of polyphenols from the food matrix, including the components of PDCF and wheat. Finally, the DIA samples, representing the fraction absorbed in the intestine, showed an increase of around 50% compared with the values of boiled pasta. As regards the specific phenolic compounds quantified in boiled pasta, only 2 out of 10 were above the limit of detection (LOD) and limit of quantitation (LOQ) in the intestinal samples of pasta with 10% PDCF: rosmarinic acid and salviaflaside. In the DIA samples they were even below the LOQ, however their detection indicates that at least a small fraction is being absorbed at this stage.

Marinelli et al. investigated the bioaccessibility of phenolic compounds in samples of pasta produced with durum wheat semolina and red grape marc, a by-product of winemaking, in combination with transglutaminase [104]. They found that the functional pasta sample showed a significantly higher concentration of bioaccessible total polyphenols than the control sample, formulated only with durum wheat semolina (5.53 vs 4.16 mg GAE/g dm, respectively).

Another study investigated the bioaccessibility and potential bioavailability of phenolics in pasta produced by substituting wheat flour (2.5% and 7.5%) with lyophilised raspberries (*Rubus idaeus* L.), boysenberries (*Rubus idaeus* × *Rubus ulmifolius*), redcurrants (*Ribes rubrum* L.) and blackcurrants (*Ribes nigrum* L.) [105]. It was observed that potentially bioaccessible polyphenols were higher in pasta enriched with fruits from *Rubus* genus than with *Ribes* fruits. Pasta fortified with raspberries and boysenberries showed an increase of 260% in polyphenols, while in samples enriched with red- and blackcurrants, the increase was 360%.

As regards the bioaccessibility of phenolics in GF pasta, Camelo-Méndez et al. investigated samples produced with flours from unripe plantain (*Musa paradisiaca* L.), chickpea and blue maize by using an in vitro model simulating gastrointestinal digestion [106]. During the oral digestion, only free polyphenols were released from the matrix, that is, those compounds not linked to other molecules, such as proteins, lipids and carbohydrates. During the gastric phase, the release of phenolic compounds was higher in samples with a higher amount of blue maize flour (i.e., 50% and 75%). The higher release was likely associated with the breakdown of complexes with proteins, fibre residues and sugars. The low pH and enzymatic activity also favour the release of phenolic compounds, mainly flavonoids, from the food matrix. After ID, the percentage of phenolic compounds released was 40% of the initial value in the samples. In detail, they observed that the bioaccessibility of the phenolic compounds in pasta was up to 80% and the highest amount was obtained with the pasta manufactured with the highest amounts of blue maize.

Palavecino et al. also studied bioaccessibility of the functional GF pasta they produced with two varieties of sorghum, and found that the white and brown sorghum pasta samples had 2.9- and 2.4-fold higher potentially bioaccessible polyphenol content than in cooked sample, respectively [41]. The antioxidant activity in sorghum pasta did not significantly vary after digestion, and it was approximately 36–48% in DIA samples.

Rocchetti et al. investigated phenolic compound bioaccessibility in six samples of commercially available pasta, formulated with black rice, chickpea, red lentil, sorghum, amaranth and quinoa [107]. They used an in vitro gastrointestinal digestion model comprising two steps: a pre-incubation step with digestive enzymes, and an in vitro large intestine fermentation process. The phenolic profile was investigated at different time points during faecal fermentation. It emerged that GF pasta samples enriched with pseudocereals or legumes were able to deliver phenolics to the large intestine, and this was likely due to the contribution of the food matrix, which acts as a carrier. In addition, once in the large intestine, the main phenolic subclasses (i.e., flavonoids, hydroxycinnamic acids, lignans and stilbenes) degraded, along with a parallel increase in low molecular weight phenolic acids (i.e., hydroxybenzoic acids), alkylphenols, hydroxybenzoketones and tyrosols. As regards phenolic compound bioaccessibility during the large intestine fermentation process, flavonoids reported values lower than 1%, regardless of the time point or matrix considered. Hydroxycinnamic acid bioaccessibility in large intestine ranged from 0.6% to 8.6% at 0 h, from 0.6% to 1.6% at 8 h, and from 0.7% to 5.5% at 24 h. Within lignans, the various classes showed differences in bioaccessibility, with furofurans having very low bioaccessibility, dibenzylbutyrolactones reached the colon in larger amounts (i.e., 2.7–12.2% of bioaccessibility); while tyrosols and alkylresorcinols were the phenolics with the highest bioaccessibility during the in vitro fermentation process.

5. Conclusions

Phenolic compounds have documented beneficial effects on human health, because of their contribution to preventing chronic diseases. Durum wheat semolina, the main ingredient of pasta, lacks phenolic compounds, since they are lost during conventional milling. Hence, several strategies have been proposed to produce functional pasta whose consumption may contribute to an increased intake of phenolic compounds. Whole grain, legume and composite flours are the main substituents of durum semolina. GF pasta has been functionalized, as well, by using ingredients rich in phenolic compounds. The use of pre-processing technologies on raw materials, such as sprouting, or modulation of extrusion-cooking conditions, may be valuable approaches to increase the phenolic content in pasta. However, a higher intake of phenolic compounds does not necessarily imply a greater bioactivity. Hence, it is pivotal to investigate bioaccessibility and bioavailability of phenolic compounds in functional pasta. Currently, few studies have been performed, and comparing results across different studies is not always reliable due to the diversity of in vitro model conditions and the lack of official methods for the determination of phenolic compound content. Hence, efforts are still needed to evaluate the contribution of functional pasta consumption to maintaining optimal health.

Author Contributions: All authors contributed to the conceptualization and design of the study. V.M. and F.M. collected available literature and jointly wrote the paper. V.M. and R.A. contributed expert opinions. All authors have read and agreed to the published version of the manuscript.

Funding: This research received no funding.

Conflicts of Interest: The authors declare no conflict of interest.

References

1. Shahidi, F.; Ambigaipalan, P. Phenolics and polyphenolics in foods, beverages and spices: Antioxidant activity and health effects—A review. *J. Funct. Foods* **2015**, *18*, 820–897. [CrossRef]

2. Luna-Guevara, M.L.; Luna-Guevara, J.J.; Hernández-Carranza, P.; Ruíz-Espinosa, H.; Ochoa-Velasco, C.E. Phenolic Compounds: A Good Choice Against Chronic Degenerative Diseases. In *Studies in Natural Products Chemistry*; Elsevier B.V.: Amsterdam, The Netherlands, 2018; Volume 59, pp. 79–108.
3. Jelena, C.H.; Giorgio, R.; Justyna, G.; Neda, M.D.; Natasa, S.; Artur, B.; Giuseppe, G. Beneficial effects of polyphenols on chronic diseases and ageing. In *Polyphenols: Properties, Recovery and Applications*; Elsevier Inc.: Amsterdam, The Netherlands, 2018; pp. 69–102. ISBN 9780128135723.
4. Călinoiu, L.F.; Vodnar, D.C. Whole grains and phenolic acids: A review on bioactivity, functionality, health benefits and bioavailability. *Nutrients* **2018**, *10*, 1615. [CrossRef] [PubMed]
5. Van Hung, P. Phenolic Compounds of Cereals and Their Antioxidant Capacity. *Crit. Rev. Food Sci. Nutr.* **2016**, *56*, 25–35. [CrossRef] [PubMed]
6. Yu, L.; Nanguet, A.L.; Beta, T. Comparison of antioxidant properties of refined and whole wheat flour and bread. *Antioxidants* **2013**, *2*, 370–383. [CrossRef] [PubMed]
7. Bach-Faig, A.; Berry, E.M.; Lairon, D.; Reguant, J.; Trichopoulou, A.; Dernini, S.; Medina, X.; Battino, M.; Belahsen, R.; Miranda, G.; et al. Mediterranean diet pyramid today. Science and cultural updates. *Public Health Nutr.* **2011**, *14*, 2274–2284. [CrossRef]
8. Available online: https://fdc.nal.usda.gov/ (accessed on 2 March 2020).
9. Atkinson, F.S.; Foster-Powell, K.; Brand-Miller, J.C. International tables of glycemic index and glycemic load values: 2008. *Diabetes Care* **2008**, *31*, 2281–2283. [CrossRef]
10. Kristensen, M.; Jensen, M.G.; Riboldi, G.; Petronio, M.; Bügel, S.; Toubro, S.; Tetens, I.; Astrup, A. Wholegrain vs. refined wheat bread and pasta. Effect on postprandial glycemia, appetite, and subsequent ad libitum energy intake in young healthy adults. *Appetite* **2010**, *54*, 163–169. [CrossRef]
11. Zou, W.; Sissons, M.; Warren, F.J.; Gidley, M.J.; Gilbert, R.G. Compact structure and proteins of pasta retard in vitro digestive evolution of branched starch molecular structure. *Carbohydr. Polym.* **2016**, *152*, 441–449. [CrossRef]
12. Korczak, R.; Timm, D.; Ahnen, R.; Thomas, W.; Slavin, J.L. High Protein Pasta is Not More Satiating than High Fiber Pasta at a Lunch Meal, Nor Does it Decrease Mid-Afternoon Snacking in Healthy Men and Women. *J. Food Sci.* **2016**, *81*, S2240–S2245. [CrossRef]
13. Fulgoni, V.L.; Bailey, R. Association of Pasta Consumption with Diet Quality and Nutrients of Public Health Concern in Adults: National Health and Nutrition Examination Survey 2009–2012. *Curr. Dev. Nutr.* **2017**, *1*, e001271. [CrossRef]
14. Bohn, T. Dietary factors affecting polyphenol bioavailability. *Nutr. Rev.* **2014**, *72*, 429–452. [CrossRef] [PubMed]
15. Vuolo, M.M.; Lima, V.S.; Maróstica Junior, M.R. Phenolic Compounds. In *Bioactive Compounds*; Elsevier: Amsterdam, The Netherlands, 2019; pp. 33–50.
16. Del Rio, D.; Rodriguez-Mateos, A.; Spencer, J.P.E.; Tognolini, M.; Borges, G.; Crozier, A. Dietary (poly) phenolics in human health: Structures, bioavailability, and evidence of protective effects against chronic diseases. *Antioxid. Redox Signal.* **2013**, *18*, 1818–1892. [CrossRef]
17. Shahidi, F.; Yeo, J.D. Insoluble-bound phenolics in food. *Molecules* **2016**, *21*, 1216. [CrossRef] [PubMed]
18. Adom, K.K.; Liu, R.H. Antioxidant activity of grains. *J. Agric. Food Chem.* **2002**, *50*, 6182–6187. [CrossRef]
19. Liyana-Pathirana, C.M.; Shahidi, F. Importance of insoluble-bound phenolics to antioxidant properties of wheat. *J. Agric. Food Chem.* **2006**, *54*, 1256–1264. [CrossRef] [PubMed]
20. Katzung, B.G. *Basic & Clinical Pharmacology*, 14th ed.; Weitz, M., Boyle, P., Eds.; McGraw Hill Education: New York, NY, USA, 2014; ISBN 978-1-260-28817-9.
21. Schönfeldt, H.C.; Pretorius, B.; Hall, N. Bioavailability of Nutrients. In *Encyclopedia of Food and Health*; Elsevier Ltd: Amsterdam, The Netherlands, 2016. [CrossRef]
22. Galanakis, C.M. *Nutraceuticals and Natural Product Pharmaceuticals*; Academic Press: Cambridge, MA, USA, 2019; ISBN 9780128164501.
23. Carbonell-Capella, J.M.; Buniowska, M.; Barba, F.J.; Esteve, M.J.; Frígola, A. Analytical Methods for Determining Bioavailability and Bioaccessibility of Bioactive Compounds from Fruits and Vegetables: A Review. *Compr. Rev. Food Sci. Food Saf.* **2014**, *13*, 155–171. [CrossRef]
24. Lafarga, T.; Villaró, S.; Bobo, G.; Simó, J.; Aguiló-Aguayo, I. Bioaccessibility and antioxidant activity of phenolic compounds in cooked pulses. *Int. J. Food Sci. Technol.* **2019**, *54*, 1816–1823. [CrossRef]

25. Zeng, Z.; Liu, C.; Luo, S.; Chen, J.; Gong, E. The profile and bioaccessibility of phenolic compounds in cereals influenced by improved extrusion cooking treatment. *PLoS ONE* **2016**, *11*, e0161086. [CrossRef]
26. Ribas-Agustí, A.; Martín-Belloso, O.; Soliva-Fortuny, R.; Elez-Martínez, P. Food processing strategies to enhance phenolic compounds bioaccessibility and bioavailability in plant-based foods. *Crit. Rev. Food Sci. Nutr.* **2018**, *58*, 2531–2548. [CrossRef]
27. Tan, J.; Li, Y.; Hou, D.X.; Wu, S. The effects and mechanisms of cyanidin-3-glucoside and its phenolic metabolites in maintaining intestinal integrity. *Antioxidants* **2019**, *8*, 479. [CrossRef]
28. Alminger, M.; Aura, A.-M.; Bohn, T.; Dufour, C.; El, S.N.; Gomes, A.; Karakaya, S.; Martínez-Cuesta, M.C.; McDougall, G.J.; Requena, T.; et al. In Vitro Models for Studying Secondary Plant Metabolite Digestion and Bioaccessibility. *Compr. Rev. Food Sci. Food Saf.* **2014**, *13*, 413–436. [CrossRef]
29. Angelino, D.; Cossu, M.; Marti, A.; Zanoletti, M.; Chiavaroli, L.; Brighenti, F.; Del Rio, D.; Martini, D. Bioaccessibility and bioavailability of phenolic compounds in bread: A review. *Food Funct.* **2017**, *8*, 2368–2393. [CrossRef] [PubMed]
30. Minekus, M.; Alminger, M.; Alvito, P.; Ballance, S.; Bohn, T.; Bourlieu, C.; Carrière, F.; Boutrou, R.; Corredig, M.; Dupont, D.; et al. A standardised static in vitro digestion method suitable for food-an international consensus. *Food Funct.* **2014**, *5*, 1113–1124. [CrossRef] [PubMed]
31. Minekus, M.; Marteau, P.; Havenaar, R.; Huis in't Veld, J.; Minekus, M.; Huis in't Veld, J.; Huisintveld, J.A. Multicompartmental Dynamic Computer-Controlled Model Simulating the Stomach and Small Intestine. *ATLA* **1995**, *23*, 197–209.
32. Nicoletti, M. Nutraceuticals and botanicals: Overview and perspectives. *Int. J. Food Sci. Nutr.* **2012**, *63*, 2–6. [CrossRef] [PubMed]
33. Wójtowicz, A.; Oniszczuk, A.; Kasprzak, K.; Olech, M.; Mitrus, M.; Oniszczuk, T. Chemical composition and selected quality characteristics of new types of precooked wheat and spelt pasta products. *Food Chem.* **2020**, *309*, 125673. [CrossRef]
34. Chen, C.Y.O.; Kamil, A.; Blumberg, J.B. Phytochemical composition and antioxidant capacity of whole wheat products. *Int. J. Food Sci. Nutr.* **2015**, *66*, 63–70. [CrossRef]
35. Hirawan, R.; Ser, W.Y.; Arntfield, S.D.; Beta, T. Antioxidant properties of commercial, regular- and whole-wheat spaghetti. *Food Chem.* **2010**, *119*, 258–264. [CrossRef]
36. Turco, I.; Bacchetti, T.; Bender, C.; Zimmermann, B.; Oboh, G.; Ferretti, G. Polyphenol content and glycemic load of pasta enriched with Faba bean flour. *Funct. Foods Heal. Dis.* **2016**, *6*, 291. [CrossRef]
37. Cota-Gastélum, A.G.; Salazar-García, M.G.; Espinoza-López, A.; Perez-Perez, L.M.; Cinco-Moroyoqui, F.J.; Martínez-Cruz, O.; Wong-Corral, F.J.; Del-Toro-Sánchez, C.L. Characterization of pasta with the addition of Cicer arietinum and Salvia hispanica flours on quality and antioxidant parameters. *Ital. J. Food Sci.* **2019**, *31*, 626–643.
38. Sęczyk, Ł.; Świeca, M.; Gawlik-Dziki, U. Effect of carob (*Ceratonia siliqua* L.) flour on the antioxidant potential, nutritional quality, and sensory characteristics of fortified durum wheat pasta. *Food Chem.* **2016**, *194*, 637–642.
39. Cárdenas-Hernández, A.; Beta, T.; Loarca-Piña, G.; Castaño-Tostado, E.; Nieto-Barrera, J.O.; Mendoza, S. Improved functional properties of pasta: Enrichment with amaranth seed flour and dried amaranth leaves. *J. Cereal Sci.* **2016**, *72*, 84–90. [CrossRef]
40. Camelo-Méndez, G.A.; Tovar, J.; Bello-Pérez, L.A. Influence of blue maize flour on gluten-free pasta quality and antioxidant retention characteristics. *J. Food Sci. Technol.* **2018**, *55*, 2739–2748. [CrossRef] [PubMed]
41. Palavecino, P.M.; Ribotta, P.D.; León, A.E.; Bustos, M.C. Gluten-free sorghum pasta: Starch digestibility and antioxidant capacity compared with commercial products. *J. Sci. Food Agric.* **2019**, *99*, 1351–1357. [CrossRef]
42. Jalgaonkar, K.; Jha, S.K.; Mahawar, M.K. Influence of incorporating defatted soy flour, carrot powder, mango peel powder, and moringa leaves powder on quality characteristics of wheat semolina-pearl millet pasta. *J. Food Process. Preserv.* **2018**, *42*, e13575. [CrossRef]
43. Lu, X.; Brennan, M.A.; Serventi, L.; Liu, J.; Guan, W.; Brennan, C.S. Addition of mushroom powder to pasta enhances the antioxidant content and modulates the predictive glycaemic response of pasta. *Food Chem.* **2018**, *264*, 199–209. [CrossRef]
44. Michalak-Majewska, M.; Teterycz, D.; Muszyński, S.; Radzki, W.; Sykut-Domańska, E. Influence of onion skin powder on nutritional and quality attributes of wheat pasta. *PLoS ONE* **2020**, *15*, e0227942. [CrossRef]

45. Padalino, L.; D'Antuono, I.; Durante, M.; Conte, A.; Cardinali, A.; Linsalata, V.; Mita, G.; Logrieco, A.; Del Nobile, M. Use of Olive Oil Industrial By-Product for Pasta Enrichment. *Antioxidants* **2018**, *7*, 59. [CrossRef]
46. Marinelli, V.; Padalino, L.; Nardiello, D.; Del Nobile, M.A.; Conte, A. New Approach to Enrich Pasta with Polyphenols from Grape Marc. *J. Chem.* **2015**. [CrossRef]
47. Pasqualone, A.; Delvecchio, L.N.; Gambacorta, G.; Laddomada, B.; Urso, V.; Mazzaglia, A.; Ruisi, P.; Di Miceli, G. Effect of Supplementation with Wheat Bran Aqueous Extracts Obtained by Ultrasound-Assisted Technologies on the Sensory Properties and the Antioxidant Activity of Dry Pasta. *Nat. Prod. Commun.* **2015**, *10*, 1739–1742. [CrossRef]
48. Menga, V.; Amato, M.; Phillips, T.D.; Angelino, D.; Morreale, F.; Fares, C. Gluten-free pasta incorporating chia (Salvia hispanica L.) as thickening agent: An approach to naturally improve the nutritional profile and the in vitro carbohydrate digestibility. *Food Chem.* **2017**, *221*, 1954–1961. [CrossRef] [PubMed]
49. Oniszczuk, A.; Wójtowicz, A.; Oniszczuk, T.; Matwijczuk, A.; Dib, A.; Markut-Miotła, E. Opuntia Fruits as Food Enriching Ingredient, the First Step towards New Functional Food Products. *Molecules* **2020**, *25*, 916. [CrossRef]
50. Oniszczuk; Widelska; Wójtowicz; Oniszczuk; Wojtunik-Kulesza; Dib; Matwijczuk Content of Phenolic Compounds and Antioxidant Activity of New Gluten-Free Pasta with the Addition of Chestnut Flour. *Molecules* **2019**, *24*, 2623. [CrossRef]
51. Abbasi Parizad, P.; Marengo, M.; Bonomi, F.; Scarafoni, A.; Cecchini, C.; Pagani, M.A.; Marti, A.; Iametti, S. Bio-Functional and Structural Properties of Pasta Enriched with a Debranning Fraction from Purple Wheat. *Foods* **2020**, *9*, 163. [CrossRef] [PubMed]
52. Zanoletti, M.; Abbasi Parizad, P.; Lavelli, V.; Cecchini, C.; Menesatti, P.; Marti, A.; Pagani, M.A. Debranning of purple wheat: Recovery of anthocyanin-rich fractions and their use in pasta production. *LWT—Food Sci. Technol.* **2017**, *75*, 663–669. [CrossRef]
53. Ciccoritti, R.; Taddei, F.; Nicoletti, I.; Gazza, L.; Corradini, D.; D'Egidio, M.G.; Martini, D. Use of bran fractions and debranned kernels for the development of pasta with high nutritional and healthy potential. *Food Chem.* **2017**, *225*, 77–86. [CrossRef] [PubMed]
54. Martini, D.; Ciccoritti, R.; Nicoletti, I.; Nocente, F.; Corradini, D.; D'Egidio, M.G.; Taddei, F. From seed to cooked pasta: Influence of traditional and non-conventional transformation processes on total antioxidant capacity and phenolic acid content. *Int. J. Food Sci. Nutr.* **2018**, *69*, 24–32. [CrossRef] [PubMed]
55. Merendino, N.; Molinari, R.; Costantini, L.; Mazzucato, A.; Pucci, A.; Bonafaccia, F.; Esti, M.; Ceccantoni, B.; Papeschi, C.; Bonafaccia, G. A new "functional" pasta containing tartary buckwheat sprouts as an ingredient improves the oxidative status and normalizes some blood pressure parameters in spontaneously hypertensive rats. *Food Funct.* **2014**, *5*, 1017–1026. [CrossRef]
56. Bruno, J.A.; Konas, D.W.; Matthews, E.L.; Feldman, C.H.; Pinsley, K.M.; Kerrihard, A.L. Sprouted and Non-Sprouted Chickpea Flours: Effects on Sensory Traits in Pasta and Antioxidant Capacity. *Polish J. Food Nutr. Sci.* **2019**, *69*, 203–209. [CrossRef]
57. Bouasla, A.; Wójtowicz, A.; Zidoune, M.N.; Olech, M.; Nowak, R.; Mitrus, M.; Oniszczuk, A. Gluten-Free Precooked Rice-Yellow Pea Pasta: Effect of Extrusion-Cooking Conditions on Phenolic Acids Composition, Selected Properties and Microstructure. *J. Food Sci.* **2016**, *81*, C1070–C1079. [CrossRef]
58. Oniszczuk, A.; Kasprzak, K.; Wójtowicz, A.; Oniszczuk, T.; Olech, M. The Impact of Processing Parameters on the Content of Phenolic Compounds in New Gluten-Free Precooked Buckwheat Pasta. *Molecules* **2019**, *24*, 1262. [CrossRef] [PubMed]
59. De Paula, R.; Rabalski, I.; Messia, M.C.; Abdel-Aal, E.S.M.; Marconi, E. Effect of processing on phenolic acids composition and radical scavenging capacity of barley pasta. *Food Res. Int.* **2017**, *102*, 136–143. [CrossRef] [PubMed]
60. Podio, N.S.; Baroni, M.V.; Pérez, G.T.; Wunderlin, D.A. Assessment of bioactive compounds and their in vitro bioaccessibility in whole-wheat flour pasta. *Food Chem.* **2019**, *293*, 408–417. [CrossRef] [PubMed]
61. Rocchetti, G.; Lucini, L.; Chiodelli, G.; Giuberti, G.; Montesano, D.; Masoero, F.; Trevisan, M. Impact of boiling on free and bound phenolic profile and antioxidant activity of commercial gluten-free pasta. *Food Res. Int.* **2017**, *100*, 69–77. [CrossRef]
62. Van Der Kamp, J.W.; Poutanen, K.; Seal, C.J.; Richardson, D.P. The HEALTHGRAIN definition of "whole grain". *Food Nutr. Res.* **2014**, *58*, 22100. [CrossRef]

63. Ross, A.B.; van der Kamp, J.W.; King, R.; Lê, K.A.; Mejborn, H.; Seal, C.J.; Thielecke, F. Perspective: A definition for whole-grain food products—Recommendations from the Healthgrain Forum. *Adv. Nutr.* **2017**, *8*, 525–531.
64. Slavin, J.; Tucker, M.; Harriman, C.; Jonnalagadda, S.S. Whole grains: Definition, dietary recommendations, and health benefits. *Cereal Foods World* **2013**, *58*, 191–198. [CrossRef]
65. Philip Karl, J.; McKeown, N.M. Whole Grains in the Prevention and Treatment of Abdominal Obesity. In *Nutrition in the Prevention and Treatment of Abdominal Obesity*; Elsevier Inc.: Amsterdam, The Netherlands, 2014; pp. 515–528. ISBN 9780124078697.
66. Kris-Etherton, P.M.; Ohlson, M.; Bagshaw, D.; Stone, N.J. Dietary Patterns for the Prevention and Treatment of Cardiovascular Disease. In *Clinical Lipidology: A Companion to Braunwald's Heart Disease*; Elsevier Inc.: Amsterdam, The Netherlands, 2009; pp. 217–231. ISBN 9781416054696.
67. Wang, L.; Sikand, G.; Wong, N.D. Nutrition, Diet Quality, and Cardiovascular Health. In *Molecular Basis of Nutrition and Aging: A Volume in the Molecular Nutrition Series*; Elsevier Inc.: Amsterdam, The Netherlands, 2016; pp. 315–330. ISBN 9780128018279.
68. Aune, D.; Keum, N.; Giovannucci, E.; Fadnes, L.T.; Boffetta, P.; Greenwood, D.C.; Tonstad, S.; Vatten, L.J.; Riboli, E.; Norat, T. Whole grain consumption and risk of cardiovascular disease, cancer, and all cause and cause specific mortality: Systematic review and dose-response meta-analysis of prospective studies. *BMJ* **2016**, *353*, i2716. [CrossRef]
69. Chandra, S.; Singh, S.; Kumari, D. Evaluation of functional properties of composite flours and sensorial attributes of composite flour biscuits. *J. Food Sci. Technol.* **2015**, *52*, 3681–3688. [CrossRef]
70. Singh, B.; Singh, J.P.; Kaur, A.; Singh, N. Phenolic composition and antioxidant potential of grain legume seeds: A review. *Food Res. Int.* **2017**, *101*, 1–16. [CrossRef]
71. Schoenlechner, R. Quinoa: Its Unique Nutritional and Health-Promoting Attributes. In *Gluten-Free Ancient Grains: Cereals, Pseudocereals, and Legumes: Sustainable, Nutritious, and Health-Promoting Foods for the 21st Century*; Elsevier Inc.: Amsterdam, The Netherlands, 2017; pp. 105–129. ISBN 9780081008911.
72. D'Amico, S.; Schoenlechner, R. Amaranth: Its Unique Nutritional and Health-Promoting Attributes. In *Gluten-Free Ancient Grains: Cereals, Pseudocereals, and Legumes: Sustainable, Nutritious, and Health-Promoting Foods for the 21st Century*; Elsevier Inc.: Amsterdam, The Netherlands, 2017; pp. 131–159. ISBN 9780081008911.
73. Alencar, N.M.M.; de Carvalho Oliveira, L. *Advances in Pseudocereals: Crop Cultivation, Food Application, and Consumer Perception*; Springer: Cham, Switzerland, 2019; pp. 1695–1713.
74. Inglett, G.E.; Chen, D.; Liu, S.X. Physical properties of gluten-free sugar cookies made from amaranth-oat composites. *LWT—Food Sci. Technol.* **2015**, *63*, 214–220. [CrossRef]
75. Chauhan, A.; Saxena, D.C.; Singh, S. Total dietary fibre and antioxidant activity of gluten free cookies made from raw and germinated amaranth (Amaranthus spp.) flour. *LWT—Food Sci. Technol.* **2015**, *63*, 939–945. [CrossRef]
76. Melini, F.; Melini, V.; Luziatelli, F.; Ruzzi, M. Current and Forward-Looking Approaches to Technological and Nutritional Improvements of Gluten-Free Bread with Legume Flours: A Critical Review. *Compr. Rev. Food Sci. Food Saf.* **2017**, *16*, 1101–1122. [CrossRef]
77. Siyuan, S.; Tong, L.; Liu, R. Corn phytochemicals and their health benefits. *Food Sci. Hum. Wellness* **2018**, *7*, 185–195. [CrossRef]
78. Girard, A.L.; Awika, J.M. Sorghum polyphenols and other bioactive components as functional and health promoting food ingredients. *J. Cereal Sci.* **2018**, *84*, 112–124. [CrossRef]
79. Althwab, S.; Carr, T.P.; Weller, C.L.; Dweikat, I.M.; Schlegel, V. Advances in grain sorghum and its co-products as a human health promoting dietary system. *Food Res. Int.* **2015**, *77*, 349–359. [CrossRef]
80. de Morais Cardoso, L.; Pinheiro, S.S.; Martino, H.S.D.; Pinheiro-Sant'Ana, H.M. Sorghum (*Sorghum bicolor* L.): Nutrients, bioactive compounds, and potential impact on human health. *Crit. Rev. Food Sci. Nutr.* **2017**, *57*, 372–390. [CrossRef]
81. Schieber, A. Side Streams of Plant Food Processing As a Source of Valuable Compounds: Selected Examples. *Annu. Rev. Food Sci. Technol.* **2017**, *8*, 97–112. [CrossRef]
82. Baiano, A. Recovery of biomolecules from food wastes—A review. *Molecules* **2014**, *19*, 14821–14842. [CrossRef]
83. Saini, A.; Panesar, P.S.; Bera, M.B. Valorization of fruits and vegetables waste through green extraction of bioactive compounds and their nanoemulsions-based delivery system. *Bioresour. Bioprocess.* **2019**, *6*, 26. [CrossRef]

84. Kumar, K.; Yadav, A.N.; Kumar, V.; Vyas, P.; Dhaliwal, H.S. Food waste: A potential bioresource for extraction of nutraceuticals and bioactive compounds. *Bioresour. Bioprocess.* **2017**, *4*, 18. [CrossRef]
85. Foschia, M.; Peressini, D.; Sensidoni, A.; Brennan, M.A.; Brennan, C.S. How combinations of dietary fibres can affect physicochemical characteristics of pasta. *LWT-Food Sci. Technol.* **2015**, *66*, 41–46. [CrossRef]
86. Pandiella, S.S.; Mousia, Z.; Laca, A.; Díaz, M.; Webb, C. DEBRANNING TECHNOLOGY TO IMPROVE CEREAL-BASED FOODS. In *Using Cereal Science and Technology for the Benefit of Consumers*; Elsevier: Amsterdam, The Netherlands, 2005; pp. 241–244.
87. Lemmens, E.; Moroni, A.V.; Pagand, J.; Heirbaut, P.; Ritala, A.; Karlen, Y.; Kim-Anne, L.; Van den Broeck, H.C.; Brouns, F.J.P.H.; De Brier, N.; et al. Impact of Cereal Seed Sprouting on Its Nutritional and Technological Properties: A Critical Review. *Compr. Rev. Food Sci. Food Saf.* **2019**, *18*, 305–328. [CrossRef]
88. Świeca, M.; Dziki, D. Improvement in sprouted wheat flour functionality: Effect of time, temperature and elicitation. *Int. J. Food Sci. Technol.* **2015**, *50*, 2135–2142. [CrossRef]
89. Ha, K.S.; Jo, S.H.; Mannam, V.; Kwon, Y.I.; Apostolidis, E. Stimulation of Phenolics, Antioxidant and α-Glucosidase Inhibitory Activities during Barley (Hordeum vulgare L.) Seed Germination. *Plant Foods Hum. Nutr.* **2016**, *71*, 211–217. [CrossRef]
90. Hithamani, G.; Srinivasan, K. Bioaccessibility of polyphenols from selected cereal grains and legumes as influenced by food acidulants. *J. Sci. Food Agric.* **2017**, *97*, 621–628. [CrossRef]
91. Pal, P.; Singh, N.; Kaur, P.; Kaur, A.; Virdi, A.S.; Parmar, N. Comparison of Composition, Protein, Pasting, and Phenolic Compounds of Brown Rice and Germinated Brown Rice from Different Cultivars. *Cereal Chem. J.* **2016**, *93*, 584–592. [CrossRef]
92. Benincasa, P.; Falcinelli, B.; Lutts, S.; Stagnari, F.; Galieni, A. Sprouted Grains: A Comprehensive Review. *Nutrients* **2019**, *11*, 421. [CrossRef]
93. Ohm, J.-B.; Lee, C.W.; Cho, K. Germinated Wheat: Phytochemical Composition and Mixing Characteristics. *Cereal Chem. J.* **2016**, *93*, 612–617. [CrossRef]
94. Ti, H.; Zhang, R.; Zhang, M.; Li, Q.; Wei, Z.; Zhang, Y.; Tang, X.; Deng, Y.; Liu, L.; Ma, Y. Dynamic changes in the free and bound phenolic compounds and antioxidant activity of brown rice at different germination stages. *Food Chem.* **2014**, *161*, 337–344. [CrossRef]
95. Erba, D.; Angelino, D.; Marti, A.; Manini, F.; Faoro, F.; Morreale, F.; Pellegrini, N.; Casiraghi, M.C. Effect of sprouting on nutritional quality of pulses. *Int. J. Food Sci. Nutr.* **2019**, *70*, 30–40. [CrossRef] [PubMed]
96. Montemurro, M.; Coda, R.; Rizzello, C.G. Recent Advances in the Use of Sourdough Biotechnology in Pasta Making. *Foods* **2019**, *8*, 129. [CrossRef] [PubMed]
97. Rashid, N.Y.A.; Jamaluddin, A.; Ghani, A.A.; Razak, D.I.A.; Jonit, J.; Mansor, A.; Manan, M.A. Quantification of phenolic compounds changes by Aspergillus oryzae on rice bran fermentation. *Food Res.* **2018**, *3*, 133–137. [CrossRef]
98. Dey, T.B.; Kuhad, R.C. Enhanced production and extraction of phenolic compounds from wheat by solid-state fermentation with Rhizopus oryzae RCK2012. *Biotechnol. Rep.* **2014**, *4*, 120–127.
99. Călinoiu, L.F.; Cătoi, A.F.; Vodnar, D.C. Solid-state yeast fermented wheat and oat bran as a route for delivery of antioxidants. *Antioxidants* **2019**, *8*, 372. [CrossRef]
100. Alam, M.S.; Kaur, J.; Khaira, H.; Gupta, K. Extrusion and Extruded Products: Changes in Quality Attributes as Affected by Extrusion Process Parameters: A Review. *Crit. Rev. Food Sci. Nutr.* **2016**, *56*, 445–473. [CrossRef]
101. Wang, T.; He, F.; Chen, G. Improving bioaccessibility and bioavailability of phenolic compounds in cereal grains through processing technologies: A concise review. *J. Funct. Foods* **2014**, *7*, 101–111. [CrossRef]
102. Acosta-Estrada, B.A.; Gutiérrez-Uribe, J.A.; Serna-Saldívar, S.O. Bound phenolics in foods, a review. *Food Chem.* **2014**, *152*, 46–55. [CrossRef]
103. Pigni, N.B.; Aranibar, C.; Lucini Mas, A.; Aguirre, A.; Borneo, R.; Wunderlin, D.; Baroni, M.V. Chemical profile and bioaccessibility of polyphenols from wheat pasta supplemented with partially-deoiled chia flour. *LWT* **2020**, *124*, 109134. [CrossRef]
104. Marinelli, V.; Padalino, L.; Conte, A.; Del Nobile, M.A.; Briviba, K. Red grape marc flour as food ingredient in durum wheat spaghetti: Nutritional evaluation and bioaccessibility of bioactive compounds. *Food Sci. Technol. Res.* **2018**, *24*, 1093–1100. [CrossRef]

105. Bustos, M.C.; Vignola, M.B.; Paesani, C.; León, A.E. Berry fruits-enriched pasta: Effect of processing and in vitro digestion on phenolics and its antioxidant activity, bioaccessibility and potential bioavailability. *Int. J. Food Sci. Technol.* **2019**. [CrossRef]
106. Camelo-Méndez, G.A.; Agama-Acevedo, E.; Rosell, C.M.; Perea-Flores, M.D.J.; Bello-Pérez, L.A. Starch and antioxidant compound release during in vitro gastrointestinal digestion of gluten-free pasta. *Food Chem.* **2018**, *263*, 201–207.
107. Rocchetti, G.; Lucini, L.; Chiodelli, G.; Giuberti, G.; Gallo, A.; Masoero, F.; Trevisan, M. Phenolic profile and fermentation patterns of different commercial gluten-free pasta during in vitro large intestine fermentation. *Food Res. Int.* **2017**, *97*, 78–86. [CrossRef] [PubMed]
108. Bustos, M.C.; Vignola, M.B.; Pérez, G.T.; León, A.E. In vitro digestion kinetics and bioaccessibility of starch in cereal food products. *J. Cereal Sci.* **2017**, *77*, 243–250. [CrossRef]

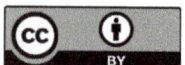

© 2020 by the authors. Licensee MDPI, Basel, Switzerland. This article is an open access article distributed under the terms and conditions of the Creative Commons Attribution (CC BY) license (http://creativecommons.org/licenses/by/4.0/).

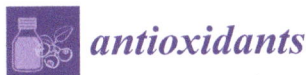

Review

The Versatility of Antioxidant Assays in Food Science and Safety—Chemistry, Applications, Strengths, and Limitations

Nabeelah Bibi Sadeer [1], Domenico Montesano [2], Stefania Albrizio [3,4,*], Gokhan Zengin [5] and Mohamad Fawzi Mahomoodally [1,*]

1. Department of Health Sciences; Faculty of Science, University of Mauritius, Réduit 80837, Mauritius; nabeelah.sadeer1@umail.uom.ac.mu
2. Department of Pharmaceutical Sciences, Section of Food Science and Nutrition, University of Perugia, via S. Costanzo, 06126 Perugia, Italy; domenico.montesano@unipg.it
3. Department of Pharmacy, University of Naples "Federico II", via D. Montesano 49, 80131 Naples, Italy
4. Consorzio Interuniversitario INBB—Viale Medaglie d'Oro, 305, I-00136 Rome, Italy
5. Department of Biology, Science Faculty, Selcuk University, 42250 Konya Campus, Turkey; gokhanzengin@selcuk.edu.tr
* Correspondence: stefania.albrizio@unina.it (S.A.); f.mahomoodally@uom.ac.mu (M.F.M.)

Received: 9 July 2020; Accepted: 31 July 2020; Published: 5 August 2020

Abstract: Currently, there is a growing interest in screening and quantifying antioxidants from biological samples in the quest for natural and effective antioxidants to combat free radical-related pathological complications. Antioxidant assays play a crucial role in high-throughput and cost-effective assessment of antioxidant capacities of natural products such as medicinal plants and food samples. However, several investigators have expressed concerns about the reliability of existing in vitro assays. Such concerns arise mainly from the poor correlation between in vitro and in vivo results. In addition, in vitro assays have the problem of reproducibility. To date, antioxidant capacities are measured using a panel of assays whereby each assay has its own advantages and limitations. This unparalleled review hotly disputes on in vitro antioxidant assays and elaborates on the chemistry behind each assay with the aim to point out respective principles/concepts. The following critical questions are also addressed: (1) What make antioxidant assays coloured? (2) What is the reason for working at a particular wavelength? (3) What are the advantages and limitations of each assay? and (4) Why is a particular colour observed in antioxidant–oxidant chemical reactions? Furthermore, this review details the chemical mechanism of reactions that occur in each assay together with a colour ribbon to illustrate changes in colour. The review ends with a critical conclusion on existing assays and suggests constructive improvements on how to develop an adequate and universal antioxidant assay.

Keywords: antioxidants; free radicals; oxidative stress; spectrophotometer; limitations; chemical reactions; colorimetry

1. Introduction

Our life relies on a well-designed and orchestrated series of naturally occurring chemical reactions. The presence of billions of cells in our body is perpetually under threat of being harmed by radicals that can lead to the development of diseases. Diseases are not developed overnight. One of the main causes of diseases is related to 'oxidative stress' involving free radicals. Oxidative stress is the most inspected stress that disturbs the normal functioning of cells. It is responsible for scads of cell damage, leading to numerous degenerative diseases including neurodegenerative disorders (Alzheimer's disease, Parkinson's disease), cancers, cardiovascular diseases, retinopathy, and dermatological diseases. As a normal defence mechanism, our body reacts to any given stress to ascertain a healthy cellular homeostasis [1]. However, antioxidant enzymes present are sometimes not enough to combat free radicals. Thus, it is vital to either consume foods rich in antioxidants or alternatively, rely on medicines for the prevention and treatment of degenerative disorders. Despite free radicals causing a panoply of diseases, it is important to remember that they also show interesting therapeutic effects, especially in antimicrobial applications. For example, the free radical-releasing system is becoming an emerging strategy to combat antibiotic resistance and biofilm formations [2]. Free radical treatment is also recognized as an effective cancer treatment [3], although in some cases free radicals could be the leading cause of cancer.

There has been an upsurge of interest in free radical chemistry since the past decades. At the time of writing, research studies conducted in various fields, regardless of whether the studies are food-related or plant-related, all samples are scrutinized for their antioxidant activities as a preliminary screening in the pursuit of novel compounds with powerful antioxidant properties [4,5]. Screening of biological samples for antioxidant capacities is done using a series of assays instead of relying on only one assay. This is because Opitz et al. [6], in their book chapter, have mentioned that one assay does not give realistic results compared to a series of assays involving different chemical reactions. It is acknowledged that published results are inconclusive and it is difficult to make comparisons between different research groups [7]. In addition, food and nutraceutical industries cannot perform strict quality control for antioxidant products [8].

The limitations and metabolism of antioxidants still represent a challenge for future research in the free radical chemistry field and thus, researchers are trying to search for alternatives or solutions to overcome such limitations. Some general limitations include: (i) In terms of neuroprotection, antioxidants do not deliver appropriate and effective protection solely due to the blood–brain barrier [9], (ii) dietary antioxidants are more sensitive in mice compared to humans. Thus, it is important to consider this fact before any clinical trials [10], (iii) Another limitation is linked with cell cultures. Sometimes during in vitro testing, antioxidants react with the reagents present in the reaction mixture, giving rise to erroneous results [7]. It is believed that the biggest problem lies in the lack of a validated and universal assay that can reliably measure the antioxidant capacities of foods and other biological samples. Interestingly, as well stressed in a review compiled by Granato et al. [11], it was mentioned that compounds measured in foods are not necessarily representative of those which are active in humans. For instance, after the consumption of blueberries, the presence of phenolic acids could be detected in the blood while noted absent in other consumers, since the compounds occurred as metabolites. Thus, it is understood that since complex interactions are involved among the intrinsic and extrinsic factors present in food and other biological matrices, antioxidant activity cannot be measured using simple chemical reactions in a test tube alone.

So far, there are piecemeal reviews on antioxidants elaborating on either one or a few assays. For instance, Re et al. [12] have reviewed an improved version of the ABTS radical cation decolorization assay. Huang, Ou, and Prior [8] have evaluated several antioxidant assays in terms of their kinetics of autoxidation. Alam et al. [13] have reviewed differences between in vivo and in vitro methods evaluating antioxidant activity. Carocho et al. [14] have compiled information on antioxidants in terms of their application in foods as preservatives. Ratnam et al. [15] have documented the role of antioxidants in a pharmaceutical perspective. Carocho and Ferreira [7] have published a review on antioxidants and pro-oxidants, including certain controversies. Kim et al. [16] have focused on the vitamin C equivalent antioxidant capacity (VCEAC) of phenolic phytochemicals, among others. After searching the existing literature, it is noticed that there is no review that systematically details the chemical reactions of each antioxidant assay. Additionally, no review has focused on the strengths and limitations of each assay or explained reasons behind the development of colours in such assays. Furthermore, consolidated improvements have not been suggested yet to develop a new and universal antioxidant assay. Therefore, such research gap has fuelled the need to present a review including all these missing aspects. The aim of the present review is not to be repetitive but attempts to provide a more informative, authoritative, and comparative coverage on the chemistry behind antioxidant assays, including a brief history on the development of different assays, explaining the principle, general concept of each assay, reasons why certain reagents are used, chemical reactions that occur are detailed, colour change developed in each assay, and the reason why absorbance is read at a particular wavelength with a spectrophotometer. The strengths and limitations of each assay are also listed, highlighting some key improvements to consider while validating a novel antioxidant method.

2. Review Methodology

The relevant literature was collected by searching scientific electronic databases, namely ScienceDirect, Scopus, PubMed, Web of Science, and Google Scholar. Keywords such as antioxidants, free radicals, antioxidants assays/methods, antioxidant enzymes, chemical reactions, mechanism of reactions, wavelength, chemical reactions, colour change, chromogens, complexes, absorption, strengths, and limitations were used in the search process. Each antioxidant assay was described in terms of who has developed the assay, when the assay was developed, the principle behind the assay, chemical reactions, a detailed mechanism of reactions, colour change, strengths, and limitations. Chemical structures presented in the mechanism of reactions were drawn with ChemDraw Ultra 12.0.

3. Chemistry of Antioxidant Methods

Generally, antioxidant assays are conducted using appropriate traditional methodologies, collecting and processing the data in terms of % inhibition or the equivalent of standards, and finally, interpreting the results. The chemistry occurring in each assay tends to be ignored. We do not know why a certain type of assays is measured at a particular wavelength (λ), why radicals/probes are coloured, or why they change colour upon reactions. The following sections attempt to answer these questions, as the current review aims to provide the chemistry behind each antioxidant (AO) reaction.

3.1. Why Are Antioxidant Assays Coloured?

Colour is the product of electronic transitions in atoms or molecules and is an indicator of the physical properties of chemical substances at the atomic level. A change in the electronic transitions results in a change in the light absorbed by the molecules and subsequently, causes a change in colour. The coloured complex formed in AO assays is called a charge–transfer (CT) complex or electron–donor–acceptor complex. A CT complex is the association of two or more molecules, or different parts of one molecule, in which a fraction of electronic charge is transferred between the molecular entities (i.e., the radical and AO). This transfer results in an electrostatic force of attraction (J) between the radical and AO providing a stabilizing force for the CT complex. For instance, in the 2,2-diphenyl-1-picrylhydrazyl (DPPH) assay, the unpaired electron in DPPH$^\bullet$ exhibits an intense deep purple colour charge–transfer band at 517 nm, however, while pairing up with another electron, a change in colour is observed resulting in pale yellow. This permits us to answer the question why there is a colour change in AO assays.

3.2. What Is the Reason for Working at a Particular Wavelength?

After receiving an electron, many complexes enter an excitation state. The excitation energy required for an electron to jump from one energy level to another often falls in the visible region of the electromagnetic spectrum, which consequently, results in the formation of intensely coloured complexes. The absorption bands are usually referred to as charge–transfer bands (CT bands). The absorption wavelength of the CT bands is distinctive in terms of the types of donor and acceptor involved. The electron donating power of the donor (E_I) is referred to as its ionization energy, which is the energy needed to remove the most loosely bound electron from a neutral atom/or molecule. On the other hand, the electron accepting power of the acceptor (E_A) is determined by its electron affinity, which is defined as the energy released when an electron is added to a neutral atom/or molecule to form an anion. The overall energy difference, denoted as ΔE, is the energy gained during the charge transfer:

$$\Delta E = E_A - E_I + J$$

where J is the electrostatic force of attraction. It is noteworthy to point out that this energy difference is directly related to a specific CT band in the electromagnetic spectrum which explains why it is important to work at a particular wavelength.

3.3. Why Is a Particular Colour Observed in an Antioxidant–Oxidant Chemical Reaction?

Light is a mixture of colours and the visible region in an electromagnetic spectrum is made up of different colours, namely red, orange, yellow, green, blue, and violet, covering a wavelength region of 400 to 750 nm, as represented by the colour wheel in Figure 1. When a molecule absorbs light at a particular wavelength, the colour that appear is the complementary colour on the colour wheel. For example, DPPH gives a deep purple appearance because it absorbs a photon of light at 515–517 nm, 2,2-azino-bis(3-ethylbenzothiazoline-6-sulfonic acid) (ABTS) absorbs at 734 nm to give a pale blue colour, and so on.

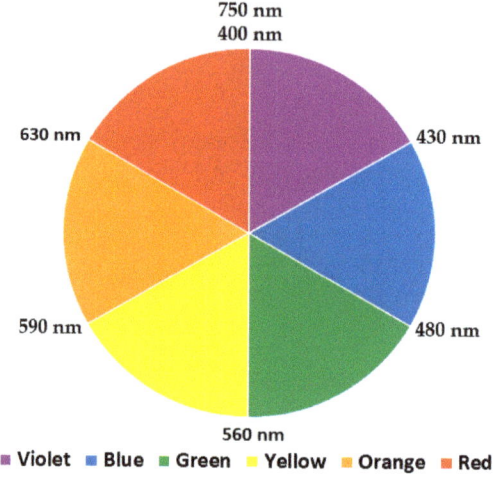

Figure 1. Colour wheel.

4. Mechanism of Action of Antioxidants

Antioxidant assays are based on a concept called total antioxidant capacity (TAC). TAC is measured as the amount of free radicals quenched by a test solution used to determine the AO capacity of a biological sample. Depending on the mechanism of chemical reactions involved, TAC assays can be further categorized as: (i) single electron transfer (SET), (ii) hydrogen atom transfer (HAT) reaction-based assays, or (iii) chelation of transition metals [17].

The single electron transfer (SET) mechanism involves a redox (reduction–oxidation) reaction with an oxidant (also known as the probe or radical) as an indicator of reaction endpoint. Hydrogen atom transfer (HAT) assays involve a synthetic radical generator, an oxidizable probe, and an antioxidant. Both SET and HAT reaction-based assays measure the radical scavenging capacity instead of the preventive capacity of a sample [8,18]. SET-based assays measure the antioxidant's reducing capacity, while HAT-based assays quantify hydrogen atom donating capacity [19]. In SET assays, AO gives an electron to the radical to stabilize it. The transfer of an electron from AO to the radical will cause a change in colour of the radical. The intensity of the colour change is proportional to the concentration of AO present in the reaction mixture. The reaction end point is reached when no change in colour is observed [8], i.e., when electron transfer has stopped.

In addition to SET and HAT mechanisms, the third type of mechanism of action of AOs is their ability to chelate transition metals, namely Zn^{2+}, Fe^{2+}, and Cu^{2+}. The chelation of transition metals can also be considered to estimate the AO capacity of an extract or compound. Several lines of evidence extracted from the recent literature have demonstrated that transition metals such as Fe^{2+} and Cu^{2+} are responsible for the pathogenesis of numerous diseases, including neurodegenerative (Alzheimer's, Parkinson's) and cardiovascular diseases [17].

Various techniques have been developed to measure antioxidant capacities of biological samples, including plant extracts and food samples. The following sections will discuss these techniques as well as various AO assays in terms of the chemical reactions involved, mechanism of each reaction, colour change of probe, strengths and limitations of each assay.

5. Different Techniques Used to Measure Antioxidant Activities

There are numerous analytical techniques available to measure the antioxidant property of samples. The different techniques fall into three main categories, namely spectrometry, electrochemical technique, and chromatography. Each one of them is discussed in Table 1. However, in this review, antioxidant assays using colorimetry as a measure of antioxidant properties are appraised, since they are the most accessible and commonly used methods to evaluate the antioxidant activities of biological samples.

Table 1. Different techniques used to measure antioxidant activity (Source: [20]).

Antioxidant Assay	Principle of Method	End Product Determination
Spectrometry		
DPPH	Antioxidant reaction with an organic radical	Colorimetry
ABTS	Antioxidant reaction with an organic radical	Colorimetry
FRAP	Antioxidant reaction with a Fe (III) complex	Colorimetry
PFRAP	Potassium ferricyanide reduction by antioxidants and subsequent reaction of potassium ferrocyanide with Fe^{3+}	Colorimetry
CUPRAC	Cu (II) reduction to Cu (I) by antioxidants	Colorimetry
ORAC	Antioxidant reaction with peroxyl radicals, induced by AAPH	Loss of fluorescence of fluorescein
HORAC	Antioxidant capacity to quench OH radicals generated by a Co (II) based Fenton-like system	Loss of fluorescence of fluorescein
TRAP	Antioxidant capacity to scavenge luminol-derived radicals, generated from AAPH decomposition	Photo chemiluminescence quenching
Fluorimetry	Emission of light by a substance that has absorbed light or other electromagnetic radiation of a different wavelength	Recording of fluorescence excitation/emission spectra

Table 1. Cont.

Antioxidant Assay	Principle of Method	End Product Determination
Electrochemical Techniques		
Cyclic voltammetry	The potential of a working electrode is linearly varied from an initial value to a final value and back, and the respective current intensity is recorded	Measurement of the intensity of the cathodic/ anodic peak
Amperometry	The potential of the working electrode is set at a fixed value with respect to a reference electrode	Measurement of the intensity of the current generated by the oxidation/reduction of an electroactive analyte
Biamperometry	The reaction of the analyte (antioxidant) with the oxidized form of a reversible indicating redox couple	Measurement of the current flowing between two identical working electrodes at a small potential difference and immersed in a solution containing the analysed sample and reversible redox couple
Chromatography		
GC	Separation of the compounds in a mixture is based on the repartition between a liquid stationary phase and a gas mobile phase	Flame ionization or thermal conductivity detection
HPLC	Separation of compounds in a mixture is based on the repartition between a solid stationary phase and a liquid mobile phase with different polarities, at high flow rate and pressure of the mobile phase	UV–vis (e.g., diode array) detection, fluorescence, mass spectrometry or electrochemical detection
TLC	Separation of compounds is based on the repartition between a solid stationary phase (silica gel) and a liquid mobile phase (mixture of acetate, formic acid and water)	Photographed under visible light

DPPH—2,2-diphenyl-1-picrylhydrazyl; ABTS—2,2-azino-bis(3-ethylbenzothiazoline-6-sulfonic acid); FRAP—Ferric reducing antioxidant power; PFRAP—Potassium ferricyanide antioxidant power; CUPRAC—Cupric reducing antioxidant capacity; ORAC—Oxygen radical absorbance capacity; HORAC—Hydroxyl radical antioxidant capacity; TRAP—Total radical trapping antioxidant parameter; GC—Gas chromatography; HPLC—High performance liquid chromatography; UV–vis—Ultraviolet–visible; TLC—Thin layer chromatography; AAPH—2,2′-azobis-2-amidino-propane.

6. Folin–Ciocalteu Assay

The Folin–Ciocalteu (F–C) assay is the most commonly used assay to determine the total phenolic content in various plant or food samples. Phenolic compounds of chemo-preventive and therapeutic values are of scientific interest in the management of countless chronic diseases since 1990. The major contributors of antioxidant capacity of fruit, vegetable, grain, or plant samples are phenolic compounds. The F–C assay is a colorimetry method based on SET reactions between the F–C reagent and phenolic compounds [21]. Phenolic compounds are good oxygen radical scavengers, since the electron reduction potential of phenolic radical is lower than that of oxygen radicals and also, phenoxyl radicals are less reactive than oxygen radicals. Thus, scavenging reactive oxygen radicals by phenolic compounds ceased further oxidative reactions [22]. The F–C assay was developed to improve the Folin–Denis (F-D) assay, which was initially designed to determine total protein concentration by measuring tryptophan and tyrosine contents. Later, it was found that F–C was more sensitive and reproducible than the F–D assay [22]. However, the F–C assay is non-specific, since other substances, namely reducing sugars and ascorbic acid which are highly abundant in plant food extracts, can reduce F–C reagent, leading to biased F–C results [22].

F–C reagent is prepared by dissolving 100 g of sodium tungstate ($Na_2WO_4 \cdot 2H_2O$) and 25 g sodium molybdate ($Na_2MoO_4 \cdot 2H_2O$) in 700 mL of distilled water. About 50 mL of concentrated HCl and 50 mL of 85% phosphoric acid are added to acidify the solution. The acidified solution is boiled for 10 h and allowed to cool before adding 150 g $Li_2SO_4 \cdot 4H_2O$. The resulting solution, which is the F–C reagent, develops an intense yellow colour [22]. The chemistry of F–C reagent is still unclear and is believed to be composed of heteropoly-phosphotungstates/molybdates [8]. During F–C assay, the reaction between F–C reagent and phenolic compounds occurs at alkaline medium (~pH 10), which is reached by adding sodium carbonate (Na_2CO_3). Under this basic condition, dissociation of a phenolic proton leads to the formation of phenolate ion, which is responsible to reduce the F–C reagent. Upon reduction, the intense yellow colour of F–C reagent turns into a blue colour [22]. The colour change is illustrated by a colour ribbon (Figure 2).

General methodology: Total phenolic content is determined using Folin–Ciocalteu reagent. To 0.2 µL sample solution (2 mg/mL), 1 mL of F–C reagent and 2 mL of Na_2CO_3 were added and mixed carefully. The resulting mixture was brought to 7 mL with deionized water and allowed to incubate at room temperature for 2 h. The absorbance is read at 765 nm. Gallic acid is usually used as a reference standard [23].

Chemical reaction:

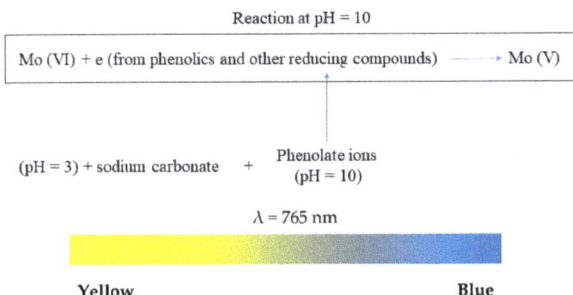

Figure 2. Folin–Ciocalteu (F–C) assay.

Strengths and Limitations

Strengths:

- Simple, rapid and reproducible [22]
- Direct correlation between phenolic compounds and antioxidant activity [24]
- Can screen many samples in a timely fashion [22]

Limitations:

- Non-specific to phenolics [22]

7. Free Radical Scavenging Antioxidant Assays

7.1. 2,2-Diphenyl-1-picrylhydrazyl Radical Scavenging Capacity (DPPH) Assay

The DPPH• radical was discovered by Goldschmidt and Renn in the 1920s. It was first developed by Blois in 1958 [25,26]. This radical is known for its remarkable stability due to the delocalization of the radical in aromatic rings. It has an intense deep purple colour [27]. In assays, the radical is neutralized by accepting either a hydrogen atom or an electron from an antioxidant species (or reducing agents) during which, it is converted into a reduced form (DPPH or DPPH-H) at the end of the process

(Figure 3). The unpaired electron of the DPPH radical absorbs strongly at 517 nm, giving rise to a deep purple colour. However, when an odd electron pairs up with another electron, the initial colour gradually decolorizes into pale yellow. Decolorization is simulated by the colour ribbon below.

General methodology: First, 50 µL of extract is added to 150 µL methanolic solution of DPPH at 0.1 mM in a 96-well plate. The mixture is then shaken vigorously in the dark at room temperature for 30 min [28]. Results are processed either as an equivalent of a standard reference (Trolox, gallic acid, ascorbic acid, BHA, BHT) or IC_{50}.

Chemical reactions:

$$DPPH^{\bullet} + ArOH \rightarrow DPPH\text{-}H + ArO^{\bullet} \quad \text{(HAT mechanism)}$$

$$DPPH^{\bullet} + ArOH \rightarrow DPPH + [ArOH]^{\bullet+} \quad \text{(SET mechanism)}$$

where ArOH: phenolic AO

Mechanism of reaction: HAT

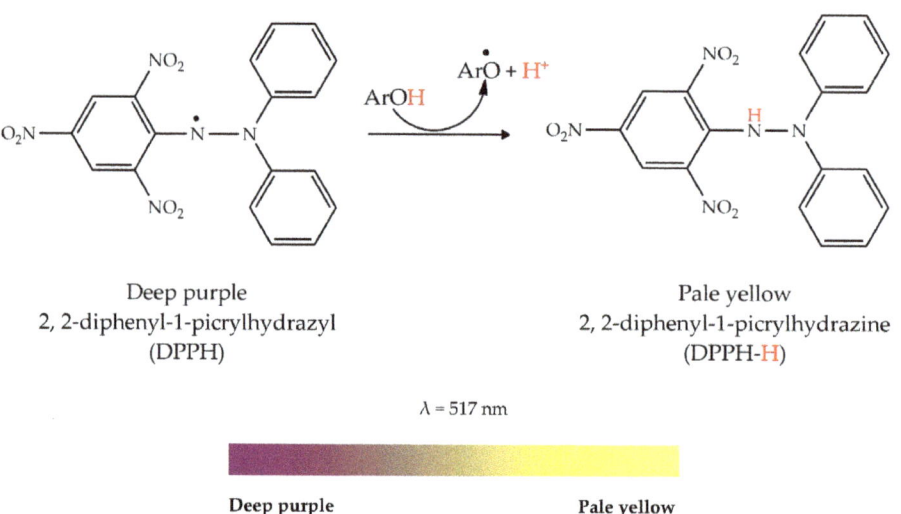

Figure 3. 2,2-diphenyl-1-picrylhydrazyl (DPPH) reaction mechanism.

Strengths and Limitations

Strengths:

- Simple, cheap and rapid, since the radical is stable and needs not be generated compared to ABTS [29]
- Can quantify antioxidants in complex biological systems [29]
- The radical scavenging time is 30 min, allowing DPPH to react efficiently, even with weak antioxidants [29]
- Results are reproducible and comparable to other radical scavenging methods [30]
- Efficient for thermally unstable compounds, since radical scavenging is measured at room temperature [31]
- Highly sensitive [16]
- Can screen many samples in a timely fashion [16]
- Good correlation is usually reported with bioactive compounds (phenols, flavonoids) with a regression factor R > 0.8

Limitations:

- DPPH radical chromogens dissolve only organic solvents (lipophilic) [16]
- DPPH tends to react with other radicals present in the tested samples [29]
- Since the nitrogen centre is highly sterically hindered by three phenyl groups, DPPH represents a poor model for radical quenching in vivo and in food samples [32]
- DPPH is sensitive to Lewis bases [33]
- Upon exposure to light, absorbance of DPPH tends to decrease, which requires analysis in the dark [34]
- Non-physiological resemblance due to the absence of DPPH free radicals in the human body [11]

7.2. Trolox Equivalent Antioxidant Capacity or 2,2'-Azino-bis (3-ethylbenzothiazoline-6-sulfonic acid) (TEAC or ABTS$^{\bullet+}$) Assay

In 1993, Miller and Rice-Evans were the first to report the ABTS$^{\bullet+}$ assay, also known as TEAC [35]. This assay was later improved by Re and Colleagues in 1999 [12]. The improvement was related to how the ABTS$^{\bullet+}$ radical was generated. Compared to DPPH, which is a stable radical by nature, the ABTS$^{\bullet+}$ radical is a radical that should be generated by chemical reactions. Originally, the generation of a radical cation (ABTS$^{\bullet+}$) was done by reacting metmyoglobin (Met-Myb) with hydrogen peroxide (H_2O_2) to produce hydroxyl radical (HO$^\bullet$). The latter radical causes the reduction of ABTS into its radical in the presence or absence of antioxidants. The reaction is illustrated in Scheme 1. However, this scheme has a major gap.

For instance, the AO can reduce the HO$^\bullet$ radical present in the system together with metmyoglobin and ABTS$^{\bullet+}$, resulting in an overestimation of the antioxidant capacity, which leads to erroneous results. To overcome this problem, an improved method is proposed by eliminating the requirement of HO$^\bullet$ radical and metmyoglobin. The improved method generates the ABTS$^{\bullet+}$ radical in only one reaction by reacting ABTS with ammonium or potassium persulfate ($(NH_4)_2 S_2O_3$ or $K_2S_2O_3$, respectively) prior to the addition of AOs. It is important to note that ABTS is in a stoichiometry ratio of 1:0.5 with persulfate salt, meaning that not all ABTSs are oxidized prior to the addition of AO [12,32,36]. The improved reaction is illustrated in Scheme 2. Oxidation of ABTS is a long reaction which takes about 12–16 h. The ABTS$^{\bullet+}$ radical solution is then diluted in ethanol/methanol until an absorbance of 0.7 ± 0.02 is reached at 734 nm. This dilution is done only before the beginning of the assay, as clearly emphasized by Re et al. [12].

Interestingly, the blue-green coloured ABTS$^{\bullet+}$ chromophore may absorb at various wavelengths, namely 645, 734, 815, and 415 nm. However, most investigators have adopted the wavelength of 734 nm because possible interferences are eliminated and sample turbidity is reduced at that wavelength [6,37]. When the ABTS$^{\bullet+}$ radical (unstable form) accepts an electron from the AO, the blue-green colour fades into a pale blue colour, which shows regeneration of ABTS (stable form). Concerning reaction time, existing studies have reported different reaction times, ranging from 1 to 30 min. Re, Pellegrini, Proteggente, Pannala, Yang, and Rice-Evans [12] have stated that completion of an ABTS reaction can be observed after the first minute itself, except for cyanidin and glutathione that show inhibitory activity even after 4 min. The mechanism of the reaction is shown in Figure 4. Decolorization is illustrated with a colour ribbon.

General methodology: The protocol initially proposed by Re et al. [12] is modified to determine the scavenging capacity against the ABTS$^{\bullet+}$ radical. First, ABTS is dissolved in water to a 7 mM concentration. Then, the ABTS$^{\bullet+}$ radical cation is generated by reacting 7 mM ABTS solution with 2.45 mM potassium persulfate in a ratio of 1:0.5. It is then allowed to stand at room temperature in the dark for 12–16 h. Before starting the assay, the ABTS solution is diluted with ethanol or methanol until an absorbance of 0.7 is reached at 734 nm. To 1 mL of extract to be tested, 2 mL of ABTS solution is added and mixed. The reaction mixture is incubated in the dark at room temperature for 30 min. Results are expressed as equivalent of a standard compound (Trolox, ascorbic acid, gallic acid, BHA, or BHT) for comparison.

Chemical reactions:

$$Met\text{-}Myb + H_2O_2 \rightarrow HO^\bullet$$
$$ABTS + HO^\bullet \rightarrow ABTS^{\bullet+} + ArOH \rightarrow ABTS + ArO^\bullet \quad \text{Scheme 1}$$

$$(NH_4)_2 S_2O_3 + ABTS \rightarrow ABTS^{\bullet+} + ArOH \rightarrow ABTS + ArO^\bullet \quad \text{Scheme 2}$$

Mechanism of reaction:

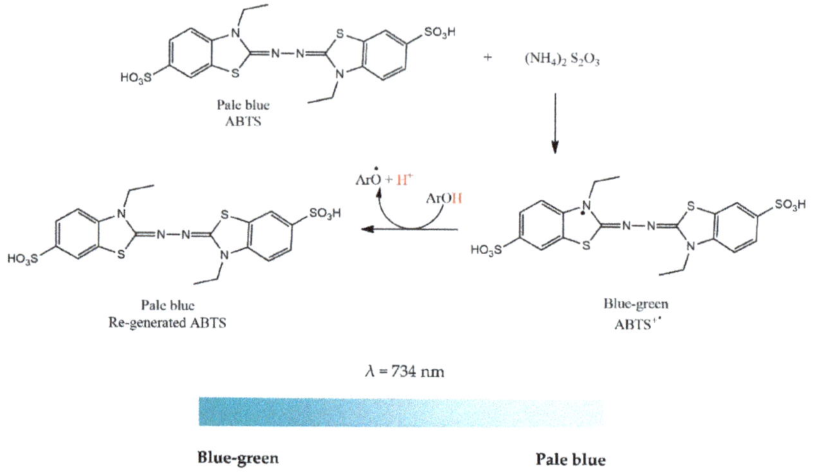

$\lambda = 734$ nm

Figure 4. 2,2′-azino-bis (3-ethylbenzothiazoline-6-sulfonic acid) (ABTS) reaction mechanism.

Strengths and Limitations

Strengths:

- The ABTS cationic radical is soluble in both organic and aqueous media in contrast to the DPPH radical, which dissolves only in organic medium. The ABTS assay can, thus, be used to screen both lipophilic and hydrophilic samples [16]
- Can be used to determine the antioxidant capacity of numerous compounds, namely carotenoids, phenolic, and plasma [12]
- The ABTS assay produces reproducible results [6]
- The ABTS$^{\bullet+}$ radical is stable for more than two days when stored in the dark at ambient temperature compared to DPPH, which has a rather short life, however, Gupta [27] stated that the radical solution is stable for a few months when stored in the refrigerator. We can say that the stability of the ABTS$^{\bullet+}$ radical solution remains debatable [12]
- Good correlation is usually reported with bioactive compounds (phenols, flavonoids), with generally, a regression factor R > 0.8

Limitations:

- The ABTS$^{\bullet+}$ assay is often criticized because the ABTS$^{\bullet+}$ radical does not exist naturally (not found in any biological system) and should be chemically generated. Thus, some literature argued that the ABTS$^{\bullet+}$ radical cannot represent in vivo system [38]
- Slow reaction for the generation of the ABTS$^{\bullet+}$ radical, which takes about 12–16 h compared to DPPH, which is readily available commercially
- Like DPPH, the ABTS$^{\bullet+}$ radical exhibits high steric hindrance around its nitrogen-centred atom and thus, does not represent a good model for highly reactive radicals, namely OH$^\bullet$, NO$^\bullet$, O$_2^{\bullet-}$ or LO(O)$^\bullet$, which are present in numerous biological samples [32]

8. Thiobarbituric Acid Reactive Species (TBARS) Assay

The hydroxyl radical (HO•) is among the most potent reactive oxygen species (ROS) present in our biological systems. It reacts with polyunsaturated fatty acid moieties that can consequently damage the cell membrane [13]. Among free radicals, OH• is the most harmful ROS which can damage cell membranes and destroy sugar groups and DNA base sequences and even causes cell apoptosis and mutations [39]. The thiobarbituric acid reactive species (TBARS) assay, developed by Kohn and Liversedge in 1944, is a way to measure lipid peroxidation in cells and tissues [40,41]. It was initially used to determine the rate of reaction between HO• and molecules having therapeutic importance. The same methodology is still used to evaluate radical activity between HO• and antioxidants with slight modifications. The protocol consists of many reagents, namely ascorbic acid (AA), deoxyribose, phosphate buffer, ferric chloride, hydrogen peroxide (H_2O_2), ethylenediamine tetraacetic acid (EDTA), trichloroacetic acid (TCA), and thiobarbituric acid (TBA). Each one of these reagents has a specific role. The assay is started by complexing EDTA with Fe^{2+} which then reacts with H_2O_2 to generate the HO• radical following a Fenton reaction, as shown in Scheme 3 [42].

The generation of the radical requires an incubation temperature of 37 °C for a duration of about 12 h. The generated HO• radical then attacks the deoxyribose sugar in the presence of AA to form a mixture of products, as presented in Scheme 4. The purpose of adding AA to the reaction mixture is to increase the rate of deoxyribose degradation by the radical. Heating the resulting mixture of products with TBA in an acidic medium at a low pH will lead to the formation of malondialdehyde (MDA). The formation of MDA can then be detected after its reaction with TBA to form a pink MDA-TBA chromogen [43,44].

The adduct $(TBA)_2$-MDA is formed according to a nucleophilic attack involving a 5-carbon of TBA with 1-carbon MDA followed by dehydration. The same reaction takes place with the second TBA molecule [42]. The proposed mechanism of chromogen formation is shown in Scheme 5. Grotto et al. [42] have stated that to prevent the formation of MDA in an assay, inhibition of deoxyribose degradation is needed. Thus, an AO can be added to the reaction mixture. The scavenging activity toward the HO• radical is measured based on inhibition of deoxyribose degradation. On the same line, we propose the addition of AOs to attack HO• radicals by donating an electron to the latter which can consequently quench the radical. In the absence of the HO• radical, the deoxyribose sugar does not undergo any degradation, thus, hindering the formation of MDA and MDA-TBA adduct, as shown by the red wavy break in Figure 5 In the absence of the MDA-TBA chromogen, the colour of the solution remains pale yellow, indicating good antioxidant activity. The colour change in the absence of an AO is illustrated by a colour ribbon. The mechanism of the reaction is shown in Figure 5.

General methodology: The hydroxyl radical is generated by mixing 0.28 mL of deoxyribose (10 mM) with 0.41 mL of phosphate buffer (pH 7.4), 0.01 mL of ferric chloride (10 mM), 0.1 mL hydrogen peroxide (10 mM), and 0.1 mL of EDTA (1 mM). Finally, 0.1 mL ascorbic acid (1mM) is added to the premixed reaction mixture containing 0.25 mL sample solution. The resulting mixture is incubated at 37 °C for 12 h. A blank is prepared similarly by mixing 0.25 mL sample solution with 1 mL of the reaction mixture without ferric chloride. Afterwards, 0.75 mL of TCA (2.8%, w/v) and 0.75 mL of TBA (1%, w/v in 50 mM NaOH) are added to the incubated sample followed by heating at 100 °C for 1 h. The absorbance of the reaction mixture is measured at 523 nm after the mixture is allowed to cool to room temperature. Results can be expressed as mannitol equivalents (e.g., mg MEs/g extract) [28].

Chemical reactions:

$$Fe^{2+}\text{-EDTA} + H_2O_2 \rightarrow Fe^{3+}\text{-EDTA} + OH^\bullet + OH^-$$ Scheme 3

$$HO^\bullet + \text{deoxyribose sugar} \xrightarrow{AA} \text{products} \xrightarrow{TBA} MDA$$ Scheme 4

$$2TBA + MDA \xrightarrow[\Delta]{TCA} MDA\text{-}TBA$$ Scheme 5

Mechanism of reaction:

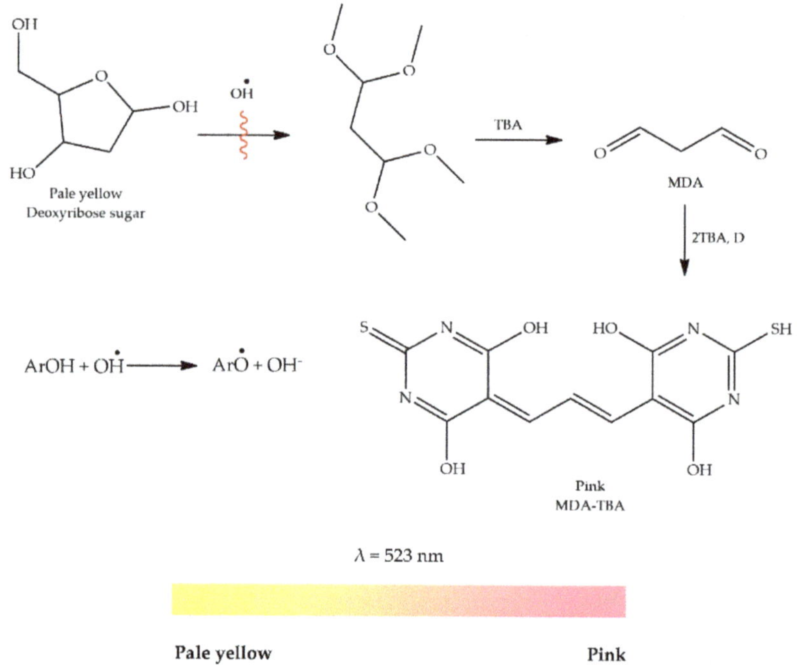

Figure 5. HO$^\bullet$ reaction mechanism.

Another way to measure the oxidative damage is by protein and DNA modifications. However, these markers can also be formed by pathways other than from free radicals. Thus, MDA remains the preferred marker to evaluate oxidative damage in tissues and cells. The determination of MDA is possible in numerous biological samples [42]. The production of TBARS occurs nearly at the end of the assay, as shown in Figure 6. This implies that an AO can be introduced into the system at any step of the process prior to the formation of TBARS. Thus, measurement of TBARS gives no indication of the mechanism of action of the antioxidant, i.e., whether it is able to interact with oxygen or metal ions, react directly with hydroperoxides, or intercept the free radicals involved in the breakdown of primary to secondary oxidation products [40].

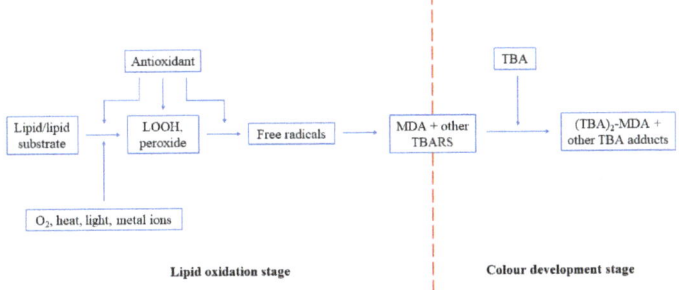

Figure 6. Steps involved in the lipid oxidation and antioxidant action in the TBARS activity assay.

Strengths and Limitations

Strengths:
• Simple, cheap, and accurate results in most cases [42]

Limitations:
• Lack of sensitivity and specificity, because TBA reacts with different compounds, namely sugars, amino acids, bilirubin, and albumin [42]
• MDA is unstable for a long period of time, since it oxidizes into alcohols and acids [42]
• Aldehydes may also react with TBA, leading to an overestimation of MDA [45]

9. Nitric Oxide Radical Scavenging Assay

In the 1980s, the team Furchgott and Zawadzki demonstrated that the endothelium released a substance that can relax blood vessels in response to muscarinic agonists. However, at that time, the chemical nature of this substance was unknown and was, thus, denoted as endothelium-derived relaxing factor (EDRF). Years later, Ignarro and Moncada independently showed that this substance was nitric oxide (NO$^\bullet$) due to the chemiluminescent product formed by NO$^\bullet$ with ozone. Nitric oxide is a free radical which is not as reactive as other radicals [46].

Nitric oxide is generated from amino acid L-arginine found in vascular endothelial cells, specific neuronal cells, and phagocytes by enzymes [47,48]. At low concentrations, NO$^\bullet$ plays an effective role in biological activities, namely antimicrobial activity, antitumor effect, vasodilation, and neuronal messenger. However, high levels of NO can cause several health complications, including inflammatory complications such as sclerosis, arthritis, and ulcerative colitis. The toxicity of NO can notably increase upon its reaction with superoxide radical to form a highly reactive anion peroxynitrite anion (ONOO$^-$). The latter anion will be discussed later. Many studies have shown that flavonoids can rapidly scavenge NO$^\bullet$ radicals [49,50].

To measure the NO$^\bullet$ radical scavenging activity, diazotization assay or Griess reaction was first developed in 1864 by a German chemist named Johann Peter Griess [51]. The modified experiment involved the reaction of nitrite (NO$_2^-$) with sulfanilic acid (SA) ($C_6H_7NO_3S$) under an acidic condition, resulting in the formation of a diazonium ion which is subsequently coupled with N-(1-naphthyl) ethylenediamine (NED) ($C_{12}H_{14}N_2$) to form a water-soluble and red-coloured azo dye ($HO_3SC_6H_4$-NN-$C_{10}H_6NH_2$) that can be measured at a wavelength of ~540 nm [52,53]. The original method required improvement in order to increase reproducibility, sensitivity, and analysis time. The modified assay shows good results on several occasions. It is now widely used for screening samples to determine their free radical scavenging activities. Interestingly, the same assay is also used to determine nitrite in water in Europe [53]. The assay is started by generating the radical (NO$^\bullet$), similar to the HO$^\bullet$ radical scavenging assay. The radical is initiated using sodium nitroprusside (SNP;

$Na_2[Fe^{III}(CN)_5(NO)]$) known to undergo spontaneous degradation in aqueous solution at physiological pH 7.2 to produce $NO^•$ (Scheme 6).

SNP is a non-ferromagnetic species that can be easily reduced to a paramagnetic species, $[Fe^{II}(CN)_5(NO)]^{3-}$, in aqueous solution [54]. Under aerobic conditions, $NO^•$ can react with O_2 to produce nitrate (NO_3^-) and nitrite (NO_2^-) as stable products that can be quantified using Griess reagent (Scheme 7). The latter reagent is prepared by mixing 1 mL of 0.33% SA with 20% glacial acetic acid. It is allowed to react for 5 min at room temperature. Then, 1 mL of NED is added to the resulting solution to form Griess reagent. The azo group, -N=N-, is the chromophore group of the azo dye compound with a molecular formula of $C_{16}H_{13}N_3SO_3$. The purpose of adding NED is to increase reproducibility, sensitivity, and solubility of the azo compound in acid and enhance coupling [53]. The absorbance of the chromophore formed can be measured at wavelengths of 546 or 548 nm depending on investigators. The colour change is illustrated with a colour ribbon. However, in the presence of an antioxidant (or absence of $NO^•$ radical), formation of NO_3^- and NO_2^- will not occur. Thus, the reaction between NO_2^- and sulfanilic acid will not take place. Consequently, no azo dye compound is formed and no red colour is observed as the solution will remain colourless. The mechanism of the reaction is shown in Figure 7.

Chemical reactions:

$Na_2[Fe^{III}(CN)_5(NO)] + RSH \rightarrow RS\text{-}NO + NO^•$ Scheme 6

$2NO^• + O_2 \rightarrow 2NO_2$

$2NO_2 \rightarrow N_2O_4$ Scheme 7

$N_2O_4 + H_2O \rightarrow NO_2^- + NO_3^- + 2H^+$

$C_6H_7NO_3S + NO_2^- \rightarrow C_{16}H_{13}N_3SO_3$ (azo dye) Scheme 8

where RSH= sulfhydryl containing compounds

Mechanism of reaction:

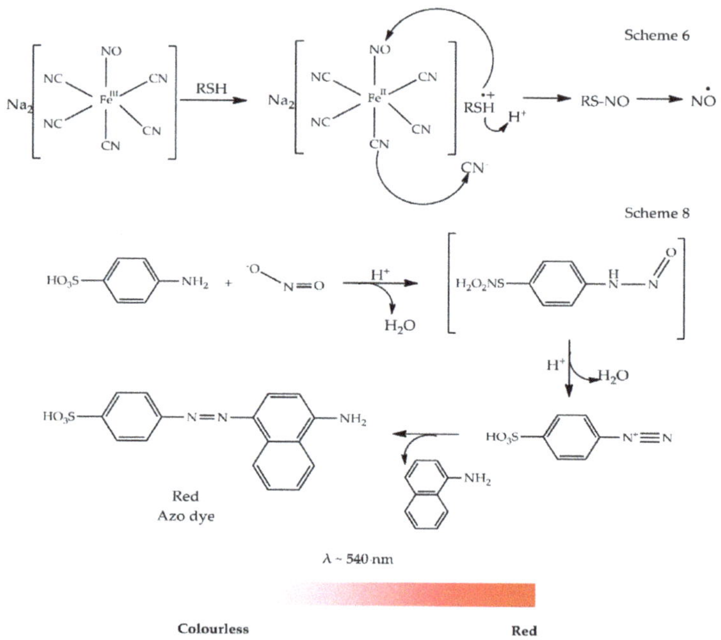

Figure 7. $NO^•$ reaction mechanism.

Strengths and Limitations

Strengths:
• Simple, cheap, sensitive, reproducible, and rapid analysis time [53]
Limitations:
• This assay may present problems due to rapid scavenging, high reactivity, and swift diffusion [52]

General methodology: SNP dissolved in aqueous solution at physiological pH 7.2 can generate nitric oxide whose level can be measured by Griess reaction. Sample solution (0.5 mL) is mixed with SNP (0.5mL, 5mM) in phosphate buffer at pH 7.4 (0.2 M), followed by an incubation at room temperature for 150 min. Similarly, a blank is prepared by adding sample solution in phosphate buffer without SNP. Griess reagent (0.33% sulfanilic acid, 20% glacial acetic acid, 0.1% NED) (1 mL) is added to the incubated sample and allowed to stand for 30 min. Absorbance values of the blank and samples are measured at 548 nm. The absorbance of the blank is then subtracted from that of the sample. Results are expressed either as %inhibition or equivalent of standard compound (e.g., Trolox) [55].

10. Peroxynitrite Scavenging Assay

Peroxynitrite ($ONOO^-$) is a strong oxidant resulting from a fast reaction between nitric oxide and superoxide ($O_2^{\bullet-}$), which occurs in vascular endothelial cells, Kupffer cells, neutrophils, and macrophages. It was first discovered in 1900 as a biological endogenous oxidant [56]. Peroxynitrite ($ONOO^-$) is not a free radical, since unpaired electrons on $NO^{\bullet}$ and $O_2^{\bullet-}$ can pair up to form a new O-N bond [57]. Although $ONOO^-$ is a stable species, its protonation can lead to the formation of a highly reactive acid (ONOOH). The presence of a notable amount of ONOOH can cause numerous problems, including apoptotic cell death, Alzheimer's disease, atherosclerosis, and rheumatoid arthritis, among others. Since endogenous enzymes for scavenging $ONOO^-$ are lacking, there is an urgent need to develop specific $ONOO^-$ scavengers [13]. $ONOO^-$ scavenging activity is measured by oxidation of dihydrorhodamine 123 (DHR 123; $CH_{20}H_{18}N_2O_3$) into a fluorescent probe, rhodamine 123 (RH 123; $CH_{21}H_{17}ClN_2O_3$), at excitation and emission wavelengths of 485 or 505 nm and 529 or 530 nm, respectively, in the presence of an AO [13,58,59]. Therefore, if the AO can successfully scavenge $ONOO^-$, no oxidation of DHR 123 will take place. Therefore, no formation of RH 123 will be observed (i.e., reduced formation of orange-red colour). The wavelength at which DHR 123 is measured can explain its red colour in appearance based on a colour wheel (Figure 1). This assay is not commonly used. It lacks information on its origin. The oxidation of DHR 123 is presented in Scheme 9. The mechanism of the reaction is shown in Figure 8.

General methodology: A stock solution of DHR 123 (5 mM) is prepared in dimethylformamide, purged with nitrogen, and kept at −80 °C. Prior to the start of the assay, the stock solution of DHR 123 is diluted to a concentration of 5 μM and placed over ice in the dark. A buffer solution containing 50 mM sodium phosphate (pH 7.4), 90 mM sodium chloride, 5 mM potassium chloride, and 100 μM diethylenetriaminepentaacetic acid (DTPA) was prepared, purged with nitrogen, and placed over ice before use. Scavenging activity of $ONOO^-$ by oxidation of DHR 123 is measured fluorometrically at excitation and emission wavelengths of 485 and 530 nm, respectively. The background and final fluorescence intensities are measured at 5 min after treatment without 3-morpholino-sydonimine (SIN-1) or authentic ($ONOO^{\bullet}$). Oxidation of DHR 123 by decomposition of SIN-1 is slowly increased. However, with authentic $ONOO^{\bullet}$, the decomposition is fast, while its final fluorescent intensity is stable with time [13,60].

Chemical reaction:

$$CH_{20}H_{18}N_2O_3 \rightarrow CH_{21}H_{17}ClN_2O_3 \qquad \text{Scheme 9}$$

Mechanism of reaction:

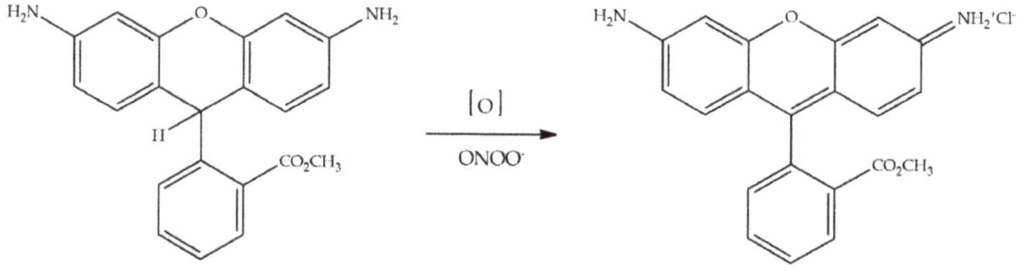

[Structure of Red DHR 123] $\xrightarrow{[O] \atop ONOO^-}$ [Structure of Orange red RH 123]

Red
DHR 123

Orange red
RH 123

Figure 8. ONOO$^-$ reaction mechanism.

Strengths and Limitations

Strengths:
• Direct physiological resemblance of peroxynitrite (ONOO-) to the human body [61]

Limitations:
• Lacks specificity. The rapid decomposition of ONOO$^-$ forms NO$^\bullet$ and $O_2^{\bullet-}$. These two species have the potential to oxidize DHR 123. Thus, it can be said that the oxidation of DHR 123 is not directly linked to ONOO$^-$ [62]
• Require expensive equipment and reagent, namely fluorescence spectrophotometer, −80 °C freezer, and DHR 123, which are not easily accessible in all laboratories

11. Superoxide Radical Scavenging Assay

The superoxide ($O_2^{\bullet-}$) radical is formed during a normal respiration process, which reduces 1–3% of the oxygen that we breath into its radical, $O_2^{\bullet-}$. The reduction of molecular oxygen (O_2) takes place intracellularly in the mitochondria under normal physiological conditions [63–66]. The AO enzyme that is responsible for quenching $O_2^{\bullet-}$ radicals is called superoxide dismutase (SOD). SOD was discovered by McCord and Fridovich in 1969 [67]. This enzyme converts $O_2^{\bullet-}$ into H_2O_2, which is further converted into O_2 and water by glutathione peroxidase and catalase [44]. The generation of the $O_2^{\bullet-}$ radical can be done using two systems: (1) a non-enzymatic system involving phenazine methosulphate (PMS; $C_{13}H_{11}N_2 \cdot CH_3SO_4$), nitroblue tetrazolium (NBT; $C_{40}H_{30}Cl_2N_{10}O_6$), and a reduced form of nicotinamide-adenine-dinucleotide (NADH; $C_{21}H_{27}N_7O_{14}P_2$); or (2) a hypoxanthine-xanthine oxidase superoxide generating system, as described by Robak and Gryglewski [68].

The scavenging activity of AOs towards $O_2^{\bullet-}$ is assessed in terms of their ability to prevent $O_2^{\bullet-}$ generation. Prior to the reduction process caused by $O_2^{\bullet-}$, NBT is a pale-yellow soluble salt. However, upon reduction occurring at a pH of 7.4, the tetrazole ring is disrupted, leading to dismutation which subsequently results in an intense blue insoluble diformazan product ($C_{40}H_{32}N_{10}O_6$), as illustrated in Scheme 10 [44,69,70]. Importantly, the addition of a potential AO will react with $O_2^{\bullet-}$ radical and inhibit the formation of diformazan. Therefore, no intense blue colour will be observed. The colour change in the absence of an AO is illustrated by the colour ribbon in Figure 9.

General methodology: Sample solution is treated with 0.05 mL phosphate buffer (250 mmol/L), 0.025 mL NADH (2 mmol/L), and 0.025 mL NBT (0.5 mmol/L). The absorbance of the resulting solution is read as a blank at 560 nm. To the resulting solution, 0.025 mL PMS (0.03 mmol/L) is added and allowed to incubate at room temperature for 5 min. The absorbance is read again at the same wavelength. Results are expressed either as %inhibition or equivalent of standard compound (e.g., gallic acid, BHA, ascorbic acid, α-tocopherol, curcumin) [71].

Chemical reactions:

$$C_{13}H_{11}N_2 \cdot CH_3SO_4 + C_{21}H_{27}N_7O_{14}P_2 \xrightarrow{O_2} O_2^{\bullet -}$$

$$C_{40}H_{30}Cl_2N_{10}O_6 \xrightarrow{O_2^{\bullet -}} C_{40}H_{32}N_{10}O_6$$

Scheme 10

Mechanism of reaction:

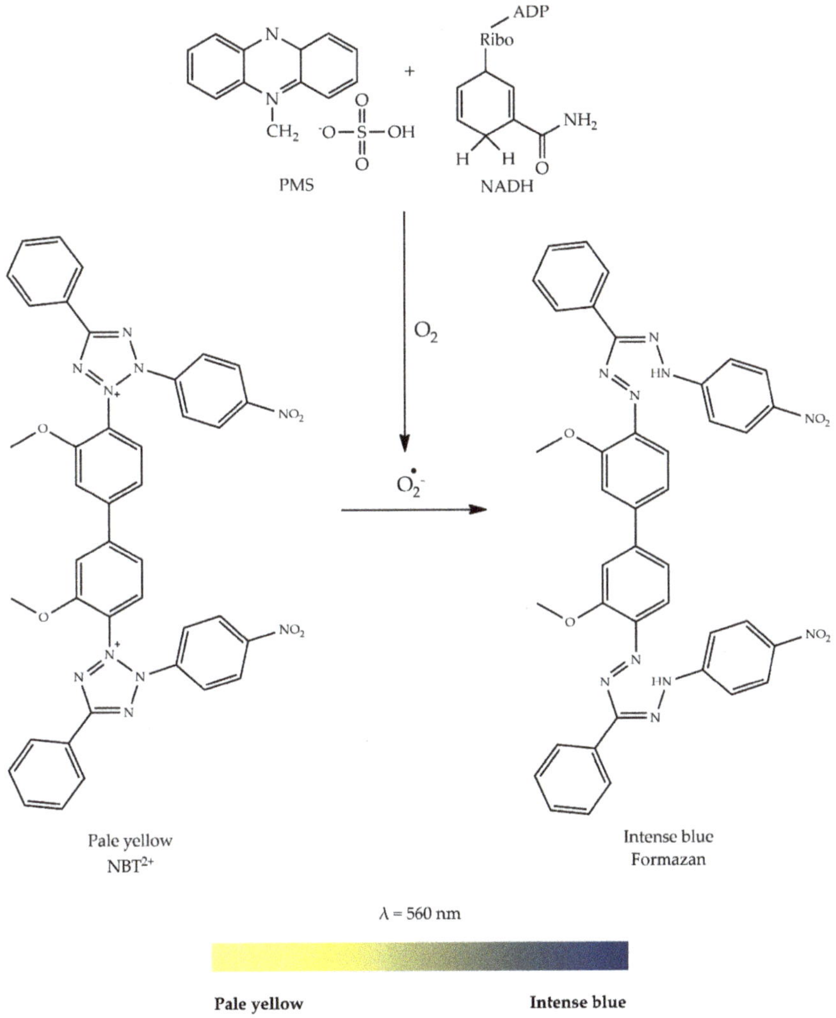

Figure 9. $O_2^{\bullet -}$ reaction mechanism.

Strengths and Limitations

Strengths:
• $O_2^{\bullet-}$ is one of the most important radicals produced inside human body. Hence, they bear resemblance to biological systems in contrast to DPPH or ABTS which are synthetic radicals

Limitations:
• Non-specific since NBT can be reduced by several reductases apart $O_2^{\bullet-}$ [69] • NBT is an expensive reagent and thus it is not affordable by all laboratories

12. Hydrogen Peroxide Scavenging Assay

After the discovery of O_2 by Lavoisier, Scheele, and Priestley in the 18th century, Thenard was the first one who reported the synthesis of H_2O_2 in 1818 [72]. Hydrogen peroxide is a major oxygen metabolite generated in vivo by activated phagocytes and oxidase enzymes. It is a good antimicrobial agent for numerous bacterial and fungal strains [59]. H_2O_2 scavenging activity is assessed based on a peroxidase system involving horseradish peroxidase (HRP), which is the most commonly used enzyme in this assay. The assay generally employs the oxidation of scopoletin by an HRP–H_2O_2 complex formed upon the addition of H_2O_2 and HRP (as illustrated in Scheme 11). Scopoletin is a 7-hydroxy-6-methoxycoumarin found in the roots of plants belonging to the genus *Scopolia*. It is a fluorescent substrate for peroxidase used for the determination of H_2O_2. It has a strong blue fluorescence under UV light [73]. The intensity of fluorescence is directly proportional to the concentration of scopoletin or inversely proportional to the concentration of oxidized scopoletin (i.e., H_2O_2 concentration) [74]. Therefore, the concentration of H_2O_2 can be measured either by monitoring the decrease in fluorescence of scopoletin or by observing the increase in fluorescence caused by the formation of oxidized scopoletin.

When H_2O_2 is mixed with HRP, scopoletin ($C_{10}H_8O_4$) is rapidly oxidized by HRP–H_2O_2 to form a blue colloidal intermediate product with a chemical formula of $C_8H_8O_4$, which absorbs light at 560 nm. The formation of this intermediate results from the loss of the blue fluorescence, since scopoletin is being consumed in the reaction. The blue intermediate is slowly oxidized into an insoluble yellow complex ($C_7H_8O_3$) on standing, which can be read either at 417–402 nm or at 385 nm, depending on different studies [63,75,76]. However, the addition of a potential AO will prevent the oxidation process to occur, thus, hindering the formation of the yellow complex. Consequently, H_2O_2 scavenging can be measured [77]. The assay is conducted at pH 4.5. The reaction is stopped with borate buffer (pH 10). After stopping the reaction, the fluorescence or absorbance is then measured. The scavenging capacity may be measured either fluorometrically or spectrophotometrically. The HRP–scopoletin-based method is preferred over the cytochrome *c* peroxidase method, since the latter method requires complex instrumentation [78]. There is not much information published on the mechanism of reaction on this assay. However, we proposed one mechanism, as shown in Figure 10, together with the colour ribbon representing the colour change in the absence of an AO.

General methodology: Sample solution (100 µL: 0.05 mg/mL) is added to 100 µL of 0.002% of hydrogen peroxide. To the resulting solution, 0.8 mL of phosphate buffer (0.1 M) and 100 mM sodium chloride are added. The reaction mixture is allowed to incubate at 37 °C for 10 min. After the incubation period, 1 mL of phenol red (0.2 mg/mL) with 0.1 mg/mL HRP in 0.1 M phosphate buffer are added. After incubation for 15 min, 50 µL sodium hydroxide (1 M) is added and the absorbance is measured at 610 nm. The hydrogen peroxide activity can be expressed as %inhibition [79].

Chemical reaction:

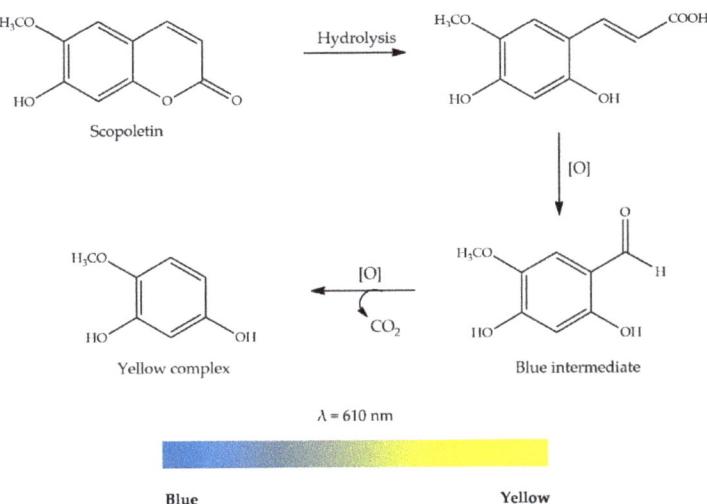

Figure 10. H_2O_2 reaction mechanism.

Strengths and Limitations

Strengths:

- Easy and sensitive [59]
- Specific [80]
- Can quantify H_2O_2 level in cells [78]
- Reagents are easily available

Limitations:

- Substrates are pH sensitive [80]
- Several reductants/or antioxidants for e.g., thiols, ascorbate can compete with scopoletin, leading to an underestimation of H_2O_2 formation [80]
- Similarly, catalase released from disruption of cells may compete with HRP for H_2O_2 [80]
- Quartz cuvettes should be used which are expensive and not affordable by all laboratories

13. Reducing Potential Antioxidant Assays

As discussed earlier, antioxidants can stabilize radicals by donating electrons. In this type of AO assay, the mechanism involves the reduction potential of transition metals, namely iron (Fe) and copper (Cu). It is acknowledged that there is a major uncertainty concerning the role of AO towards free radicals in the presence of metal ions, namely Cu (II) and Fe (III). The role of AO is uncertain in the presence of these metal ions because it is still unclear whether the AO will scavenge the free radicals or chelate with metal ions [81]. Additionally, working with coloured radicals can be problematic, since it is difficult to generate them. In addition, it is hard to maintain their stability (e.g., ABTS or

DPPH) [82]. The antioxidant capacity of a biological sample cannot be evaluated by a single assay, since many factors are not taken into consideration. For instance, not all methods can be used to screen both lipophilic and hydrophilic samples. Possible interferences in reaction mixtures can lead to underestimation or overestimation. We will discuss each reducing potential assay in greater detail in the next sections.

13.1. Ferric Ion Reducing Antioxidant Power (FRAP)

The ferric ion reducing antioxidant power or ferric reducing ability of plasma, abbreviated as FRAP, was developed by Iris Benzie and J. J. Strain [83]. The FRAP method is based on the reduction of ferric-tripyridyltriazine $[Fe^{III}(TPTZ)]^{3+}$, forming an intense blue coloured ferrous complex $[Fe^{II}(TPTZ)]^{2+}$ under acidic conditions (pH 3.6). The chemical reaction is presented in Scheme 12. The colour developed in this assay is intense blue, which is the complementary colour of orange, as shown in the colour wheel in Figure 1. This explains why the absorbance is read at 593 nm. This method was developed in such a way that it could be conducted in every laboratory due to its simplicity, high reproducibility, and simple instrumentation [83]. The redox potential of Fe (III) is approximately 0.70V, which is comparable to the redox potential of $ABTS^{\bullet+}$ (0.68 V) according to the review compiled by Huang et al. (2005). Interestingly, there is a thin line between $ABTS^{\bullet+}$ and FRAP methods except that the ABTS assay is conducted at neutral pH while FRAP is carried out under acidic conditions [8]. However, this assay is non-specific. This is because if any species present in the reaction mixture possesses a redox potential lower than that of Fe (III) (<0.70 V), that species will be responsible for the reduction in $[Fe^{III}(TPTZ)_2]^{3+}$ [83], leading to an underestimation. Importantly, while preparing FRAP reagent, it is essential to add reagents in a specific order. For instance, acetate buffer is added first. $FeCl_3$ is then added, while TPTZ is added last. This order is vital to prevent the reduction of $FeCl_3$ by TPTZ. Colour change and mechanism of reaction are presented in Figure 11.

General methodology: FRAP reagent is prepared by mixing 0.3 M acetate buffer (pH 3.6) and 10 mM 2,4,6-tris(2-pyridyl)-S-triazine in 40 mM hydrochloric acid and ferric chloride (20 mM) at a ratio of 10:1:1 (v/v/v). The sample solution (0.1 mL) is added to 2 mL premixed FRAP reagent and allowed to incubate at room temperature for 30 min. The sample absorbance is then read at 593 nm. FRAP activity can be expressed as equivalents of Trolox, gallic acid, ascorbic acid, quercetin, or α-tocopherol [28].

Chemical reaction:

$[Fe^{III}(TPTZ)_2]^{3+} + ArOH \rightarrow [Fe^{II}(TPTZ)]^{2+} + ArO^{\bullet} + H^+$ Scheme 12

Mechanism of reaction:

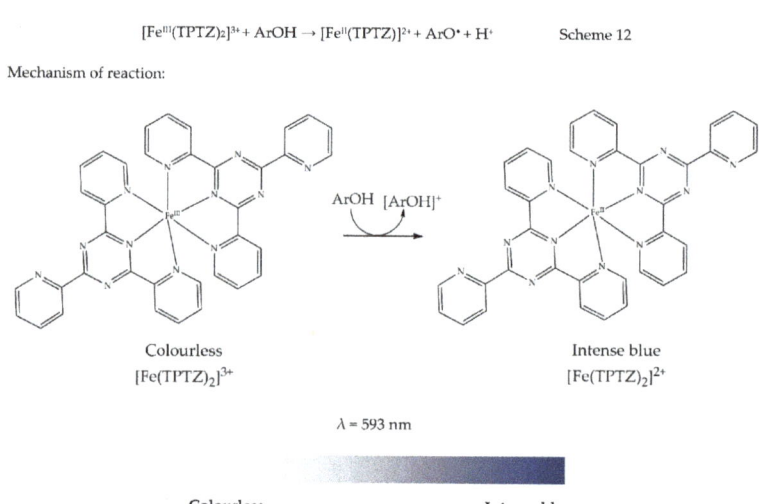

Figure 11. Ferric reducing antioxidant power (FRAP) reaction mechanism.

Strengths and Limitations

Strengths:

- Simple and inexpensive instrumentation [84]
- Highly reproducible and sensitive [83]
- Can screen a wide spectrum of biological samples including plasma, blood, serum, saliva, tears, urine, cerebrospinal fluid, exudates, transudates, and aqueous and organic extracts of drugs, foods, and plants [85]
- Good correlation is usually observed with H_2O_2 scavenging assay [86]

Limitations:

- Non-specific [83]

13.2. Cupric Reducing Antioxidant Capacity (CUPRAC)

The CUPRAC method was developed by Apak, Guclu, Ozyurek, and Karademir [82] from the Analytical Chemistry Department of Istanbul University, seven years after the FRAP method was developed. The sole reason for developing this assay was to bring forward a method that could express the 'total antioxidant' as a nutritional index for food labelling due to the lack of a standard quantitation method. Indeed, this method has been proven to be effective for many polyphenols (namely, phenolic acids, hydroxycinnamic acids, flavonoids, carotenoids, and anthocyanins) in addition to thiols, synthetic AOs, and vitamins C and E. It has been used by many investigators in different laboratories over the last few years since its development. The chromogen used in this assay is bis(neocuproine) copper (II) cation $[Cu (Nc)_2^{2+}]$. Upon its reduction by an AO, the light blue chromophore is reduced into an orange-yellow bis(neocuproine) copper (I) chelate $[Cu (Nc)_2^+]$ that can be read at 450 nm. Reaction time to reach the completion may vary between 30 and 60 min, depending on how fast the AO is. According to a comprehensive review compiled by Özyürek et al. [87], it is essential to allow completion of CUPRAC reaction. If an AO develops colour at a slow pace, an incubation at 50 °C in a water bath for 20 min may be needed, which is viewed as a limitation. While conducting the CUPRAC assay, a sample blank without copper (II) chloride ($CuCl_2$) should be prepared, since absorbance is measured between 400 and 500 nm. However, in the FRAP assay, no sample blank is required, since the absorbance falls after 500 nm. The mechanism of the reaction and the colour change are illustrated by the colour ribbon shown in Figure 12. The chemical reaction is presented in Scheme 13.

General methodology: A reaction mixture containing $CuCl_2$ (1 mL, 10 mM), neocuproine (1 mL, 7.5 mM), and ammonium acetate aqueous buffer at pH 7 (1 mL, 1 M) is prepared. The sample solution (0.5 mL) is added to the premixed reaction mixture. A blank is prepared in a similar manner by adding a 0.5 mL sample solution to 3 mL premixed reaction mixture without $CuCl_2$. The sample and the blank are allowed to incubate at room temperature for 30 min. Their absorbance values are then read at 450 nm. CUPRAC capacity can be expressed either as %inhibition or equivalent of a standard compound, namely Trolox, gallic acid, ascorbic acid, quercetin, or α-tocopherol [28].

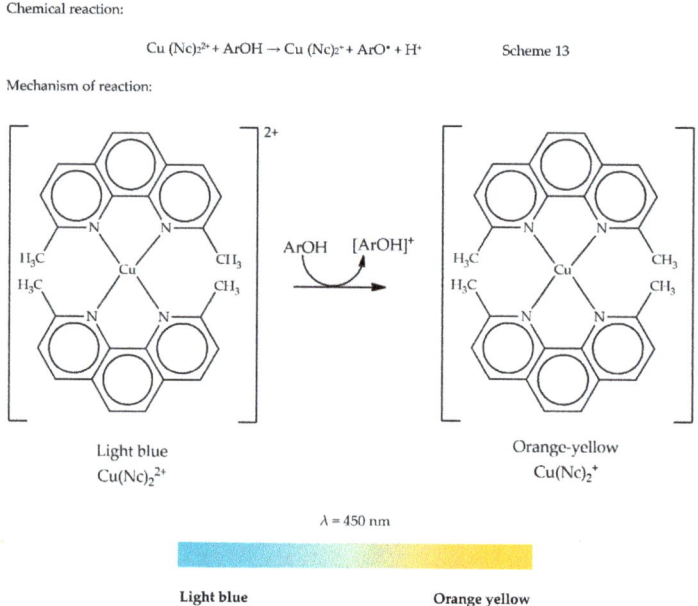

Figure 12. Cupric reducing antioxidant capacity (CUPRAC) reaction mechanism.

Strengths and Limitations

Strengths:

- Reagents are cheap, relatively stable, and more accessible than DPPH and ABTS reagents [81]
- Rapid colour development [81]
- Can screen both lipophilic and hydrophilic samples [81]
- The assay is performed at pH 7, which is close to the physiological pH in contrast to the unrealistic acidic pH 3.6 of FRAP [81]
- Effective for evaluating the AO capacity of synthetic mixtures [81]
- It can detect glutathione and thiol-type AO in contrary to FRAP. The reason lies behind the fact that Fe (III) has a half-filled d orbital which contribute to its chemical inertness, while the electronic structure of Cu (II) triggers fast kinetics [87]
- Simple instrumentation required
- No interferences from chemicals found in solutions reported yet
- Shows good correlation with numerous polyphenolics namely flavonoids, phenolic acids and also, with other AO methods, namely ABTS
- A linear correlation is usually observed with the phosphomolybdenum assay

Limitations:

- Unable to measure antioxidant enzymes [81]
- Depending on CUPRAC version, longer times of measurement may be required [81]
- Sometimes requires incubation at 50 °C in a water bath for 20 min for compounds which develop color slowly namely naringin and naringenin [82]

14. Potassium Ferricyanide Assay

The potassium ferricyanide assay is another type of FRAP method based on the reduction of Fe (III) to Fe (II), usually abbreviated as PFRAP. It can be used to measure the reducing capacity of AO. In addition, it has several other usages such as for the determination of reducing sugars in plants [88], the estimation of pravastatin sodium [89], the determination of dopamine hydrochloride in serum or pharmaceutical samples [90], and the detection of catalase isozymes in either plants or animals [91]. It is noteworthy to point out that this assay can form different coloured complexes upon reaction of the sample of interest with potassium ferricyanide-Fe (III). For instance, in the determination of pravastatin sodium drug, a green chromogen is formed, which exhibits a maximum absorption at 737 nm [89]. However, in the determination of dopamine hydrochloride, a Prussian blue complex is formed, exhibiting a maximal absorption at 735 nm [90]. Thus, it can be said that the colour of the chromogen formed in this AO assay depends on the sample under investigation. In this review, we are interested in biological samples derived from plant materials. Thus, the methodology, colour ribbon, and principle are focused on for the formation of a Prussian blue complex.

The potassium ferricyanide ($K_4[Fe(CN)_6]^{3-}$) assay was originally developed to study the rate of sugar oxidation by Ariyama and Shaffer in 1928. Later, it was implemented in blood sugar analysis [92]. After this, the authors in [93] used this method for the determination of reducing sugars present in plants. Potassium ferricyanide with chemical formula $K_4[Fe(CN)_6]^{3-}$ is a bright red salt that contains octahedrally coordinated ion $[Fe(CN)_6]^{3-}$.

As highlighted in Section 3.1, the colour of a complex results from a change in its electronic transitions. Before explaining the important theory behind the colour change of potassium ferricyanide-Fe (III), some basic chemistry knowledge will be provided. To start with, we need to understand that coordination compounds (often called complexes) are molecules that contain covalent bonds between a transition metal ion and one or more ligands. Such coordinate covalent bonds are formed when the metal ion acts as a Lewis acid (electron-pair acceptor) and ligands act as Lewis bases (electron-pair donors). The covalent bond is formed when the molecular orbital consisting of the lone pair of electrons present on ligands overlap with d-orbitals of the metal ion. These d-orbitals are the frontier orbitals of transition metal complexes. Numerous physical properties of coordination compounds (or complexes), such as colour, shape, reactivity, and stability, are related to the electron occupancy of d-orbitals of the metal ion. Crystal Field Theory (CFT) is the simplest model to explain the structure and properties of transition metal complexes. CFT focuses on the interaction of five d-orbitals of the transition metal ion with ligands surrounding it. According to CFT, an octahedral complex is formed due to electrostatic interaction of the transition metal ion with six negatively charged ligands. To clearly understand CFT, we should know that in the absence of ligands, these five d-orbitals are at the same energy level (degenerate). However, when the metal ion is in the proximity of ligands, those d-orbitals will split into two groups of different energy levels, namely e_g and t_{2g}, due to repulsion caused by the ligands. These e_g orbitals now have two orbitals ($d_{x^2-y^2}$, d_{z^2}) at a higher energy level than the other three t_{2g} orbitals (d_{xy}, d_{xz}, d_{yz}). The energy difference between the e_g and t_{2g} orbitals is denoted as Δ_O, as illustrated in Figure 13. The energy difference depends on the nature of the ligands. In the case of potassium ferricyanide, cyanide (CN^-) is considered as a strong field ligand that causes a big splitting. The value Δ_O increases as the oxidation state of the metal ion increases. In this assay, Fe (III) is reduced to Fe (II). Thus, Δ_O is decreased. Energy (Δ_O) is related to wavelength with the following equation: $E(\Delta_O) = hc/\lambda$, where h is Planck's constant and c is the speed of light [94].

The reduced Fe (II) is read at 700 nm, meaning that a photon at wavelength of 700 nm is absorbed, promoting an electron from a t_{2g} to an e_g orbital, which makes the Fe (II) enter an excitation state (unstable). When the electron returns to its ground state (stable), the energy emitted is equal to the energy corresponding to the red region in a colour wheel. This explains why the reduced form of potassium ferricyanide-Fe (II) appears Prussian blue (dark blue) in colour.

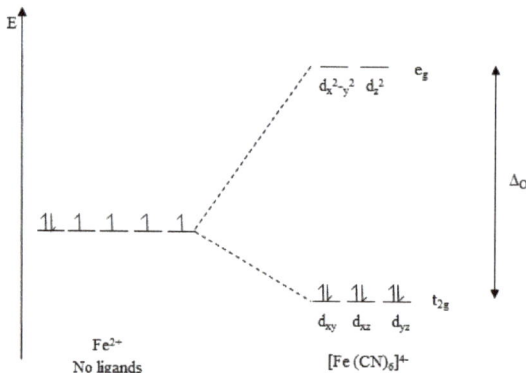

Figure 13. Fe (II) complexes have six electrons in the 5-d orbitals. In the absence of a crystal field (ligands), the orbitals are degenerate. In the presence of ligands (CN$^-$), the d-orbitals split into e_g and t_{2g} orbitals with an energy difference of Δ_O.

The purpose of heating the resulting solution containing sample, buffer, and potassium ferricyanide at 50 °C for 20 min, as proposed in the general methodology of this assay, is to reduce the maximum amount of potassium ferricyanide [88]. The mechanism of the reaction and the colour change are illustrated by the colour ribbon, as shown in Figure 14.

General methodology: Briefly, sample solution (0.5 mL) is mixed with 0.5 mL phosphate buffer (0.2 M, pH 6.6) and 0.5 mL potassium ferricyanide (1%). The resulting mixture is incubated at 50 °C for 20 min. After the incubation period, 0.5 mL trichloroacetic acid (10%), 2.5 mL deionized water, and 0.5 mL ferric chloride (0.1%) are added to the mixture. The sample absorbance is read at 700 nm. The reduction of Fe (III) to Fe (II) can be expressed as %inhibition or equivalent of a standard compound (e.g., Trolox) [28].

Chemical reaction:

$$4FeCl_3 + 3K_4[Fe(CN)_6]^{3-} \rightarrow Fe_4[Fe(CN)_6]_3{}^+ + 12KCl$$

Mechanism of reaction:

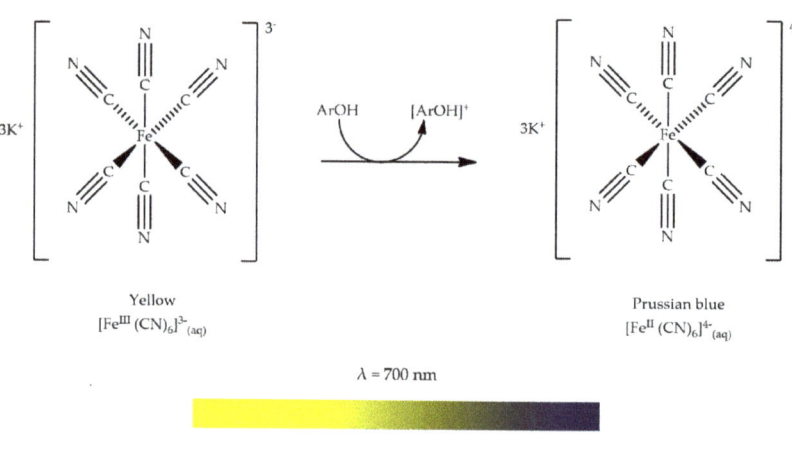

Figure 14. Potassium ferricyanide reaction mechanism.

Strengths and Limitations

Strengths:
• Cheap, simple, and reliable method [88]
• Since absorbance is read at a high wavelength, possible interference from the reaction mixture is minimized [90]
• Simple instrumentation is used

Limitations:
• If the samples are very active, pellets can be observed in tubes. Thus, centrifugation will be needed
• The assay cannot be performed in microplates which can be time-consuming and tiring while screening many samples
• If samples have a high level of protein, precipitation with trichloroacetic acid may be hard

15. Phosphomolybdenum Assay

The phosphomolybdenum assay is a quantitative method developed by Prieto et al. [95]. This assay was originally used to quantify vitamin E in seeds. Considering simplicity and sensitivity, its application has been extended to plant extracts [95]. The assay is widely used by many investigators. The phosphomolybdenum method follows either an ET or HAT mechanism, causing the reduction of molybdenum (VI) to molybdenum (V). The absorbance of the greenish-blue complex can be read at 695 nm [96]. The chemical reaction is presented in Scheme 14.

A reaction endpoint of about 90 min is enough for complete formation of the greenish-blue phosphomolybdenum complex. The greenish-blue colour results from the reduction of ammonium molybdate into an oxide known as the Keggin ion $[H_3PO_4(MoO_3)_{12}]$ under acidic conditions. The resulting Keggin ion is then reduced into $[H_4PMo_8^{VI}Mo_4^{V}O_{40}]^{3-}$ in the presence of an AO [97,98].

The formation of the phosphomolybdenum complex is possible at room temperature. However, the rate of reaction is very slow, and the yield of the complex is low. Generally, to increase the rate of a chemical reaction, we either increase the concentration, temperature, or the surface area of the reactant or by adding a catalyst to the reaction. In the case of phosphomolybdenum assay, Prieto, Pineda, and Aguilar [95] have reported that the formation of the complex is temperature-dependent. Indeed, an increase in temperature of 95 °C has accelerated the reaction rate and increased the yield of the green phosphomolybdenum complex [95]. To determine the precision of this assay, a comparison was made with a standard HPLC method. Statistical results from Student's t-test showed no significant difference between the phosphomolybdenum assay and the HPLC method at a confidence level of 95% [95].

The colour developed in this assay is green or greenish-blue, which is the complementary color of red, as shown in the colour wheel (Figure 1). This explains why the absorbance is read at 695 nm. Furthermore, this assay does not require any blank since the maximum absorbance is read after 500 nm, similar to the FRAP assay. The phosphomolybdenum assay has many pros and cons as all other AO assays. One of its main limitations is for screening essential oil samples. For instance, if an essential oil sample does not show good DPPH activity, significant TAC can be observed with the phosphomolybdenum assay, showing pronounced absorbance values which then require dilution of the sample. The reason behind this inconsistency is related to complex chemical compositions of essential oils. Essential oils are complex biological samples containing multiple compounds, mainly terpenoids, thymol, carvacrol, and menthol that are strong reducing agents. Interestingly, the correlation between phosphomolybdenum assay and other AO assays remains debatable, since some studies have reported a correlation between phosphomolybdenum assay and free radical scavenging activity [96], while other studies have denied such correlation [99]. Similarly, one study has suggested a good correlation between phosphomolybdenum assay and reducing capacity assays (FRAP, CUPRAC) [100], while another study has reported a weak correlation between FRAP and CUPRAC assays [101]. Prieto, Pineda, and Aguilar [95] have highlighted that DPPH and ABTS$^{\bullet+}$ can detect AOs such as flavonoids and phenols, while phosphomolybdenum can generally detect AOs, namely ascorbic acid, some phenolics, α-tocopherol, and carotenoids. This may explain why a high polyphenolic content does not reflect a significant TAC in the phosphomolybdenum assay. The colour change and mechanism of reaction are presented in Figure 15.

General methodology: Phosphomolybdenum reagent solution is prepared by mixing 0.6 M sulfuric acid, 28 mM sodium phosphate, and 4 mM ammonium molybdate. The sample solution (0.3 mL) is added to the premixed phosphomolybdenum reagent solution and allowed to incubate at 95 °C for 90 min. The sample absorbance is read at 695 nm. Results can be expressed either as %inhibition or equivalent of a standard compound, namely ascorbic acid [28,95].

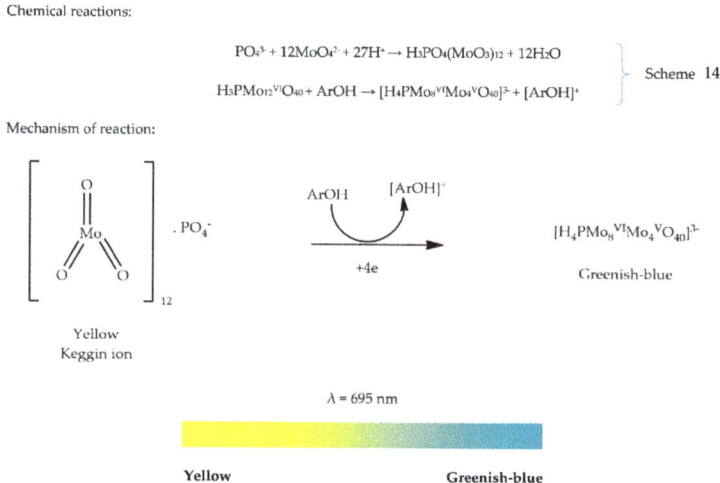

Figure 15. Phosphomolybdenum reaction mechanism.

Strengths and Limitations

Strengths:

- Formation of the phosphomolybdenum complex is independent of the different organic solvents (hexane, methanol, ethanol, and dimethyl sulfoxide) used to prepare AO or extract stock solution [95]
- Simple, sensitive, and cheap reagents are used [95]
- Can screen a wide spectrum of samples, including lipophilic plant extracts, vegetal oils, butter, serum, pharmaceutical, and cosmeceutical samples [95]

Limitations:

- Bad correlation is observed with bioactive compounds (phenolics, flavonoids) [86]
- A weak correlation is usually reported with free radical scavenging assays, namely DPPH [99]
- Time-consuming. Since high temperature (95 °C) is required, the assay should be performed in test tubes instead of microplates, which could be problematic while screening a large number of samples
- Bad correlation with bioactive compounds in essential oil samples due to their complex chemical composition
- Non-specific, since the assay does not detect only phenolics but also ascorbic acid, carotenoids and α-tocopherol [95]

16. Metal Chelating (Ferrous Ion Chelating) Assay

Free radicals can also originate from heavy and transition metals, namely mercury, lead, arsenic, and iron, leading to diseases associated with oxidative stress. To eliminate these noxious metals, chelation therapy is applied. Unfailingly, AOs once again have proven their worth in radical chemistry. One of the possible mechanisms followed by AOs is chelation of transition metals [102]. Basically, chelation therapy is a treatment that uses medicine (drugs) to remove these toxic metals from our body via excretion (urine). Arsenic is one of the oldest poisonous agents known. Long exposure to arsenic may lead to numerous health complications, including neurodegenerative diseases, cardiovascular diseases, and skin cancer [103]. Another metal ion involved in chelation therapy is iron. Although iron takes part in every cell function, it is frequently responsible for several pathological diseases, namely liver and heart problems, cancer, neurodegenerative diseases, and diabetes. Treatment of iron toxicity involves decontamination of gastrointestinal and administration of chelating agents [104]. The removal of iron, copper, and lead from the central nervous system is a slow process, since penetration of chelators across the blood–brain barrier is restricted [103]. To improve the efficacy of chelation therapy, Flora and Pachauri [104] have suggested the use of a combination therapy consisting of more than one chelating agent or the use of AOs or nutraceuticals.

The ferrous ion chelating assay is performed according to the method described by Dinis et al. [105]. Under mild acidic conditions (pH 6), phenolic compounds (Ph-OH) can only bind with a fraction of Fe^{2+}, while the remaining Fe^{2+} ions can react with ferrozine ($C_{20}H_{12}N_4Na_2O_6S_2$) to form a ferrous ion–ferrozine complex which is stable, water-soluble and red or deep purple in colour. The chemical reaction is presented in Scheme 15. In the presence of a chelator/extract/AO, the formation of the complex is hindered, leading to a loss in the red or deep purple colour. The chemical reaction is presented in Scheme 16. Measurement of this decrease in colour by spectrophotometry gives an estimation of the binding ability of the chelator/extract/AO. The ferrous ion–ferrozine complex shows maximum absorbance at 562 nm. The higher the absorbance value at 562 nm, the higher the concentration of the ferrous ion–ferrozine complex and the lower the binding ability of the chelator/extract/AO [17,106]. The mechanism of the reaction and the colour change are illustrated by the colour ribbon in the absence of an AO, as shown in Figure 16.

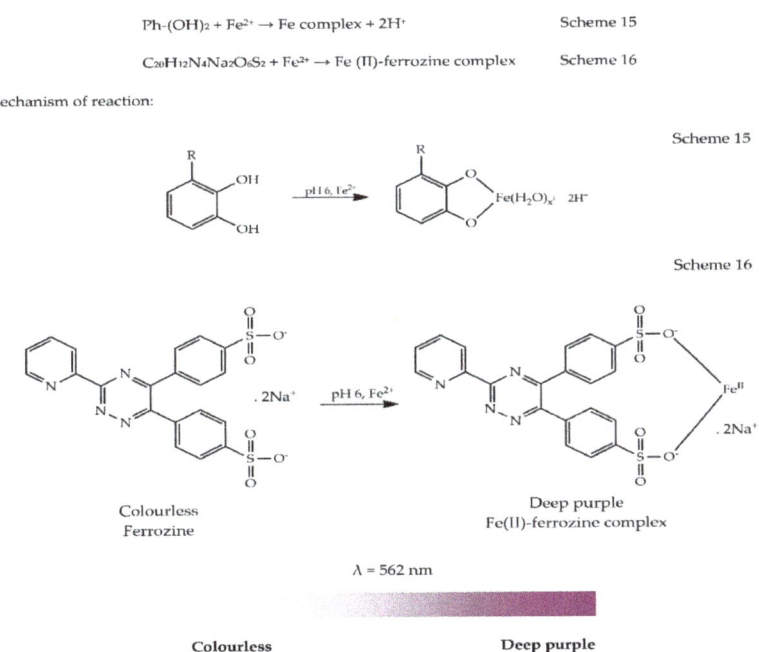

Figure 16. Metal chelating reaction mechanism.

Strengths and Limitations

Strengths:
• Easily available and cheap reagents [17] • Simple instrumentation is used • Good repeatability and reproducibility [17] • Assay can be carried out in both test tubes and 96-well microplates
Limitations:
• Non-specific, since this assay does not only react with phenolic compounds but also with peptides and sulphates present in the medium • Sometimes, results from total bioactive components (phenolic, flavonoids) assay do not correlate with the results of metal chelating • Bad correlation with FRAP, CUPRAC, ABTS, and DPPH assays

General methodology: Briefly, sample solution (2 mL) is added to 0.05 mL $FeCl_2$ solution (2 mM). The reaction is initiated by adding 0.2 mL ferrozine (5 mM). A blank is prepared without ferrozine (i.e., to 2 mL sample solution, 0.05 mL $FeCl_2$ (2 mM), and 0.2 mL water are added). The reaction mixture is incubated at room temperature for 10 min. The sample and blank absorbances are read at 562 nm. The absorbance of the blank is subtracted from that of the sample to obtain real absorbance. Results are expressed as either %inhibition or an equivalent of a standard compound. EDTA or BHA can be used a positive control [28,105].

17. β-Carotene Bleaching Assay

Antioxidant capacity determined by the β-carotene bleaching assay involves a different scenario compared to the other AO assays discussed above. This assay measures the rate of oxidative destruction of β-carotene by free radicals generated from oxidized linoleic acid in an emulsion system. In the presence of an AO, bleaching of β-carotene occurs [107]. Since an emulsion system is involved in this AO method, the famous theory called 'Polar paradox theory' is directly applied. William. L. Porter introduced this theory in 1980. According to this theory, polar (hydrophilic) AOs are more effective in less polar media (bulk oils) while non-polar (lipophilic) AOs are more effective in more polar media (emulsions), solely based on the different polarities in which AOs are present [108]. However, the authors in [109] have suggested that this theory should be re-evaluated, since the theory suffers some contradictions based on several studies conducted. For instance, in addition to the polarity of media, molecular size, and concentration of AOs should be taken into consideration. A non-linear relationship (a bell-shaped curve) between AO activity and polarity has been observed due to interference of the molecular size of AO in this relationship, as illustrated in Figure 17. This curve explains that as the size of chain lengths of phenolic AOs increases, the lipophilicity also increases, resulting in an increase in AO activity until a threshold is reached. After a certain chain length, a drastic drop in AO activity is observed. This threshold phenomenon is referred to as the cut-off effect. Reasons behind such cut-off effect have been discussed in detail in the review of Shahidi and Zhong [109].

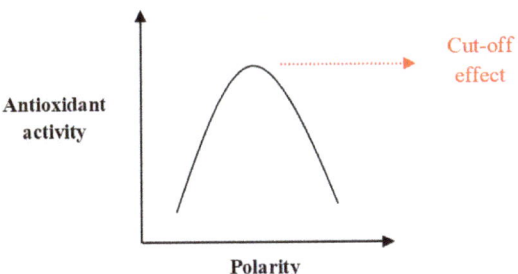

Figure 17. Cut-off effect of antioxidant activity with respect to polarity (Adapted from Shahidi and Zhong [109]).

Based on the polar paradox theory, derivatives with high lipophilicity exhibit a stronger inhibitory effect on β-carotene bleaching. It is common to observe a high surface-to-volume ratio of oil-in-water emulsions in food systems. Consequently, it is important to determine the effectiveness of AOs in oil-in-water emulsions to evaluate their AO properties before their application in food systems [110]. The prevention of autooxidation of emulsified linoleic acid in extracts was first evaluated using the method developed by Marco [111]. The protocol was modified over the years for convenience while minimizing its weakness. The modified method is highly reproducible compared to the original one. It can quantify both AOs and pro-oxidants. Although the modified method has been accepted as a method for screening various food and biological samples, it is not considered as a universal method [112]. According to published literature, the level of reproducibility of this assay differed. For instance, Prieto et al. [112] reported high reproducibility, while Mikami et al. [113] defined the rate of reproducibility as low. The β-carotene–linoleic acid method involves decolorization of the orange-yellow or dark yellow β-carotene solution caused by radicals generated (lipid or lipid peroxyl radicals) by instantaneous oxidation of fatty acids present in an aqueous emulsion of linoleic acid ($C_{18}H_{32}O_2$) and β-carotene ($C_{40}H_{56}$) (lipophilic oxidizable substrate). Lipids or lipid peroxyl radicals are generated from linoleic acid upon exposure to oxygenated distilled water. Once lipids or lipid peroxyl radicals are formed, they are attacked by β-carotene, causing decolorization of β-carotene. The decolorization is due to the breaking of π-conjugation by the addition reaction of radicals into a C=C bond of β-carotene. Chemical reactions are presented in Schemes 17 and 18. In the presence of an AO, the decolorization is slowed down because AO will compete with β-carotene to quench radicals. Quantification of the AO is based on the different rates that β-carotene decays, usually measured at 490–470 nm [112,114,115]. The mechanism of the reaction and the colour change are illustrated by the colour ribbon in the absence of an AO, as shown in Figure 18.

General methodology: The β-carotene–linoleic acid model system is prepared by dissolving 0.5 mg β-carotene in 1 mL chloroform followed by the addition of 25 mL linoleic acid and 200 mg Tween 40. A rotary evaporator is used to completely evaporate the chloroform added into the system. To the resulting solution, 100 mL of oxygenated distilled water is added followed by vigorous shaking. To the test tube containing 0.5 mL sample solution (1 mg/mL), 1.5 mL of the reaction mixture is added. The emulsion system is then incubated at 50 °C for 2 h. Blank and standard solutions are similarly prepared. Absorbance values of the sample and the blank are then read at 490 nm. The measurement of the absorbance is continued until the colour of β-carotene disappears [28,112]. The bleaching rate (R) of β-carotene is calculated using Equation (1):

$$R = \left[\frac{ln(a|b)}{t}\right] \quad (1)$$

where ln = natural log, a = absorbance at time 0, b = absorbance at time t (30, 60, 90, and 120 min). The antioxidant activity (AA) is calculated in terms of % inhibition with respect to the control using Equation (2):

$$AA = \left(\frac{Rcontrol - Rsample}{Rcontrol}\right) \times 100 \qquad (2)$$

Chemical reactions:

$$C_{18}H_{32}O_2 \rightarrow C_{18}H_{32}O_2{}^\bullet \rightarrow C_{18}H_{32}O_2\text{-OO}^\bullet \qquad \text{Scheme 17}$$
$$\text{Linoleic acid} \quad \text{Lipid radical} \quad (\text{LOO}^\bullet)$$

$$C_{40}H_{56} \rightarrow C_{40}H_{56}\text{-OO}^\bullet \qquad \text{Scheme 18}$$

Mechanism of reaction:

Scheme 17

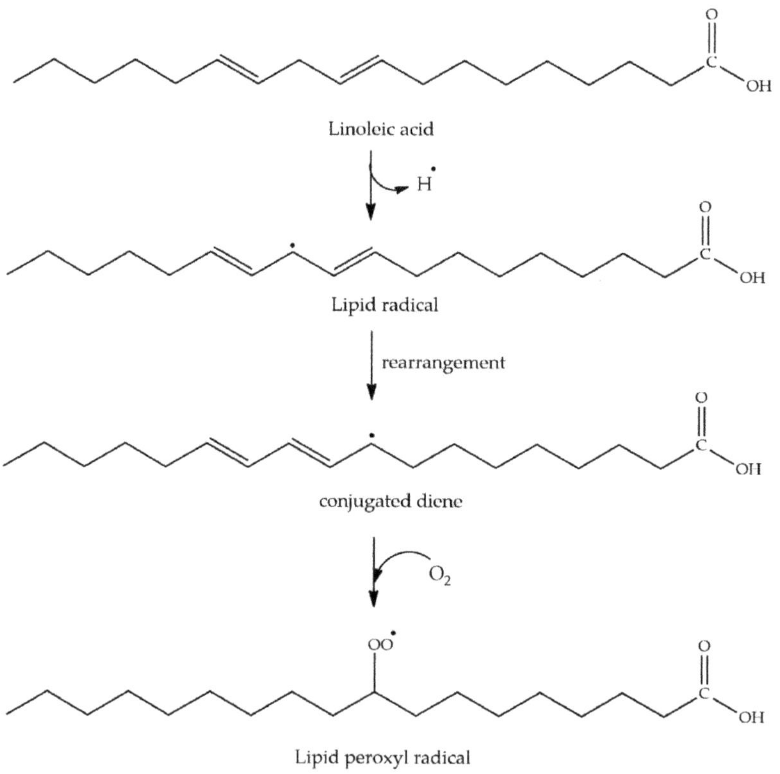

Linoleic acid

Lipid radical

rearrangement

conjugated diene

O_2

Lipid peroxyl radical

Figure 18. *Cont.*

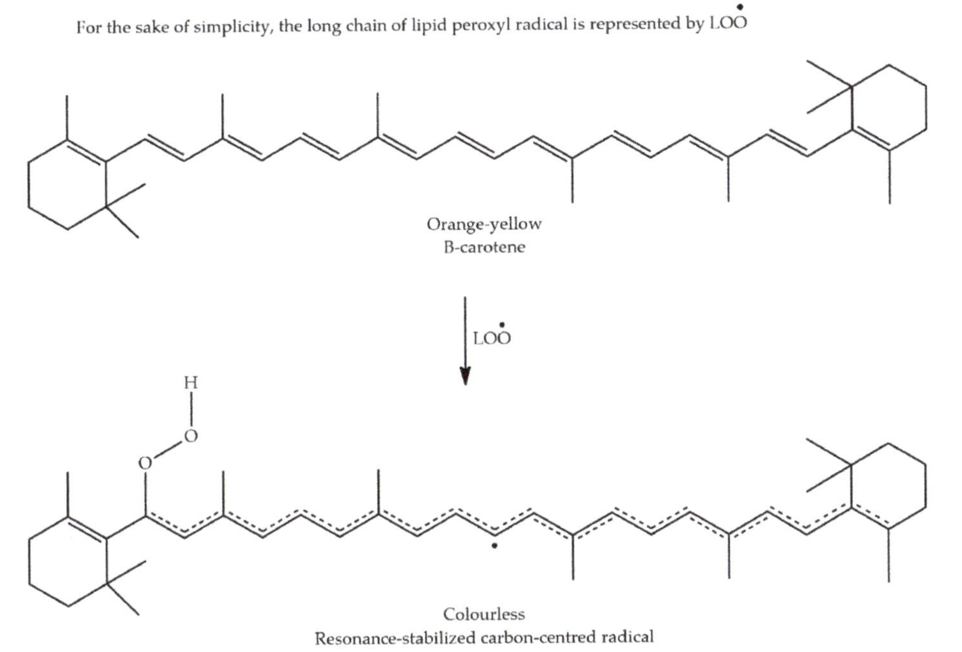

For the sake of simplicity, the long chain of lipid peroxyl radical is represented by LOO•

Orange-yellow
β-carotene

↓ LOO•

Colourless
Resonance-stabilized carbon-centred radical

Figure 18. β-carotene reaction mechanism.

Strengths and Limitations

Strengths:

- Highly reproducible [112]
- Can screen both lipophilic and hydrophilic samples [114]

Limitations:

- Time-consuming
- Sometimes, the results from total bioactive components (phenolic, flavonoids) assay do not correlate with the results of this assay
- Bad correlation with numerous assays, namely FRAP, CUPRAC, ABTS, and DPPH
- Difficulty in interpreting results in the presence of bad correlations
- Low reproducibility [113]
- Sensitive to oxygen, pH, temperature, and solvent effects [111,112]

18. Conclusions

The science community is always avid for new technologies, new solutions, new applications, new methodologies, new products, and so on. This keen interest is for better advancement to provide more reliable and efficient results. After conducting a thorough literature search for the compilation of this present review, we noticed that the existing in vitro antioxidant assays possessed numerous controversies affecting their reliability. Presently, a universal and optimized protocol for the determination of antioxidant capacities is lacking. We do not have a standard assay that can give us an overall image of the antioxidant capacity that a test sample possesses. However, a combination of a few assays (minimum three) must be carried out to have a realistic assessment of the antioxidant capacity that a sample exhibit. This has been found to be time-consuming and expensive, since many reagents are needed.

As discussed earlier in this review, different assays follow either the HAT or the SET mechanism or chelation of metal ions. Interestingly, a few antioxidant methods involve specific theories in addition to the type of mechanism they follow. For instance, the β-carotene assay is directly linked to the Polar Paradox Theory, since the assay is conducted in an emulsified medium and the potassium ferricyanide assay is related to the Crystal Field Theory (CFT) due to its octahedral structure surrounded by ligands (CN^-). As expected, antioxidant assays hold a lot of chemistry. During the last few years, shreds of evidence have piled up against the methods used to measure antioxidant activity in biological samples. Several reviews have been published with considerably different opinions. It seems that there is no consensus of opinions among scientists, most probably because the area of antioxidants is such a complex topic. Since a standardized and thoroughly validated assay is lacking, it is difficult to make a comparison between results gathered by different research groups. It is also difficult to conduct suitable quality control for antioxidant products in food and nutraceutical industries [8]. In addition, existing published results remain questionable and inconclusive. Usually, after a preliminary screening (in vitro analysis) is performed, scientists tend to embark on in vivo testing and later, in clinical research. In that sense, if there is a serious shortfall in in vitro results, the following in vivo analysis together with advanced clinical research can be compromised, which represents a major hurdle.

Based on the existing literature, the current antioxidant assays have been reported to possess several strengths such as simple procedure, rapid analysis time, screening of many samples in a timely fashion, cheap reagents, and simple instrumentation being used. These strengths are generally good but not strong enough to support the efficacy and reliability of these assays as they are seriously flawed. Overall, antioxidant methods are non-specific, non-sensitive, bear no resemblance to biological systems, have bad correlation with bioactive compounds, and reaction of other species to react with the oxidant leading to overestimation is possible, to cite a few. To be able to develop a universal and reliable antioxidant assay, these limitations can be addressed by answering the following questions: (1) What are the real protective properties of antioxidants? (2) What type of species in these antioxidant assays can provide protection or which substrates are being oxidized and what products will inhibit the oxidation? (3) Is there any possible effect caused by other chemical species present in the system under investigation? (4) What can be done to improve the similarity of these antioxidant assays to biological systems, i.e., how to reduce the gap between in vitro methods and in vivo experiments? (5) Under which conditions we should work to improve the sensitivity and specificity? (6) How can underestimation and overestimation of antioxidants be prevented? (7) How can poor correlation between bioactive components (phenolic, flavonoid) and antioxidants be solved? Huang, Ou, and Prior [8] have mentioned that if we claim antioxidant activity of tested samples solely based on assays such as DPPH, ABTS, FRAP, and CUPRAC, it would be unscientific, exaggerated, and out of context, since they bear no similarity to biological systems.

In conclusion, it is of paramount importance to develop a proper and universal antioxidant method emphasizing the fundamental chemistry rather than concentrating on the development of an easy, simple, economical, and rapid assay with the aim to better elucidate radical quenching, reducing capacity or metal chelation ability of different groups of compounds present in biological samples. Figure 19 illustrates a flowchart showing important steps in the development of a universal antioxidant assay in a sequential order. Finally, we must learn how to exploit this information for a more effective application in the clinical context.

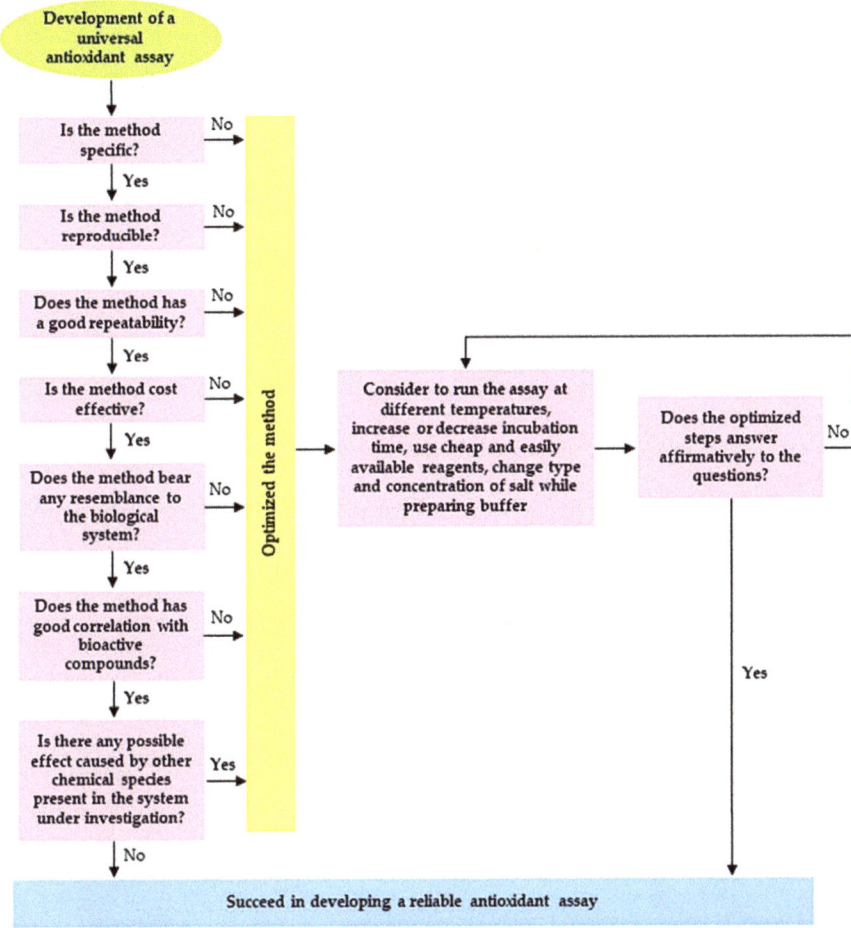

Figure 19. Flowchart with proposed steps to follow in order to develop a universal antioxidant assay.

Author Contributions: Conceptualization, N.B.S., M.F.M., and D.M.; formal analysis, M.F.M., N.B.S., G.Z.; project administration, M.F.M. validation, M.F.M. and N.B.S.; writing—original draft, M.F.M. and N.B.S.; writing—review and editing, M.F.M., N.B.S., D.M., S.A. and G.Z. All authors have read and agreed to the published version of the manuscript.

Funding: This research received no external funding.

Conflicts of Interest: All the authors declare that there is no conflict of interest.

References

1. Mozahheb, N.; Arefian, E.; Amoozegar, M.A. Designing a whole cell bioreporter to show antioxidant activities of agents that work by promotion of the KEAP1–NRF2 signaling pathway. *Sci. Rep.* **2019**, *9*, 3248. [CrossRef] [PubMed]
2. Fasiku, V.; Omolo, C.A.; Govender, T. Free radical-releasing systems for targeting biofilms. *J. Control. Release* **2020**, *322*, 248–273. [CrossRef] [PubMed]

3. Thirunavukkarasu, G.K.; Nirmal, G.R.; Lee, H.; Lee, M.; Park, I.; Lee, J.Y. On-demand generation of heat and free radicals for dual cancer therapy using thermal initiator- and gold nanorod-embedded PLGA nanocomplexes. *J. Ind. Eng. Chem.* **2019**, *69*, 405–413. [CrossRef]
4. Nguyen, V.B.; Wang, S.-L.; Nguyen, A.D.; Lin, Z.-H.; Doan, C.T.; Tran, T.N.; Huang, H.T.; Kuo, Y.-H. Bioactivity-guided purification of novel herbal antioxidant and anti-NO compounds from *Euonymus laxiflorus* champ. *Molecules* **2018**, *24*, 120. [CrossRef] [PubMed]
5. Yahia, Y.; Benabderrahim, M.A.; Tlili, N.; Bagues, M.; Nagaz, K. Bioactive compounds, antioxidant and antimicrobial activities of extracts from different plant parts of two *Ziziphus* Mill. species. *PLoS ONE* **2020**, *15*, e0232599. [CrossRef]
6. Opitz, S.E.W.; Smrke, S.; Goodman, B.A.; Yeretzian, C. Chapter 26—Methodology for the measurement of antioxidant capacity of coffee: A validated platform composed of three complementary antioxidant assays. In *Processing and Impact on Antioxidants in Beverages*; Preedy, V., Ed.; Academic Press: San Diego, CA, USA, 2014; pp. 253–264. [CrossRef]
7. Carocho, M.; Ferreira, I.C. A review on antioxidants, prooxidants and related controversy: Natural and synthetic compounds, screening and analysis methodologies and future perspectives. *Food Chem. Toxicol.* **2013**, *51*, 15–25. [CrossRef]
8. Huang, D.; Ou, B.; Prior, R.L. The chemistry behind antioxidant capacity assays. *J. Agric. Food Chem.* **2005**, *53*, 1841–1856. [CrossRef]
9. Fortalezas, S.; Tavares, L.; Pimpão, R.; Tyagi, M.; Pontes, V.; Alves, M.P.; McDougall, G.; Stewart, D.; Ferreira, B.R.; Santos, N.C. Antioxidant properties and neuroprotective capacity of strawberry tree fruit (*Arbutus unedo*). *Nutrients* **2010**, *2*, 214–229. [CrossRef]
10. Halliwell, B. Free radicals and antioxidants—Quo Vadis? *Trends Pharmacol. Sci.* **2011**, *32*, 125–130. [CrossRef]
11. Granato, D.; Shahidi, F.; Wrolstad, R.; Kilmartin, P.; Melton, L.D.; Hidalgo, F.J.; Miyashita, K.; van Camp, J.; Alasalvar, C.; Ismail, A.B.; et al. Antioxidant activity, total phenolics and flavonoids contents: Should we ban in vitro screening methods? *Food Chem.* **2018**, *264*, 471–475. [CrossRef]
12. Re, R.; Pellegrini, N.; Proteggente, A.; Pannala, A.; Yang, M.; Rice-Evans, C. Antioxidant activity applying an improved ABTS radical cation decolorization assay. *Free Radic. Biol. Med.* **1999**, *26*, 1231–1237. [CrossRef]
13. Alam, M.N.; Bristi, N.J.; Rafiquzzaman, M. Review on in vivo and in vitro methods evaluation of antioxidant activity. *Saudi Pharm. J.* **2013**, *21*, 143–152. [CrossRef] [PubMed]
14. Carocho, M.; Morales, P.; Ferreira, I.C.F.R. Antioxidants: Reviewing the chemistry, food applications, legislation and role as preservatives. *Trends Food Sci. Technol.* **2018**, *71*, 107–120. [CrossRef]
15. Ratnam, D.V.; Ankola, D.D.; Bhardwaj, V.; Sahana, D.K.; Kumar, M.N. Role of antioxidants in prophylaxis and therapy: A pharmaceutical perspective. *J. Control. Release* **2006**, *113*, 189–207. [CrossRef]
16. Kim, D.-O.; Lee, K.W.; Lee, H.J.; Lee, C.Y. Vitamin C equivalent antioxidant capacity (VCEAC) of phenolic phytochemicals. *J. Agric. Food Chem.* **2002**, *50*, 3713–3717. [CrossRef]
17. Santos, J.S.; Alvarenga Brizola, V.R.; Granato, D. High-throughput assay comparison and standardization for metal chelating capacity screening: A proposal and application. *Food Chem.* **2017**, *214*, 515–522. [CrossRef]
18. Rubio, C.P.; Hernández-Ruiz, J.; Martinez-Subiela, S.; Tvarijonaviciute, A.; Ceron, J.J. Spectrophotometric assays for total antioxidant capacity (TAC) in dog serum: An update. *BMC Vet. Res.* **2016**, *12*, 166. [CrossRef]
19. Apak, R.; Güçlü, K.; Özyürek, M.; Çelik, S.E. Mechanism of antioxidant capacity assays and the CUPRAC (cupric ion reducing antioxidant capacity) assay. *Microchim. Acta* **2008**, *160*, 413–419. [CrossRef]
20. Moharram, H.; Youssef, M. Methods for determining the antioxidant activity: A review. *Alex. J. Food Sci. Technol.* **2014**, *11*, 31–42.
21. Sánchez-Rangel, J.C.; Benavides, J.; Heredia, J.B.; Cisneros-Zevallos, L.; Jacobo-Velázquez, D.A. The Folin–Ciocalteu assay revisited: Improvement of its specificity for total phenolic content determination. *Anal. Methods* **2013**, *5*, 5990–5999. [CrossRef]
22. Ainsworth, E.A.; Gillespie, K.M. Estimation of total phenolic content and other oxidation substrates in plant tissues using Folin–Ciocalteu reagent. *Nat. Protoc.* **2007**, *2*, 875–877. [CrossRef] [PubMed]
23. Aktumsek, A.; Zengin, G.; Guler, G.O.; Cakmak, Y.S.; Duran, A. Screening for in vitro antioxidant properties and fatty acid profiles of five *Centaurea* L. species from Turkey flora. *Food Chem. Toxicol.* **2011**, *49*, 2914–2920. [CrossRef] [PubMed]

24. Bastola, K.P.; Guragain, Y.N.; Bhadriraju, V.; Vadlani, P.V. Evaluation of standards and interfering compounds in the determination of phenolics by Folin–Ciocalteu assay method for effective bioprocessing of biomass. *Am. J. Chem.* **2017**, *8*, 416–431. [CrossRef]
25. Blois, M.S. Antioxidant determinations by the use of a stable free radical. *Nature* **1958**, *181*, 1199–1200. [CrossRef]
26. Foti, M.C. Use and abuse of the DPPH• radical. *J. Agric. Food Chem.* **2015**, *63*, 8765–8776. [CrossRef] [PubMed]
27. Gupta, D. Methods for determination of antioxidant capacity: A review. *Int. J. Pharm. Sci. Res.* **2015**, *6*, 546–566.
28. Zengin, G.; Sarikurkcu, C.; Uyar, P.; Aktumsek, A.; Uysal, S.; Kocak, M.S.; Ceylan, R. *Crepis foetida* L. subsp. rhoeadifolia (Bieb.) Celak. As a source of multifunctional agents: Cytotoxic and phytochemical evaluation. *J. Funct. Foods* **2015**, *17*, 698–708. [CrossRef]
29. Kedare, S.B.; Singh, R.P. Genesis and development of DPPH method of antioxidant assay. *J. Food Sci. Technol.* **2011**, *48*, 412–422. [CrossRef]
30. Gil, M.I.; Tomas-Barberan, F.A.; Hess-Pierce, B.; Holcroft, D.M.; Kader, A.A. Antioxidant activity of pomegranate juice and its relationship with phenolic composition and processing. *J. Agric. Food Chem.* **2000**, *48*, 4581–4589. [CrossRef]
31. Bondet, V.; Brand-Williams, W.; Berset, C. Kinetics and Mechanisms of antioxidant activity using the DPPH• free radical method. *LWT Food Sci. Technol.* **1997**, *30*, 609–615. [CrossRef]
32. Schaich, K.M.; Tian, X.; Xie, J. Hurdles and pitfalls in measuring antioxidant efficacy: A critical evaluation of ABTS, DPPH, and ORAC assays. *J. Funct. Foods* **2015**, *14*, 111–125. [CrossRef]
33. Ancerewicz, J.; Migliavacca, E.; Carrupt, P.A.; Testa, B.; Bree, F.; Zini, R.; Tillement, J.P.; Labidalle, S.; Guyot, D.; Chauvet-Monges, A.M.; et al. Structure-property relationships of trimetazidine derivatives and model compounds as potential antioxidants. *Free Radic. Biol. Med.* **1998**, *25*, 113–120. [CrossRef]
34. Min, D.B.; Boff, J.M. Lipid oxidation of edible oil. In *Food Lipids: Chemistry, Nutrition and Biotechnology*; Marcel Dekker: New York, NY, USA, 2002; pp. 335–363. [CrossRef]
35. Miller, N.J.; Rice-Evans, C.; Davies, M.J.; Gopinathan, V.; Milner, A. A novel method for measuring antioxidant capacity and its application to monitoring the antioxidant status in premature neonates. *Clin. Sci.* **1993**, *84*, 407–412. [CrossRef]
36. Miller, N.J.; Rice-Evans, C.A. Factors influencing the antioxidant activity determined by the ABTS•+ radical cation assay. *Free Radic. Res.* **1997**, *26*, 195–199. [CrossRef] [PubMed]
37. Cerretani, L.; Bendini, A. Chapter 67—Rapid assays to evaluate the antioxidant capacity of phenols in virgin olive oil. In *Olives and Olive Oil in Health and Disease Prevention*; Preedy, V.R., Watson, R.R., Eds.; Academic Press: San Diego, CA, USA, 2010; pp. 625–635. [CrossRef]
38. Magalhães, L.M.; Segundo, M.A.; Reis, S.; Lima, J.L.F.C. Methodological aspects about in vitro evaluation of antioxidant properties. *Anal. Chim. Acta* **2008**, *613*, 1–19. [CrossRef] [PubMed]
39. Taihua, M. *Sweet Potato Processing Technology*; Academic Press: London, UK, 2017.
40. Ghani, M.A.; Barril, C.; Bedgood, D.R.; Prenzler, P.D. Measurement of antioxidant activity with the thiobarbituric acid reactive substances assay. *Food Chem.* **2017**, *230*, 195–207. [CrossRef]
41. Kohn, H.I.; Liversedge, M. On a new aerobic metabolite whose production by brain is inhibited by apomorphine, emetine, ergotamine, epinephrine, and menadione. *J. Pharmacol. Exp. Ther.* **1944**, *82*, 292–300.
42. Grotto, D.; Maria, L.S.; Valentini, J.; Paniz, C.; Schmitt, G.; Garcia, S.C.; Pomblum, V.J.; Rocha, J.B.T.; Farina, M. Importance of the lipid peroxidation biomarkers and methodological aspects FOR malondialdehyde quantification. *Quím. Nova* **2009**, *32*, 169–174. [CrossRef]
43. Halliwell, B.; Gutteridge, J.M.C.; Aruoma, O.I. The deoxyribose method: A simple "test-tube" assay for determination of rate constants for reactions of hydroxyl radicals. *Anal. Biochem.* **1987**, *165*, 215–219. [CrossRef]
44. Nimse, S.B.; Pal, D. Free radicals, natural antioxidants, and their reaction mechanisms. *RSC Adv.* **2015**, *5*, 27986–28006. [CrossRef]
45. Templar, J.; Kon, S.P.; Milligan, T.P.; Newman, D.J.; Raftery, M.J. Increased plasma malondialdehyde levels in glomerular disease as determined by a fully validated HPLC method. *Nephrol. Dial. Transplant.* **1999**, *14*, 946–951. [CrossRef]

46. Loscalzo, J. The identification of nitric oxide as endothelium-derived relaxing factor. *Circ. Res.* **2013**, *113*, 100–103. [CrossRef] [PubMed]
47. Boora, F.; Chirisa, E.; Mukanganyama, S. Evaluation of nitrite radical scavenging properties of selected Zimbabwean plant extracts and their phytoconstituents. *J. Food Process.* **2014**, *2014*, 918018. [CrossRef]
48. Thomas, D.D. Breathing new life into nitric oxide signaling: A brief overview of the interplay between oxygen and nitric oxide. *Redox Biol.* **2015**, *5*, 225–233. [CrossRef] [PubMed]
49. Bhaskar, H.; Balakrishnan, N. In vitro antioxidant property of laticiferous plant species from Western Ghats Tamilnadu, India. *Int. J. Health Res.* **2009**, *2*, 163–170. [CrossRef]
50. Lakhanpal, P.; Rai, D.K. Quercetin: A versatile flavonoid. *IJMU* **2007**, *2*, 22–37. [CrossRef]
51. Griess, J.P., XVIII. On a new series of bodies in which nitrogen substituted for hydrogen. *Philos. Trans. R. Soc. Lond.* **1864**, *154*, 667–731. [CrossRef]
52. Hetrick, E.M.; Schoenfisch, M.H. Analytical chemistry of nitric oxide. *Annu. Rev. Anal. Chem.* **2009**, *2*, 409–433. [CrossRef]
53. Tsikas, D. Analysis of nitrite and nitrate in biological fluids by assays based on the Griess reaction: Appraisal of the Griess reaction in the L-arginine/nitric oxide area of research. *J. Chromatogr. B* **2007**, *851*, 51–70. [CrossRef]
54. Grossi, L.; D'Angelo, S. Sodium Nitroprusside: Mechanism of NO Release Mediated by Sulfhydryl-Containing Molecules. *J. Med. Chem.* **2005**, *48*, 2622–2626. [CrossRef]
55. Zengin, G.; Sarikurkcu, C.; Aktumsek, A.; Ceylan, R.; Ceylan, O. A comprehensive study on phytochemical characterization of *Haplophyllum myrtifolium* Boiss. endemic to Turkey and its inhibitory potential against key enzymes involved in Alzheimer, skin diseases and type II diabetes. *Ind. Crops Prod.* **2014**, *53*, 244–251. [CrossRef]
56. Beckman, J.S.; Beckman, T.W.; Chen, J.; Marshall, P.A.; Freeman, B.A. Apparent hydroxyl radical production by peroxynitrite: Implications for endothelial injury from nitric oxide and superoxide. *Proc. Natl. Acad. Sci. USA* **1990**, *87*, 1620–1624. [CrossRef] [PubMed]
57. Beckman, J.S.; Chen, J.; Ischiropoulos, H.; Crow, J.P. [23] Oxidative chemistry of peroxynitrite. In *Methods in Enzymology*; Academic Press: Cambridge, MA, USA, 1994; Volume 233, pp. 229–240.
58. Costa, D.; Fernandes, E.; Santos, J.L.; Pinto, D.C.; Silva, A.M.; Lima, J.L. New noncellular fluorescence microplate screening assay for scavenging activity against singlet oxygen. *Anal. Bioanal. Chem.* **2007**, *387*, 2071–2081. [CrossRef] [PubMed]
59. Sánchez-Moreno, C. Review: Methods Used to Evaluate the Free Radical Scavenging Activity in Foods and Biological Systems. *Food Sci. Technol. Int.* **2002**, *8*, 121–137. [CrossRef]
60. Kooy, N.W.; Royall, J.A.; Ischiropoulos, H.; Beckman, J.S. Peroxynitrite-mediated oxidation of dihydrorhodamine 123. *Free Radic. Biol. Med.* **1994**, *16*, 149–156. [CrossRef]
61. Pacher, P.; Beckman, J.S.; Liaudet, L. Nitric Oxide and peroxynitrite in health and disease. *Physiol. Rev.* **2007**, *87*, 315–424. [CrossRef]
62. Kalyanaraman, B.; Darley-Usmar, V.; Davies, K.J.A.; Dennery, P.A.; Forman, H.J.; Grisham, M.B.; Mann, G.E.; Moore, K.; Roberts, L.J., II; Ischiropoulos, H. Measuring reactive oxygen and nitrogen species with fluorescent probes: Challenges and limitations. *Free Radic. Biol. Med.* **2012**, *52*, 1–6. [CrossRef]
63. Boveris, A.; Cadenas, E. Mitochondria: Source and Target of Free Radicals. In *Encyclopedia of Biological Chemistry*, 2nd ed.; Lennarz, W.J., Lane, M.D., Eds.; Academic Press: Waltham, MA, USA, 2013; pp. 168–175. [CrossRef]
64. Kehrer, J.P.; Robertson, J.D.; Smith, C.V. 1.14. Free Radicals and Reactive Oxygen Species. In *Comprehensive Toxicology*, 2nd ed.; McQueen, C.A., Ed.; Elsevier: Oxford, UK, 2010; pp. 277–307. [CrossRef]
65. O-Uchi, J.; Jhun, B.S.; Mishra, J.; Sheu, S.-S. Organellar Ion Channels and Transporters. In *Cardiac Electrophysiology: From Cell to Bedside*, 7th ed.; Zipes, D.P., Jalife, J., Stevenson, W.G., Eds.; Elsevier: Amsterdam, The Netherlands, 2018; pp. 66–79. [CrossRef]
66. O-Uchi, J.; Jhun, B.S.; Sheu, S.-S. Structural and Molecular Bases of Mitochondrial Ion Channel Function. In *Cardiac Electrophysiology: From Cell to Bedside*, 6th ed.; Zipes, D.P., Jalife, J., Eds.; W.B. Saunders: Philadelphia, PA, USA, 2014; pp. 71–84. [CrossRef]
67. Koppenol, W.H. The basic chemistry of nitrogen monoxide and peroxynitrite. *Free Radic. Biol. Med.* **1998**, *25*, 385–391. [CrossRef]
68. Robak, J.; Gryglewski, R.J. Flavonoids are scavengers of superoxide anions. *Biochem. Pharmacol.* **1988**, *37*, 837–841. [CrossRef]

69. Miller, F.J.; Griendling, K.K. Functional evaluation of nonphagocytic NAD(P)H oxidases. In *Methods in Enzymology*; Sen, C.K., Packer, L., Eds.; Academic Press: Cambridge, MA, USA, 2002; Volume 353, pp. 220–233.
70. Volk, A.P.D.; Moreland, J.G. Chapter Thirteen—ROS-Containing Endosomal Compartments: Implications for Signaling. In *Methods in Enzymology*; Conn, P.M., Ed.; Academic Press: Cambridge, MA, USA, 2014; Volume 535, pp. 201–224.
71. Goto, M.; Kuda, T.; Shikano, A.; Charrouf, Z.; Yamauchi, K.; Yokozawa, M.; Takahashi, H.; Kimura, B. Induction of superoxide anion radical-scavenging capacity in an argan press cake-suspension by fermentation using Lactobacillus plantarum Argan-L1. *LWT* **2019**, *100*, 56–61. [CrossRef]
72. Sies, H. Hydrogen peroxide as a central redox signaling molecule in physiological oxidative stress: Oxidative eustress. *Redox Biol.* **2017**, *11*, 613–619. [CrossRef] [PubMed]
73. Gnonlonfin, B.; Sanni, A.; Brimer, L. Review Scopoletin—A Coumarin Phytoalexin with Medicinal Properties. *Crit. Rev. Plant Sci.* **2012**, *31*, 47–56. [CrossRef]
74. Corbett, J.T. The scopoletin assay for hydrogen peroxide—A review and a better method. *J. Biochem. Biophys. Methods* **1989**, *18*, 297–307. [CrossRef]
75. Marquez, L.A.; Dunford, H.B. Transient and Steady-State Kinetics of the Oxidation of Scopoletin by Horseradish Peroxidase Compounds I, II and III in the Presence of NADH. *Eur. J. Biochem.* **1995**, *233*, 364–371. [CrossRef] [PubMed]
76. Miller, R.W.; Sirois, J.C.; Morita, H. The reaction of coumarins with horseradish peroxidase. *Plant Physiol.* **1975**, *55*, 35–41. [CrossRef]
77. Halliwell, B. How to characterize a biological antioxidant. *Free Radic. Res.* **1990**, *9*, 1–32. [CrossRef]
78. Boveris, A.; Martino, E.; Stoppani, A.O.M. Evaluation of the horseradish peroxidase-scopoletin method for the measurement of hydrogen peroxide formation in biological systems. *Anal. Biochem.* **1977**, *80*, 145–158. [CrossRef]
79. Sroka, Z.; Cisowski, W. Hydrogen peroxide scavenging, antioxidant and anti-radical activity of some phenolic acids. *Food Chem. Toxicol.* **2003**, *41*, 753–758. [CrossRef]
80. Grisham, M.B. Methods to detect hydrogen peroxide in living cells: Possibilities and pitfalls. *Comp. Biochem. Physiol. A Mol. Integr. Physiol.* **2013**, *165*, 429–438. [CrossRef]
81. Apak, R.; Guclu, K.; Ozyurek, M.; Karademir, S.E.; Altun, M. Total antioxidant capacity assay of human serum using copper(II)-neocuproine as chromogenic oxidant: The CUPRAC method. *Free Radic. Res.* **2005**, *39*, 949–961. [CrossRef]
82. Apak, R.; Guclu, K.; Ozyurek, M.; Karademir, S.E. Novel total antioxidant capacity index for dietary polyphenols and vitamins C and E, using their cupric ion reducing capability in the presence of neocuproine: CUPRAC method. *J. Agric. Food Chem.* **2004**, *52*, 7970–7981. [CrossRef] [PubMed]
83. Benzie, I.F.; Strain, J.J. The ferric reducing ability of plasma (FRAP) as a measure of "antioxidant power": The FRAP assay. *Anal. Biochem.* **1996**, *239*, 70–76. [CrossRef] [PubMed]
84. Berker, K.I.; Guclu, K.; Tor, I.; Apak, R. Comparative evaluation of Fe(III) reducing power-based antioxidant capacity assays in the presence of phenanthroline, batho-phenanthroline, tripyridyltriazine (FRAP), and ferricyanide reagents. *Talanta* **2007**, *72*, 1157–1165. [CrossRef] [PubMed]
85. Benzie, I.F.F.; Strain, J.J. [2] Ferric reducing/antioxidant power assay: Direct measure of total antioxidant activity of biological fluids and modified version for simultaneous measurement of total antioxidant power and ascorbic acid concentration. In *Methods in Enzymology*; Academic Press: Cambridge, MA, USA, 1999; Volume 299, pp. 15–27.
86. Choirunnisa, A. Comparison of five antioxidant assays for estimating antioxidant capacity from three Solanum sp. extracts. *Asian J. Pharm. Clin. Res.* **2016**, *9*, 123–128.
87. Özyürek, M.; Güçlü, K.; Tütem, E.; Sözgen Başkan, K.; Erçağ, E.; Karademir Çelik, S.; Baki, S.; Yıldız, L.; Karaman, Ş.; Apak, R. A comprehensive review of CUPRAC methodology. *Anal. Methods* **2011**, *3*, 2439–2453. [CrossRef]
88. Prado, F.; González, J.; Boero, C.; Sampietro, A. A simple and sensitive method for determining reducing sugars in plant tissues. *Application to quantify the sugar content in quinoa* (Chenopodium quinoa Willd.) seedlings. *Phytochem. Anal.* **1998**, *9*, 58–62.
89. Al-Badr, A.A.; Mostafa, G.A.E. Chapter Eight—Pravastatin Sodium. In *Profiles of Drug Substances, Excipients and Related Methodology*; Brittain, H.G., Ed.; Academic Press: Cambridge, MA, USA, 2014; Volume 39, pp. 433–513.

90. Guo, L.; Zhang, Y.; Li, Q. Spectrophotometric determination of dopamine hydrochloride in pharmaceutical, banana, urine and serum samples by potassium ferricyanide-Fe(III). *Anal. Sci.* **2009**, *25*, 1451–1455. [CrossRef]
91. Woodbury, W.; Spencer, A.; Stahmann, M. An improved procedure using ferricyanide for detecting catalase isozymes. *Anal. Biochem.* **1971**, *44*, 301–305. [CrossRef]
92. Shaffer, P.A.; Williams, R.D. Sugar determination by the ferricyanide electrode. *J. Biol.* **1935**, *111*, 707–723.
93. Hassid, W.Z. Determination of sugars in plants. *Ind. Eng. Chem. Anal.* **1937**, *9*, 228–229. [CrossRef]
94. Atkins, P.; Overton, T.; Rourke, J.; Weller, M.; Armstrong, F.; Hagerman, M. *Inorganic Chemistry*, 5th ed.; W. H. Freeman and Company: New York, NY, USA, 2009.
95. Prieto, P.; Pineda, M.; Aguilar, M. Spectrophotometric quantitation of antioxidant capacity through the formation of a phosphomolybdenum complex: Specific application to the determination of Vitamin E. *Anal. Biochem.* **1999**, *269*, 337–341. [CrossRef] [PubMed]
96. Thangaraj, P. *Medicinal Plants: Promising Future for Health and New Drugs*, 1st ed.; CRC Press: Boca Raton, FL, USA, 2018; 382p.
97. Miller, C.; Taylor, A. On reduction of ammonium molybdate in acid solution. *J. Biol.* **1914**, *17*, 531–535.
98. Nagul, E.A.; McKelvie, I.D.; Worsfold, P.; Kolev, S.D. The molybdenum blue reaction for the determination of orthophosphate revisited: Opening the black box. *Anal. Chim. Acta* **2015**, *890*, 60–82. [CrossRef] [PubMed]
99. Grigore, A.; Paraschiv, I.; Mihul, A.; Corina, B.; Draghici, E.; Ichim, M. Chemical composition and antioxidant activity of *Thymus vulgaris* L. volatile oil obtained by two different methods. *Rom. Biotechnol. Lett.* **2010**, *15*, 5436–5443.
100. Phatak, R.S.; Hendre, A.S. Total antioxidant capacity (TAC) of fresh leaves of *Kalanchoe pinnata*. *J. Pharmacogn. Phytochem.* **2014**, *2*, 32–35.
101. Diwan, R.; Shinde, A.; Malpathak, N. Phytochemical composition and antioxidant potential of *Ruta graveolens* L. in vitro culture lines. *J. Bot.* **2012**, *2012*, 685427. [CrossRef]
102. Viuda-Martos, M.; Ruiz Navajas, Y.; Sánchez Zapata, E.; Fernández-López, J.; Pérez-Álvarez, J.A. Antioxidant activity of essential oils of five spice plants widely used in a Mediterranean diet. *Flavour Fragr. J.* **2010**, *25*, 13–19. [CrossRef]
103. Aaseth, J.; Skaug, M.A.; Cao, Y.; Andersen, O. Chelation in metal intoxication—Principles and paradigms. *J. Trace Elem. Med. Biol.* **2015**, *31*, 260–266. [CrossRef]
104. Flora, S.J.S.; Pachauri, V. Chelation in metal intoxication. *Int. J. Environ. Res. Public Health* **2010**, *7*, 2745–2788. [CrossRef]
105. Dinis, T.C.P.; Madeira, V.M.C.; Almeida, L.M. Action of phenolic derivatives (Acetaminophen, Salicylate, and 5-Aminosalicylate) as inhibitors of membrane lipid peroxidation and as peroxyl radical scavengers. *Arch. Biochem. Biophys.* **1994**, *315*, 161–169. [CrossRef]
106. Aparadh, V.; Naik, V.; Karadge, B. Antioxidative properties (TPC, DPPH, FRAP, metal chelating ability, reducing power and TAC) within some Cleome species. *Ann. Bot.* **2012**, *2*, 49–56.
107. Akanbi, T.O.; Barrow, C.J. Lipase-produced hydroxytyrosyl eicosapentaenoate is an excellent antioxidant for the stabilization of omega-3 bulk oils, emulsions and microcapsules. *Molecules* **2018**, *23*, 275. [CrossRef] [PubMed]
108. Porter, W.L.; Black, E.D.; Drolet, A.M. Use of polyamide oxidative fluorescence test on lipid emulsions: Contrast in relative effectiveness of antioxidants in bulk versus dispersed systems. *J. Agric. Food Chem.* **1989**, *37*, 615–624. [CrossRef]
109. Shahidi, F.; Zhong, Y. Revisiting the polar paradox theory: A critical overview. *J. Agric. Food Chem.* **2011**, *59*, 3499–3504. [CrossRef] [PubMed]
110. Wang, J.; Shahidi, F. Acidolysis of p-coumaric acid with omega-3 oils and antioxidant activity of phenolipid products in in vitro and biological model systems. *J. Agric. Food Chem.* **2014**, *62*, 454–461. [CrossRef] [PubMed]
111. Marco, G. A rapid method for evaluation of antioxidants. *J. Am. Oil Chem. Soc.* **1968**, *45*, 594–598. [CrossRef]
112. Prieto, M.A.; Rodríguez-Amado, I.; Vázquez, J.A.; Murado, M.A. β-carotene assay revisited. Application to characterize and quantify antioxidant and prooxidant activities in a microplate. *J. Agric. Food Chem.* **2012**, *60*, 8983–8993. [CrossRef]
113. Mikami, I.; Yamaguchi, M.; Shinmoto, H.; Tsushida, T. Development and validation of a microplate-based β-carotene bleaching assay and comparison of antioxidant activity (AOA) in several crops measured by β-carotene bleaching, DPPH and ORAC assays. *Food Sci. Technol. Res.* **2009**, *15*, 171–178. [CrossRef]

114. Lage, M.Á.P.; García, M.A.M.; Álvarez, J.A.V.; Anders, Y.; Curran, T.P. A new microplate procedure for simultaneous assessment of lipophilic and hydrophilic antioxidants and pro-oxidants, using crocin and β-carotene bleaching methods in a single combined assay: Tea extracts as a case study. *Food Res. Int.* **2013**, *53*, 836–846. [CrossRef]
115. Ueno, H.; Yamakura, S.; Arastoo, R.S.; Oshima, T.; Kokubo, K. Systematic evaluation and mechanistic investigation of antioxidant activity of fullerenols using β-carotene bleaching assay. *J. Nanomater.* **2014**, *2014*, 802596. [CrossRef]

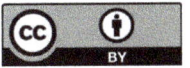

© 2020 by the authors. Licensee MDPI, Basel, Switzerland. This article is an open access article distributed under the terms and conditions of the Creative Commons Attribution (CC BY) license (http://creativecommons.org/licenses/by/4.0/).

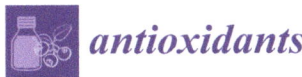

Review

Lycopene as a Natural Antioxidant Used to Prevent Human Health Disorders

Muhammad Imran [1], Fereshteh Ghorat [2], Iahtisham Ul-Haq [3], Habib Ur-Rehman [4], Farhan Aslam [5], Mojtaba Heydari [6], Mohammad Ali Shariati [7], Eleonora Okuskhanova [8], Zhanibek Yessimbekov [8], Muthu Thiruvengadam [9,*], Mohammad Hashem Hashempur [10,11,*] and Maksim Rebezov [12,13]

[1] University Institute of Diet and Nutritional Sciences, Faculty of Allied Health Sciences, The University of Lahore, Lahore 54000, Pakistan; muhammad.imran8@dnsc.uol.edu.pk
[2] Non-Communicable Diseases Research Center, Sabzevar University of Medical Sciences, Sabzevar 9617913112, Iran; f-ghorat@alumnus.tums.ac.ir
[3] Department of Diet and Nutritional Sciences, Faculty of Health and Allied Sciences, Imperial College of Business Studies, Lahore 53720, Pakistan; hod.ddns@imperial.edu.pk
[4] Department of Clinical Nutrition, NUR International University, Lahore 54000, Pakistan; habib.rehman@niu.edu.pk
[5] Department of Food Science and Human Nutrition, University of Veterinary and Animal Sciences, Lahore Syed Abdul Qadir Jillani (Out Fall) Road, Lahore 54000, Pakistan; foodandnutrition1983@gmail.com
[6] Poostchi Ophthalmology Research Center, Shiraz University of Medical Sciences, Shiraz 7134845794, Iran; mheydari@sums.ac.ir
[7] Department of Technology of Food Products, K.G. Razumovsky Moscow State University of Technologies and Management (the First Cossack University), 109004 Moscow, Russia; m.ali.sh@semgu.kz
[8] Food Science and Technology Department, Shakarim State University of Semey, Semey 071412, Kazakhstan; eokuskhanova@gmail.com (E.O.); zyessimbekov@semgu.kz (Z.Y.)
[9] Department of Crop Science, College of Sanghuh Life Science, Konkuk University, Seoul 05029, Korea
[10] Noncommunicable Diseases Research Center, Fasa University of Medical Sciences, Fasa 7461686688, Iran
[11] Department of Persian Medicine, Fasa University of Medical Sciences, Fasa 7461686688, Iran
[12] V.M. Gorbatov Federal Research Center for Food Systems of Russian Academy of Sciences, Moscow 109029, Russia; rebezov@ya.ru
[13] K.G. Razumovsky Moscow State University of Technologies and Management (the First Cossack University), Moscow 109004, Russia
* Correspondence: muthu@konkuk.ac.kr (M.T.); hashempur@gmail.com (M.H.H.); Tel.: +82-02450-0577 (M.T.); +98-71-53314076 (M.H.H.)

Received: 12 June 2020; Accepted: 30 July 2020; Published: 4 August 2020

Abstract: Lycopene, belonging to the carotenoids, is a tetraterpene compound abundantly found in tomato and tomato-based products. It is fundamentally recognized as a potent antioxidant and a non-pro-vitamin A carotenoid. Lycopene has been found to be efficient in ameliorating cancer insurgences, diabetes mellitus, cardiac complications, oxidative stress-mediated malfunctions, inflammatory events, skin and bone diseases, hepatic, neural and reproductive disorders. This review summarizes information regarding its sources and uses amongst different societies, its biochemistry aspects, and the potential utilization of lycopene and possible mechanisms involved in alleviating the abovementioned disorders. Furthermore, future directions with the possible use of this nutraceutical against lifestyle-related disorders are emphasized. Its protective effects against recommended doses of toxic agents and toxicity and safety are also discussed.

Keywords: lycopene; antioxidants; oxidative stress; cancer; diabetes; cardiovascular diseases; skin disorders

1. Introduction

Lycopene is a phytochemical mainly found in tomato and tomato-based products. It is a tetraterpene compound consisting of eight isoprene units and 11 double linear bonds. Lycopene is a non-pro-vitamin A carotenoid [1,2]. However, it is mentioned as an intermediate of carotenoid synthesis in plants [3]. Some fruits' and vegetables' red and orange coloration is attributed to this liposoluble pigment [2]. Despite this, it is found in some non-red or non-orange plants, such as asparagus and parsley [4]. It should be noted that lycopene cannot be synthesized in the human body. Therefore, it must be consumed in a daily diet [5]. The absorbed lycopene is mostly stored in the liver, adrenals, and prostate. Moreover, it can be found in other body parts (e.g., brain and skin) in a lower concentration [6]. Lycopene bioavailability can be decreased by ageing, and some of the pathological states, such as cardiovascular diseases (CVDs) [7]. Therefore, its supplementation—through various means, such as pasteurized watermelon juice—has been suggested to increase its circulating serum level in populations in need [8,9].

Interestingly, carotenoids have the highest concentration in the serum and tissues between different natural antioxidants. In addition, according to one study on a United States population, lycopene is the leading carotenoid in plasma and tissues [10]. Furthermore, second to astaxanthin (amongst different carotenoids), lycopene is the most potent antioxidant. It is an important deactivator of reactive oxygen species (ROS). For instance, it can remove singlet oxygen two and ten times more than beta-carotene and alpha-tocopherol, respectively [11]. In recent years, there has been an ever-increasing interest in lycopene's health benefits. It is not only a potent antioxidant; its beneficial effects in the prevention and treatment of a wide variety of diseases have been assessed and approved by many systematic reviews and meta-analysis studies [12].

For instance, it has been shown that a higher dietary intake and circulating concentration of lycopene have protective effects against prostate cancer (PCa), in a dose-dependent way [13]. The findings approve this effect for the whole tomato, cooked tomato, and sauces consumption [14]. In addition, lycopene's inhibitory effect on the proliferation and progression of the colorectal cancer cells has been investigated [15]. Moreover, the protective role of lycopene in metabolic syndrome has been well-studied. It seems that different metabolic syndrome components can be improved by lycopene supplementation *"rather than demonstrating consistent improvement in a single component"* [16]. Lycopene can be used in different CVDs, too [17]. It can improve ventricular remodeling, and vascular and endothelial function. In addition, it is useful in the reduction in atherosclerotic plaque size, and arterial stiffness. Therefore, it can be concluded that this nutraceutical has a vital role in the primary and secondary prevention of CVDs [3]. In addition, lycopene is a natural neuroprotective agent. It seems that this carotenoid contributes to cognitive longevity [18] and the treatment of several neuronal diseases, including cerebral ischemia, Parkinson's disease (PD), Alzheimer's disease (AD), subarachnoid haemorrhage, epilepsy, Huntington's disease, and depression [19]. There are several other clinical applications for this available phytochemical. It can be used in different skin [20], oral, and dental diseases, too [21]. This paper aims to make a comprehensive review on lycopene, from its sources and uses amongst different societies, to its biochemistry and its different biological effects. Furthermore, its protective effect against various toxins, its recommended dose, and toxicity and side effects were discussed separately.

2. Natural Sources of Lycopene and Its Use Amongst Different Societies

Tomato and tomato-based products are the major dietary sources of lycopene and account for approximately 80% of the consumption of lycopene in western countries. It is also present in a high amount in watermelon, guava, pink grapefruit, rosehips, papaya, and apricot [22]. Table 1 shows its amount in different sources [23–25]. Lycopene contents significantly differ in diverse varieties of tomato and other fruits and vegetables. Its content depends on several factors: 1, the degree of maturity; 2, the weather temperature (lycopene is transformed to beta-carotene at temperatures higher than 35 °C);

and 3, the soil quality (conditioners including necessary microorganisms may cause lycopene content to be increased about 36%) [26].

Table 1. Lycopene content in different sources.

Food Sources	Contents (mg/100 g)
Fresh tomatoes	0.72–4.2
Cooked tomatoes	3.70
Tomato sauce	6.20
Tomato paste	5.40–150
Ketchup	9.90–13.44
Pumpkin	0.38–0.46
Sweet potato	0.02–0.11
Pink grapefruit	0.35–3.36
Carrot	0.65–0.78
Pink guava	5.23–5.5
Watermelon	2.30–7.20
Apricot	0.01–0.05
Papaya	0.11–5.3
Rosehip	0.68–0.71

Lycopene intake is also varied among different people in different regions [25]. In the population of European countries, lycopene consumption from natural sources is varied from approximately 0.5 to 5 mg/day. Nevertheless, variation in lycopene consumption was reported, where adults in Spain consume less lycopene (1.64 mg/day) compared to adults from France, and the UK, where the intake was from 4.43 to 5.01 mg/day [27,28]. In the United States, daily intake is more than 7 mg/day [29]. Higher utilization of fruits and vegetables, especially tomato-based products, may result in occasional intakes of 20 mg lycopene/day. Approximately 50–65% of the total exposure to lycopene was produced from natural sources. Some of the important daily sources of lycopene are tomatoes, soups, pasta dishes, tomato sauces and ketchup [30].

3. Biochemistry of Lycopene

In nature, there are more than 600 carotenoids which are mostly colored, produced by plants, fungi and bacteria. Carotenoids have two main groups: (i) the highly unsaturated hydrocarbons (α, β-, and γ-carotene, lycopene), (ii) xanthophylls (lutein, β-cryptoxanthin, and zeaxanthin). Xanthophylls possess a minimum of an oxygenated group on their end rings, while unsaturated hydrocarbon carotenoids contain just carbon and hydrogen atoms with no oxygen [31]. Modified carotenoid structures, such as the cyclization of terminal groups and inserting oxygen, are linked with diverse forms of carotenoids resulting in color alterations and also various antioxidant properties [32].

Lycopene (C40H56), as a hydrocarbon carotenoid, includes an acyclic open chain structure containing 13 double bonds that are subjected to isomerization and differed *cis* isomers, such as 5, 9, 13, and 15 observed in plants and blood plasma [33]. Naturally, lycopene can be found in all the *trans* isomers, but the *cis* isomers are the most typical type in tissue and plasma [34]. This takes place during food pretreatment, preparation, processing, storage and transportation, as well as during metabolism in the body [35]. The conversion of *cis* to *trans* isomerization takes place in enterocytes, liver and stomach [36,37]. The absorption of lycopene in the intestine is aided by scavenger receptor CD36 and B1 [38,39]. Partial metabolism can be seen in the enterocyte assisted by two enzymes: 15′-oxygenase-1, β-carotene 15, which is linked with blood lycopene level, and 10′ oxygenase-2, β-carotene-9 [40,41].

Furthermore, there is limited research on labelled lycopene molecules. For instance, a study conducted by Ross et al. on 14C-labelled lycopene (92% *trans*-lycopene) revealed that the *trans*-lycopene was completely isomerized (5-*cis*, 9-*cis*, 13-*cis*, and 15-*cis* lycopene isomers) following dosing and quickly metabolized into polar metabolites entered in the urine [42]. The quick exclusion of $14CO_2$ indicated sufficient oxidization of the ingested lycopene. In the compartmental model research,

13C-labelled lycopene was used. No significant differences were found in the bioavailability of *cis*- and *trans*-lycopene (24.5 vs. 23.2%, respectively). Moreover, it was confirmed that post-absorptive *trans*-to-*cis* isomerization affects tissue and plasma isomeric profiles [43]. The most thermodynamical lycopene firm configuration has shown the all-*trans*-isomer. Light, heat, or many chemical reactions may cause isomerization from the *trans*-isomer toward several mono- or poly-*cis* types, of which two types are non-conjugated. In comparison, 11 types are conjugated double bonds, forming a chromophore involved in visible ruby color, as well as lycopene antioxidant activities [23]. Figure 1 shows the molecular structures of lycopene and its derivatives and isomers.

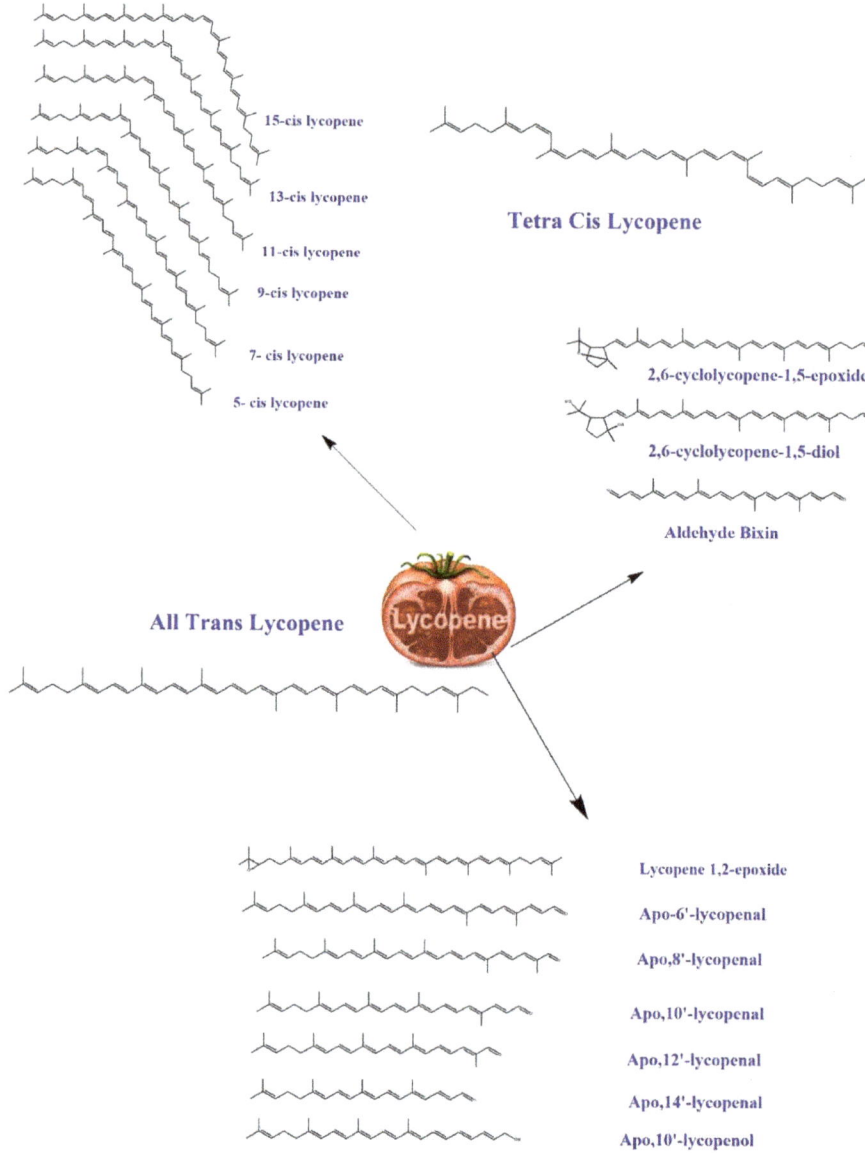

Figure 1. The molecular structures of lycopene and its derivatives and isomers.

4. Biological Effects

There is a wide variety of pharmacological actions and clinical applications which have been attributed to the lycopene by a chain of researches worldwide. Table 2 summarizes these insights by discussing different mechanisms of action briefly.

Table 2. Various mechanisms for lycopene's biological effects.

Biological Effect	Mechanisms of Action	References
Anticancer	Reduced nuclear factor-kappa B (NF-κB) expression, serum level of oxidative stress marker malondialdehyde (MDA) Improved nuclear factor erythroid 2 expressions Reduced the expression of signal transducer and activator of transcription 3 (STAT3) Induced the protein inhibitor of activated STAT3 expression	[44,45]
	Induced cell cycle arrest and modified the potential of mitochondrial membrane, DNA fragmentation	[46,47]
	Treatment of HGC-27 cells with lycopene exhibited significant improvement in LC3-I, Phosphorylated Extracellular Signal-Regulated Kinase (p-ERK) proteins expressions	[48]
	Reduced NADPH oxidase (NOX) 4 activity Lowered invasion, migration, and adhesion, NOX activity, matrix metalloproteinase (MMP)-9, MMP-2 activities and NOX4 protein expression	[49]
	Reduced metastatic load and inhibited cancer antigen 125 (CA125) expression Down-regulated expression of Integrin beta-1 (ITGB1), MMP9, Integrin alpha-5 (ITGA5), Focal Adhesion Kinase (FAK), integrin-linked kinase (ILK) and EMT markers Decreased activity of mitogen-activated protein kinase (MAPK) and inhibited integrin α5 protein expression	[50]
Antidiabetic	Lowered MDA levels, and increased antioxidant enzyme activities	[51]
	Decreased the glycated haemoglobin (HbA1c) and C-reactive protein (CRP)	[52,53]
	Enhanced antioxidant enzymes activities (i.e., superoxide dismutase (SOD), glutathione peroxidase (GPx), catalase (CAT), glutathione-S-transferase)	[54]
	Lowered the expression of BCL2-associated X protein (BAX), but improved B-cell lymphoma-extra large (Bcl-xL) levels and B-cell lymphoma 2 (Bcl-2)	[55]
	Downregulated RAGE expression and declined NF-κB and MMP-2 expressions	[56]
	Reduced levels of serum nitrate-nitrite level	[57]

Table 2. Cont.

Biological Effect	Mechanisms of Action	References
Cardioprotective	Decreased low-density lipoprotein-cholesterol (LDL), total cholesterol (TC), and thiobarbituric acid-reacting substances	[58]
	Lowered very-low-density lipoprotein-cholesterol (VLDL), triglycerides (TG) and increased high-density lipoprotein-cholesterol (HDL) level	[59]
	Decreased inflammatory factors (CRP, interleukin (IL)-6), pulse wave velocity, adhesion molecules and endothelial function	[60]
	Lowered the expression of Rho-associated protein kinase (ROCK)1, Ki-67, intercellular adhesion molecule-1 (ICAM-1) and ROCK2 Improved the expression of endothelial nitric oxide synthase (eNOS) implanted arteries and cGMP plasma concentration	[61]
Antioxidant	Increased CAT, glutathione (GSH) and SOD activities and mRNAs antioxidant enzyme Reduced age-related neuroinflammatory disorders by decreasing microgliosis (Ionized calcium-binding adaptor protein-1 (IBA-1)) Down regulate the accumulation of amyloid beta (Aβ)$_{1\text{-}42}$ in the old CD-1 mice's brain.	[62]
	Decreased Aβ accumulation, amyloid precursor protein (APP) Reduced the expression of neuronal β-secretase (BACE)1 Improved the expressions of α-secretase A Disintegrin And Metalloproteinase (ADAM)10 Suppressed IBA-1 (a marker of microglial activation) expression, inflammatory mediators Inhibited NF-κB, phosphorylation of MAPKs and Nuclear factor erythroid 2-related factor 2 (Nrf2) activity	[63]
	Decreased myeloperoxidase (MPO) activity, tumor necrosis factor-alpha (TNF-α) Down-regulated gene expression of inducible nitric oxide synthase (iNOS)	[64]
	Decreased inflammatory cytokines Improved antioxidant enzymes NAD(P)H: quinone oxidoreductase (NQO1) and heme oxygenase-1 (HO-1) mRNA expressions Downregulated inflammatory cytokines TNF-α and IL-1β Improved the glial cells inflammatory markers glial fibrillary acidic protein (GFAP) and IBA-1 expression	[65]
Antiinflammatory	Up-regulated the HO-1 mRNA Gene expression suppression of the TNF-α and lipopolysaccharide (LPS)-stimulated cyclooxygenase-2 (COX-2), nitric oxide synthase 2 (NOS2)	[66]
	Lowered the IL-1β, TNF-α, IL-6β serum level and increased the NF-κB p65 mRNA, Toll-like receptor 4 (TLR4) and protein expressions	[67]
	Inhibited COX-2, iNOS and NF-κB Reduced the leukocytes migration	[68]

Table 2. Cont.

Biological Effect	Mechanisms of Action	References
Hepatoprotective	Lowered aspartate aminotransferase, alanine aminotransferase, free fatty acid, MDA and LDL Increased the SOD, GSH condensation Down-regulated the expression of Cytochrome P450 2E1 (CYP2E1), TNF-α	[69]
	Enhanced the S-adenosyl-homocysteine hydrolase, hepatic cystathionine beta-synthase activities	[70]
	Reduced nitric oxide (NO) and MDA levels	[71]
Against dermatologic diseases	Decreased Ultraviolet (UV) B-induced cell growth and increased apoptosis Prevented from Forkhead box O3 (FOXO3) phosphorylation when exposing to UVB radiation and cytoplasm sequestering Decreased cyclin-dependent kinase 4 (CDK4) and CDK2 Increased in the expression of Poly (ADP-ribose) polymerase (PARP), BAX and cell apoptosis Inhibited UVA1- and UVA/B-induced upregulation of HO-1	[72]
Neuroprotective	Suppressing 4 aminopyridines (4-AP) evoked glutamate release and elevated intrasynaptosomal Ca^{2+} level Suppressing release of 4-AP-evoked glutamate	[73]
	Improved mitochondrial enzymatic activities, kindling score, oxidative stress	[74]
	Decreased impairment in biochemical, behavioral, neuroinflammatory and neurochemical markers	[75]
Boneprotective	Osteoblasts differentiation improved	[76]
	Modified the biomarkers of serum osteocalcin, bone metabolism, crosslinked carboxyterminal telopeptides and N-terminal propeptide of type 1 collagen in serum Downregulated the osteoclast differentiation concurrent Up-regulated the osteoblasts alongside GPx, SOD, and CAT activities	[77]
Targeting reproductive disorders	Reduced lipid peroxidation and sperm DNA fragmentation	[78]
	Improved the sperm motility and sperm count Improved mitochondrial enzymatic activity, i.e., CAT, SOD, glucocorticoid receptor (GR), GPx and alcohol dehydrogenase (ADH)) and non-enzymatic antioxidant level (GSH and ascorbate)	[79]

4.1. Anticancer

Inflammation is known as one of the most important key points in cancer. Therefore, lycopene, as one of the most potent antiinflammatory nutraceuticals, is under research in many preclinical and clinical cancer studies. Epidemiological studies showed a reverse relation between its serum level and cancer occurrence [80]. In addition, increased consumption of lycopene (from each source) has been reported to be associated with a decreased risk of a wide variety of cancers, such as breast, lung, ovary, prostate, stomach, and ovary [81].

In laying hens, supplementation (200 to 400 mg lycopene/kg diet) significantly reduced ovarian tumor occurrence, and also the tumors' size and number. Moreover, supplementation with lycopene reduced the STAT3 expression in ovarian tissues via the induction of the protein inhibitor of activated STAT3 expression [44,45]. The lycopene extract (dose: 400 and 800 µg/mL) reduced the risk of human breast adenocarcinoma cells (MCF-7). It could modify the mitochondrial membrane potential, DNA fragmentation and also affected the granularity and size of the MCF-7 cell. Additionally, it does not result in noticeable damage to the cell membrane, necrosis and regular apoptosis [46,47]. Treatment of HGC-27 cells with lycopene exhibited significant improvement in LC3-I, p-ERK proteins expressions [48].

Moreover, in vitro and in vivo investigations exhibited that lycopene (dose: 0.1–5 µM) affected human liver adenocarcinoma (SK-Hep-1) cells and indicated a substantial reduction in NOX activity. Moreover, it inhibits the protein expression of NOX4, NOX4 mRNA and ROS intracellular amounts. The transforming growth factor-β (TGF-β)-related effects were antagonized via the lycopene (2.5 µM) incubation with SK-Hep-1 cells. Through small interfering RNA (siRNA) transient transfection against NOX4, the results reveal that NOX4 downregulation could mimic lycopene via the inhibition of cell migration and MMP-9 and MMP-2 activities in incubating with/without TGF-β on SK-Hep-1 cells [49].

In another study, lycopene consumption markedly decreased the metastatic load in a tumor-bearing rat model of ovarian carcinoma. Lycopene has anti-tumorigenic effects on paclitaxel and carboplatin. Its consumption further inhibits biomarkers for ovarian cancer, such as *CA125* expression. The anti-proliferative and anti-metastatic impacts were complemented via *ITGB1, MMP9, ITGA5, FAK, ILK* and *EMT* markers' down-regulated expression, decreasing the MAPK activity and inhibiting integrin α5 protein expression [50].

FOXO3a is crucial to modify cell death genes expression. Treatment with lycopene reduced cell hyperproliferation induced by UVB and ultimately promoted apoptosis and reduced CDK2 and CDK4 complex in SKH-1 hairless mice and human keratinocytes. It is sequestered in cytoplasm and can phosphorylate against UVB irradiation, although pretreatment with lycopene reduced all these activities. *FOXO3a* gene ablation reduced lycopene-caused attenuation in cell hyper-proliferation, CDK2, and CDK4 complex. *FOXO3a* siRNA transfection prevents lycopene-related elevation in cell apoptosis, cleaved PARP expression and BAX. Furthermore, protein kinase B (AKT) loss can induce more lycopene-caused *FOXO3a* dephosphorylation, whereas losing the mechanistic target of rapamycin complex 2 (mTORC2) via transfection with a rapamycin-insensitive companion of mammalian target of rapamycin (RICTOR) siRNA induces AKT phosphorylation to amounts like the levels gained by lycopene. On the other hand, AKT/mTORC2 overexpression decreases the lycopene impact on the *FOXO3a* expression and AKT phosphorylation, indicating the link between lycopene and the mTORC2/AKT signaling negative modulation [82]. Interestingly, lycopene treatment for human breast carcinoma cell line MCF-7 in vitro, leading to cell shrinkage and breakage, is dependent on the dose and time. Moreover, lycopene treatment up-regulates Bax mRNAs and p53 expression [83].

Lycopene doses of 0, 10, 20, and 30 µM were used to treat human colorectal cancer cells. Lycopene's effect on cell proliferation was evaluated through the 3-(4,5-dimethylthiazol-2-yl)-2,5-diphenyl tetrazolium bromide (MTT) method. Prostaglandin E2 (PGE2), and NO levels declined after lycopene administration [84].

Treatment of human PCa cells was done with lycopene extracts (5 mg/mL) and indicated a significant drop in cell viability and apoptotic cell population [85]. In addition, lycopene nanoparticles (in lipid-based wall material in MCF-7 cells), in a time- and concentration-dependent fashion, significantly reduced cell viability and cell survival [86]. Regarding human trails, in head and neck squamous cell carcinoma, a lycopene concentration of >10 µM for a period of 24 h prevents Cal27 and FaDu cell growth, dependent on the dose and time. Lycopene doses of 25 µM decrease invasion abilities and have significant inhibitory effects. Moreover, lycopene consumption up-regulates B cell lymphoma linked with X protein, a pro-apoptotic protein, and results in inhibiting mitogen-activated and B-protein kinase signaling route [87,88].

In another study on PCa, lycopene, or its metabolite (i.e., apo-10-lycopene), enhanced β, β-carotene-9′, 10′-oxygenase 2 (BCO2) expression, while decreasing cell proliferation in androgen-sensitive cells. However, lycopene cannot modify BCO2 expression and cell development in androgen-resistant cells. The mutant (enzymatically inactive)/wild-type BCO2 exogenous expression in PCa cells decreased NF-κB function, DNA binding and reduced NF-κB translocation in the nucleus [89]. In hepatocellular carcinoma, lycopene supplementation (lycopene dose: 6.6 mg/kg BW/day) inhibited NNK-related α7 nicotinic acetylcholine receptor expression (lung), NF-κB and CYP2E1 (liver) and reduced NNK-related death and pathological abrasions in ferrets' livers and lungs [90]. However, cell invasion, proliferation and migration showed no alteration in a dose-dependent fashion. In another research, lycopene intake is protective against PCa in 46,719 men. It seems that this effect is via decreasing the gene fusion transmembrane protease, serine 2 (TMPRSS2): v-ets avian erythroblastosis virus E26 oncogene homolog (ERG) [91].

4.2. Antidiabetic

There is scientific evidence which supports the beneficial role of lycopene against diabetes. Regarding animal studies and epidemiological surveys, it can be used for both the prevention and treatment of diabetes [92]. In a diabetic rat model (streptozotocin (STZ)-induced), lycopene decreased diabetes-associated pancreas injury and urine and blood glucose levels. In addition, it increased serum insulin levels [93]. The interactions between advanced glycation end products (AGEs) and their receptors (RAGEs) induce oxidative stress-like conditions. Moreover, in vitro and in vivo investigations revealed that lycopene slows down ribose-related forming of AGE in HK-2 cells, while in vivo studies showed that in kidneys, it down-regulates RAGE expression. HK-2 cells with reduced amounts of RAGE indicated reduced NF-κB and MMP 2 expressions [56]. Lycopene supplementation significantly reduced serum nitrate–nitrite levels in diabetic Wistar rats [57].

In addition, lycopene exhibited some effects on histological alterations and also Bcl-2 family gene expression in the STZ-induced diabetic rats' hippocampus. Lycopene (dose: 4 mg/day/kg) decreased the Bax expression. However, it improved Bcl-xL amounts and Bcl-2 [55].

In addition, lycopene considerably controlled high-fat diet (HFD)-related elevation of glucose, insulin level, fasting blood glucose, insulin intolerance and decrease hepatic glycogen level. Lycopene decreases the fatty acid synthase (FAS), sterol regulatory element-binding protein 1c (SREBP-1c), and Acetyl-CoA carboxylase (ACC1) expression in HFD mice. The consumption of lycopene considerably decreases the phosphorylation and STAT3 expression in livers in HFD mice. The adenovirus treatment with lycopene noticeably inhibited a reduction in SREBP-1c expression. Moreover, an increase in STAT3 motioning via adenovirus noticeably blocked a decrease in fasting blood insulin as well as glucose amount [94].

4.3. Cardioprotective

Lycopene is a cardioprotective nutraceutical. Different research showed a protective effect against atherosclerosis and several CVDs [58,95]. It can scavenge some of the potent oxidants that are known to be associated with atherosclerosis. Moreover, lycopene reduces oxidation of cholesterols. Therefore, the early steps in atherosclerosis are prohibited [96]. In hypercholesteremic rats, lycopene administration (50 mg/kg) significantly decreased low-density lipoprotein-cholesterol (LDL), total cholesterol (TC), thiobarbituric acid reactive substances (TBARS), very low-density lipoprotein-cholesterol (VLDL), triglycerides (TG), and increased high-density lipoprotein-cholesterol (HDL) level [59,97]. Furthermore, lycopene was studied for its positive health benefits on some important inflammatory factors (e.g., CRP, IL-6), lowering blood pressure, pulse wave velocity, adhesion molecules (ICAM-1) and endothelial function (flow-mediated dilation) [60]. Moreover, lycopene was found to protect grafted vessels by regulating the expression of key proteins which are essential in arteriosclerosis. It remarkably lessened the expression of ROCK1, Ki-67, ICAM-1 and ROCK2, whereas it improved the expression of eNOS-implanted arteries and cGMP plasma concentration. In summary, lycopene is able to improve the vascular arteriosclerosis in the case of allograft transplantation by downregulating the expression of Rho-related kinases and by regulation of the NO/cGMP pathways expression, as well [61].

Importantly, lycopene consumption protects the heart from Atrazine (ATZ) exposure and also prevents ATZ-induced damage [98]. The results reveal that oral intake of lycopene also prevents myocardial ischemia-reperfusion (I/R) injury. Lycopene use (1 µM) prior to the incidence of re-oxygenation significantly prevents hypoxia/reoxygenation (H/R)-induced cardiomyocyte death. Lycopene (1 µM, intravenous) considerably inhibited myocardial infarction (MI), production of ROS and c-Jun N-terminal Kinase (JNK) phosphorylation in I/R mice [7,99]. Moreover, lycopene has a protective effect against the apoptosis mediated by endoplasmic reticulum stress (ERS), which is due to H/R in H9C2 cardiomyocytes. In I/R myocardium, lycopene dose (10 µM) diminished the lactic dehydrogenase, apoptosis ratio and protein expression of 78 kDa glucose-regulated protein (GRP78). It can be associated with phosphorylated JNK (pJNK), C/EBP homologous protein (CHOP) and Caspase-12 routes [100].

It also improved ERS caused by apoptosis that can be observed via decreasing the expression of CHOP/growth arrest and DNA damage-inducible gene (GADD153), Bax/Bcl-2, caspase-3, caspase-12 activity in H/R-treated cardiomyocytes. It was also reported that lycopene is capable of preventing thapsigargin (THG)-related ERS through a reduction in the GRP78 and CHOP/GADD153 protein expression in the THG group, considerably enhancing cell viability which is caused by THG. It also inhibited apoptosis in THG-treated cardiomyocytes [35,101,102]. Another study reported that lycopene (dose: 10 mg/day/kg) in mice with post-MI ventricular remodeling notably reduced the expression of TGF-β1, collagen III, collagen I, IL-1β, TNF-α, caspase-3, caspase-8 and caspase-9, and reduced NF-κB activity. The administration of lycopene also decreased the level of ventricular remodeling post-MI [103]. Moreover, lycopene supplementation improves the endothelial function in patients with CVD diseases [104].

4.4. Antioxidative

Lycopene is a well-known antioxidant. It can protect DNA, proteins, and lipids against oxidation. In addition, "*lycopene can act on other free radicals such as hydrogen peroxide, nitrogen dioxide and hydroxyl radicals*" [105].

Oxidative stress, as well as inflammation, is essential in acute pancreatitis (AP) pathogenesis. Lycopene (50 mg/kg) significantly prevented AP by a substantial decrease in MPO activity, TNF-α and down-regulating *iNOS* gene expression along with decreasing NO level, increasing pancreatic glutathione (GSH), decreasing serum α-amylase and lipase functions in Wistar rats [64]. Fluorosis can induce oxidative stress by activating MAPK cascade that can cause cell apoptosis. The combination of vitamin E and lycopene prevented fluoride-induced spermatogenic cell apoptosis in rats. Both decreased the expression of rescued clustering and toxicity induced by fluorosis. As well as this, it also decreased the improved JNK and also phosphorylation of the ERK [106].

Another study showed the lycopene role via down-regulating the expression rate of the proprotein convertase subtilisin/kexin type-9 (PCSK-9) by inhibiting hepatocyte nuclear factor-1α, improving LDL-receptor, and sterol regulatory element-binding protein-2. Lycopene reduces Apo-CIII to assemble with lipoprotein lipase (LPL) bonding, too. Likewise, lycopene improved LPS-induced oxidative stress by increasing total antioxidant and HDL-related PON-1 function as well as down-regulating the plasma level and inflammatory mediators expression [107].

Interestingly, lycopene intake (50 mg/kg BW/day) improved D-galactose in CD-1 male mice having cognitive defects. It also improved histopathological injury and repaired brain-derived neurotrophic factor (BDNF) amounts in mice's hippocampal area. Lycopene considerably increased antioxidant enzymatic activity and decreased inflammatory cytokines in D-galactose-administrated mice serum. Furthermore, lycopene supplementation improves mRNA expressions of the NQO-1 and HO-1 as antioxidant enzymes. It was also found to downregulate inflammatory cytokines (i.e., TNF-α, and IL-1β) in the hippocampus of the mice. Lycopene noticeably improves the *GFAP* and Iba-1 expression as the glial cells' inflammatory makers. Lycopene decreased neuronal oxidative damage by activating Nrf2, as well as by inactivating NF-κB translocation in H_2O_2-related SH-SY5Y cell model [65]. Moreover, in a rat model of colitis, it significantly reduced the malondialdehyde (MDA), overall sialic acid, DNA fragmentation concentration, and improved the function of the antioxidant enzyme [108]. In addition, lycopene has significant effects against pathological findings caused by carbofuran on oxidative and biochemical stress biomarkers. It (18 mg/kg BW) markedly improved the serum acetylcholinesterase, albumin, protein and lipids. Furthermore, it improved the catalase (CAT), superoxide dismutase (SOD), and GSH levels, and antioxidant capacity [109].

Lycopene administration considerably improved cognitive defects, noticeably reduced MDA levels and elevated GSH-Px activity, and remarkably reduced tau (or τ proteins) hyperphosphorylation at Thr231/Ser235, Ser262, and Ser396 in P301L transgenic mice's brains [109] (104). In a study conducted on an animal model, in which male mice (C57BL/6) were orally administrated (lycopene dose; 10 or 100 mg/kg), the results reveal that lycopene significantly reduced ROS synthesis in SK-Hep-1 cells while inhibiting NADPH oxidase, which was carried by the protein kinase C (PKC) pathway. Lycopene was also found to be effective against hepatotoxicity by acting as an antioxidant, regulating total glutathione (tGSH) and CAT concentrations, reducing glutathione disulfide (GSSG) and oxidative damage via reducing protein carbonylation. It also elevated MMP-2 down-regulation [110]. Regarding regulator of calcineurin 1 (RCAN1), lycopene reduced mitochondrial ROS and intracellular concentrations, NF-κB activity, Nucling expression, while decreasing the respiration per mitochondrion, MMP and glycolytic activity in RCAN1-overexpressing cells. It suppressed cell death, caspase-3 activation, DNA fragmentation, and cytochrome-c secretion in RCAN1-overexpressing cell lines [111].

The antioxidative role of lycopene was tested in the field of nephrology, also. In gentamicin-induced nephrotoxicity, intake of lycopene and rosmarinic acid could reduce the elevated level of blood urea N2, serum creatinine, renal MDA and immune expression autophagic marker protein (LC3/B), proapoptotic protein (Bax), autophagic marker protein (LC3/B), iNOS and autophagic marker protein (LC3/B). They also increased lower SOD level, GSH, GPx, and antiapoptotic protein (Bcl-2) immunoexpression [112]. In addition, previous researchers found that lycopene (10 mg/kg) attenuated fluoride toxicity via decreasing caspase-3 and caspase-9, and Bax gene expression functions, while improving the activities of GPX and SOD and Bcl-2 gene expression in rats. Ferrous ascorbate administration decreased spermatozoa mobility, viability and spermatozoa antioxidant capacity. It enhanced superoxide production, ROS generation and lipid peroxidation (ferrous ascorbate (FeAA)). On the other hand, the administration of lycopene prevented these changes and has significant antioxidant properties and ROS-scavenging activity in the case of male reproductive cells [113].

It is also able to reduce Aβ-induced oxidative stress due to the lower production of intracellular ROS and superoxide obtained by mitochondria. Moreover, it showed improved Aβ-related mitochondrial morphological modifications, releasing cytochrome-c and opening of mitochondrial transition pores. Lycopene was also found to be effective in restoring ATP in Aβ-treated neurons and improved mitochondrial complex activities. In vivo studies also revealed that in mitochondria, lycopene significantly prevented DNA damage and enhanced transcription factor A level [114].

4.5. Anti-Inflammatory Activity

Lycopene not only quenches singlet ROS, but also prevents lipid peroxidation, too. It has been shown that lycopene (50 and 100 μM) upregulated the HO-1 mRNA. However, it cannot regulate the *NOS2* mRNA and COX-2 expression. Such concentrations also suppressed the LPS-stimulated COX-2, NOS2 and TNF-α gene expression in RAW264.7 cells [66]. Moreover, lycopene has a protective role in β-amyloid-induced inflammation. β-amyloid increased the serum IL-1β, TNF-α, IL-6β levels, and upregulated the expressions of NF-κB p65 mRNA, TLR4 and protein at the choroid plexus. Lycopene supplementation decreased the inflammatory cytokines and reversed the Aβ1-42-related expression and up-regulation of NF-κB p65 mRNA, TLR4 and protein at the choroid plexus [67].

Lycopene supplementation (12.5 mg/kg BW) in carrageenan-induced inflammation considerably decreased edema in Swiss mice via various phlogistic compounds and immunostaining for COX-2, iNOS and NF-κB. It also decreased the migration of leukocytes in paw tissue and peritoneal cavity, lowered the concentration of MPO, while increasing the GSH levels [68]. Furthermore, lycopene has been investigated in different doses (i.e., 0.5, 1.0, 2.0, 4.0, 8.0, 10.0 and 25 µM) for the prevention of cigarette smoking-induced inflammation. Lycopene inhibited the increase in interferon-γ, TNF-α and interleukin-10 concentrations [115]. In a recent study, induction of endotoxin-induced uveitis was performed in Sprague–Dawley rats by LPS single injection (200 µg). The lycopene intraperitoneal administration (10 mg/kg) noticeably lowered the elevated levels of infiltrating cell number, total protein concentration, and NO, TNF-α, and IL-6 induced via LPS [116].

Lycopene is also effective against the treatment of mitochondrial dysfunctioning caused by Aβ1-42 accompanied by TGF-β, increased proinflammatory cytokines, TNF-α and IL-1β and also NF-κB and caspase-3 function in the brain of rats [117]. Lycopene from tomato juice significantly lowered the ICAM-1, and vascular cell adhesion molecule 1 (VCAM-1) level [118]. Lycopene also protects rats against acute lung injury due to LPS by reducing the IL-6 and TNF-α level, suppressing MAPK activity and NF-κB transcription factor. As a result, normal metabolism is retrieved [119]. In LPS-challenge inflammation and depression, lycopene treatment (60 mg/kg/day, orally) for 7 days and also an intraperitoneal injection of LPS (1 mg/kg) was effective. In addition, lycopene improved neuronal cell damage in the hippocampal CA1 region. It reduced HO-1 and IL-1β LPS-related expression in the hippocampus as well as reducing TNF-α and IL-6 in the plasma [120,121].

In the case of THP1 cells, lycopene (2 µM for 2 h) strengthened pro-inflammatory gene expression. The effectiveness of lycopene dose is associated with using a pro-inflammatory stimulus (i.e., LPS, PMA or TNF). At higher concentrations (>2 Mm), lycopene improved metalloprotease secretion, which is a c-AMP-dependent process, by reducing the production of ROS. Cell culture media, PMA-treated monocytes and moved on CaCo-2 epithelial cells could induce proinflammation in these cells. Such inflammation was overcome by treating the cells with lycopene within 12 h. At a lower level of lycopene (<2 µM), it promotes an inflammatory condition not associated with the modulation of ROS. When the concentration of lycopene increases (5 to 20 µM), it was noted that ROS production decreases and consequently, an antiinflammatory effect was produced [122].

4.6. Hepatoprotective

Functional mitochondria perturbation is related to fulminant hepatic failure. Recently, in a study conducted on animal models, d-GalN/LPS (dose: 300 mg/kg and 30 µg/kg BW) induced several instabilities in mitochondrial functioning by increasing H_2O_2 and lipid peroxide levels, decreasing the antioxidant activities of mitochondria, disturbing enzymatic functions of the electron transport chain, tricarboxylic acid cycle and adenosine triphosphate content in cells. Lycopene (10 mg/kg BW, through 6 days) reduced lipid peroxidation and limited excessive H_2O_2 production. Lycopene consumption also regulated d-GalN/LPS-related disturbance in ATP synthesis and elevated enzymatic functions [123]. In addition, pre-treatment with lycopene (5, 10, and 20 mg/kg) has a protective role in a rat model of non-alcoholic fatty liver disease through lowering the liver enzymes levels, like aspartate transaminase (AST), alanine transaminase (ALT), LDL, free fatty acid, and MDA. Furthermore, its role was conducted via an increase in the SOD and GSH concentrations in liver tissue, down-regulating the CYP2E1 and TNF-α expression and reducing the penetration of liver fats [69]. In another study by Yefsah-Idres et al. (2016), it was shown that lycopene administration ameliorated liver injury. It decreased the levels of ALT, serum homocysteine, and AST. In addition, its hepatoprotective effect was performed by enhancing the S-adenosyl-homocysteine hydrolase, hepatic cystathionine beta-synthase activities and decreasing the level of hepatic MDA [70]. Moreover, tomato powder has been shown to have a protective agent against alcohol-induced hepatic injury by inducing cytochrome p450 2E1 [80]. The lycopene treatment considerably improved liver functioning in case of rats with bile duct ligation (BDL). It reduced NO and MDA levels and improved reduced enzymatic level (i.e., CAT, GSTs, GSH, and SOD) in the BDL rat. In addition, lycopene decreased DNA damage [71].

The efficacy of lycopene (40 mg/kg) with proanthocyanidins (450 mg/kg) against mercuric chloride-induced hepatotoxicity was assessed in an animal model. It has been revealed that they inhibited ROS production, protected antioxidant enzymes, and reversed hepatotoxicity in rats' liver [124]. In another study, carbon tetrachloride-caused hepatotoxicity was done in male Wistar rats via intraperitoneal injection (dose; 0.1 mL/kg BW, 14 days). Then, the *Portulaca oleracea* aqueous extract with lycopene (dose; 50 mg/kg body weight) exhibited a hepatoprotective effect against carbon tetrachloride-induced hepatotoxicity. The results also reveal that lycopene significantly restores serum enzyme level to the normal amount in rats [125].

In a study on methotrexate-induced liver injury (20 mg/kg), histopathologic examination of the rats showed that inflammatory cell infiltration, sinusoidal dilatation and congestion were improved significantly by lycopene consumption (10 mg/kg). According to the results, IL-1β, and TNF-α concentrations in the liver tissue were reduced significantly compared to the control group. At the same time, a reduction in oxidative stress index (OSI) was non-significant [126]. In another study on acetaminophen-induced liver damage in C57BL/6 mice, lycopene treatment improved redox imbalance, decreased IL-1β expression, thiobarbituric acid reactive species level and MMP-2 activity [127]. Another study on the hepatoprotective role of lycopene focused on ATZ-induced hepatotoxicity. ATZ (50 and 200 mg/kg) induced hepatotoxicity, whereas lycopene (5 mg/kg) significantly reduced the total cytochrome b5 (Cyt b5) and CYP450 contents. In addition, it prevented from CYP450s stimulation activity (erythromycin N-demethylase (ERND), aniline-4-hydroxylase (AH), aminopyrine N-demethylase (APND), and NADPH-cytochrome c reductase (NCR)) in microsomes of the liver. Lycopene administration effectively modulates CYP450s activities and contents and also normalizes the four CYP450s genes expression, including CYP2a4, CYP2E1, CYP1b1, and 4A14 [128,129].

Furthermore, lycopene (10 mg/kg BW/day, intraperitoneal administration) markedly prevented oxidative damage in experimental hepatitis due to D-galactosamine/LPS. It improved the enzymatic antioxidants levels (i.e., CAT, GPx, SOD, and GSTs) as well as non-enzymatic antioxidants (i.e., vitamin C and E, and GHS). Moreover, lycopene reduced the high level of lipid peroxides and decreased the DNA strand breaks [130]. Additionally, D-Gal/LPS could induce hepatitis in experimental rats, and lycopene significantly reduced the lipid metabolizing enzymatic activity (i.e., LPL, lecithin-cholesterol acyltransferase (LCAT), hepatic triglyceride lipase (HTGL), and increase in the HDL level [131]).

4.7. Against Dermatologic Diseases

Treatment with lycopene decreased UVB-caused cell proliferation while increasing apoptosis via declining CDK2 and CDK4 in hairless SKH-1 mice and human keratinocytes [82]. Moreover, the study conducted on volunteers revealed that lycopene decreased the expression of UVA1 radiation-inducible genes HO-1 upregulation caused by UVA1 and UVA/B [72].

4.8. Neuroprotective

The lycopene consumption relieved cognitive defects, age-related memory loss, neuronal damage, and synaptic dysfunction of the brain. Furthermore, lycopene consumption considerably reduced age-related neuroinflammatory disorders by decreasing microgliosis (IBA-1), as well as down-regulating inflammatory mediators. In addition, a study revealed that lycopene down-regulates the Aβ1-42 accumulation in the brains of aged CD-1 mice [62]. Similarly, lycopene (0.03% w/w) has been found to inhibit the LPS (0.25 mg/kg)-induced memory loss in 3-month old male C57BL/6J mice by reducing Aβ accumulation, APP, reducing the expression of neuronal β-secretase beta-site amyloid precursor protein cleaving enzyme 1 (BACE1), and improving the α-secretase A disintegrin and metalloproteinase 10 (ADAM10) expressions. In addition, it suppressed IBA-1 expression as the marker of microglia activation, inflammatory mediators and also decreased oxidative stress (among mice treated with LPS). Furthermore, lycopene inhibited NF-κB, MAPKs and Nrf2 activity phosphorylation in BV2 microglial cells (LPS treated) [63].

Lycopene suppressed the 4-AP-invoked release of glutamate and elevated intra-synaptosomal Ca^{2+} level. The studies revealed that the inhibitory impact of lycopene on 4-AP-evoked glutamate secretion decreased the presence of Cav2.1 (P/Q-type) and Cav2.2 (N-type) channel blocker ω-conotoxin MVIIC noticeably. However, it did not affect the inhibitors of CGP37157 and intracellular Ca^{2+} release. Moreover, lycopene's effect on evoked glutamate secretion was protected via PKC inhibitors Go6976 and GF109203X [73]. Wang et al. reported that rats that were fed on HFD with lycopene (4 mg/kg, oral administration) had considerably reduced cognitive defects and improved learning abilities through the prevention of a decrease in dendritic spine density [132]. In another study, lycopene administration (5, 10 mg/kg, oral) significantly decreased impairment in biochemical, behavioral, neuroinflammatory and neurochemical markers in rats with haloperidol-induced orofacial dyskinesia [75].

Lycopene's neuroprotective effect was also studied for pentylenetetrazol (PTZ)-induced kindling epilepsy in rats treated with lycopene at the concentrations of 2.5, 5, and 10 mg/kg, sodium valproate through 29 days, and 40 mg/kg of PTZ (intraperitoneal) with alternate days. Rats were assessed for various behavioral and biochemical parameters (SOD, lipid peroxidation, CAT, decreased GSH and nitrite) and activities of the enzymes of mitochondria (I, II, and IV) in the brain. Based on the findings, lycopene (5, 10 mg/kg) considerably improved mitochondrial enzymatic activities, kindling score, and oxidative stress as compared to control [74]. The neuroprotective role of lycopene was also studied in a male C57BL/6 mice model of bilateral common carotid artery occlusion (BCCAO). The Nrf2/HO 1 signaling route function via increasing the Nrf2 HO 1 expression was also seen. The results indicate that the Nrf2/HO 1 signaling route is associated with lycopene's neuroprotective impact [133].

Regarding AD, lycopene considerably prevents paralysis in Aβ1-42-transgenic *Caenorhabditis elegans* strain GMC101. Treating with lycopene inhibited Aβ1-42 release in SH-SY5Y cells by the overexpression of the Swedish mutant type of human APP (APPsw). Additionally, lycopene can effectively down-regulate APP expression in APPsw cells. Furthermore, treating with lycopene did not affect endogenous ROS amount and apoptosis in case of APPsw cells. It significantly improved the neurological scores in BCCAO mouse. It reduced neuronal apoptosis via TUNEL staining and decreased oxidative stress due to global brain ischemia [134]. Interestingly, it has a neuroprotective effect against PD caused by 1-methyl-4-phenyl-1,2,3,6-tetrahydropyridine (MPTP) in mice. Treating with lycopene (5, 10 and 20 mg/kg/day, oral administration) prevented PD by MPTP in a concentration-dependent fashion. It also reduced MPTP-caused motor abnormalities and oxidative stress [135]. Chronic consumption of lycopene can effectively improve cognitive abilities, decrease mitochondrial-oxidative damage, inhibit neuroinflammation and repair BDNF concentration in β-A1-42-treated rats [136].

The lycopene neuroprotective effect on oxidative stress, as well as neurobehavioral disorders in PD of adult C57BL/6 mice due to rotenone, was studied in a recent study. Lycopene treatment (10 mg/kg BW, oral administration) in the rotenone-treated animals enhanced GSH-Px, SOD and CAT activities and reduced MDA concentrations. It also elevated the number of tyrosine hydroxylase-, enhanced alpha-synuclein (alpha-SYN)- and microtubule-associated protein 3 light chain (LC3-B)-positive neurons [137]. Lycopene provides protection against neurotoxicity through methylmercury (MeHg) induced in cultured rat cerebellar granule neurons (CGNs). Lycopene prevented the loss of cell viability and release of LDH. Lycopene also protected from the inhibition of mitochondrial complexes III and IV enzyme activities and decreased the production of ATP and mtDNA (copy, transcript levels) [138].

There is an in vivo study on rat's treatment using rotenone (3 mg/kg BW, intraperitoneal) for 30 days. NADH dehydrogenase as a marker of rotenone action was markedly suppressed (35%) in treated animals' striatum. On the other hand, oral administration of lycopene (10 mg/kg) to the rotenone-treated animals for 30 days elevated the activity by 39% compared to the animals treated with rotenone. Rotenone treatment enhanced the MDA concentrations (75.15%) in the striatum, while lycopene treatment reduced its concentrations by 24.33%. This was associated with cognitive and motor impairments in rotenone-treated animals that were reversed on lycopene administration. Finally, lycopene administration inhibited the cytochrome c release from mitochondria [139].

4.9. Bone Protective

Lycopene has several molecular and cellular effects on human osteoblasts and osteoclasts. It reduced osteoclast differentiation, whereas it did not change cell survival/cell density; calcium-phosphate resorbing was also reduced. In addition, osteoblast proliferation (reduction on apoptosis) and differentiation were improved by lycopene [76,140]. Moreover, lycopene supplementation has an effective role in postmenopausal osteoporosis [80]. Lycopene administration inhibited the ovariectomized (OVX)-related increase in bone turnover, such as modification in biomarkers of serum osteocalcin, serum cross-linked carboxyterminal telopeptides, bone metabolism, serum N-terminal propeptide of type 1 collagen, and urinary deoxypyridinoline. Remarkable upgrading in OVX-related loss of bone mass, microarchitectural deterioration and bone strength was witnessed in lycopene-administrated OVX animals. These observations were more prominent in areas full of trabecular bone and low level of cortical bone. In these six-week-old Sprague–Dawley female rats, the bone mineral density of the tibial proximal metaphysis and lumbar spine increased via lycopene treatment dependent on the dose. Lycopene administration also down-regulated the osteoclast differentiation along with up-regulation of the osteoblast and GPx CAT and SOD activities [77,141]. Daily lycopene consumption reduces the risk of bone resorption in postmenopausal female cases by oxidation prevention [142].

4.10. Targeting Reproductive Disorders

Lycopene can decrease sperm DNA fragmentation, as well as lipid peroxidation by its antioxidant activity in normospermic infertile men [78,105]. It (4 mg/kg/day, orally) improved the sperm count and motility by decreasing H_2O_2 and lipid peroxidation, and improving mitochondrial enzymatic activity (i.e., CAT, SOD, GR, GPx, and ADH) and non-enzymatic antioxidant level (GSH and ascorbate). In addition, lycopene showed a significant improvement in the testicular mitochondria's enzymatic activities of tricarboxylic (i.e., isocitrate dehydrogenase, succinate dehydrogenase, fumarase and malate dehydrogenase) [79].

Lycopene (4 mg/kg) ameliorated adriamycin (ADR) (10 mg/kg)-induced reductions in Sprague–Dawley rats' epididymis and testes weights. The sperm morphology and motility were noticeably normalized by lycopene treatment. While the testosterone amount was reduced in the ADR group, no significant effect was found in the treated group. Interestingly, pretreatment with lycopene significantly reformed MDA and decreased GSH levels. Moreover, ADR-induced histopathological changes were reversed by the lycopene treatment [143].

Lycopene has protective effects against cisplatin-induced spermiotoxicity, too. Lycopene (4 mg/kg) showed significant results in decreasing total abnormal sperms, improving sperm viability and motility. In addition, lycopene decreased testicular MDA concentration and increased GPx activity [144]. Another study revealed a protective effect of lycopene (1.5 mg/0.5 mL Tween; 80/100 g BW) in cyproterone acetate-induced infertility in rats. Lycopene made a significant retrieval effect on sperm count, viability, and motility, hypo-osmotic swelling tail to coil spermatozoa, testicular functions of 17β- hydroxysteroid dehydrogenase (HSD), CAT, 3β-HSD and SOD, conjugated diene level, MDA, serum testosterone, and testicular cholesterol [145]. Figure 2 illustrates some of the common signaling pathways which are mentioned in this section. The figure was designed and modified based on Trejo-Solís and co-authors' paper [146].

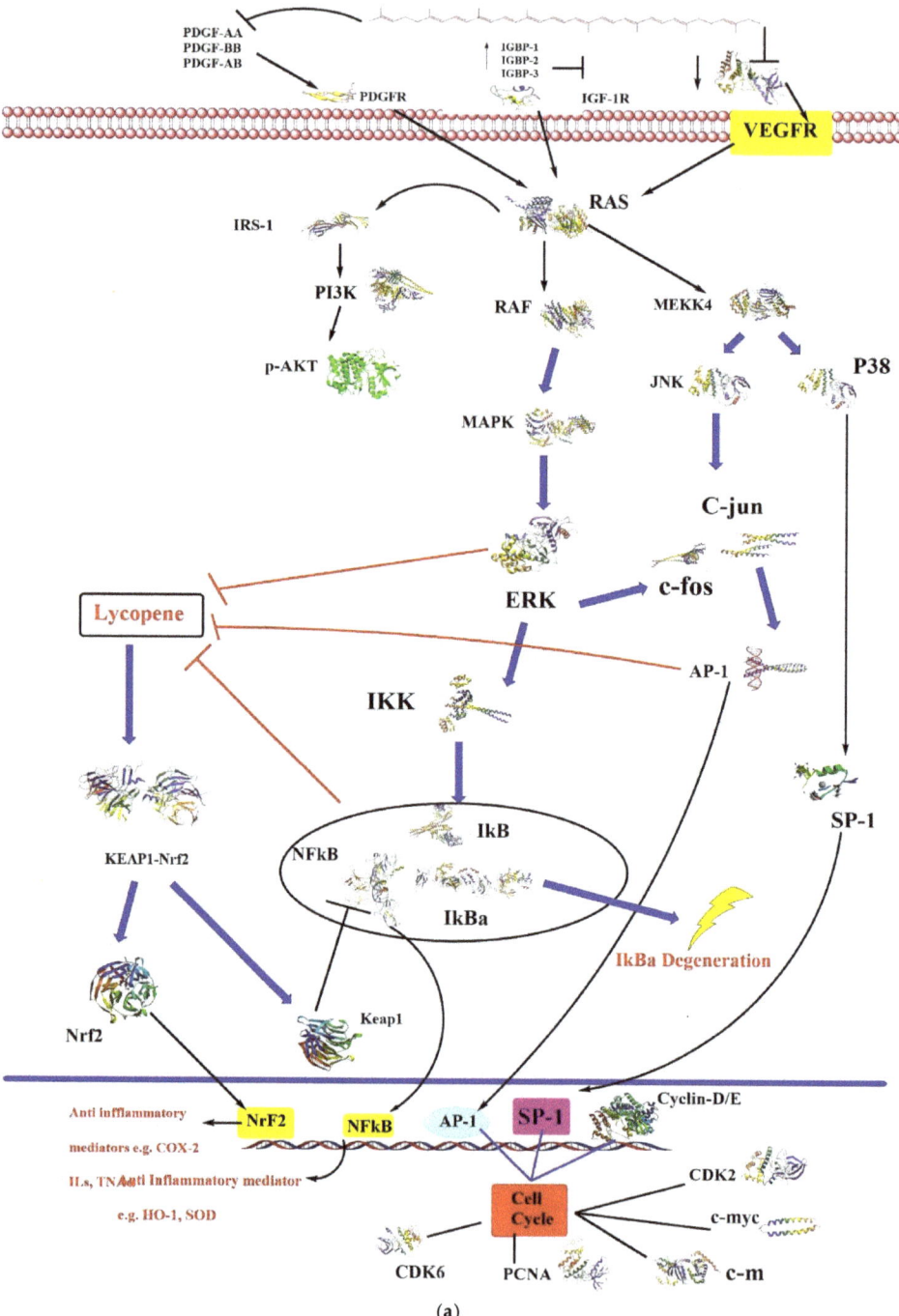

(a)

Figure 2. Cont.

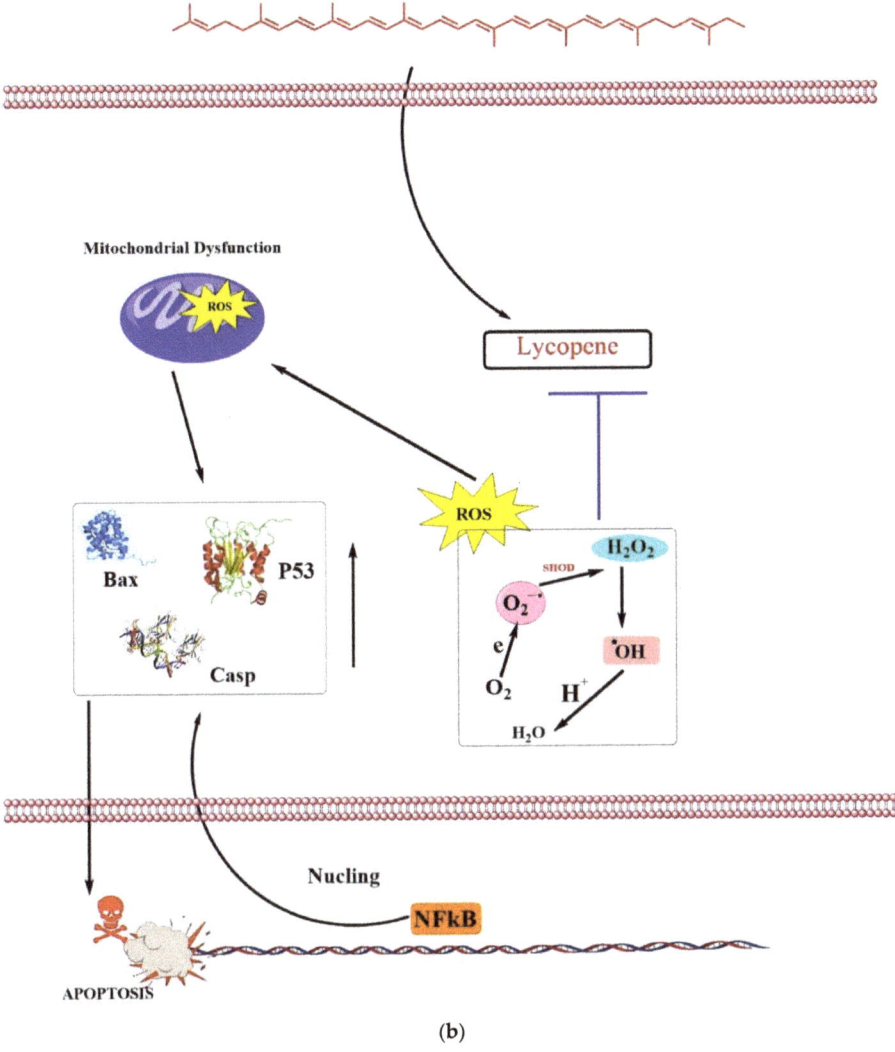

Figure 2. (**a**). Effect of lycopene on PDGFR-, IGF-IR-, and VEGFR-mediated signal pathways. (**b**) Effect of Lycopene on Reactive Oxygen Species (modified from [146]).

VEGF: vascular endothelial growth factor; AP-1: activator protein-1; CASP: caspase; ERK1/2: kinase regulated by extracellular signals; IGF: insulin-like growth factor; IKK: IκB kinase; IRS: insulin-1 receptor substrate; Keap1: Kelch-like ECH-associated protein 1; PCNA: proliferating cell nuclear antigen; PDGF: platelet-derived growth factor; PI3K: phosphoinositide 3-kinase; RAF: proto-oncogene serine/threonine-protein kinase; SP-1: specificity protein 1.

5. Protective Effects of Lycopene Against Different Toxins

Besides the aforementioned anti-toxicity effects of lycopene, this action should be briefly discussed. Previous studies suggested its significant protection against a wide variety of natural and chemical toxins. Different chemical agents with known neurotoxicity, hepatotoxicity, nephrotoxicity, and cardiotoxicity are inhibited by lycopene. Lycopene's main properties which are believed to be necessary for this action are anti-oxidative, chelating, free-radical scavenging and antiapoptotic activities. This miracle pigment prevents bacterial toxins, mycotoxins, fluoride, metals, and pesticides from exerting their toxicities against the human body [4].

6. Recommended Dose

It should be noted that there is no ideal dose for daily lycopene consumption. Although previous studies only give ideas about lycopene intake at a different level, that would be helpful. For example, an in vivo study revealed that lycopene (6.5 mg/day) was effective against cancer in men [147]. However, lycopene dose should be increased up to 10 mg/day, in the case of advanced PCa. In another study, lycopene supplementation (15 mg/day, for 12 weeks) in an old aged population improved immune function through increasing natural killer cell activity by 28% [148]. Therefore, it seems that different lycopene doses and duration of supplementation can be suggested for various health purposes. Finally, according to different epidemiological studies, daily lycopene intake can be suggested to be 2 to 20 mg per day [10].

7. Safety and Toxicity

Safety monitoring should be considered as an important issue about medicinal plants and plant-derived phytochemicals [149,150]. There are several in vitro and in vivo studies on the possible toxicity of lycopene. For instance, it has been shown that lycopene (up to 10 µM) has no toxicity on the rat's cultured cerebellar granule neurons viability [138]. Another research on cultured rat hippocampal neurons showed no significant toxic effects of lycopene when it was applied to these cells [151], even though it seems that carotenoids in some certain settings at high tissue concentrations may show a pro-oxidant effect [152]. A toxicological study on rats showed the no-observed-adverse-effect level at the highest examined dose (i.e., 1.0% in the diet) [153]. It should be noted that different lycopene forms (i.e., lycopene extracted from tomato, synthetic lycopene, and its crystallized extract) are generally recognized as safe when used in different food products [154]. There are no reports on adverse events from lycopene use at normal and ordinary doses [155]. Human studies suggested the no-observed-adverse-effect level for lycopene as 3 g per day/kg of body weight. Daily lycopene intake has been estimated as being significantly less than this level. Even the 99th percentile for its intake is 123 mg per day [156]. It seems that the expression of cytochrome P450 2E1 can be induced by high doses of lycopene and alcohol. Therefore, their high dose of concomitant use should be avoided [157]. In addition, regarding lycopene's potent antioxidative effect, precautions should be kept in mind for patients under chemo and radiation therapy [158]. A case report described lycopenemia in a woman who had ingested about 2 liters of tomato juice every day and for several years. She had lycopene deposits in the liver (with no evidence of hepatic dysfunction) and deep orange discoloration of the skin. The lycopenodermia disappeared 3 weeks after stopping tomato juice consumption [159]. In addition, there is a chain of studies in which the lycopene mutagenicity was assessed. The results indicate that formulated lycopene has no mutagenic effects, although crystalline lycopene showed some mutagenic activity when degraded under exposure to light and air [160].

8. Conclusions

Lycopene possesses potent anticancer, antioxidant, antiinflammatory, and antidiabetic potential. In addition, it is a nutraceutical which protects against a wide variety of heart, liver, bone, skin, nervous, and reproductive systems diseases, as evident from numerous studies. However, further investigations are necessary to unveil the underlying mechanisms of actions, with a special emphasis on gene expression studies. Additionally, the recommended and effective doses of this functional food need to be further investigated. Safety concerns about its genotoxicity, maternal toxicity, and teratogenic effects should also be inquired.

Author Contributions: M.I., F.G., I.U.-H., H.U.-R., F.A., M.A.S., and M.H.H. conceived the review idea and focus, drafted the article, and critically revised the article. M.R., M.H., E.O., Z.Y. and M.T. were involved in the reference collection, writing the article. All authors have read and agreed to the published version of the manuscript.

Funding: This paper was supported by the KU Research Professor Program of Konkuk University, Seoul, South Korea.

Conflicts of Interest: The authors declare no conflict of interest.

References

1. Pennathur, S.; Maitra, D.; Byun, J.; Sliskovic, I.; Abdulhamid, I.; Saed, G.M.; Diamond, M.P.; Abu-Soud, H.M. Potent antioxidative activity of lycopene: A potential role in scavenging hypochlorous acid. *Free Radic. Biol. Med.* **2010**, *49*, 205–213. [CrossRef]
2. Yin, Y.; Zheng, Z.; Jiang, Z. Effects of lycopene on metabolism of glycolipid in type 2 diabetic rats. *Biomed. Pharmacother.* **2019**, *109*, 2070–2077. [CrossRef] [PubMed]
3. Mozos, I.; Stoian, D.; Caraba, A.; Malainer, C.; Horbańczuk, J.O.; Atanasov, A.G. Lycopene and vascular health. *Front. Pharmacol.* **2018**, *9*, 521. [CrossRef] [PubMed]
4. Hedayati, N.; Naeini, M.B.; Nezami, A.; Hosseinzadeh, H.; Wallace Hayes, A.; Hosseini, S.; Imenshahidi, M.; Karimi, G. Protective effect of lycopene against chemical and natural toxins: A review. *BioFactors* **2019**, *45*, 5–23. [CrossRef] [PubMed]
5. Woodside, J.V.; McGrath, A.J.; Lyner, N.; McKinley, M.C. Carotenoids and health in older people. *Maturitas* **2015**, *80*, 63–68. [CrossRef] [PubMed]
6. Moran, N.E.; Erdman, J.W., Jr.; Clinton, S.K. Complex interactions between dietary and genetic factors impact lycopene metabolism and distribution. *Arch. Biochem. Biophys.* **2013**, *539*, 171–180. [CrossRef] [PubMed]
7. Petyaev, I.M. Lycopene deficiency in ageing and cardiovascular disease. *Oxidative Med. Cell. Longev.* **2016**, *2016*, 3218605. [CrossRef] [PubMed]
8. Ellis, A.C.; Dudenbostel, T.; Crowe-White, K. Watermelon juice: A novel functional food to increase circulating lycopene in older adult women. *Plant Foods Hum. Nutr.* **2019**, *74*, 200–203. [CrossRef]
9. Naviglio, D.; Sapio, L.; Langilla, C.; Ragone, A.; Illiano, M.; Naviglio, S.; Gallo, M. Beneficial Effects and Perspective Strategies for Lycopene Food Enrichment: A Systematic Review. *Syst. Rev. Pharm.* **2019**, *10*, 383–392.
10. Saini, R.K.; Rengasamy, K.R.; Mahomoodally, F.M.; Keum, Y.-S. Protective effects of lycopene in cancer, cardiovascular, and neurodegenerative diseases: An update on epidemiological and mechanistic perspectives. *Pharmacol. Res.* **2020**, *155*, 104730. [CrossRef]
11. Przybylska, S. Lycopene–a bioactive carotenoid offering multiple health benefits: A review. *Int. J. Food Sci. Technol.* **2020**, *55*, 11–32. [CrossRef]
12. Joshi, B.; Kar, S.K.; Yadav, P.K.; Yadav, S.; Shrestha, L.; Bera, T.K. Therapeutic and medicinal uses of lycopene: A systematic review. *Int. J. Res. Med Sci.* **2020**, *8*, 1195. [CrossRef]
13. Rowles, J.; Ranard, K.; Smith, J.; An, R.; Erdman, J. Increased dietary and circulating lycopene are associated with reduced prostate cancer risk: A systematic review and meta-analysis. *Prostate Cancer Prostatic Dis.* **2017**, *20*, 361–377. [CrossRef] [PubMed]
14. Rowles, J.L.; Ranard, K.M.; Applegate, C.C.; Jeon, S.; An, R.; Erdman, J.W. Processed and raw tomato consumption and risk of prostate cancer: A systematic review and dose–response meta-analysis. *Prostate Cancer Prostatic Dis.* **2018**, *21*, 319–336. [CrossRef] [PubMed]
15. Carini, F.; David, S.; Tomasello, G.; Mazzola, M.; Damiani, P.; Rappa, F.; Battaglia, L.; Cappello, F.; Jurjus, A.; Geagea, A.G. Colorectal cancer: An update on the effects of lycopene on tumor progression and cell proliferation. *J. Biol. Regul. Homeost. Agents* **2017**, *31*, 769–774.
16. Senkus, K.E.; Tan, L.; Crowe-White, K.M. Lycopene and metabolic syndrome: A systematic review of the literature. *Adv. Nutr.* **2019**, *10*, 19–29. [CrossRef]
17. Kwatra, B. A review on potential properties and therapeutic applications of lycopene. *Int. J. Med Biomed. Stud.* **2020**, *4*. [CrossRef]
18. Crowe-White, K.M.; Phillips, T.A.; Ellis, A.C. Lycopene and cognitive function. *J. Nutr. Sci.* **2019**, *8*. [CrossRef]
19. Chen, D.; Huang, C.; Chen, Z. A review for the pharmacological effect of lycopene in central nervous system disorders. *Biomed. Pharmacother.* **2019**, *111*, 791–801. [CrossRef]

20. Chernyshova, M.P.; Pristenskiy, D.V.; Lozbiakova, M.V.; Chalyk, N.E.; Bandaletova, T.Y.; Petyaev, I.M. Systemic and skin-targeting beneficial effects of lycopene-enriched ice cream: A pilot study. *J. Dairy Sci.* **2019**, *102*, 14–25. [CrossRef]
21. Salehi, B.; Lopez-Jornet, P.; Pons-Fuster López, E.; Calina, D.; Sharifi-Rad, M.; Ramírez-Alarcón, K.; Forman, K.; Fernández, M.; Martorell, M.; Setzer, W.N. Plant-derived bioactives in oral mucosal lesions: A key emphasis to curcumin, lycopene, chamomile, aloe vera, green tea and coffee properties. *Biomolecules* **2019**, *9*, 106. [CrossRef] [PubMed]
22. Maiani, G.; Periago Castón, M.J.; Catasta, G.; Toti, E.; Cambrodón, I.G.; Bysted, A.; Granado-Lorencio, F.; Olmedilla-Alonso, B.; Knuthsen, P.; Valoti, M. Carotenoids: Actual knowledge on food sources, intakes, stability and bioavailability and their protective role in humans. *Mol. Nutr. Food Res.* **2009**, *53*, S194–S218. [CrossRef] [PubMed]
23. Shi, J.; Maguer, M.L. Lycopene in tomatoes: Chemical and physical properties affected by food processing. *Crit. Rev. Food Sci. Nutr.* **2000**, *40*, 1–42. [CrossRef] [PubMed]
24. Bramley, P.M. Is lycopene beneficial to human health? *Phytochemistry* **2000**, *54*, 233–236. [CrossRef]
25. Barber, N.; Barber, J. Lycopene and prostate cancer. *Prostate Cancer Prostatic Dis.* **2002**, *5*, 6–12. [CrossRef]
26. Grabowska, M.; Wawrzyniak, D.; Rolle, K.; Chomczyński, P.; Oziewicz, S.; Jurga, S.; Barciszewski, J. Let food be your medicine: Nutraceutical properties of lycopene. *Food Funct.* **2019**, *10*, 3090–3102. [CrossRef]
27. O'Neill, M.; Carroll, Y.; Corridan, B.; Olmedilla, B.; Granado, F.; Blanco, I.; Van den Berg, H.; Hininger, I.; Rousell, A.-M.; Chopra, M. A European carotenoid database to assess carotenoid intakes and its use in a five-country comparative study. *Br. J. Nutr.* **2001**, *85*, 499–507. [CrossRef]
28. Porrini, M.; Riso, P. What are typical lycopene intakes? *J. Nutr.* **2005**, *135*, 2042S–2045S. [CrossRef]
29. Jacques, P.F.; Lyass, A.; Massaro, J.M.; Vasan, R.S.; D'Agostino Sr, R.B. Relationship of lycopene intake and consumption of tomato products to incident CVD. *Br. J. Nutr.* **2013**, *110*, 545–551. [CrossRef]
30. Authority, E.F.S. Revised exposure assessment for lycopene as a food colour. *EFSA J.* **2010**, *8*, 1444. [CrossRef]
31. Holzapfel, N.P.; Holzapfel, B.M.; Champ, S.; Feldthusen, J.; Clements, J.; Hutmacher, D.W. The potential role of lycopene for the prevention and therapy of prostate cancer: From molecular mechanisms to clinical evidence. *Int. J. Mol. Sci.* **2013**, *14*, 14620–14646. [CrossRef] [PubMed]
32. Agarwal, S.; Rao, A. Carotenoids and chronic diseases. *Drug Metab. Drug Interact.* **2000**, *17*, 189–210. [CrossRef] [PubMed]
33. Canene-Adams, K.; Campbell, J.K.; Zaripheh, S.; Jeffery, E.H.; Erdman, J.W., Jr. The tomato as a functional food. *J. Nutr.* **2005**, *135*, 1226–1230. [CrossRef] [PubMed]
34. Walfisch, Y.; Walfisch, S.; Agbaria, R.; Levy, J.; Sharoni, Y. Lycopene in serum, skin and adipose tissues after tomato-oleoresin supplementation in patients undergoing haemorrhoidectomy or peri-anal fistulotomy. *Br. J. Nutr.* **2003**, *90*, 759–766. [CrossRef] [PubMed]
35. Burton-Freeman, B.M.; Sesso, H.D. Whole food versus supplement: Comparing the clinical evidence of tomato intake and lycopene supplementation on cardiovascular risk factors. *Adv. Nutr.* **2014**, *5*, 457–485. [CrossRef]
36. Richelle, M.; Sanchez, B.; Tavazzi, I.; Lambelet, P.; Bortlik, K.; Williamson, G. Lycopene isomerisation takes place within enterocytes during absorption in human subjects. *Br. J. Nutr.* **2010**, *103*, 1800–1807. [CrossRef]
37. Teodoro, A.J.; Perrone, D.; Martucci, R.B.; Borojevic, R. Lycopene isomerisation and storage in an in vitro model of murine hepatic stellate cells. *Eur. J. Nutr.* **2009**, *48*, 261–268. [CrossRef]
38. Moussa, M.; Landrier, J.-F.; Reboul, E.; Ghiringhelli, O.; Coméra, C.; Collet, X.; Fröhlich, K.; Böhm, V.; Borel, P. Lycopene absorption in human intestinal cells and in mice involves scavenger receptor class B type I but not Niemann-Pick C1-like 1. *J. Nutr.* **2008**, *138*, 1432–1436. [CrossRef]
39. Moussa, M.; Gouranton, E.; Gleize, B.; Yazidi, C.E.; Niot, I.; Besnard, P.; Borel, P.; Landrier, J.F. CD36 is involved in lycopene and lutein uptake by adipocytes and adipose tissue cultures. *Mol. Nutr. Food Res.* **2011**, *55*, 578–584. [CrossRef]
40. Ferrucci, L.; Perry, J.R.; Matteini, A.; Perola, M.; Tanaka, T.; Silander, K.; Rice, N.; Melzer, D.; Murray, A.; Cluett, C. Common variation in the β-carotene 15, 15′-monooxygenase 1 gene affects circulating levels of carotenoids: A genome-wide association study. *Am. J. Hum. Genet.* **2009**, *84*, 123–133. [CrossRef]
41. Lindshield, B.L.; Canene-Adams, K.; Erdman, J.W., Jr. Lycopenoids: Are lycopene metabolites bioactive? *Arch. Biochem. Biophys.* **2007**, *458*, 136–140. [CrossRef] [PubMed]

42. Ross, A.B.; Vuong, L.T.; Ruckle, J.; Synal, H.A.; Schulze-König, T.; Wertz, K.; Rümbeli, R.; Liberman, R.G.; Skipper, P.L.; Tannenbaum, S.R. Lycopene bioavailability and metabolism in humans: An accelerator mass spectrometry study. *Am. J. Clin. Nutr.* **2011**, *93*, 1263–1273. [CrossRef] [PubMed]
43. Moran, N.E.; Cichon, M.J.; Riedl, K.M.; Grainger, E.M.; Schwartz, S.J.; Novotny, J.A.; Erdman, J.W., Jr.; Clinton, S.K. Compartmental and noncompartmental modeling of 13C-lycopene absorption, isomerization, and distribution kinetics in healthy adults. *Am. J. Clin. Nutr.* **2015**, *102*, 1436–1449. [CrossRef] [PubMed]
44. Sahin, K.; Yenice, E.; Tuzcu, M.; Orhan, C.; Mizrak, C.; Ozercan, I.H.; Sahin, N.; Yilmaz, B.; Bilir, B.; Ozpolat, B. Lycopene protects against spontaneous ovarian cancer formation in laying hens. *J. Cancer Prev.* **2018**, *23*, 25. [CrossRef] [PubMed]
45. Cataño, J.G.; Trujillo, C.G.; Caicedo, J.I.; Bravo-Balado, A.; Robledo, D.; Mariño-Alvarez, A.M.; Pedraza, A.; Arcila, M.J.; Plata, M. Efficacy of lycopene intake in primary prevention of prostate cancer: A systematic review of the literature and meta-analysis. *Arch. Esp. Urol.* **2018**, *71*, 187–197.
46. Dos Santos, R.C.; Ombredane, A.S.; Souza, J.M.T.; Vasconcelos, A.G.; Plácido, A.; das GN Amorim, A.; Barbosa, E.A.; Lima, F.C.; Ropke, C.D.; Alves, M.M. Lycopene-rich extract from red guava (Psidium guajava L.) displays cytotoxic effect against human breast adenocarcinoma cell line MCF-7 via an apoptotic-like pathway. *Food Res. Int.* **2018**, *105*, 184–196. [CrossRef]
47. Morgia, G.; Voce, S.; Palmieri, F.; Gentile, M.; Iapicca, G.; Giannantoni, A.; Blefari, F.; Carini, M.; Vespasiani, G.; Santelli, G. Association between selenium and lycopene supplementation and incidence of prostate cancer: Results from the post-hoc analysis of the procomb trial. *Phytomedicine* **2017**, *34*, 1–5. [CrossRef]
48. Zhou, S.; Zhang, R.; Bi, T.; Lu, Y.; Jiang, L. Inhibitory effect of lycopene against the growth of human gastric cancer cells. *Afr. J. Tradit. Complement. Altern. Med.* **2016**, *13*, 184–190. [CrossRef]
49. Jhou, B.-Y.; Song, T.-Y.; Lee, I.; Hu, M.-L.; Yang, N.-C. Lycopene inhibits metastasis of human liver adenocarcinoma SK-Hep-1 cells by downregulation of NADPH oxidase 4 protein expression. *J. Agric. Food Chem.* **2017**, *65*, 6893–6903. [CrossRef]
50. Holzapfel, N.P.; Shokoohmand, A.; Wagner, F.; Landgraf, M.; Champ, S.; Holzapfel, B.M.; Clements, J.A.; Hutmacher, D.W.; Loessner, D. Lycopene reduces ovarian tumor growth and intraperitoneal metastatic load. *Am. J. Cancer Res.* **2017**, *7*, 1322.
51. Baş, H.; Pandır, D. Protective effects of lycopene on furantreated diabetic and non-diabetic rat lung. *Biomed. Environ. Sci.* **2016**, *29*, 143–147.
52. Reddy, P.V.N.; Ambati, M.; Koduganti, R. Systemic lycopene as an adjunct to scaling and root planing in chronic periodontitis patients with type 2 diabetes mellitus. *J. Int. Soc. Prev. Community Dent.* **2015**, *5*, S25. [PubMed]
53. Sandikci, M.; Karagenc, L.; Yildiz, M. Changes in the Pancreas in Experimental Diabetes and the Effect of Lycopene on These Changes: Proliferating, Apoptotic, and Estrogen Receptor α Positive Cells. *Anat. Rec.* **2017**, *300*, 2000–2007. [CrossRef] [PubMed]
54. Uçar, S.; Pandir, D. Furan induced ovarian damage in non-diabetic and diabetic rats and cellular protective role of lycopene. *Arch. Gynaecol. Obstet.* **2017**, *296*, 1027–1037. [CrossRef]
55. Soleymaninejad, M.; Joursaraei, S.G.; Feizi, F.; Jafari Anarkooli, I. The effects of lycopene and insulin on histological changes and the expression level of Bcl-2 family genes in the hippocampus of streptozotocin-induced diabetic rats. *J. Diabetes Res.* **2017**, *2017*, 4650939. [CrossRef] [PubMed]
56. Tabrez, S.; Al-Shali, K.Z.; Ahmad, S. Lycopene powers the inhibition of glycation-induced diabetic nephropathy: A novel approach to halt the AGE-RAGE axis menace. *Biofactors* **2015**, *41*, 372–381. [CrossRef]
57. Yegın, S.Ç.; Yur, F.; Çetın, S.; Güder, A. Effect of lycopene on serum nitrite-nitrate levels in diabetic rats. *Indian J. Pharm. Sci.* **2015**, *77*, 357. [CrossRef]
58. Costa-Rodrigues, J.; Pinho, O.; Monteiro, P. Can lycopene be considered an effective protection against cardiovascular disease? *Food Chem.* **2018**, *245*, 1148–1153. [CrossRef]
59. Kumar, R.; Salwe, K.J.; Kumarappan, M. Evaluation of antioxidant, hypolipidemic, and antiatherogenic property of lycopene and astaxanthin in atherosclerosis-induced rats. *Pharmacogn. Res.* **2017**, *9*, 161.
60. Cheng, H.M.; Koutsidis, G.; Lodge, J.K.; Ashor, A.; Siervo, M.; Lara, J. Tomato and lycopene supplementation and cardiovascular risk factors: A systematic review and meta-analysis. *Atherosclerosis* **2017**, *257*, 100–108. [CrossRef]

61. He, Y.; Xia, P.; Jin, H.; Zhang, Y.; Chen, B.; Xu, Z. Lycopene Ameliorates Transplant Arteriosclerosis in Vascular Allograft Transplantation by Regulating the NO/cGMP Pathways and Rho-Associated Kinases Expression. *Oxidative Med. Cell. Longev.* **2016**, *2016*, 3128280. [CrossRef] [PubMed]
62. Zhao, B.; Liu, H.; Wang, J.; Liu, P.; Tan, X.; Ren, B.; Liu, Z.; Liu, X. Lycopene supplementation attenuates oxidative stress, neuroinflammation, and cognitive impairment in aged CD-1 mice. *J. Agric. Food Chem.* **2018**, *66*, 3127–3136. [CrossRef] [PubMed]
63. Wang, J.; Li, L.; Wang, Z.; Cui, Y.; Tan, X.; Yuan, T.; Liu, Q.; Liu, Z.; Liu, X. Supplementation of lycopene attenuates lipopolysaccharide-induced amyloidogenesis and cognitive impairments via mediating neuroinflammation and oxidative stress. *J. Nutr. Biochem.* **2018**, *56*, 16–25. [CrossRef] [PubMed]
64. El-Ashmawy, N.E.; Khedr, N.F.; El-Bahrawy, H.A.; Hamada, O.B. Suppression of inducible nitric oxide synthase and tumor necrosis factor-alpha level by lycopene is comparable to methylprednisolone in acute pancreatitis. *Dig. Liver Dis.* **2018**, *50*, 601–607. [CrossRef]
65. Zhao, B.; Ren, B.; Guo, R.; Zhang, W.; Ma, S.; Yao, Y.; Yuan, T.; Liu, Z.; Liu, X. Supplementation of lycopene attenuates oxidative stress induced neuroinflammation and cognitive impairment via Nrf2/NF-κB transcriptional pathway. *Food Chem. Toxicol.* **2017**, *109*, 505–516. [CrossRef]
66. Kawata, A.; Murakami, Y.; Suzuki, S.; Fujisawa, S. Anti-inflammatory activity of β-Carotene, lycopene and tri-n-butylborane, a scavenger of reactive oxygen species. *Vivo* **2018**, *32*, 255–264.
67. Liu, C.-B.; Wang, R.; Yi, Y.-F.; Gao, Z.; Chen, Y.-Z. Lycopene mitigates β-amyloid induced inflammatory response and inhibits NF-κB signaling at the choroid plexus in early stages of Alzheimer's disease rats. *J. Nutr. Biochem.* **2018**, *53*, 66–71. [CrossRef]
68. Vasconcelos, A.G.; das GN Amorim, A.; dos Santos, R.C.; Souza, J.M.T.; de Souza, L.K.M.; de SL Araújo, T.; Nicolau, L.A.D.; de Lima Carvalho, L.; de Aquino, P.E.A.; da Silva Martins, C. Lycopene rich extract from red guava (Psidium guajava L.) displays anti-inflammatory and antioxidant profile by reducing suggestive hallmarks of acute inflammatory response in mice. *Food Res. Int.* **2017**, *99*, 959–968. [CrossRef]
69. Jiang, W.; Guo, M.-H.; Hai, X. Hepatoprotective and antioxidant effects of lycopene on non-alcoholic fatty liver disease in rat. *World J. Gastroenterol.* **2016**, *22*, 10180. [CrossRef]
70. Yefsah-Idres, A.; Benazzoug, Y.; Otman, A.; Latour, A.; Middendorp, S.; Janel, N. Hepatoprotective effects of lycopene on liver enzymes involved in methionine and xenobiotic metabolism in hyperhomocysteinemic rats. *Food Funct.* **2016**, *7*, 2862–2869. [CrossRef]
71. Tokaç, M.; Aydin, S.; Taner, G.; Özkardeş, A.B.; Taşlipinar, M.Y.; Doğan, M.; Dündar, H.Z.; Kilic, M.; Başaran, A.A.; Başaran, A.N. Hepatoprotective and antioxidant effects of lycopene in acute cholestasis. *Turk. J. Med Sci.* **2015**, *45*, 857–864. [CrossRef] [PubMed]
72. Grether-Beck, S.; Marini, A.; Jaenicke, T.; Stahl, W.; Krutmann, J. Molecular evidence that oral supplementation with lycopene or lutein protects human skin against ultraviolet radiation: Results from a double-blinded, placebo-controlled, crossover study. *Br. J. Dermatol.* **2017**, *176*, 1231–1240. [CrossRef]
73. Lu, C.-W.; Hung, C.-F.; Jean, W.-H.; Lin, T.-Y.; Huang, S.-K.; Wang, S.-J. Lycopene depresses glutamate release through inhibition of voltage-dependent Ca2+ entry and protein kinase C in rat cerebrocortical nerve terminals. *Can. J. Physiol. Pharmacol.* **2017**, *96*, 479–484. [CrossRef] [PubMed]
74. Bhardwaj, M.; Kumar, A. Neuroprotective effect of lycopene against PTZ-induced kindling seizures in mice: Possible behavioural, biochemical and mitochondrial dysfunction. *Phytother. Res.* **2016**, *30*, 306–313. [CrossRef] [PubMed]
75. Datta, S.; Jamwal, S.; Deshmukh, R.; Kumar, P. Beneficial effects of lycopene against haloperidol induced orofacial dyskinesia in rats: Possible neurotransmitters and neuroinflammation modulation. *Eur. J. Pharmacol.* **2016**, *771*, 229–235. [CrossRef] [PubMed]
76. Costa-Rodrigues, J.; Fernandes, M.H.; Pinho, O.; Monteiro, P.R.R. Modulation of human osteoclastogenesis and osteoblastogenesis by lycopene. *J. Nutr. Biochem.* **2018**, *57*, 26–34. [CrossRef] [PubMed]
77. Ardawi, M.-S.M.; Badawoud, M.H.; Hassan, S.M.; Rouzi, A.A.; Ardawi, J.M.; AlNosani, N.M.; Qari, M.H.; Mousa, S.A. Lycopene treatment against loss of bone mass, microarchitecture and strength in relation to regulatory mechanisms in a postmenopausal osteoporosis model. *Bone* **2016**, *83*, 127–140. [CrossRef]
78. Ghyasvand, T.; Goodarzi, M.T.; Amiri, I.; Karimi, J.; Ghorbani, M. Serum levels of lycopene, beta-carotene, and retinol and their correlation with sperm DNA damage in normospermic and infertile men. *Int. J. Reprod. Biomed.* **2015**, *13*, 787. [CrossRef]

79. Aly, H.A.; El-Beshbishy, H.A.; Banjar, Z.M. Mitochondrial dysfunction induced impairment of spermatogenesis in LPS-treated rats: Modulatory role of lycopene. *Eur. J. Pharmacol.* **2012**, *677*, 31–38. [CrossRef]
80. Nedamani, A.R.; Nedamani, E.R.; Salimi, A. The role of lycopene in human health as a natural colorant. *Nutr. Food Sci.* **2019**, *49*, 284–298.
81. Ghadage, S.; Mane, K.; Agrawal, R.; Pawar, V. Tomato lycopene: Potential health benefits. *Pharma Innov. J.* **2019**, *8*, 1245–1248.
82. Chen, P.; Xu, S.; Qu, J. Lycopene protects keratinocytes against UVB radiation-induced carcinogenesis via negative regulation of FOXO3a through the mTORC2/AKT signaling pathway. *J. Cell. Biochem.* **2018**, *119*, 366–377. [CrossRef] [PubMed]
83. Peng, S.; Li, J.; Zhou, Y.; Tuo, M.; Qin, X.; Yu, Q.; Cheng, H.; Li, Y. In vitro effects and mechanisms of lycopene in MCF-7 human breast cancer cells. *Genet. Mol. Res.* **2017**, *16*, 13. [CrossRef]
84. Cha, J.H.; Kim, W.K.; Ha, A.W.; Kim, M.H.; Chang, M.J. Anti-inflammatory effect of lycopene in SW480 human colorectal cancer cells. *Nutr. Res. Pract.* **2017**, *11*, 90–96. [CrossRef] [PubMed]
85. Soares, N.D.C.P.; Machado, C.L.; Trindade, B.B.; do Canto Lima, I.C.; Gimba, E.R.P.; Teodoro, A.J.; Takiya, C.; Borojevic, R. Lycopene extracts from different tomato-based food products induce apoptosis in cultured human primary prostate cancer cells and regulate TP53, Bax and Bcl-2 transcript expression. *Asian Pac. J. Cancer Prev. APJCP* **2017**, *18*, 339. [PubMed]
86. Jain, A.; Sharma, G.; Kushwah, V.; Thakur, K.; Ghoshal, G.; Singh, B.; Jain, S.; Shivhare, U.; Katare, O. Fabrication and functional attributes of lipidic nanoconstructs of lycopene: An innovative endeavour for enhanced cytotoxicity in MCF-7 breast cancer cells. *Colloids Surf. B Biointerfaces* **2017**, *152*, 482–491. [CrossRef]
87. Ye, M.; Wu, Q.; Zhang, M.; Huang, J. Lycopene inhibits the cell proliferation and invasion of human head and neck squamous cell carcinoma. *Mol. Med. Rep.* **2016**, *14*, 2953–2958. [CrossRef]
88. Wang, X.; Yang, H.-H.; Liu, Y.; Zhou, Q.; Chen, Z.-H. Lycopene consumption and risk of colorectal cancer: A meta-analysis of observational studies. *Nutr. Cancer* **2016**, *68*, 1083–1096. [CrossRef]
89. Gong, X.; Marisiddaiah, R.; Zaripheh, S.; Wiener, D.; Rubin, L.P. Mitochondrial β-carotene 9′, 10′ oxygenase modulates prostate cancer growth via NF-κB inhibition: A lycopene-independent function. *Mol. Cancer Res.* **2016**, *14*, 966–975. [CrossRef]
90. Aizawa, K.; Liu, C.; Tang, S.; Veeramachaneni, S.; Hu, K.Q.; Smith, D.E.; Wang, X.D. Tobacco carcinogen induces both lung cancer and non-alcoholic steatohepatitis and hepatocellular carcinomas in ferrets which can be attenuated by lycopene supplementation. *Int. J. Cancer* **2016**, *139*, 1171–1181. [CrossRef]
91. Graff, R.E.; Pettersson, A.; Lis, R.T.; Ahearn, T.U.; Markt, S.C.; Wilson, K.M.; Rider, J.R.; Fiorentino, M.; Finn, S.; Kenfield, S.A. Dietary lycopene intake and risk of prostate cancer defined by ERG protein expression. *Am. J. Clin. Nutr.* **2016**, *103*, 851–860. [CrossRef] [PubMed]
92. Zhu, R.; Chen, B.; Bai, Y.; Miao, T.; Rui, L.; Zhang, H.; Xia, B.; Li, Y.; Gao, S.; Wang, X.-D. Lycopene in protection against obesity and diabetes: A mechanistic review. *Pharmacol. Res.* **2020**, *159*, 104966. [CrossRef] [PubMed]
93. Ozmen, O.; Topsakal, S.; Haligur, M.; Aydogan, A.; Dincoglu, D. Effects of caffeine and lycopene in experimentally induced diabetes mellitus. *Pancreas* **2016**, *45*, 579–583. [CrossRef] [PubMed]
94. Zeng, Y.-C.; Peng, L.-S.; Zou, L.; Huang, S.-F.; Xie, Y.; Mu, G.-P.; Zeng, X.-H.; Zhou, X.-L.; Zeng, Y.-C. Protective effect and mechanism of lycopene on endothelial progenitor cells (EPCs) from type 2 diabetes mellitus rats. *Biomed. Pharmacother.* **2017**, *92*, 86–94. [CrossRef] [PubMed]
95. Hasan, T.; Sultana, M. Lycopene and Cardiovascular Diseases: A Review of the Literature. *Int. J. Res. Rev.* **2017**, *4*, 73–86.
96. Sen, S. The chemistry and biology of lycopene: Antioxidant for human health. *Int. J. Adv. Life Sci. Res.* **2019**, *2*, 8–14. [CrossRef]
97. Song, B.; Liu, K.; Gao, Y.; Zhao, L.; Fang, H.; Li, Y.; Pei, L.; Xu, Y. Lycopene and risk of cardiovascular diseases: A meta-analysis of observational studies. *Mol. Nutr. Food Res.* **2017**, *61*, 1601009. [CrossRef]
98. Lin, J.; Li, H.-X.; Xia, J.; Li, X.-N.; Jiang, X.-Q.; Zhu, S.-Y.; Ge, J.; Li, J.-L. The chemopreventive potential of lycopene against atrazine-induced cardiotoxicity: Modulation of ionic homeostasis. *Sci. Rep.* **2016**, *6*, 24855. [CrossRef]

99. Tong, C.; Peng, C.; Wang, L.; Zhang, L.; Yang, X.; Xu, P.; Li, J.; Delplancke, T.; Zhang, H.; Qi, H. Intravenous administration of lycopene, a tomato extract, protects against myocardial ischemia-reperfusion injury. *Nutrients* **2016**, *8*, 138. [CrossRef]
100. Gao, Y.; Jia, P.; Shu, W.; Jia, D. The protective effect of lycopene on hypoxia/reoxygenation-induced endoplasmic reticulum stress in H9C2 cardiomyocytes. *Eur. J. Pharmacol.* **2016**, *774*, 71–79. [CrossRef]
101. Müller, L.; Caris-Veyrat, C.; Lowe, G.; Böhm, V. Lycopene and its antioxidant role in the prevention of cardiovascular diseases—A critical review. *Crit. Rev. Food Sci. Nutr.* **2016**, *56*, 1868–1879. [CrossRef] [PubMed]
102. Xu, J.; Hu, H.; Chen, B.; Yue, R.; Zhou, Z.; Liu, Y.; Zhang, S.; Xu, L.; Wang, H.; Yu, Z. Lycopene protects against hypoxia/reoxygenation injury by alleviating ER stress induced apoptosis in neonatal mouse cardiomyocytes. *PLoS ONE* **2015**, *10*, e0136443. [CrossRef] [PubMed]
103. He, Q.; Zhou, W.; Xiong, C.; Tan, G.; Chen, M. Lycopene attenuates inflammation and apoptosis in post-myocardial infarction remodeling by inhibiting the nuclear factor-κB signaling pathway. *Mol. Med. Rep.* **2015**, *11*, 374–378. [CrossRef] [PubMed]
104. Gajendragadkar, P.R.; Hubsch, A.; Mäki-Petäjä, K.M.; Serg, M.; Wilkinson, I.B.; Cheriyan, J. Effects of oral lycopene supplementation on vascular function in patients with cardiovascular disease and healthy volunteers: A randomised controlled trial. *PLoS ONE* **2014**, *9*, e99070. [CrossRef] [PubMed]
105. Caseiro, M.; Ascenso, A.; Costa, A.; Creagh-Flynn, J.; Johnson, M.; Simões, S. Lycopene in human health. *LWT* **2020**, *127*, 109323. [CrossRef]
106. Tian, Y.; Xiao, Y.; Wang, B.; Sun, C.; Tang, K.; Sun, F. Vitamin E and lycopene reduce coal burning fluorosis-induced spermatogenic cell apoptosis via oxidative stress-mediated JNK and ERK signaling pathways. *Biosci. Rep.* **2018**, *38*. [CrossRef]
107. Alvi, S.S.; Ansari, I.A.; Ahmad, M.K.; Iqbal, J.; Khan, M.S. Lycopene amends LPS induced oxidative stress and hypertriglyceridemia via modulating PCSK-9 expression and Apo-CIII mediated lipoprotein lipase activity. *Biomed. Pharmacother.* **2017**, *96*, 1082–1093. [CrossRef]
108. Baykalir, B.G.; Aksit, D.; Dogru, M.S.; Yay, A.H.; Aksit, H.; Seyrek, K.; Atessahin, A. Lycopene ameliorates experimental colitis in rats via reducing apoptosis and oxidative stress. *Int. J. Vitam Nutr. Res* **2016**, *86*, 27–35. [CrossRef]
109. Yu, L.; Wang, W.; Pang, W.; Xiao, Z.; Jiang, Y.; Hong, Y. Dietary lycopene supplementation improves cognitive performances in tau transgenic mice expressing P301L mutation via inhibiting oxidative stress and tau hyperphosphorylation. *J. Alzheimer's Dis.* **2017**, *57*, 475–482. [CrossRef]
110. Bandeira, A.C.B.; da Silva, T.P.; de Araujo, G.R.; Araujo, C.M.; da Silva, R.C.; Lima, W.G.; Bezerra, F.S.; Costa, D.C. Lycopene inhibits reactive oxygen species production in SK-Hep-1 cells and attenuates acetaminophen-induced liver injury in C57BL/6 mice. *Chem. -Biol. Interact.* **2017**, *263*, 7–17. [CrossRef]
111. Lim, S.; Hwang, S.; Yu, J.H.; Lim, J.W.; Kim, H. Lycopene inhibits regulator of calcineurin 1-mediated apoptosis by reducing oxidative stress and down-regulating Nucling in neuronal cells. *Mol. Nutr. Food Res.* **2017**, *61*, 1600530. [CrossRef]
112. Bayomy, N.A.; Elbakary, R.H.; Ibrahim, M.A.; Abdelaziz, E.Z. Effect of lycopene and rosmarinic acid on gentamicin induced renal cortical oxidative stress, apoptosis, and autophagy in adult male albino rat. *Anat. Rec.* **2017**, *300*, 1137–1149. [CrossRef] [PubMed]
113. Tvrdá, E.; Kováčik, A.; Tušimová, E.; Paál, D.; Mackovich, A.; Alimov, J.; Lukáč, N. Antioxidant efficiency of lycopene on oxidative stress-induced damage in bovine spermatozoa. *J. Anim. Sci. Biotechnol.* **2016**, *7*, 50. [CrossRef] [PubMed]
114. Qu, M.; Jiang, Z.; Liao, Y.; Song, Z.; Nan, X. Lycopene prevents amyloid [beta]-induced mitochondrial oxidative stress and dysfunctions in cultured rat cortical neurons. *Neurochem. Res.* **2016**, *41*, 1354–1364. [CrossRef] [PubMed]
115. Campos, K.K.D.; Araújo, G.R.; Martins, T.L.; Bandeira, A.C.B.; de Paula Costa, G.; Talvani, A.; Garcia, C.C.M.; Oliveira, L.A.M.; Costa, D.C.; Bezerra, F.S. The antioxidant and anti-inflammatory properties of lycopene in mice lungs exposed to cigarette smoke. *J. Nutr. Biochem.* **2017**, *48*, 9–20. [CrossRef]
116. Göncü, T.; Oğuz, E.; Sezen, H.; Koçarslan, S.; Oğuz, H.; Akal, A.; Adıbelli, F.M.; Çakmak, S.; Aksoy, N. Anti-inflammatory effect of lycopene on endotoxin-induced uveitis in rats. *Arq. Bras. Oftalmol.* **2016**, *79*, 357–362. [CrossRef]

117. Sachdeva, A.K.; Chopra, K. Lycopene abrogates Aβ(1-42)-mediated neuroinflammatory cascade in an experimental model of Alzheimer's disease. *J. Nutr. Biochem.* **2015**, *26*, 736–744. [CrossRef]
118. Colmán-Martínez, M.; Martínez-Huélamo, M.; Valderas-Martínez, P.; Arranz-Martínez, S.; Almanza-Aguilera, E.; Corella, D.; Estruch, R.; Lamuela-Raventós, R.M. trans-Lycopene from tomato juice attenuates inflammatory biomarkers in human plasma samples: An intervention trial. *Mol. Nutr. Food Res.* **2017**, *61*, 1600993. [CrossRef]
119. Liu, T.Y.; Chen, S.B. Sarcandra glabra combined with lycopene protect rats from lipopolysaccharide induced acute lung injury via reducing inflammatory response. *Biomed. Pharmacother.* **2016**, *84*, 34–41. [CrossRef]
120. Li, Y.F.; Chang, Y.Y.; Huang, H.C.; Wu, Y.C.; Yang, M.D.; Chao, P.M. Tomato juice supplementation in young women reduces inflammatory adipokine levels independently of body fat reduction. *Nutrition* **2015**, *31*, 691–696. [CrossRef]
121. Zhang, F.; Fu, Y.; Zhou, X.; Pan, W.; Shi, Y.; Wang, M.; Zhang, X.; Qi, D.; Li, L.; Ma, K.; et al. Depression-like behaviors and heme oxygenase-1 are regulated by lycopene in lipopolysaccharide-induced neuroinflammation. *J. Neuroimmunol.* **2016**, *298*, 1–8. [CrossRef] [PubMed]
122. Makon-Sébastien, N.; Francis, F.; Eric, S.; Henri, V.P.; François, L.J.; Laurent, P.; Yves, B.; Serge, C. Lycopene modulates THP1 and Caco2 cells inflammatory state through transcriptional and nontranscriptional processes. *Mediat. Inflamm.* **2014**, *2014*, 507272. [CrossRef] [PubMed]
123. Sheriff, S.A.; Shaik Ibrahim, S.; Devaki, T.; Chakraborty, S.; Agarwal, S.; Pérez-Sánchez, H. Lycopene Prevents mitochondrial dysfunction during d-galactosamine/lipopolysaccharide-induced fulminant hepatic failure in albino rats. *J. Proteome Res.* **2017**, *16*, 3190–3199. [CrossRef] [PubMed]
124. Deng, Y.; Xu, Z.; Liu, W.; Yang, H.; Xu, B.; Wei, Y. Effects of lycopene and proanthocyanidins on hepatotoxicity induced by mercuric chloride in rats. *Biol. Trace Elem. Res.* **2012**, *146*, 213–223. [CrossRef] [PubMed]
125. Anusha, M.; Venkateswarlu, M.; Prabhakaran, V.; Taj, S.S.; Kumari, B.P.; Ranganayakulu, D. Hepatoprotective activity of aqueous extract of *Portulaca oleracea* in combination with lycopene in rats. *Indian J. Pharmacol.* **2011**, *43*, 563–567. [CrossRef] [PubMed]
126. Yucel, Y.; Oguz, E.; Kocarslan, S.; Tatli, F.; Gozeneli, O.; Seker, A.; Sezen, H.; Buyukaslan, H.; Aktumen, A.; Ozgonul, A.; et al. The effects of lycopene on methotrexate-induced liver injury in rats. *Bratisl. Lek. Listy* **2017**, *118*, 212–216. [CrossRef]
127. Bandeira, A.C.B.; da Silva, R.C.; Rossoni, J.V.J.; Figueiredo, V.P.; Talvani, A.; Cangussú, S.D.; Bezerra, F.S.; Costa, D.C. Lycopene pretreatment improves hepatotoxicity induced by acetaminophen in C57BL/6 mice. *Bioorg. Med. Chem.* **2017**, *25*, 1057–1065. [CrossRef]
128. Bayramoglu, G.; Bayramoglu, A.; Altuner, Y.; Uyanoglu, M.; Colak, S. The effects of lycopene on hepatic ischemia/reperfusion injury in rats. *Cytotechnology* **2015**, *67*, 487–491. [CrossRef]
129. Xia, J.; Lin, J.; Zhu, S.Y.; Du, Z.H.; Guo, J.A.; Han, Z.X.; Li, J.L.; Zhang, Y. Lycopene protects against atrazine-induced hepatotoxicity through modifications of cytochrome P450 enzyme system in microsomes. *Exp. Toxicol. Pathol.* **2016**, *68*, 223–231. [CrossRef]
130. Sheik Abdulazeez, S.; Thiruvengadam, D. Effect of lycopene on oxidative stress induced during D-galactosamine/lipopolysaccharide-sensitized liver injury in rats. *Pharm. Biol.* **2013**, *51*, 1592–1599. [CrossRef]
131. Sheriff, S.A.; Devaki, T. Lycopene stabilizes lipoprotein levels during D-galactosamine/lipopolysaccharide induced hepatitis in experimental rats. *Asian Pac. J. Trop. Biomed.* **2012**, *2*, 975–980. [CrossRef]
132. Wang, Z.; Fan, J.; Wang, J.; Li, Y.; Xiao, L.; Duan, D.; Wang, Q. Protective effect of lycopene on high-fat diet-induced cognitive impairment in rats. *Neurosci. Lett.* **2016**, *627*, 185–191. [CrossRef] [PubMed]
133. Lei, X.; Lei, L.; Zhang, Z.; Cheng, Y. Neuroprotective effects of lycopene pretreatment on transient global cerebral ischemia-reperfusion in rats: The role of the Nrf2/HO-1 signaling pathway. *Mol. Med. Rep.* **2016**, *13*, 412–418. [CrossRef]
134. Chen, W.; Mao, L.; Xing, H.; Xu, L.; Fu, X.; Huang, L.; Huang, D.; Pu, Z.; Li, Q. Lycopene attenuates Aβ1-42 secretion and its toxicity in human cell and *Caenorhabditis elegans* models of Alzheimer disease. *Neurosci. Lett.* **2015**, *608*, 28–33. [CrossRef]
135. Prema, A.; Janakiraman, U.; Manivasagam, T.; Thenmozhi, A.J. Neuroprotective effect of lycopene against MPTP induced experimental Parkinson's disease in mice. *Neurosci. Lett.* **2015**, *599*, 12–19. [CrossRef]
136. Prakash, A.; Kumar, A. Implicating the role of lycopene in restoration of mitochondrial enzymes and BDNF levels in β-amyloid induced Alzheimer's disease. *Eur. J. Pharm.* **2014**, *741*, 104–111. [CrossRef] [PubMed]

137. Liu, C.B.; Wang, R.; Pan, H.B.; Ding, Q.F.; Lu, F.B. Effect of lycopene on oxidative stress and behavioral deficits in rotenone induced model of Parkinson's disease. *Zhongguo Ying Yong Sheng Li Xue Za Zhi = Zhongguo Yingyong Shenglixue Zazhi = Chin. J. Appl. Physiol.* **2013**, *29*, 380–384.

138. Qu, M.; Nan, X.; Gao, Z.; Guo, B.; Liu, B.; Chen, Z. Protective effects of lycopene against methylmercury-induced neurotoxicity in cultured rat cerebellar granule neurons. *Brain Res.* **2013**, *1540*, 92–102. [CrossRef]

139. Kaur, H.; Chauhan, S.; Sandhir, R. Protective effect of lycopene on oxidative stress and cognitive decline in rotenone induced model of Parkinson's disease. *Neurochem. Res.* **2011**, *36*, 1435–1443. [CrossRef]

140. Hayhoe, R.P.G.; Lentjes, M.A.H.; Mulligan, A.A.; Luben, R.N.; Khaw, K.T.; Welch, A.A. Carotenoid dietary intakes and plasma concentrations are associated with heel bone ultrasound attenuation and osteoporotic fracture risk in the European Prospective Investigation into Cancer and Nutrition (EPIC)-Norfolk cohort. *Br. J. Nutr.* **2017**, *117*, 1439–1453. [CrossRef]

141. Sahni, S.; Hannan, M.T.; Blumberg, J.; Cupples, L.A.; Kiel, D.P.; Tucker, K.L. Protective effect of total carotenoid and lycopene intake on the risk of hip fracture: A 17-year follow-up from the Framingham Osteoporosis Study. *J. Bone Miner. Res.* **2009**, *24*, 1086–1096. [CrossRef]

142. Mackinnon, E.S.; Rao, A.V.; Rao, L.G. Dietary restriction of lycopene for a period of one month resulted in significantly increased biomarkers of oxidative stress and bone resorption in postmenopausal women. *J. Nutr. Health Aging* **2011**, *15*, 133–138. [CrossRef] [PubMed]

143. Ateşşahin, A.; Türk, G.; Karahan, I.; Yilmaz, S.; Ceribaşi, A.O.; Bulmuş, O. Lycopene prevents adriamycin-induced testicular toxicity in rats. *Fertil. Steril.* **2006**, *85* (Suppl. 1), 1216–1222. [CrossRef]

144. Ateşşahin, A.; Karahan, I.; Türk, G.; Gür, S.; Yilmaz, S.; Ceribaşi, A.O. Protective role of lycopene on cisplatin-induced changes in sperm characteristics, testicular damage and oxidative stress in rats. *Reprod. Toxicol.* **2006**, *21*, 42–47. [CrossRef] [PubMed]

145. Tripathy, A.; Ghosh, A.; Dey, A.; Pakhira, B.P.; Ghosh, D. Attenuation of the cyproterone acetate-induced testicular hypofunction by a novel nutraceutical lycopene: A genomic approach. *Andrologia* **2017**, *49*, e12709. [CrossRef] [PubMed]

146. Trejo-Solís, C.; Pedraza-Chaverrí, J.; Torres-Ramos, M.; Jiménez-Farfán, D.; Cruz Salgado, A.; Serrano-García, N.; Osorio-Rico, L.; Sotelo, J. Multiple molecular and cellular mechanisms of action of lycopene in cancer inhibition. *Evid. -Based Complement. Altern. Med. eCAM* **2013**, *2013*, 705152. [CrossRef]

147. Giovannucci, E.; Ascherio, A.; Rimm, E.B.; Stampfer, M.J.; Colditz, G.A.; Willett, W.C. Intake of carotenoids and retinol in relation to risk of prostate cancer. *J. Natl. Cancer Inst.* **1995**, *87*, 1767–1776. [CrossRef]

148. Corridan, B.; O'Donohue, M.; Morrissey, P. Carotenoids and immune response in elderly people. In *Proceedings of Proceedings-Nutrition Society of London*; Cambridge University Press: Cambridge, UK, 1998; p. 4A.

149. Khiveh, A.; Hashempur, M.H.; Shakiba, M.; Lotfi, M.H.; Shakeri, A.; Kazemeini, S.; Mousavi, Z.; Jabbari, M.; Kamalinejad, M.; Emtiazy, M. Effects of rhubarb (*Rheum ribes* L.) syrup on dysenteric diarrhea in children: A randomized, double-blind, placebo-controlled trial. *J. Integr. Med.* **2017**, *15*, 365–372. [CrossRef]

150. Shakeri, A.; Hashempur, M.H.; Mojibian, M.; Aliasl, F.; Bioos, S.; Nejatbakhsh, F. A comparative study of ranitidine and quince (*Cydonia oblonga* Mill) sauce on gastroesophageal reflux disease (GERD) in pregnancy: A randomised, open-label, active-controlled clinical trial. *J. Obstet. Gynaecol.* **2018**, *38*, 899–905. [CrossRef]

151. Qu, M.; Zhou, Z.; Chen, C.; Li, M.; Pei, L.; Chu, F.; Yang, J.; Wang, Y.; Li, L.; Liu, C.; et al. Lycopene protects against trimethyltin-induced neurotoxicity in primary cultured rat hippocampal neurons by inhibiting the mitochondrial apoptotic pathway. *Neurochem. Int.* **2011**, *59*, 1095–1103. [CrossRef]

152. Wang, X.-D. *Carotenoid Oxidative/Degradative Products and Their Biological Activities*; Marcel Dekker: New York, NY, USA, 2004.

153. Jonker, D.; Kuper, C.F.; Fraile, N.; Estrella, A.; Rodríguez Otero, C. Ninety-day oral toxicity study of lycopene from *Blakeslea trispora* in rats. *Regul. Toxicol. Pharmacol. RTP* **2003**, *37*, 396–406. [CrossRef]

154. Trumbo, P.R. Are there adverse effects of lycopene exposure? *J. Nutr.* **2005**, *135*, 2060s–2061s. [CrossRef] [PubMed]

155. Krinsky, N.I.; Beecher, G.; Burk, R.; Chan, A.; Erdman, j.J.; Jacob, R.; Jialal, I.; Kolonel, L.; Marshall, J.; Taylor Mayne, P.R. Dietary reference intakes for vitamin C, vitamin E, selenium, and carotenoids. *Inst. Med.* **2000**. [CrossRef]

156. Trumbo, P.; Yates, A.A.; Schlicker, S.; Poos, M. Dietary reference intakes: Vitamin A, vitamin K, arsenic, boron, chromium, copper, iodine, iron, manganese, molybdenum, nickel, silicon, vanadium, and zinc. *J. Acad. Nutr. Diet.* **2001**, *101*, 294.
157. Veeramachaneni, S.; Ausman, L.M.; Choi, S.W.; Russell, R.M.; Wang, X.D. High dose lycopene supplementation increases hepatic cytochrome P4502E1 protein and inflammation in alcohol-fed rats. *J. Nutr.* **2008**, *138*, 1329–1335. [CrossRef]
158. Cassileth, B. Lycopene. *Oncology* **2010**, *24*, 296.
159. Reich, P.; Shwachman, H.; Craig, J.M. Lycopenemia: A variant of carotenemia. *N. Engl. J. Med.* **1960**, *262*, 263–269. [CrossRef]
160. Michael McClain, R.; Bausch, J. Summary of safety studies conducted with synthetic lycopene. *Regul. Toxicol. Pharmacol. RTP* **2003**, *37*, 274–285. [CrossRef]

© 2020 by the authors. Licensee MDPI, Basel, Switzerland. This article is an open access article distributed under the terms and conditions of the Creative Commons Attribution (CC BY) license (http://creativecommons.org/licenses/by/4.0/).

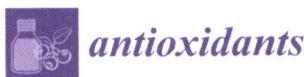

Article

Inhibition of Osteoclast Differentiation by Carotenoid Derivatives through Inhibition of the NF-κB Pathway

Shlomit Odes-Barth [1,†], Marina Khanin [1], Karin Linnewiel-Hermoni [1,‡], Yifat Miller [2,3], Karina Abramov [2,3], Joseph Levy [1] and Yoav Sharoni [1,*]

[1] Clinical Biochemistry and Pharmacology, Faculty of Health Sciences, Ben-Gurion University of the Negev, Beer-Sheva 84105, Israel; shlomitbarth@post.bgu.ac.il (S.O.-B.); hanin@bgu.ac.il (M.K.); Karin.Hermoni@lycored.com (K.L.-H.); lyossi@bgu.ac.il (J.L.)
[2] Department of Chemistry, Ben-Gurion University of the Negev, Beer-Sheva 84105, Israel; ymiller@bgu.ac.il (Y.M.); karinaab@post.bgu.ac.il (K.A.)
[3] Ilse Katz Institute for Nanoscale Science and Technology, Ben-Gurion University of the Negev, Beer-Sheva 84105, Israel
* Correspondence: yoav@bgu.ac.il; Tel.: +972-52-483-0883
† Deceased.
‡ Current address: Lycored, Secaucus, NJ 08876, USA.

Received: 12 October 2020; Accepted: 20 November 2020; Published: 23 November 2020

Abstract: The bone protective effects of carotenoids have been demonstrated in several studies, and the inhibition of RANKL-induced osteoclast differentiation by lycopene has also been demonstrated. We previously reported that carotenoid oxidation products are the active mediators in the activation of the transcription factor Nrf2 and the inhibition of the NF-κB transcription system by carotenoids. Here, we demonstrate that lycopene oxidation products are more potent than intact lycopene in inhibiting osteoclast differentiation. We analyzed the structure–activity relationship of a series of dialdehyde carotenoid derivatives (diapocarotene-dials) in inhibiting osteoclastogenesis. We found that the degree of inhibition depends on the electron density of the carbon atom that determines the reactivity of the conjugated double bond in reactions such as Michael addition to thiol groups in proteins. Moreover, the carotenoid derivatives attenuated the NF-κB signal through inhibition of IκB phosphorylation and NF-κB translocation to the nucleus. In addition, we show a synergistic inhibition of osteoclast differentiation by combinations of an active carotenoid derivative with the polyphenols curcumin and carnosic acid with combination index (CI) values < 1. Our findings suggest that carotenoid derivatives inhibit osteoclast differentiation, partially by inhibiting the NF-κB pathway. In addition, carotenoid derivatives can synergistically inhibit osteoclast differentiation with curcumin and carnosic acid.

Keywords: apo-carotenals; lycopene; polyphenols; bone; osteoclasts; NFκB; synergy

1. Introduction

Several epidemiological studies imply that fruit and vegetable consumption decreases morbidity and has a beneficial effect on bone health [1–3]. Carotenoids, a major group of micronutrients in a fruit and vegetable-rich diet, are fat soluble and pigmented phytochemicals produced by bacteria, fungi, algae, and plants [4]. From the more than 600 natural carotenoids that have been identified, nearly 50 are consumed by humans [5], whereas about 20 appear in human tissues and blood [6]. β-carotene, lycopene, and lutein compose the major plasma carotenoids [7]. Lycopene is derived mainly from tomatoes and tomato products, and its content in tomatoes is 0.7–20 mg/100 g wet weight [8]. The sources of other carotenoids are more diverse; for example, β-carotene is rich in orange-yellow vegetables and fruits, but it is also found in leafy vegetables. Humans appear to absorb carotenoids in a relatively non-specific fashion and, thus, their plasma and tissue concentrations reflect their individual dietary habits [7]. The relative abundance of each of the five major carotenoids in the diet are similar to their distribution in plasma.

The role of carotenoids has been investigated in epidemiological and interventional studies. Lycopene supplementation to postmenopausal women for four months significantly decreased oxidative stress parameters and the bone resorption marker n-telopeptide of type I collagen. This was accompanied by a significant increase in serum lycopene. Most adult bone diseases are due to excess osteoclastic activity, which results in an imbalance in bone remodeling which favors resorption by osteoclasts over building by osteoblasts [9]. Animal and cellular studies on the role of fruits and dietary phytochemicals in bone protection were reviewed by Shen et al. [10]. An in-vivo study showed that a supplement containing tomatoes improved bone health in ovariectomized osteoporotic rats [11]. The effect of carotenoids on bone has also been studied in cell culture. Rao et al. showed that the carotenoid lycopene stimulates osteoblast cell proliferation and alkaline phosphatase activity in SaOS-2 cells, inhibiting osteoclast formation and mineral resorption mediated by reactive oxygen species in cells from rat bone marrow [12,13]. Costa-Rodrigues et al. studied the effects of lycopene on differentiation and function in human osteoclasts and osteoblasts. They found that lycopene decreased osteoclast differentiation and resorbing activity, and increased osteoblast proliferation and differentiation [14]. Using signaling inhibitors, they tried to identify the pathways involved in lycopene action but were unable to show an effect on NF-κB in osteoclasts even though such an effect was found in osteoblasts.

Identification of the osteoclastogenesis inducer, RANKL, expressed mainly in osteoblasts; its cognate receptor, RANK, expressed on osteoclast progenitors; and its decoy receptor osteoprotegerin has contributed to understanding of the molecular mechanisms of osteoclast differentiation and activity [15]. One of the early molecular events induced by RANK is NF-κB activation [16,17]. In non-stimulated cells, NF-κB proteins are found in the cytoplasm, but enter the nucleus upon cell stimulation. The NF-κB pathway is composed of two distinct pathways: the canonical and the alternative. Both are shown to be essential in osteoclastogenesis [17–20]. NF-κB transcription factor activity is the hallmark of inflammation. In this respect, the role of lycopene as an anti-inflammatory agent was studied. Joo et al. [21] demonstrated that tomato lycopene extract inhibits NF-κB signaling, leading to reduced-lipopolysaccharide-induced pro-inflammatory gene expression in rat small intestinal epithelial cells. A similar anti-inflammatory effect of lycopene was shown in lipopolysaccharide-induced peritoneal macrophages [22]. These findings were supported by a study showing that lycopene regulates cigarette smoke-driven inflammation by inhibition of macrophage NF-κB activity [23]. However, whether inhibition of NF-κB signaling is involved in lycopene's effect in osteoclasts is not yet known.

In several types of cell including bone osteoblasts, we have previously shown that carotenoid oxidation products, and not the intact carotenoid, stimulate the electrophile/antioxidant response element (ARE/Nrf2) transcription system [24] and inhibit the NF-κB transcription system [25]. Similar opposing effects on these two transcription systems were obtained with synthetic dialdehyde carotenoid derivatives (diapocarotene-dials), which can be formed by spontaneous oxidation [26] or after chemical [27] or enzymatic [28] catalyzed oxidation of various carotenoids. Although such diapocarotene-dials have not been identified in human or animal samples, mono-apocarotenals, that have similar, but lower activities [24], have been documented in raw tomatoes [29]. The synthetic diapocarotene-dials also inhibited estrogen signaling in breast cancer cells but did not inhibit and even stimulated it in osteoblast bone cells [30]. In addition, we demonstrated that the activity of individual diapocarotene-dials in inducing the ARE/Nrf2 transcription system and inhibiting the NF-κB transcription system depends on the reactivity of the conjugated double bond in reactions such as Michael addition. This reactivity is determined by the electron density around the reactive carbon atoms (the fourth atom from each side of the molecule; see Table 1) [25]. We hypothesized that oxidized derivatives of lycopene and other carotenoids also act as the active mediators in inhibiting osteoclast differentiation.

Table 1. Structures, Mulliken population values, and HOMO-LUMO energy gap of the synthetic derivatives.

Derivative [1]	Structure	Mulliken Population Values (Electron Density)		HOMO-LUMO [2] Energy Gap (kcal/mol)
		Left	Right	
6,14′		6.16	6.10	189.51
10,10′		6.17	6.17	191.39
8,8′		6.21	6.21	178.21
8,12′		6.23	6.22	210.84
12,12′		6.24	6.24	214.61

[1] The abbreviated names of the derivatives are derived from the putative position of oxidative cleavage in the carotenoid backbone, which could lead to the formation of these derivatives, Full names: 6,14′-diapocarotene-6,14′-dial (6,14′); 10,10′-diapocarotene-10,10′-dial (10,10′); 8,8′-diapocarotene-8,8′-dial (8,8′); 8,12′-diapocarotene-8,12′-dial (8,12′); 12,12′-diapocarotene-12,12′-dial (12,12′). [2] HOMO: High Occupied Molecular Orbitals; LUMO: Low Unoccupied Molecular Orbitals.

The aim of the current work was to determine if intact lycopene or its oxidized derivatives inhibit RANKL-induced osteoclast differentiation in RAW264.7 osteoclast progenitor cells. In addition, we determined the relative inhibition of osteoclast differentiation by various diapocarotene-dials in order to evaluate if the structure–activity relationship is similar to that of NF-κB inhibition [25]. After establishing this similarity, we aimed to verify if oxidized lycopene and the carotenoid derivatives interfere in the NF-κB pathway.

It is well accepted that the health benefits of a fruit and vegetable-based diet reside, at least in part, in additive or synergistic activities of their phytonutrients. We hypothesized that this is true also for the inhibition of osteoclast differentiation; thus, another aim of this study was to look for synergy between carotenoid derivatives and other phytonutrients. To check this possibility, we compared the inhibition of osteoclastogenesis by a carotenoid derivative alone to its combination with phytochemicals belonging to the large family of polyphenols, several of which are known to have beneficial effects on bone health. Polyphenols are present in many foods of plant origin and are characterized by having one or several phenolic groups in their chemical structure. There are over 500 different polyphenols in foods, and the mean intake of all of them is about 1 g per day, which is split between many specific polyphenols [31]. From the various polyphenols, we selected two which affect osteoclasts—curcumin [32,33] and carnosic acid [34,35]—and studied their cooperativity with carotenoid derivatives in inhibiting osteoclast activity.

2. Materials and Methods

2.1. Materials

Crystalline lycopene preparations, purified from tomato extract (>97%), were supplied by Lycored Ltd. (Beer Sheva, Israel). Tetrahydrofuran (THF), containing 0.025% butylated hydroxytoluene (BHT) as an antioxidant, was purchased from Aldrich (Milwaukee, WI, USA). fetal calf serum (FCS), sodium pyruvate, and Ca^{2+}/Mg^{2+}-free PBS were purchased from Biological Industries (Beth Haemek, Israel). DMEM medium was purchased from Gibco (Grand Island, NY, USA). α-MEM medium, Dimethyl sulfoxide (DMSO), P-nitrophenyl phosphate and acid phosphatase leukocyte kit (387A) were purchased from Sigma Chemicals. Curcumin was purchased from Cayman Chemicals (Ann Arbor, MI, USA). Carnosic acid was purchased from Alexis Biochemicals (Läufenfingen, Switzerland).

2.2. Ethanolic Extract of Lycopene

An ethanolic extract was prepared from a crystalline lycopene preparation that was stored at −20 °C for about a year. 27.2 mg of this partially oxidized lycopene were extracted with ethanol and then evaporated under a vacuum, yielding 24 mg (~88% of the original lycopene). The extract was dissolved in 1.8 mL ethanol, and the resulting solution contained no detectable lycopene, as verified by measuring the absorption spectrum at 250–600 nm (not shown). The lycopene crystals that remained after the ethanol extraction (3.2 mg) were defined as intact lycopene based on the characteristic absorption spectrum (Figure 1b).

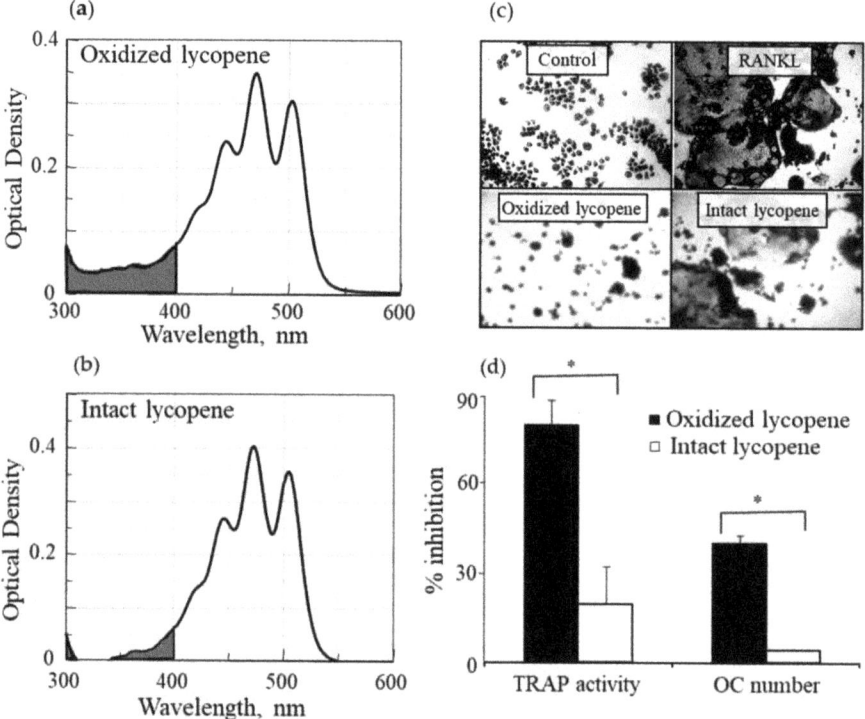

Figure 1. Oxidized lycopene inhibits osteoclast differentiation. Characteristic absorption spectrum of the oxidized lycopene (**a**) and intact lycopene (**b**) used in the experiment. (**c**,**d**) RAW264.7 cells (4×10^4 cells/well) were incubated either alone or in the presence of RANKL (20 ng/mL) without lycopene or with one of its two types at a concentration of 10 µM. (**c**) Photographs of cells after staining for tartrate resistant acid phosphatase- (TRAP)-positive cells (original magnification × 100). (**d**) Counting of multinucleated TRAP-positive cells and measurement of TRAP activity. Values are the means ± SD of three experiments, each performed in triplicate. * $p < 0.01$ for the difference between the % inhibition with oxidized lycopene vs. intact lycopene.

2.3. Synthetic Carotenoid Derivatives

Synthetic carotenoid derivatives, shown in Table 1 (>99% purity), were synthesized and provided by BASF (Dr. Hansgeorg Ernst, Ludwigshafen, Germany). The compounds, characterized using UV/VIS spectroscopy, HPLC, and 1H and 13C NMR, proved to be in an all-E-configuration.

2.4. Energy Calculations

The electronic structure method Restricted Hartree-Fock (RHF) was applied to resolve the chemical optimized structures [36] using the GAMESS suite of programs [37]. The basis set DZV was used to model all molecular orbitals. Atomic charges were computed using the Mulliken scheme, in which the atomic orbitals and molecular orbital coefficients were converted to an orthogonal set. These calculations provide electron populations that are less sensitive to basis set type [38]. In each molecule, there are two reactive carbon atoms in the conjugated chain. The Mulliken analysis was achieved for the two reactive carbon atoms (fourth position from both sides of the molecule, Table 1).

2.5. Solubilization of the Test Compounds

The synthetic derivatives were dissolved at 2 mM in THF and stored at −20°C. Before experiments, the absorption spectra of the compounds were checked for stability. Spectrophotometric analysis was performed at 250–600 nm using the V 530 UV/VIS spectrophotometer (Jasco, Easton, MD, USA). The THF stock solutions of each derivative were diluted in chloroform, and the concentrations were calculated according to the absorption values at the characteristic peaks [24]. The concentration of carotenoid solutions in the THF were calculated from the absorption after dilution in n-hexane: dichlomethane (5:1) containing 1.2 mM BHT.

Stock solutions were added to the cell culture medium under vigorous stirring and nitrogen flow to prevent oxidation. The final concentration of the carotenoids in the medium was measured by spectrophotometry after extraction in 2-propanol and n-hexane-dichloromethane. Stock solutions of curcumin (10 mM) were prepared in DMSO. Carnosic acid (30 mM) was dissolved in absolute ethanol. All procedures were done under reduced lighting, and the final concentrations of THF, ethanol, and DMSO in the medium were 0.75%, 0.15%, and 0.2%, respectively. The vehicles had no effect on the measured parameters.

2.6. Cell Culture

RAW264.7, murine monocyte-macrophage-like cells purchased from American Type Culture Collection (Manassas, VA, USA), were kindly provided by Dr. Bennie Gaiger (Weizmann Institute of Science, Rehovot, Israel). Cells were grown in DMEM (Gibco) with penicillin (500 units/mL), streptomycin (0.5 mg/mL), and 10% FCS. In all experiments, the cells were grown in α-MEM medium containing the same supplements, as well as RANKL (R&D systems, Minneapolis, MN, USA). Cells were grown in a humidified atmosphere of 95% air and 5% CO_2, at 37 °C.

2.7. Differentiation Assays

Cells were seeded in 96-well plates (40,000 cells/mL), and test compounds were added 7–16 h later. In order to evaluate osteoclast differentiation, both TRAP activity and the number of TRAP-positive multinucleated cells were examined. TRAP activity in the cells was determined after 2–3 days by fixation with formaldehyde for 5 min (3.7% v/v) and washing with ethanol (95% v/v) for one min, followed by incubating the cells with 10–20 mM p-nitrophenyl phosphate (Sigma-Aldrich, St. Louis, MO, USA) in the presence of 10 mM sodium tartrate. The reaction was stopped with 0.1 M NaOH, and absorbance was measured at 410 nm. TRAP levels were corrected to cell number using crystal violet. Briefly, after fixation, cells were incubated for 15 min with crystal violet (0.5%) and washed thoroughly in tap water. After drying overnight, the dye was dissolved in sodium citrate, and absorbance was measured at 550 nm. It should be noted that the values of crystal violet staining, after treatment of cells with the various dietary compounds, did not differ by more than 20% from the value measured with RANKL alone. After 4 days, cells were fixed and stained for TRAP using a Leukocyte Acid Phosphatase kit (Sigma-Aldrich, St. Louis, MO, USA). The number of TRAP-positive multinucleated (>5 nucleus) cells was counted under a light microscope.

2.8. Cell Fractionation

Cells were seeded in 100-mm plates (3×10^6 cells per plate). 16 h later, the test compounds were added for 3 h of pre-incubation. Then RANKL was added for 40 min. Cells were lysed with ice-cold cytosolic lysis buffer containing 10 mM NaCl, 10 mM Tris HCl (pH 7.4), 0.1 mM NP-40, 3 mM $MgCl_2$, 1 mM EDTA, 2 mM sodium orthovanadate, 50 mM NaF, 0.2 mM DTT, and 1:25 Complete™ protease-inhibitor cocktail, and centrifuged at $310\times g$ for 10 min at 4 °C. Supernatant samples were then centrifuged at $20,000\times g$ for 10 min at 4 °C (cytosolic fraction). The pellet was resuspended with cytosolic lysis buffer and centrifuged ($310\times g$ for 10 min at 4 °C) twice. The nucleus pellet was lysed with nuclear lysis buffer containing 20 mM Hepes KOH (pH = 7.9), 1:4 glycerol, 420 mM NaCl, 1.5 mM $MgCl_2$, 0.2 mM EDTA, 2 mM sodium orthovanadate, 50 mM NaF, 0.2 mM DTT, and 1:25 Complete™ protease-inhibitor cocktail, and incubated on ice for 20 min. The samples were centrifuged at $20,000\times g$ for 10 min at 4 °C (nuclear fraction). Both fractions were further treated as described for Western blotting using the following antibodies: rabbit polyclonal IgG anti-p65 (#3034) (Cell Signaling Technology, Danvers, MA, USA), mouse monoclonal IgG anti-NF-κB p52 (sc-7386), goat polyclonal IgG anti-lamin B (sc-6216), rabbit polyclonal anti-b-tubulin (sc-9104) (Santa Cruz Biotechnology, Santa Cruz, CA, USA), and peroxidase-conjugated donkey anti-rabbit IgG (711-035-152) (Jackson Immunoresearch Laboratories, Inc. West Grove, PA, USA.).

2.9. Western Blotting

RAW264.7 cells were seeded in 100-mm plates (3×10^6 cells per plate). 16 h later, the test compounds were added for 3 h of pre-incubation. Then RANKL was added for 15 min. Next, whole cell extracts were prepared. Briefly, cells were lysed in ice-cold lysis buffer containing 50 mM, HEPES (pH 7.5), 150 mM NaCl, 10% (v/v) glycerol, 1% (v/v) Triton X-100, 1.5 mM EGTA, 2 mM sodium orthovanadate, 20 mM sodium pyrophosphate, 50 mM NaF, 1 mM DTT, and 1:25 Complete™ protease-inhibitor cocktail (Roche Molecular Biochemicals, Mannheim, Germany), and centrifuged at $20,000\times g$ for 10 min at 4 °C. 50 µg protein of the supernatants were separated by SDS-PAGE, and then blotted into nitrocellulose membrane (Whatman, Dassel, Germany). The membranes were blocked with 5% milk for 2 h and incubated with primary antibodies overnight at 4 °C, followed by incubation with peroxidase–conjugated secondary antibodies (Promega, Madison, WI, USA) for 2 h. The protein bands were visualized using Western Lightning™ Chemiluminescence Reagent Plus (PerkinElmer Life Sciences, Inc., Boston, MA, USA). The blots were stripped and re-probed for the constitutively present protein calreticulin, which served as the loading control. The optical density (OD) of each band was quantitated using ImageQuant TL7.0 (GE Healthcare, Chicago, IL, USA). The following antibodies were used: mouse monoclonal IgG anti-phospho-IκBα Ser32/36 (#9246) (cell signaling technology), mouse monoclonal IgG anti-IκB (OP142) (Oncogene Research Products, La Jolla, CA, USA), and rabbit polyclonal IgG anti-calreticulin (PA3-900) from Affinity BioReagent (Golden, CO, USA).

2.10. Statistical Analysis

All experiments were repeated at least three times. The significance of the differences between the means of the various subgroups was assessed by a two-tailed Student's t test using Microsoft Excel. Statistically significant differences among the multiple groups were analyzed by a one-way ANOVA, followed by a Newman–Keuls multiple comparison test using the GraphPad Prizm 5.0 program (GraphPad Software, San Diego, CA, USA). $p < 0.05$ was considered statistically significant. The interaction between the polyphenols and the carotenoid derivatives in inhibiting TRAP activity was assessed by CI analysis using Calcusyn version 2.1, (BIOSOFT, Cambridge, Great Britain). The CI values were calculated based on the % inhibition by each agent individually and by the combinations at a constant ratio.

3. Results

3.1. Oxidized Lycopene Is More Potent than Intact Lycopene in Inhibiting RANKL-Induced Osteoclast Differentiation

Using a partially oxidized lycopene, we separated the hydrophobic intact lycopene, which is not soluble in ethanol, from its more hydrophilic oxidation products by ethanol extraction. The hydrophilic fraction comprised about 89% by weight of the oxidized lycopene preparation. The spectral absorption of the non-extracted oxidized lycopene preparation (Figure 1a) showed higher absorption in the 300–400 nm range than that of the intact lycopene preparation (Figure 1b), suggesting that the latter does not contain a considerable amount of oxidized derivatives. We examined the effect of these intact and oxidized preparations of lycopene in the inhibition of RANKL-induced osteoclast differentiation in RAW264.7 cells. The picture in Figure 1c shows small monocytes in the control and large multinucleated osteoclasts in the RANKL-treated cells. Similar osteoclasts are seen in cells treated with RANKL and intact lycopene, in contrast to cells treated with RANKL and oxidized lycopene that showed no multinucleated osteoclasts, suggesting that the oxidized lycopene inhibited osteoclast differentiation. A quantitative analysis showed that the oxidized lycopene preparation was much more potent in inhibiting TRAP activity and formation of TRAP+ multinucleated osteoclasts than the intact lycopene (Figure 1d). To evaluate whether the treatment of cells with oxidized or intact lycopene affect cell survival, the values of cell protein, measured by crystal violet staining (used to normalize TRAP results), was compared to that of cells treated with RANKL alone. The average of four experiments, each performed in triplicate was 46,700 ± 2000, 44,600 ± 4300, and 49,100 ± 5400 for RANKL alone, RANKL with oxidized lycopene, and RANKL with intact lycopene, respectively. Thus, the results presented in Figure 1d represent inhibition of osteoclast differentiation and are not attributed to cell death.

3.2. Diapocarotene-Dials Inhibition of RANKL-Induced Osteoclast Differentiation Depends on the Electron Density around the Reactive Carbon Atoms of the Molecules

To determine the effect of diapocarotene-dials on RANKL-induced osteoclast differentiation in RAW264.7 cells, we incubated these cells with RANKL and with different concentrations of 6,14'-diapocarotene-6,14'-dial (6,14'), and assessed TRAP activity and the formation of multinucleated TRAP+ cells. The percent inhibition by 6,14' was similar for the two measured parameters. The inhibition of osteoclast differentiation by this derivative was dose dependent, and almost complete inhibition was observed at 10 µM (Figure 2a). We measured TRAP activity and the formation of multinucleated TRAP+ cells with 10 µM of two different diapocarotene-dials (6,14' and 10,10'). The percent inhibition by each compound was similar for the two measured parameters, and 6,14' was more active than 10,10' (Figure 2b). Treatment of cells with diapocarotene-dials alone without RANKL did not result in any response (data not shown). Different diapocarotene-dials inhibited osteoclast differentiation to different extents (Figure 2c). In previous work, we have shown that the activity of individual carotenoid derivatives in inhibiting the NF-κB reporter gene activity [25] depends on the electron density around the reactive carbon atoms (the fourth atom from each side of the molecule). Since NF-κB is known to partially mediate RANKL signaling, we assumed that RANKL-induced osteoclast differentiation would similarly depend on the structure of the diapocarotene-dials. Indeed, a strong correlation ($R^2 = 0.938$) exists between the electron density at the reactive C-atom of the various diapocarotene-dials (Table 1) and the % inhibition of TRAP activity (Figure 2c). The results strengthen the evidence that the potency of these derivatives depends on the electron density around the reactive carbon atoms.

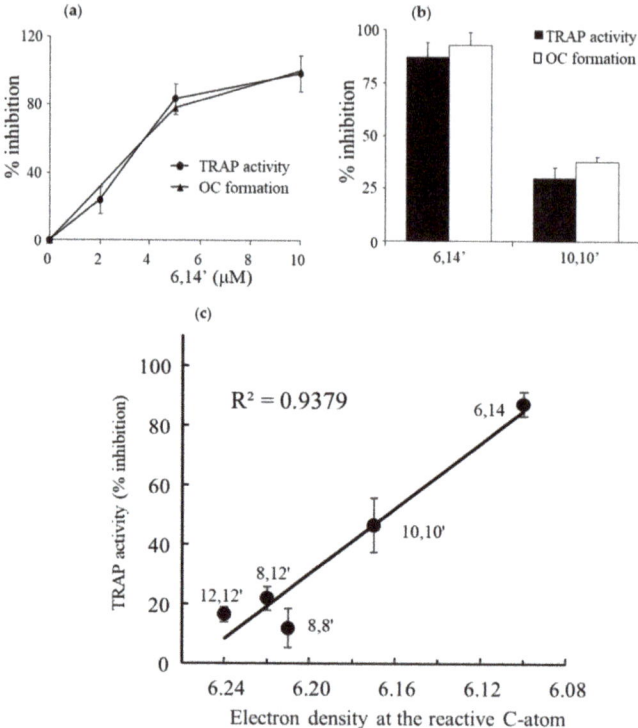

Figure 2. Diapocarotene-dials inhibit RANKL-induced osteoclastogenesis. Osteoclast differentiation was measured as described in the Materials and Methods section and in Figure 1. Cell were incubated with RANKL alone or with (**a**) different concentrations of the diapocarotene-dial 6,14′ or (**b,c**) with 10 µM different diapocarete-dials. Inhibition is shown in relation to positive control with RANKL. (**b**) Comparison of the inhibition by 6,14′ and 10,10′. Values are the means ± SE of 3–14 experiments, each performed in triplicate, $p < 0.01$ for the difference between the % inhibition with 6,14′ vs. 10,10′. (**c**) Correlation between the electron density at the reactive C-atom of the various diapocarotene-dials and the % inhibition of osteoclast TRAP activity. Values are the means ± SE of 3–11 independent experiments, each performed in triplicate. The results are statistically significant (ANOVA test) $p < 0.05$.

3.3. Diapocarotene-Dials Inhibit RANKL-Induced NF-κB Activation in Osteoclast Precursors

Activation of NF-κB is comprised of two pathways: the canonical and the alternative or non-canonical. Phosphorylation and degradation of its inhibitory subunit IκBα is an essential step in activating the canonical pathway. Western blot analysis revealed that the active diapocarotene-dials 6,14′ and 10,10′ significantly inhibit RANKL-induced IκBα phosphorylation and degradation, as opposed to the inactive diapocarotene-dial 8,8′ and 12,12′ (Figure 3a,b), in accordance with the structure-activity relationship described above. It is noticeable in Figure 3a that the level of pIκB in the 6,14′-treated sample was greater than with RANKL alone; however, quantitating the pIκB:IκB ratio (Figure 3b, corrected to calreticulin) clearly shows that 6,14′ treatment reduced this ratio by more than 30%, which indicates downregulation of IκBα phosphorylation and inhibition of RANKL-induced degradation of IκBα. IκBα degradation enables the translocation of p65 to the nucleus. Fractionation analysis of nuclear p65 (Figure 3c,d) shows some reduction in the nucleus after treatment with lycopene or its active derivatives; however, this reduction was not statistically significant, but may suggest that the active derivatives attenuate the canonical pathway of NF-κB.

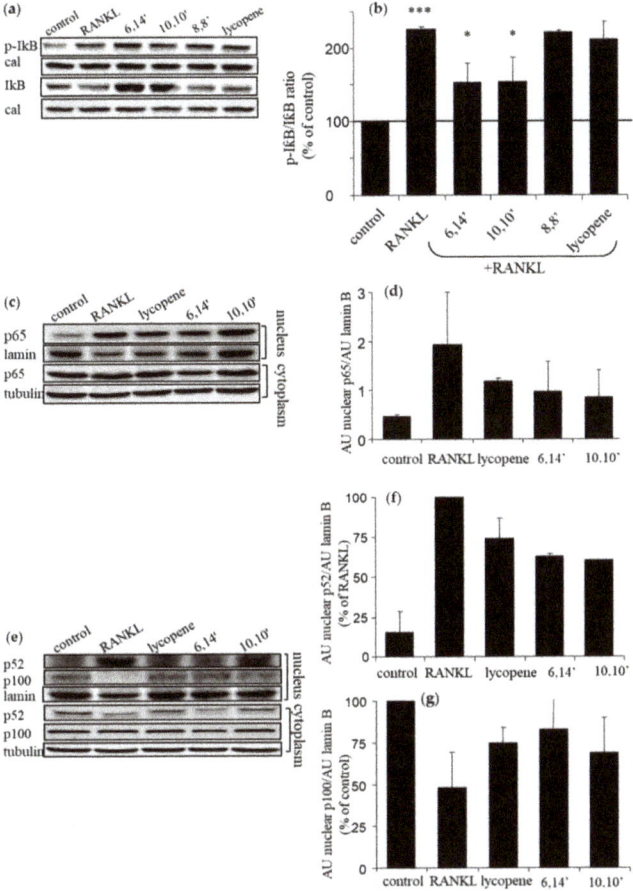

Figure 3. Diapocarotene-dials attenuate the NF-κB signal in RANKL-activated RAW264.7 cells. 5×10^6 cells in 100-mm plates were either incubated alone or in the presence of the indicated diapocarotene-dials (10 μM) or lycopene (10 μM) for 2 h, and then treated with RANKL (40 ng/mL) for 15 min (**a,b**) and 40 min (**c–g**). Whole cell lysates (**a,b**) and cytoplasmatic and nuclear fractions (**c–g**) were prepared and analyzed by Western blotting, as described in Materials and Methods. Values are the means ± SE of three independent experiments. (**a**) Blots of IκBα and pIκB. (**b**) The ratio of p-IκB:IκB after normalization with calreticulin (cal) is presented as the % of the control without RANKL. *** $p < 0.001$ for the difference between RANKL to the control. * $p < 0.05$ for the difference between RANKL to 6,14′ and 10,10′. (**c**) Blots of nuclear and cytosolic p65. (**d**) Nuclear p65 levels normalized to laminin B. (**e**) Blots of nuclear and cytosolic p52 and p100. (**f**) Nuclear p52 levels normalized to laminin B. Results are % of RANKL. (**g**) Nuclear p100 levels normalized to laminin B. Results are % of control.

Degradation of the precursor p100 to the active NF-κB component p52 is essential in activating the alternative pathway. RANKL reduced the nuclear level of p100 and increased that of p52 (Figure 3e–g). Treatment with lycopene, 6,14′ and 10,10′ suggests inhibition of the RANKL-induced conversion of p100 to p52, but the changes were not significant. In addition, these compounds preserved the cytosolic levels of p52 and prevented its translocation to the nucleus (Figure 3e). These results may suggest that active diapocarotene-dials inhibit both pathways in RANKL-induced NF-κB activation in RAW264.7 cells.

3.4. Active Diapocarotene-Dials Inhibit RANKL-Induced TRAP Activity Synergistically with Curcumin and with Carnosic Acid

RAW264.7 cells were incubated with combinations of the diapocarotene-dial 6,14′, with the polyphenols curcumin and carnosic acid. At low concentrations of each agent, these combinations produced a synergistic anti-differentiative effect in RANKL-induced cells. Synergistic effects were evaluated using Calcusyn Software for Dose Effect Analysis. Dose effect curves and CI values for the combination of 6,14′ with curcumin (Figure 4a,b) and 6,14′ with carnosic acid (Figure 4c,d) are presented. Most CI values are below 1.0, indicating some synergy at most of the tested concentrations. However, CI values at low concentrations, resulting in 20–40% inhibition, are smaller than 0.5, indicating a strong synergistic effect at concentrations that can be found in human blood.

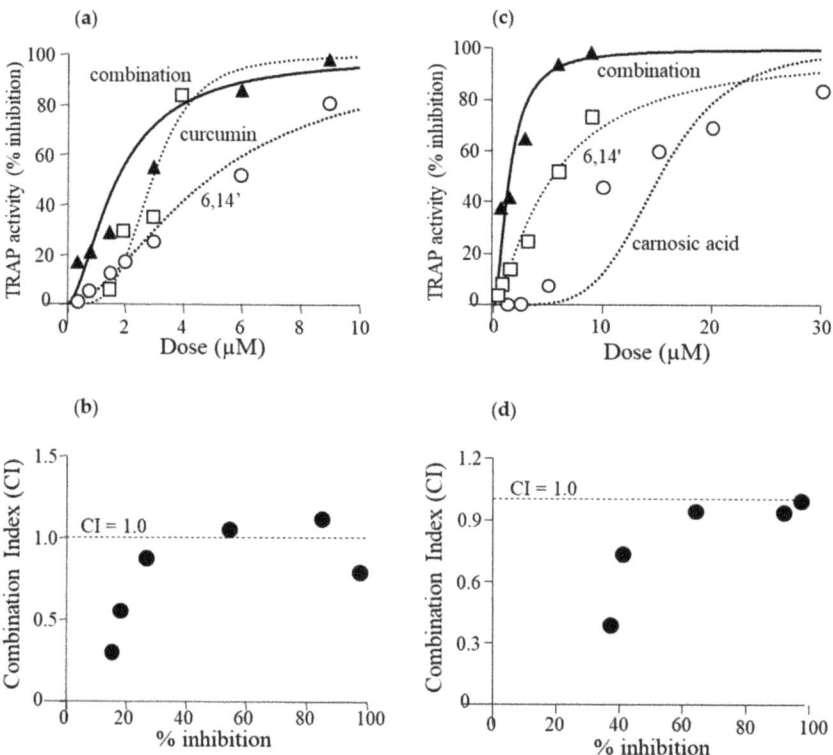

Figure 4. Synergistic effect of 6,14′ with curcumin or carnosic acid. Osteoclast differentiation was measured as described in the Materials and Methods section and in Figure 1. Cell were incubated with RANKL alone or in the presence of different concentrations of 6,14′ with curcumin or with carnosic acid at constant concentration ratios. Values are the means of 3–4 experiments, each performed in triplicate. (**a**) The dose effect curve of the combinations of 6,14′ with curcumin at a ratio of 1:1. (**b**) Combination index (CI) values for the combinations of 6,14′ with curcumin. (**c**) The dose effect curve of the combinations of 6,14′ with carnosic acid at a ratio of 1:3. (**d**) CI values for the combinations of 6,14′ with carnosic acid.

4. Discussion

The main finding of the current study is that the inhibition of RANKL-induced osteoclast differentiation by partially oxidized lycopene is mediated by the hydrophilic oxidation products, and not by the intact lycopene molecule. Two different approaches led us to this conclusion. (a) We separated the spontaneously oxidized derivatives from the intact carotenoid using an ethanolic extraction of a partially oxidized lycopene preparation, and found that the oxidized lycopene inhibited osteoclast differentiation, whereas the parent molecule was nearly ineffective. (b) Using a series of fully characterized synthetic diapocarotene-dials, we found that these compounds inhibited osteoclast differentiation, and the inhibition efficiency correlated with the reactivity of the α,β-unsaturated carbonyl groups in reactions such as Michael addition. This reactivity was estimated by calculating the electron density around the reactive carbon atoms, as shown in Table 1. The relative effectiveness of the diapocarotene-dials in the inhibition of osteoclastogenesis was similar to that found for activation of the ARE/Nrf2 transcription system [24] and for inhibition of TNFα-induced NFκB activity [25] by carotenoid derivatives. Thus, it is suggested that the inhibition of RANKL-induced osteoclast differentiation resulted, at least partially, from inhibition of the RANKL-activated NF-κB activity. In support of this suggestion, we found that the effective diapocarotene-dials reduced activation of the canonical NFκB pathway by RANKL. This was evident from the reduction of IκBα phosphorylation and degradation, and of p65 nuclear translocation that are essential stages in the canonical pathway. The active diapocarotene-dials and lycopene also reduced the nuclear translocation of p52, suggesting inhibition of the non-canonical NFκB pathway that is known to be involved in RANKL-induced osteoclast differentiation [17,20].

Several proteins that take part in the NFκB pathway (e.g., IκB kinase) and the NFκB subunits (e.g., p65) contain cysteine residues which regulate NFκB activity [39,40]. The interaction of electrophiles with these cysteine thiols leads to NFκB pathway inhibition [39]. Similarly, it was shown that sulforaphane, its analogs [41], and other electrophiles such as carnosic acid [42], interact with reactive cysteine thiols in the Keap1 protein, leading to activation of the ARE/Nrf2 transcription system. Hydrophobic carotenoids such as lycopene and beta carotene are devoid of electrophilic groups which can interact with these cysteines; however, we previously demonstrated that apo-carotenal derivatives interact directly with thiol groups of IκB kinase [25]. In addition, we previously suggested, although did not directly prove, that carotenoid-oxidized derivatives activate the Nrf2 transcription system by interaction with such reactive cysteines in the Keap1 protein [24]. Since NFκB is involved in RANKL activation of osteoclast differentiation, and reduction of RANKL-induced ROS generation through activation of ARE/Nrf2 was suggested to inhibit this differentiation [35], we propose that the interaction of carotenoid derivatives with thiol groups in proteins critically involved in NFκB and ARE/Nrf2 pathways may be part of the mechanism for the inhibition of osteoclast differentiation by oxidized derivatives of lycopene and other carotenoids.

As all the effects of carotenoid derivatives were obtained in in-vitro cellular systems, an important question is whether such effects can also be obtained in-vivo. Although this question is difficult to answer directly, what we can try to resolve is whether such apo-carotenals can be found in mammalian blood and tissues, and what their potential sources are. It is possible that the derivatives are consumed with the carotenoids from foods or formed inside the body. Diapocarotene-dials similar to those used in the current study were only rarely found in plants, most likely because they are reactive and instable molecules, which makes them difficult to detect in biological samples [43]. Recently, Jia et al. identified in Arabidopsis a presumed carotenoid-derived dialdehyde, anchorene, (12,12′-diapocaroten-12,12′-dial according to our nomenclature) that promotes the development of anchor roots [44]. However, such rare plant metabolites probably have no importance in the human diet and, thus, it is not surprising that diapocarotene-dials have not been detected in mammalian samples. In contrast, mono-apocarotenals, both, β-apo-carotenals [45] and lycopenals [46], were identified in both human and plant samples. Specifically, apolycopenals including apo-10′-, apo-12′-, apo-14′-, and apo-15′-lycopenal were found in foods that are rich in lycopene such as raw tomatoes, red grapefruit, and watermelon. These lycopenals were also detected in the plasma of individuals who had consumed tomato juice for 8 weeks [46]. Similar compounds, apo-8′- and apo-12′-lycopenals, were detected in rat livers [47], and in a recent study, additional apo-carotenals were detected, including β-apo-12′-carotenal and several apo-zeaxanthinals and apo-luteinals [48]. The concentration of these apo-lycopenals in foods is very low, and is about 500 times lower than that of lycopene [49], with similar relative concentrations found in human plasma. However, it is not clear if apo-carotenals are absorbed from foods or produced in the body since it was found that 4-week supplementation of high-β-carotene and high-lycopene tomato juice did not lead to detectable concentrations of most β-apocarotenals or lycopenals that were present in the juice [50]. It is not certain if the accessibility of these compounds to bone and other cells in-vivo is sufficient to achieve the beneficial effects. Another alternative is that the apo-carotenals are formed inside the cells from the intact carotenoids, close to the site of their activity. Carotenoids are cleaved in the cells by the central cleavage enzyme 15,15′-β-carotene oxygenase 1 (BCO1) and by the eccentric cleavage enzyme β,β-carotene-9′,10′-oxygenase 2 (BCO2). The latter enzyme exhibits broad substrate specificity and cleaves both carotenes, such as lycopene, and xanthophylls like lutein [51]. The cleavage at the 9,10 double bond results in the formation of apo-10′-carotenals and 10,10′-diapocarotenals [52]. The 10,10′-diapocaroten-10,10′-dial was formed in vitro by incubation of β-carotene, as well as other carotenoids, with a recombinant BCO2 [53], but they were not detected in mammalian samples perhaps because of their high reactivity in biological systems [24]. Although, in the current study, we analyzed the activity of only the diapocarotenal, the reactivity of the apo-10′-lycopenals in the activation of the ARE/Nrf2 transcription system was only 1.5–2.5 fold lower than that of the 10,10′-diapocaroten-10,10′-dial [24]. Thus, it is possible that formation inside the osteoclasts may result in high enough local concentrations to lead to the inhibition of osteoclast differentiation.

Similar to carotenoid derivatives, other phyto-nutrients are known to inhibit osteoclast differentiation. These include flavonoids such as quercetin [54], polyphenols such as curcumin [55], and resveratrol [56], sulforaphane [57], and other isothiocyanates [58]. Although these nutrients have different chemical structures, they, and the carotenoid derivatives, all have electrophilic groups in common that can interact with thiol groups of reactive proteins of the NFκB system [39,40] or other signaling pathways involved in osteoclast differentiation. A significant inhibition of osteoclastogenesis by the two polyphenols and by the carotenoid derivatives tested in the current study occur at high concentrations (6,14′ and curcumin—above 2 µM; carnosic acid—above 10 µM). Since, usually, these concentrations cannot be achieved in-vivo, we tested if their combination would result in activity at concentrations that could be achieved. We found a strong synergy between the polyphenols and the carotenoid derivative, 6,14′, leading to significant inhibition at concentrations below 1 µM. However, understanding the mechanism of this synergy would require extensive research to explore whether it results from synergistic inhibition of NFκB at different elements of the pathways or from interference in other pathways leading to osteoclast differentiation. For example, curcumin has been shown to inhibit the differentiation of human monocytes to osteoclasts by reducing phosphorylation and activation of mitogen-activated protein kinase (MAPK) proteins, such as ERK, p38, and JNK, which leads to reduced expression of c-Fos and NFATc1 that are essential for differentiation of osteoclasts [59]. Similar reduction of the phosphorylation of ERK, p38, and JNK MAPKs by carnosic acid was evident in RANKL-induced RAW264.7 cells, followed by a decrease in expression of c-Fos and NFATc1 and inhibition of osteoclastogenesis [35]. Thus, inhibition of MAPKs by the polyphenols, curcumin and carnosic acid, can increase the inhibitory effect of carotenoid derivatives that reduce RANKL-induced NFκB activation. Thummuri, et al. have shown in RAW264.7 cells and in mouse bone marrow macrophages that activation of ARE/Nrf2 and reduction of RANKL-induced ROS generation is one of the mechanisms for carnosic acid inhibition of osteoclastogenesis [35]. This is another possible explanation for the synergy we presented between the polyphenols and the carotenoid derivatives, as we have recently shown a strong synergy in ARE/Nrf2 activation in human keratinocytes by combinations of lycopene or tomato extract with carnosic acid or curcumin [60].

5. Conclusions

The current paper suggests that the protective effect of lycopene and other carotenoids on bone health, as shown in population and animal studies, is at least partially related to the inhibition of osteoclast differentiation and activity. This inhibition is possibly associated with that of the NFκB transcriptional system. Although most previous studies were done with carotenoids in foods or with pure carotenoids, we suggest that the osteoclasts are actually affected by the apo-carotenal carotenoid derivatives and not by the intact molecules.

Author Contributions: Conceptualization, S.O.-B., K.L.-H., J.L. and Y.S.; Formal analysis, S.O.-B., M.K., Y.M., K.A. and Y.S.; Funding acquisition, J.L. and Y.S.; Investigation, S.O.-B. and M.K.; Methodology, S.O.-B., M.K., K.L.-H., J.L. and Y.S.; Project administration, J.L. and Y.S.; Supervision, J.L. and Y.S.; Visualization, S.O.-B., M.K., K.L.-H., J.L. and Y.S.; Writing—original draft, S.O.-B., Y.M., J.L. and Y.S.; Writing—review & editing, J.L. and Y.S. All authors have read and agreed to the published version of the manuscript.

Funding: This research was funded by Lycored Ltd., Beer Sheva, Israel (to Y.S. and J.L.) (899646).

Acknowledgments: We thank Hansgeorg Ernst (BASF, Ludwigshafen, Germany) and the late, Catherine Caris-Veyrat (INRA, Avignon University, Avignon, France) for their help in designing the synthetic carotenoid derivatives, and Hansgeorg Ernst for preparing and donating the carotenoid derivatives. We thank Tanya Svedlov, Lycored Ltd., Beer Sheva, Israel for donating purified lycopene and for the extraction of lycopene, and Robin Miller for English editing.

Conflicts of Interest: J.L. and Y.S. are consultants for Lycored Ltd., Beer Sheva, Israel. K.L.-H. is currently employed by Lycored, but at the time of conducting the experiments was a Ph.D. student at the laboratory of JL and Y.S. J.L. and Y.S. received research funding from Lycored. All other authors declare no conflict of interest. Lycored is a supplier to the dietary supplement and functional food industries worldwide. Lycored Ltd. had no role in the design of the study; in the collection, analyses, or interpretation of data; in the writing of the manuscript, or in the decision to publish the results.

References

1. Tucker, K.L.; Hannan, M.T.; Chen, H.; Cupples, L.A.; Wilson, P.W.; Kiel, D.P. Potassium, magnesium, and fruit and vegetable intakes are associated with greater bone mineral density in elderly men and women. *Am. J. Clin. Nutr.* **1999**, *69*, 727–736. [CrossRef]
2. Muhlbauer, R.C.; Li, F. Effect of vegetables on bone metabolism. *Nature* **1999**, *401*, 343–344. [CrossRef] [PubMed]
3. New, S.A.; Robins, S.P.; Campbell, M.K.; Martin, J.C.; Garton, M.J.; Bolton-Smith, C.; Grubb, D.A.; Lee, S.J.; Reid, D.M. Dietary influences on bone mass and bone metabolism: Further evidence of a positive link between fruit and vegetable consumption and bone health? *Am. J. Clin. Nutr.* **2000**, *71*, 142–151. [CrossRef] [PubMed]
4. Arscott, S.A. Food sources of carotenoids. In *Carotenoids and Human Health*; Tanumihardjo, S.A., Ed.; Springer: New York, NY, USA, 2013; pp. 1–331. [CrossRef]
5. Khachik, F. Distribution and metabolism of dietary carotenoids in humans as a criterion for development of nutritional supplements. *Pure Appl. Chem.* **2006**, *78*, 1551–1557. [CrossRef]
6. Parker, R.S. Carotenoids in human blood and tissues. *J. Nutr.* **1989**, *119*, 101–104. [CrossRef]
7. El-Sohemy, A.; Baylin, A.; Kabagambe, E.; Ascherio, A.; Spiegelman, D.; Campos, H. Individual carotenoid concentrations in adipose tissue and plasma as biomarkers of dietary intake. *Am. J. Clin. Nutr.* **2002**, *76*, 172–179. [CrossRef]
8. Shi, J.; Le Maguer, M. Lycopene in tomatoes: Chemical and physical properties affected by food processing. *Crit. Rev. Biotechnol.* **2000**, *20*, 293–334. [CrossRef]
9. Boyle, W.J.; Simonet, W.S.; Lacey, D.L. Osteoclast differentiation and activation. *Nature* **2003**, *423*, 337–342. [CrossRef]
10. Shen, C.L.; Von Bergen, V.; Chyu, M.C.; Jenkins, M.R.; Mo, H.; Chen, C.H.; Kwun, I.S. Fruits and dietary phytochemicals in bone protection. *Nutr. Res.* **2012**, *32*, 897–910. [CrossRef]
11. Cheong, S.H.; Chang, K.J. The preventive effect of fermented milk supplement containing tomato (*Lycopersion esculentum*) and taurine on bone loss in ovariectomized rats. *Adv. Exp. Med. Biol.* **2009**, *643*, 333–340. [CrossRef]
12. Rao, L.G.; Krishnadev, N.; Banasikowska, K.; Rao, A.V. Lycopene I—Effect on osteoclasts: Lycopene inhibits basal and parathyroid hormone-stimulated osteoclast formation and mineral resorption mediated by reactive oxygen species in rat bone marrow cultures. *J. Med. Food* **2003**, *6*, 69–78. [CrossRef] [PubMed]

13. Kim, L.; Rao, A.V.; Rao, L.G. Lycopene II—Effect on osteoblasts: The carotenoid lycopene stimulates cell proliferation and alkaline phosphatase activity of SaOS-2 cells. *J. Med. Food* **2003**, *6*, 79–86. [CrossRef] [PubMed]
14. Costa-Rodrigues, J.; Fernandes, M.H.; Pinho, O.; Monteiro, P.R.R. Modulation of human osteoclastogenesis and osteoblastogenesis by lycopene. *J. Nutr. Biochem.* **2018**, *57*, 26–34. [CrossRef] [PubMed]
15. Suda, T.; Takahashi, N.; Udagawa, N.; Jimi, E.; Gillespie, M.T.; Martin, T.J. Modulation of osteoclast differentiation and function by the new members of the tumor necrosis factor receptor and ligand families. *Endocr. Rev.* **1999**, *20*, 345–357. [CrossRef]
16. Yavropoulou, M.P.; Yovos, J.G. Osteoclastogenesis—Current knowledge and future perspectives. *J. Musculoskelet. Neuronal Interact.* **2008**, *8*, 204–216.
17. Boyce, B.F.; Xiu, Y.; Li, J.; Xing, L.; Yao, Z. NF-κB-mediated regulation of osteoclastogenesis. *Endocrinol. Metab.* **2015**, *30*, 35–44. [CrossRef]
18. Asagiri, M.; Takayanagi, H. The molecular understanding of osteoclast differentiation. *Bone* **2007**, *40*, 251–264. [CrossRef]
19. Franzoso, G.; Carlson, L.; Xing, L.; Poljak, L.; Shores, E.W.; Brown, K.D.; Leonardi, A.; Tran, T.; Boyce, B.F.; Siebenlist, U. Requirement for NF-κB in osteoclast and B-cell development. *Genes Dev.* **1997**, *11*, 3482–3496. [CrossRef]
20. Maruyama, T.; Fukushima, H.; Nakao, K.; Shin, M.; Yasuda, H.; Weih, F.; Doi, T.; Aoki, K.; Alles, N.; Ohya, K.; et al. Processing of the NF-κB2 precursor p100 to p52 is critical for RANKL-induced osteoclast differentiation. *J. Bone Miner. Res.* **2010**, *25*, 1058–1067.
21. Joo, Y.E.; Karrasch, T.; Muhlbauer, M.; Allard, B.; Narula, A.; Herfarth, H.H.; Jobin, C. Tomato lycopene extract prevents lipopolysaccharide-induced NF-κB signaling but worsens dextran sulfate sodium-induced colitis in NF-κBEGFP mice. *PLoS ONE* **2009**, *4*, e4562. [CrossRef]
22. Hadad, N.; Levy, R. The synergistic anti-inflammatory effects of lycopene, lutein, beta-carotene, and carnosic acid combinations via redox-based inhibition of NF-κB signaling. *Free Radic. Biol. Med.* **2012**, *53*, 1381–1391. [CrossRef] [PubMed]
23. Simone, R.E.; Russo, M.; Catalano, A.; Monego, G.; Froehlich, K.; Boehm, V.; Palozza, P. Lycopene inhibits NF-kB-mediated IL-8 expression and changes redox and PPARgamma signalling in cigarette smoke-stimulated macrophages. *PLoS ONE* **2011**, *6*, e19652. [CrossRef] [PubMed]
24. Linnewiel, K.; Ernst, H.; Caris-Veyrat, C.; Ben-Dor, A.; Kampf, A.; Salman, H.; Danilenko, M.; Levy, J.; Sharoni, Y. Structure activity relationship of carotenoid derivatives in activation of the electrophile/antioxidant response element transcription system. *Free Radic. Biol. Med.* **2009**, *47*, 659–667. [CrossRef] [PubMed]
25. Linnewiel-Hermoni, K.; Motro, Y.; Miller, Y.; Levy, J.; Sharoni, Y. Carotenoid derivatives inhibit nuclear factor κB activity in bone and cancer cells by targeting key thiol groups. *Free Radic. Biol. Med.* **2014**, *75*, 105–120. [CrossRef] [PubMed]
26. Nara, E.; Hayashi, H.; Kotake, M.; Miyashita, K.; Nagao, A. Acyclic carotenoids and their oxidation mixtures inhibit the growth of HL-60 human promyelocytic leukemia cells. *Nutr. Cancer* **2001**, *39*, 273–283. [CrossRef]
27. Caris-Veyrat, C.; Schmid, A.; Carail, M.; Bohm, V. Cleavage products of lycopene produced by in vitro oxidations: Characterization and mechanisms of formation. *J. Agric. Food Chem.* **2003**, *51*, 7318–7325. [CrossRef]
28. Giuliano, G.; Al-Babili, S.; Von Lintig, J. Carotenoid oxygenases: Cleave it or leave it. *Trends Plant. Sci.* **2003**, *8*, 145–149. [CrossRef]
29. Ben-Aziz, A.; Britton, G.; Goodwin, T.W. Carotene epoxides of Lycopersicon esculentum. *Phytochemistry* **1973**, *12*, 2759–2764. [CrossRef]
30. Veprik, A.; Khanin, M.; Linnewiel-Hermoni, K.; Danilenko, M.; Levy, J.; Sharoni, Y. Polyphenols, isothiocyanates, and carotenoid derivatives enhance estrogenic activity in bone cells but inhibit it in breast cancer cells. *Am. J. Physiol. Endocrinol. Metab.* **2012**, *303*, E815–E824. [CrossRef]
31. Pérez-Jiménez, J.; Neveu, V.; Vos, F.; Scalbert, A. Identification of the 100 richest dietary sources of polyphenols: An application of the Phenol-Explorer database. *Eur. J. Clin. Nutr.* **2010**, *64*, S112–S120. [CrossRef]
32. Cao, F.; Liu, T.; Xu, Y.; Xu, D.; Feng, S. Curcumin inhibits cell proliferation and promotes apoptosis in human osteoclastoma cell through MMP-9, NF-κB and JNK signaling pathways. *Int. J. Clin. Exp. Pathol.* **2015**, *8*, 6037–6045. [PubMed]

33. Cheng, T.; Zhao, Y.; Li, B.; Cheng, M.; Wang, J.; Zhang, X. Curcumin attenuation of wear particle-induced osteolysis via RANKL signaling pathway suppression in mouse calvarial model. *Mediat. Inflamm.* **2017**, *2017*, 5784374. [CrossRef] [PubMed]
34. Liu, M.; Zhou, X.; Zhou, L.; Liu, Z.; Yuan, J.; Cheng, J.; Zhao, J.; Wu, L.; Li, H.; Qiu, H.; et al. Carnosic acid inhibits inflammation response and joint destruction on osteoclasts, fibroblast-like synoviocytes, and collagen-induced arthritis rats. *J. Cell. Physiol.* **2018**, *233*, 6291–6303. [CrossRef] [PubMed]
35. Thummuri, D.; Naidu, V.G.M.; Chaudhari, P. Carnosic acid attenuates RANKL-induced oxidative stress and osteoclastogenesis via induction of Nrf2 and suppression of NF-κB and MAPK signalling. *J. Mol. Med.* **2017**, *95*, 1065–1076. [CrossRef]
36. Schmidt, M.W.; Baldridge, K.K.; Boatz, J.A.; Elbert, S.T.; Gordon, M.S.; Jensen, J.H.; Koseki, S.; Matsunaga, N.; Nguyen, K.A.; Su, S.; et al. General atomic and molecular electronic structure system. *J. Comput. Chem.* **1993**, *14*, 1347–1363. [CrossRef]
37. Mark Gordon's Quantum Theory Group. Available online: http://www.msg.ameslab.gov/GAMESS/GAMESS.html (accessed on 2 November 2020).
38. Mulliken, R.S. Electronic population analysis on LCAO–MO molecular wave functions. I. *J. Chem. Phys.* **1955**, *23*, 1833–1840. [CrossRef]
39. Na, H.K.; Surh, Y.J. Transcriptional regulation via cysteine thiol modification: A novel molecular strategy for chemoprevention and cytoprotection. *Mol. Carcinog.* **2006**, *45*, 368–380. [CrossRef] [PubMed]
40. Pande, V.; Sousa, S.F.; Ramos, M.J. Direct covalent modification as a strategy to inhibit nuclear factor-κB. *Curr. Med. Chem.* **2009**, *16*, 4261–4273. [CrossRef] [PubMed]
41. Dinkova-Kostova, A.T.; Holtzclaw, W.D.; Cole, R.N.; Itoh, K.; Wakabayashi, N.; Katoh, Y.; Yamamoto, M.; Talalay, P. Direct evidence that sulfhydryl groups of Keap1 are the sensors regulating induction of phase 2 enzymes that protect against carcinogens and oxidants. *Proc. Natl. Acad. Sci. USA* **2002**, *99*, 11908–11913. [CrossRef] [PubMed]
42. Satoh, T.; Kosaka, K.; Itoh, K.; Kobayashi, A.; Yamamoto, M.; Shimojo, Y.; Kitajima, C.; Cui, J.; Kamins, J.; Okamoto, S.; et al. Carnosic acid, a catechol-type electrophilic compound, protects neurons both in vitro and in vivo through activation of the Keap1/Nrf2 pathway via S-alkylation of targeted cysteines on Keap1. *J. Neurochem.* **2008**, *104*, 1116–1131. [CrossRef] [PubMed]
43. Felemban, A.; Braguy, J.; Zurbriggen, M.D.; Al-Babili, S. Apocarotenoids involved in plant development and stress response. *Front. Plant Sci.* **2019**, *10*, 1168. [CrossRef] [PubMed]
44. Jia, K.-P.; Dickinson, A.J.; Mi, J.; Cui, G.; Kharbatia, N.M.; Guo, X.; Sugiono, E.; Aranda, M.; Rueping, M.; Benfey, P.N.; et al. Anchorene is an endogenous diapocarotenoid required for anchor root formation in *Arabidopsis*. *bioRxiv* **2018**. [CrossRef]
45. Harrison, E.H.; dela Sena, C.; Eroglu, A.; Fleshman, M.K. The formation, occurrence, and function of beta-apocarotenoids: Beta-carotene metabolites that may modulate nuclear receptor signaling. *Am. J. Clin. Nutr.* **2012**, *96*, 1189S–1192S. [CrossRef] [PubMed]
46. Kopec, R.E.; Riedl, K.M.; Harrison, E.H.; Curley, R.W., Jr.; Hruszkewycz, D.P.; Clinton, S.K.; Schwartz, S.J. Identification and quantification of apo-lycopenals in fruits, vegetables, and human plasma. *J. Agric. Food Chem.* **2010**, *58*, 3290–3296. [CrossRef] [PubMed]
47. Gajic, M.; Zaripheh, S.; Sun, F.; Erdman, J.W., Jr. Apo-8′-lycopenal and apo-12′-lycopenal are metabolic products of lycopene in rat liver. *J. Nutr.* **2006**, *136*, 1552–1557. [CrossRef] [PubMed]
48. Zoccali, M.; Giuffrida, D.; Salafia, F.; Giofrè, S.V.; Mondello, L. Carotenoids and apocarotenoids determination in intact human blood samples by online supercritical fluid extraction-supercritical fluid chromatography-tandem mass spectrometry. *Anal. Chim. Acta* **2018**, *1032*, 40–47. [CrossRef]
49. Eroglu, A.; Harrison, E.H. Carotenoid metabolism in mammals, including man: Formation, occurrence, and function of apocarotenoids. *J. Lipid Res.* **2013**, *54*, 1719–1730. [CrossRef]
50. Cooperstone, J.L.; Novotny, J.A.; Riedl, K.M.; Cichon, M.J.; Francis, D.M.; Curley, R.W., Jr.; Schwartz, S.J.; Harrison, E.H. Limited appearance of apocarotenoids is observed in plasma after consumption of tomato juices: A randomized human clinical trial. *Am. J. Clin. Nutr.* **2018**, *108*, 784–792. [CrossRef]
51. Lobo, G.P.; Amengual, J.; Palczewski, G.; Babino, D.; von Lintig, J. Mammalian carotenoid-oxygenases: Key players for carotenoid function and homeostasis. *Biochim. Biophys. Acta* **2012**, *1821*, 78–87. [CrossRef]

52. Kiefer, C.; Hessel, S.; Lampert, J.M.; Vogt, K.; Lederer, M.O.; Breithaupt, D.E.; von Lintig, J. Identification and characterization of a mammalian enzyme catalyzing the asymmetric oxidative cleavage of provitamin A. *J. Biol. Chem.* **2001**, *276*, 14110–14116. [CrossRef]
53. Amengual, J.; Lobo, G.P.; Golczak, M.; Li, H.N.; Klimova, T.; Hoppel, C.L.; Wyss, A.; Palczewski, K.; von Lintig, J. A mitochondrial enzyme degrades carotenoids and protects against oxidative stress. *FASEB J.* **2011**, *25*, 948–959. [CrossRef] [PubMed]
54. Pang, J.L.; Ricupero, D.A.; Huang, S.; Fatma, N.; Singh, D.P.; Romero, J.R.; Chattopadhyay, N. Differential activity of kaempferol and quercetin in attenuating tumor necrosis factor receptor family signaling in bone cells. *Biochem. Pharmacol.* **2006**, *71*, 818–826. [CrossRef] [PubMed]
55. Bharti, A.C.; Takada, Y.; Aggarwal, B.B. Curcumin (diferuloylmethane) inhibits receptor activator of NF-κB ligand-induced NF-κB activation in osteoclast precursors and suppresses osteoclastogenesis. *J. Immunol.* **2004**, *172*, 5940–5947. [CrossRef] [PubMed]
56. He, X.; Andersson, G.; Lindgren, U.; Li, Y. Resveratrol prevents RANKL-induced osteoclast differentiation of murine osteoclast progenitor RAW 264.7 cells through inhibition of ROS production. *Biochem. Biophys. Res. Commun.* **2010**, *401*, 356–362. [CrossRef]
57. Kim, S.J.; Kang, S.Y.; Shin, H.H.; Choi, H.S. Sulforaphane inhibits osteoclastogenesis by inhibiting nuclear factor-κB. *Mol. Cells* **2005**, *20*, 364–370.
58. Murakami, A.; Song, M.; Ohigashi, H. Phenethyl isothiocyanate suppresses receptor activator of NF-κB ligand (RANKL)-induced osteoclastogenesis by blocking activation of ERK1/2 and p38 MAPK in RAW264.7 macrophages. *BioFactors* **2007**, *30*, 1–11. [CrossRef]
59. Shang, W.; Zhao, L.J.; Dong, X.L.; Zhao, Z.M.; Li, J.; Zhang, B.B.; Cai, H. Curcumin inhibits osteoclastogenic potential in PBMCs from rheumatoid arthritis patients via the suppression of MAPK/RANK/c-Fos/NFATc1 signaling pathways. *Mol. Med. Rep.* **2016**, *14*, 3620–3626. [CrossRef]
60. Calniquer, G.; Khanin, M.; Ovadia, H.; Linnewiel-Hermoni, K.; Stepensky, D.; Trachtenberg, A.; Levy, J.; Sharoni, Y. Combined effects of carotenoids and polyphenols in balancing the response of skin cells to UV irradiation. *Eur. J. Nutr.* **2020**, submitted.

Publisher's Note: MDPI stays neutral with regard to jurisdictional claims in published maps and institutional affiliations.

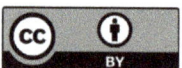

© 2020 by the authors. Licensee MDPI, Basel, Switzerland. This article is an open access article distributed under the terms and conditions of the Creative Commons Attribution (CC BY) license (http://creativecommons.org/licenses/by/4.0/).

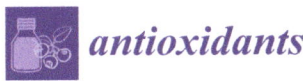

Article

Effects of Food Processing on In Vivo Antioxidant and Hepatoprotective Properties of Green Tea Extracts

Xiao-Yu Xu [1], Jie Zheng [1], Jin-Ming Meng [1], Ren-You Gan [2,3,*], Qian-Qian Mao [1], Ao Shang [1], Bang-Yan Li [1], Xin-Lin Wei [3] and Hua-Bin Li [1,*]

[1] Guangdong Provincial Key Laboratory of Food, Nutrition and Health, Department of Nutrition, School of Public Health, Sun Yat-Sen University, Guangzhou 510080, China; xuxy53@mail2.sysu.edu.cn (X.-Y.X.); zhengj37@mail2.sysu.edu.cn (J.Z.); mengjm@mail2.sysu.edu.cn (J.-M.M.); maoqq@mail2.sysu.edu.cn (Q.-Q.M.); shangao@mail2.sysu.edu.cn (A.S.); liby35@mail2.sysu.edu.cn (B.-Y.L.)
[2] Institute of Urban Agriculture, Chinese Academy of Agricultural Sciences, Chengdu 610213, China
[3] Department of Food Science & Technology, School of Agriculture and Biology, Shanghai Jiao Tong University, Shanghai 200240, China; weixinlin@sjtu.edu.cn
* Correspondence: ganrenyou@caas.cn (R.-Y.G.); lihuabin@mail.sysu.edu.cn (H.-B.L.); Tel.: +86-28-8020-3191 (R.-Y.G.); +86-20-8733-2391 (H.-B.L.)

Received: 24 October 2019; Accepted: 19 November 2019; Published: 21 November 2019

Abstract: Food processing can affect the nutrition and safety of foods. A previous study showed that tannase and ultrasound treatment could significantly increase the antioxidant activities of green tea extracts according to in vitro evaluation methods. Since the results from in vitro and in vivo experiments may be inconsistent, the in vivo antioxidant activities of the extracts were studied using a mouse model of alcohol-induced acute liver injury in this study. Results showed that all the extracts decreased the levels of aspartate transaminase and alanine aminotransferase in serum, reduced the levels of malondialdehyde and triacylglycerol in the liver, and increased the levels of catalase and glutathione in the liver, which can alleviate hepatic oxidative injury. In addition, the differences between treated and original extracts were not significant in vivo. In some cases, the food processing can have a negative effect on in vivo antioxidant activities. That is, although tannase and ultrasound treatment can significantly increase the antioxidant activities of green tea extracts in vitro, it cannot improve the in vivo antioxidant activities, which indicates that some food processing might not always have positive effects on products for human benefits.

Keywords: green tea extract; food processing; tannase; ultrasound; antioxidant activity; liver injury

1. Introduction

The antioxidant properties of food include the capacities of reducing, scavenging radicals, chelating metal ions, inhibiting oxidative enzymes, and activities as antioxidative enzymes [1–6]. Many methods have been developed for the evaluation of in vitro antioxidant activities of natural products, and some of them showed strong antioxidant activities, such as vegetables, fruits, cereals, algae, and tea [7–16].

Oxidative stress can be caused in the human body due to the overproduction of reactive oxygen species (ROS) over the capability of cells to present an effective antioxidant response [17,18]. The oxidative stress results in cellular dysfunction and is involved in various chronic disease initiation and progression, such as diabetes, cancer, neurodegeneration, aging, cardiovascular diseases, and liver diseases [19–21]. Due to strong in vitro antioxidant activities, some natural products have been regarded as effective agents for the prevention and management of several chronic diseases [22–25]. On the other hand, the formation of ROS in vivo can be stimulated due to alcohol metabolism [26,27]. The animal model with acute alcohol administration has been used to investigate the in vivo antioxidant activities of food [28,29], and it often occurs accompanied by liver injury, which can be used for hepatoprotection studies [30]. Hence, we used an animal model with acute alcohol-induced liver injury to evaluate the in vivo antioxidant and hepatoprotective activities of green tea extracts with different processing in this study.

Green tea (*Camellia sinensis* L.) has been reported to show multiple bioactivities with health benefits, such as antioxidant, anti-inflammation, hepatoprotection, cardiovascular protection, neuroprotection, and anti-cancer [31–36]. The epidemiological studies showed that green tea consumption can result in a decreased risk of metabolic syndrome, but there is not enough evidence to draw a strong conclusion regarding tea and non-alcoholic fatty liver [37]. Moreover, accumulating in vivo evidence suggested that green tea showed hepatoprotective effects, which can ameliorate the liver injury induced by alcohol, cholesterol, chemicals, or drugs [38–41]. These benefits are mainly due to the richness of bioactive compounds like polyphenols, polysaccharides, and amino acids [42–45]. The major polyphenols in green tea include catechins and phenolic acids [46]. Catechins are mainly composed of (−)-epicatechin (EC), (−)-epigallocatechin (EGC), (−)-epicatechin gallate (ECG), and (−)-epigallocatechin gallate (EGCG), and phenolic acids include gallic, coumaric, caffeic acids, etc. [47,48]. Furthermore, many findings have demonstrated that the catechins and phenolic acids are responsible for the antioxidant properties of green tea, which has protective effects against many diseases, such as diabetes, cancer, hypertension, and cardiovascular diseases [49–53]. However, there is potential hepatotoxicity induced by the overdose of EGCG [54,55]. Hence, food processing, such as enzymatic treatment, is used to reduce the content of EGCG in green tea extracts to eliminate its negative effects [56].

Numerous types of enzymes are currently used in food processing to meet the demands of a broad variety of food products [57,58]. Additionally, the use of enzymes in foods produces other substances from enzymatic hydrolysis and improves the quality of food products [59–62]. Due to its capacities in catalyzing hydrolysis of gallic acid esters and hydrolysable tannins, tannase (tannin acyl hydrolase EC 3.1.1.20) is widely used in the production of gallic acid [63,64]. On the other hand, ultrasound has been extensively used in food processing, improving the quality and safety of products [62,65,66]. Also, ultrasound creates cavitation and promotes heat and mass transfer, which accelerates chemical reactions, such as enzymatic reactions [67–69]. However, some compounds in products have been changed during food processing, and they might pose negative effects on the quality and health benefits of foods [70]. Most present studies use in vitro methods to evaluate antioxidant properties of food after they are treated with different processing methods. But fewer studies were found about the in vivo antioxidant activities of processed and original products. Our previous study revealed that tannase and ultrasound treatments markedly increase the antioxidant activities of green tea extracts based on the results of in vitro assays. In this study, we aim to investigate the in vivo effects of green tea extracts processed by tannase and ultrasound against oxidative stress and liver injury induced by alcohol.

2. Materials and Methods

2.1. Chemicals and Reagents

Tannase (200 U/g) was bought from Yuanye Biological Technology Co., Ltd. (Shanghai, China). All the other chemicals or reagents were of analytical grade. The kits of aspartate transaminase (AST), alanine aminotransferase (ALT), triglyceride (TG), malondialdehyde (MDA), glutathione (GSH), superoxide dismutase (SOD), catalase (CAT), and total protein were purchased from Nanjing Jiancheng Bioengineering Institute (Nanjing, China). The deionized water was used for all experiments.

2.2. Preparation of Green Tea Extracts

Green tea was purchased from the local market of Guangzhou, China, and was ground into powder which was filtered through a 100 mesh sieve. The deionized water was used to mix with the powder (50 g/L, *w/v*), and then the mixture was heated at 85 °C for 30 min in a water bath and centrifugated at 4200× g for 30 min. The supernatants were collected as the green tea extracts for further experiments.

According to the previous study, the green tea extracts showed the highest antioxidant activities in vitro under the optimal extraction conditions with 0.1 M citrate-phosphate buffer (pH 4.62), ultrasonic temperature of 44.12 °C, ultrasonic time of 12.17 min, tannase concentration of 1 mg/mL, and ultrasonic power of 360 W [71]. The green tea extracts were divided into four groups with different treatments. For the first group, the treatment of ultrasound and tannase (UST) was conducted by mixing the green tea extract with 1 mg/mL tannase in 0.1 M citrate-phosphate buffer (pH 4.62) and using an ultrasonic device (Kejin Ultrasonic Equipment Factory, Guangzhou, China) for 12.17 min at 44.12 °C under 360 W. For the second group, the ultrasound treatment (US) was carried out by mixing the extract with 0.1 M citrate-phosphate buffer (pH 4.62) without tannase and treating with ultrasound for 12.17 min at 44.12 °C under 360 W. For the next group, the only tannase (TAN) treatment was mixed with 1 mg/mL tannase in 0.1 M citrate-phosphate buffer (pH 4.62), and placed in a water bath at 44.12 °C for 12.17 min. The group with the green tea extract (GTE) had a treatment which included the dilution of original extract with the same buffer solution. After the completion of treatment, the mixtures were fully mingled by a vortexing machine. Then they were placed in the water bath at 100 °C for 10 min to inactivate tannase and cooled down to room temperature. The mixture was centrifugated at 4200× g for 10 min, and the supernatant was collected for further experiments.

The extracts from UST, US, TAN, and GTE groups were later dried via the vacuum rotary evaporator. The dried crude extracts were collected and dissolved in deionized water for the animal study.

2.3. Animal Study

Male Kunming mice (20–25 g) were obtained from the Experimental Animal Center of Sun Yat-Sen University, Guangzhou, China. All procedures were strictly carried out according to the principles of "laboratory animal care and use" approved by School of Public Health, Sun Yat-Sen University (No. 2019-002; 28 February 2019). The mice were fed in a specific pathogen free (SPF) animal room under a temperature of 22 ± 0.5 °C, relative humidity of 40–60%, and 12 h light/dark cycle. After the mice had acclimated for one week, they were randomly divided into different groups (6 mice in each group), including control, model, and treatment groups. The treatment groups were fed intragastrically with the solutions of US (50 mg/kg body weight), TAN (50 mg/kg body weight), GTE (50 mg/kg body weight), and UST (50, 100, 200 mg/kg body weight) for 7 days. The model and control groups received the deionized water. On the seventh day, all treatment and model groups were fed intragastrically with 52% alcohol (v/v, 10 mL/kg body weight) 30 min after the last administration, while the control group received the deionized water. After 6 h fasting following the last administration of alcohol, all mice were weighed and anaesthetized to sacrifice. Then the blood samples were collected and centrifuged at 3000× g for 10 min. The serum was isolated for AST and ALT evaluation which followed the instructions of the commercial kits. The liver was harvested and weighed. In order to control potential oxidation of the sample, the low temperature condition was adopted. That is, the 10% (w/v) liver homogenate was prepared by mixing the liver and ice-cold 0.9% normal saline solution in a glass tube that was put in the ice box and the liver was grinded with a glass grinder [29,72,73]. The homogenate of liver was centrifuged at 2500× g for 10 min to obtain the supernatant which was used for the biochemical assays.

2.4. Biochemical Assays

The determination of SOD, CAT, GSH, MDA, TG, and total protein followed the instructions of the Nanjing Jiancheng commercial kits produced by Nanjing Jiancheng Bioengineering Institute, Nanjing, China [29,72–76]. (1) Determination of SOD activity: the xanthine and xanthine oxidase reacted to produce superoxide radicals. The radicals oxidated hydroxylamine to induce nitrite that reacted with a color developing agent to produce a purple-red compound. When the sample contained SOD, it reduced the production of nitrite, which was reflected on a decrease in absorbance. The liver homogenate was diluted by ice-cold saline solution to 0.25% (w/v), and the 50 µL was mixed with reagents. The mixture was placed in room temperature for 10 min. The absorbance was detected at 550 nm using a spectrophotometer. (2) Determination of CAT activity: CAT catalyzed the H_2O_2 decomposition, and the remaining H_2O_2 reacted with ammonium molybdate to produce a light yellow compound. The activity of CAT was calculated based on the change in absorbance. The liver homogenate was diluted by ice-cold saline solution to 0.5% (w/v), and the 50 µL was mixed with reagents. The absorbance of mixture was detected at 405 nm using the microplate reader. (3) Determination of GSH content: The reaction of GSH and 5,5'-dithiobis-(2-nitrobenzoic acid) (DTNB) produced a yellow compound. The GSH content was determined by the colorimetry. The 100 µL liver homogenate (10%, w/v) was mixed with 0.1 mL precipitant, and the mixture was centrifuged at 3500× g for 20 min to obtain the supernatant. The 100 µL supernatant was mixed with reagents, and placed in room temperature for 5 min. The absorbance of mixture was determined at 405 nm using the microplate reader. (4) Determination of MDA content: The reaction of MDA with thiobarbituric acid (TBA) led to a red product that had an absorbance peak at 532 nm. The 100 µL liver homogenate (10%, w/v) was mixed with reagents, and put in a water bath at 95 °C for 40 min. After the mixture was cooled down, it was centrifuged at 4000× g for 10 min. The absorbance of the supernatant was detected at 532 nm using a spectrophotometer. (5) Determination of TG content: TG was hydrolyzed into glycerol and fatty acids by the lipase. The reaction of glycerol and adenosine triphosphate (ATP) was catalyzed by glycerol kinase (GK) and produced glycerol-3-phosphate, which was further oxidized into H_2O_2 and dihydroxyacetone phosphate by glycerophosphate oxidase. H_2O_2 reacted with 4-aminoantipyrine (4-AAP) and p-chlorophenol under the catalysis of peroxidase to produce a red quinone compound, and its color was proportional to the TG content. The 2.5 µL liver homogenate (10%, w/v) was mixed with reagents and placed in the water bath at 37 °C for 10 min. The absorbance of mixture was detected at 510 nm using the microplate reader. (6) Determination of AST activity: AST could act on α-ketoglutaric acid and aspartic acid to produce oxaloacetic acid and glutamic acid. The oxaloacetic acid decarboxylated into pyruvate acid that reacted with 2,4-dinitrophenylhydrazine (DNPH) to produce 2,4-dinitrophenylhydrazone which was a reddish brown compound under alkaline conditions. The 5 µL serum was mixed with the reagents and placed at room temperature for 15 min. The absorbance was detected at 510 nm using a microplate reader. (7) Determination of ALT activity: Under the condition of 37 °C and pH 7.4, ALT acted on alanine and α-ketoglutaric acid to produce pyruvate acid and glutamic acid. After 30 min, DNPH in hydrochloric acid solution was added to form acetone phenylhydrazone that was a reddish brown compound under alkaline conditions. The 5 µL serum was mixed with the reagents and placed at room temperature for 15 min. The absorbance was recorded at 510 nm using the microplate reader. (7) Determination of total protein: The protein reduced Cu^{2+} to Cu^+ under the alkaline conditions, and Cu^+ reacted with the bicinchoninic acid (BCA) reagent to form a purple complex compound that had an absorbance peak at 562 nm. The absorbance was proportional to the concentration of total protein. The liver homogenate was diluted by ice-cold saline solution to 0.5% (w/v), and the 10 µL diluted liver homogenate was mixed with the reagents. The mixture was placed at 37 °C for 30 min and the microplate reader was used to detect the absorbance at 562 nm.

2.5. Statistical Analysis

All experiments were conducted independently three times, and the results were presented as mean ± standard deviation (SD). The statistical analysis was performed by using SPSS 19.0 (IBM SPSS Statistics, IBM Corp, Somers, NY, USA). One-way ANOVA plus a post hoc least-significant difference (LSD) test was utilized to analyze the significance of differences for each group, and the statistical significance was defined at $p < 0.05$.

3. Results and Discussion

3.1. Effects of Extracts on Antioxidant Enzymes, GSH, and MDA in the Liver

The animal experiments were conducted with the model of alcohol-induced liver injury to assess antioxidant activities of the extracts in vivo. The alcohol administration was observed to induce oxidative stress in mice. Compared with the control group, the model group showed an obvious decrease in CAT and SOD activities as well as GSH content, and an increase in MDA content in the mouse liver ($p < 0.05$, Figure 1).

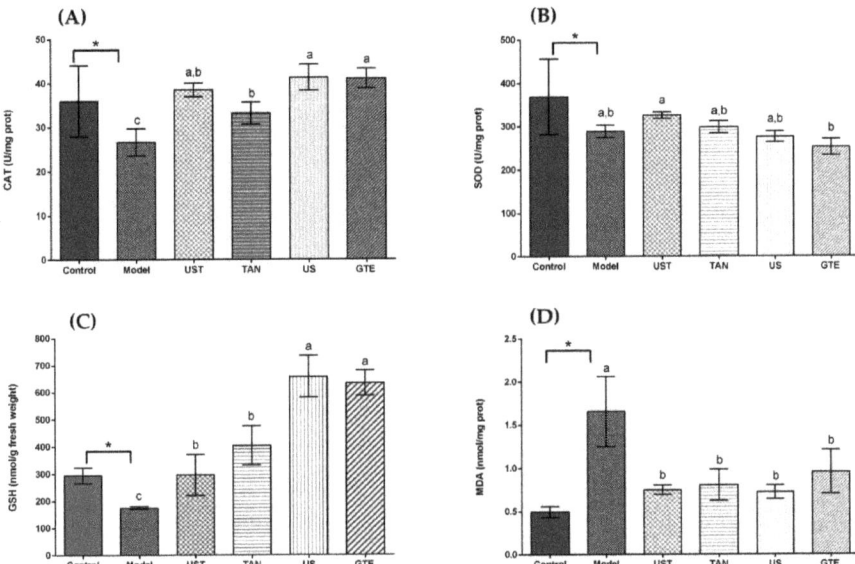

Figure 1. Effects of different extracts on catalase (CAT), superoxide dismutase (SOD), glutathione (GSH), and malondialdehyde (MDA) in the liver. (**A**) CAT, (**B**) SOD, (**C**) GSH, and (**D**) MDA: extracts from different methods (50 mg/kg body weight). One unit of CAT activity is defined as the amount of protein which decomposes 1 μmol H_2O_2 per second. One unit for SOD activity is defined as the amount of protein necessary to inhibit 50% of the SOD reaction where superoxide radicals oxidize hydroxylamine to produce nitrite. UST, the group treated with ultrasound and tannase; TAN, the group treated with only tannase; US, the group treated with only ultrasound; green tea extract (GTE), the group treated without ultrasound and tannase. The values are presented as means ± SD. Bars with different letters (a–c) are significantly different ($p < 0.05$). * $p < 0.05$, the model group vs. the control group.

As displayed in Figure 1A, all treatment groups at the same dose (50 mg/kg body weight) significantly increased the CAT activity in comparison with the model group. In addition, there was no significant difference in CAT activity among the UST, US, and GTE groups. However, the TAN group showed a negative effect on CAT activity compared with the GTE group. This is because tannase might induce the degradation of some related bioactive compounds [71]. Seen from Figure 1B, although the activity of SOD in the UST group was significantly higher than that of the GTE group, all treatment groups did not increase SOD activity compared with the model group. However, treatment with 200 mg/kg body weight could increase SOD activity (Figure 2B). Therefore, the dose of 50 mg/kg body weight was too low to increase the SOD activity. From Figure 1C, all treatment groups improved GSH content significantly when they were compared with the model group. In addition, there was no marked difference in the levels of GSH between the US and GTE groups. However, the UST and

TAN groups showed significantly lower levels of GSH than the GTE groups. These results suggest that tannase treatment might pose negative effects on the in vivo antioxidant activities of green tea extract. As shown in Figure 1D, green tea extracts by different methods reversed the alcohol-induced increase in the level of hepatic MDA, but the differences between groups were not significant. For another thing, the effects of UST at different doses (50, 100, and 200 mg/kg body weight) were shown in Figure 2, and they all increased the activities of CAT and SOD as well as GSH content and lowered the level of MDA. There was no distinct dose-dependent response for the levels of CAT, SOD, and MDA. However, a higher dose showed a stronger effect on GSH content.

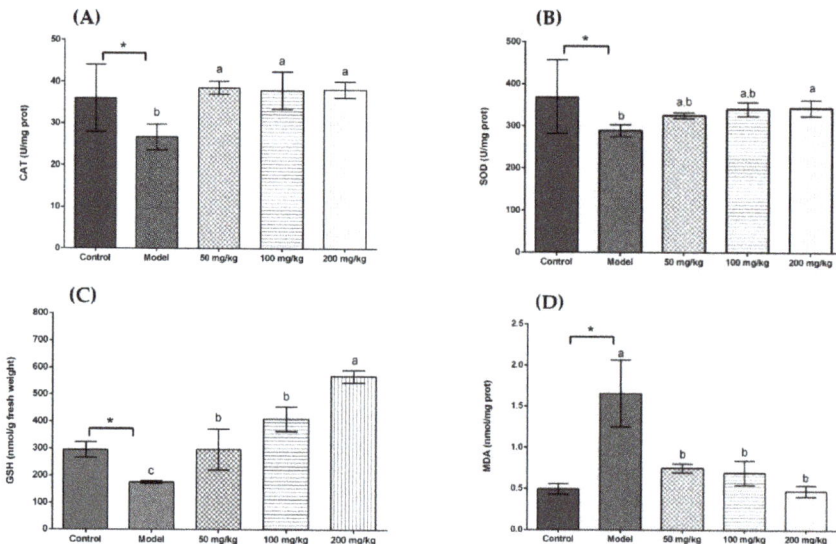

Figure 2. Effects of different doses of UST extracts on CAT, SOD, GSH, and MDA in liver. (**A**) CAT, (**B**) SOD, (**C**) GSH, and (**D**) MDA: UST extract (50, 100, and 200 mg/kg body weight). One unit of CAT activity is defined as the amount of protein which decomposes 1 μmol H_2O_2 per second. One unit for SOD activity is defined as the amount of protein necessary to inhibit 50% of the SOD reaction where superoxide radicals oxidize hydrosylamine to produce nitrite. UST, the group treated with ultrasound and tannase; TAN, the group treated with only tannase; US, the group treated with only ultrasound; GTE, the group treated without ultrasound and tannase. The values are presented as means ± SD. Bars with different letters (a–c) are significantly different ($p < 0.05$). * $p < 0.05$, the model group vs. the control group.

Acute alcohol consumption has been reported to induce oxidative stress and stimulate lipid peroxidation, leading to hepatic dysfunction [77]. It produces free radicals and promotes the development of liver diseases. Thus, the activation of antioxidant enzymes for scavenging free radicals is essential for the protection against alcoholic liver disease. SOD and CAT are important antioxidant enzymes in the defence against oxidative damage. SOD acts on removing superoxide, and CAT catalyses the decomposition of hydrogen peroxide [30]. The contents of GSH are also a crucial indicator reflecting the antioxidant and oxidant status in vivo [78]. MDA is an important product of lipid peroxidation, and its content shows the degree of interaction of ROS with polyunsaturated fatty acid [79].

The present study showed that the administration of extracts increased the levels of CAT, SOD, and GSH, and decreased the contents of MDA in the liver as compared to the model group. However, the differences among groups were not significant in the assays of SOD and MDA. On the other hand, the groups with tannase treatment showed low CAT activity and GSH content, indicating that tannase might degrade some other compounds and affect antioxidant activity negatively in vivo. Overall, the tannase and ultrasound treatment had no significant beneficial effects on the antioxidant enzymes and MDA compared with GTE groups, even posing negative effects on the GSH content.

3.2. Effects of Extracts on AST and ALT in Serum

The activities of serum aspartate transaminase (AST) and alanine transaminase (ALT) were measured to investigate the effects of extracts on liver injury induced by acute alcohol intake. In Figure 3, the serum AST and ALT activities were increased in the model group compared with the control group ($p < 0.05$). All treatment groups significantly decreased the serum AST activities in comparison with the model group, but there was no significance among the treatment groups. On the other hand, all treatment groups non-significantly decreased the serum ALT activities compared with the model group. As shown in Figure 3C,D, the ingestion of UST extracts significantly ameliorated the alcohol-induced increase in AST activities, but the dose-dependent effect was not significant. For the ALT activity, the highest dose of UST extracts decreased significantly the activity of ALT in comparison with the model group.

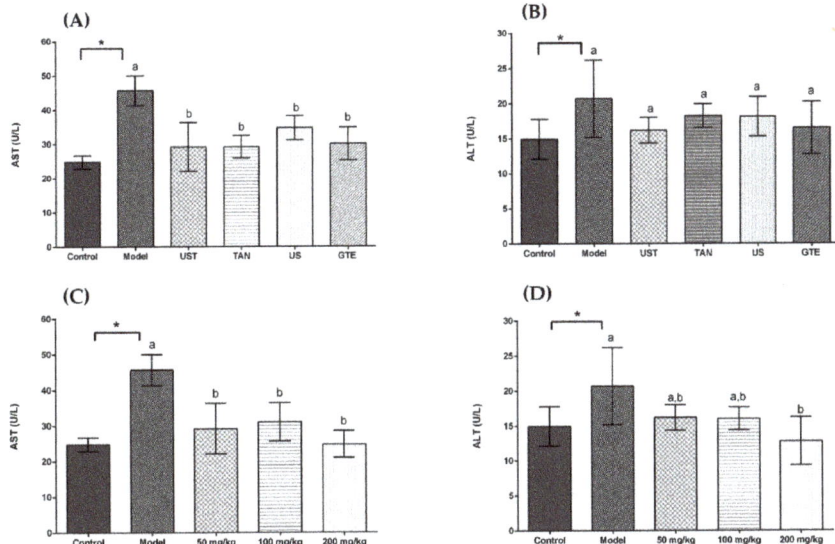

Figure 3. Effects of different extracts on serum aspartate transaminase (AST) and alanine aminotransferase (ALT) activities. (**A**) AST and (**B**) ALT: extracts from different methods (50 mg/kg body weight). (**C**) AST and (**D**) ALT: UST extracts (50, 100, and 200 mg/kg body weight). UST, the group treated with ultrasound and tannase; TAN, the group treated with only tannase; US, the group treated with only ultrasound; GTE, the group treated without ultrasound and tannase. The values are presented as means ± SD. Bars with different letters (a,b) are significantly different ($p < 0.05$). * $p < 0.05$, the model group vs. the control group.

AST and ALT are known as effective markers for liver function. In response to liver damage, AST and ALT are released to plasma from hepatocytes, and the levels of serum AST and ALT are enhanced [80]. In this study, the model groups showed higher serum AST and ALT activities than the control group, which indicated the injury in the liver. The extracts with different methods reduced the serum AST and ALT activities, but the differences among groups were not significant. It indicated that the treatment of ultrasound or tannase contributed little to the reduction in serum ALT and AST activities compared with GTE group. In addition, treatment groups decreased non-significantly the

ALT activity in the comparison with the model group. It might be because the doses of extracts were too small to produce a significant effect. In the dose-dependent experiment, a higher dose of UST extract showed a more potent effect on attenuating the abnormal increase in serum ALT activities (Figure 3D). It suggested that using appropriate doses of extracts obtained from the combined treatment of ultrasound and tannase in green tea could diminish the liver dysfunction induced by alcohol in vivo.

3.3. Effects of Extracts on TG in Liver

Acute alcohol intake resulted in disturbed lipid metabolism with an increase in hepatic TG. Figure 4 displays the effects of extracts on TG level in liver tissue, and a significant elevation in the level of TG was observed in the model group ($p < 0.05$). The administration of extracts from different methods non-significantly decreased the level of TG in liver tissue compared with the model group. In addition, the results showed that high doses of UST extract could lower the hepatic TG significantly compared with the model group in Figure 4B, but the dose-dependent effect was not obvious.

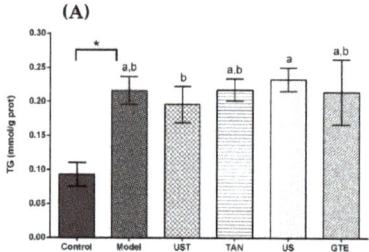
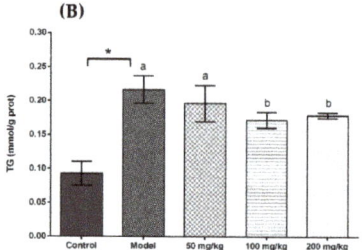

Figure 4. Effects of different extracts on the levels of triglyceride (TG). (**A**) Extracts from different methods (50 mg/kg body weight). (**B**) UST extracts (50, 100, and 200 mg/kg body weight). UST, the group treated with ultrasound and tannase; TAN, the group treated with only tannase; US, the group treated with only ultrasound; GTE, the group treated without ultrasound and tannase. The values are presented as means ± SD. Bars with different letters (a,b) are significantly different ($p < 0.05$). * $p < 0.05$, the model group vs. the control group.

Excessive drinking can lead to lipid production in the liver, and the accumulation of adipose in liver tissue promotes the progress of relevant diseases [81]. The results revealed that the ultrasound and tannase treatment had little effect in reducing lipid accumulation, and there was no significant difference compared with the GTE group. On the other hand, a high dose of UST extracts could significantly reduce the level of TG in the liver. These results indicated that a certain dose of UST extract could be effective in reducing lipids in the liver.

In our previous study, the treated extracts showed stronger in vitro antioxidant activities than the original extracts, and the contents of several compounds were determined using the HPLC method [71]. HPLC results revealed that tannase and ultrasound treatment increased gallic acid content, while the original extract had a higher EGCG content than the treated extracts. It indicated that the in vitro antioxidant activities of UST and TAN were mainly attributed to the content of gallic acid, while the antioxidant properties of US and GTE mainly depended on the contents of EGCG. On the other hand, this study showed that the differences between treated and original extracts were not significant in vivo, and to our surprise, the food processing even posed a negative effect on in vivo antioxidant activities in some cases. Therefore, the results from in vivo and in vitro studies on antioxidant activities were inconsistent, suggesting that some food processing might not always have positive effects on health benefits. This study also indicated that in the future, the effects of food processing on the quality of products should not be evaluated only using in vitro methods, and in vivo evaluation methods should be adopted.

3.4. Histopathological Observation

The histopathological analysis on hematoxylin and eosin (H&E)-stained liver tissue slices further confirmed the protective effects of all treatment groups against acute alcohol liver injury (Figure 5). The model group showed obvious pathologic changes such as disordered cell arrangement and lipid droplets accumulation, while the control group had no significant damage (Figure 5A,B). All treatment groups presented less steatosis than the model group (Figure 5C–F), which indicated that the lesion induced by acute alcohol administration was attenuated by green tea extracts from different treatment methods. In addition, there was no obvious difference among different treatment groups.

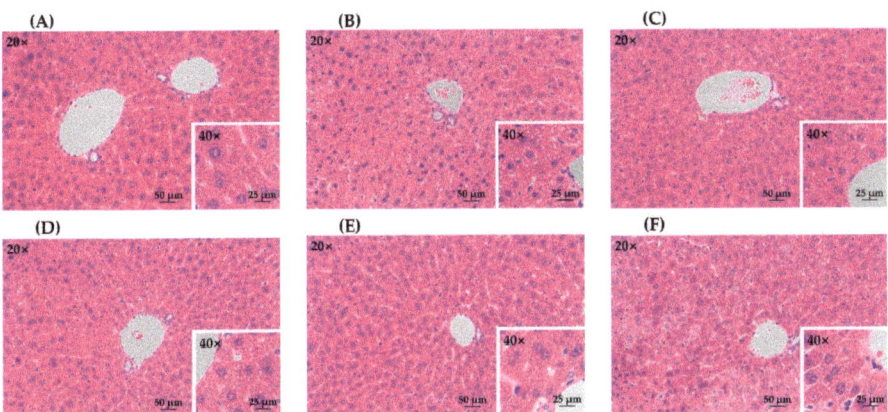

Figure 5. The histopathological observation of hematoxylin and eosin (H&E)-stained liver tissue slices. (**A**) control group; (**B**) model group; (**C**) UST group (50 mg/kg body weight); (**D**) TAN group (50 mg/kg body weight); (**E**) US group (50 mg/kg body weight); (**F**) GTE group (50 mg/kg body weight). UST, the group treated with ultrasound and tannase; TAN, the group treated with only tannase; US, the group treated with only ultrasound; GTE, the group treated without ultrasound and tannase.

4. Conclusions

This study investigated the effects of food processing (tannase and ultrasound treatments) on in vivo antioxidant and hepatoprotective properties of green tea extracts. Results showed that green tea extracts with ultrasound and tannase treatment could attenuate the oxidative stress induced by acute alcohol administration. It increased the activities of antioxidant enzymes, such as SOD and CAT, and the content of antioxidants such as GSH, and reduced the level of MDA. However, there was no significant difference between the treated and original extracts. To our surprise, the tannase treatment even had negative effects on the in vivo antioxidant activities of extracts, which might be related to its degradation of some compounds. In addition, the dose-effect relationship was not significant in green tea extracts with tannase and ultrasound treatment. Thus, it was indicated that the in vitro and in vivo antioxidant activities could be inconsistent, which might be affected by many other factors, such as metabolism and bioavailability. Moreover, the effects of food processing on properties of products should not be evaluated only using in vitro methods, and more in vivo evaluation methods should be carried out. Also, further studies are needed on the necessity of using different food processing methods to produce functional compounds.

Author Contributions: Conceptualization, X.-Y.X., R.-Y.G., and H.-B.L.; data curation, X.-Y.X., and J.-M.M.; formal analysis, X.-Y.X., and J.-M.M.; funding acquisition, X.-Y.X., R.-Y.G., and H.-B.L.; investigation, X.-Y.X., J.-M.M., Q.-Q.M., A.S., and B.-Y.L.; methodology, X.-Y.X., J.Z., Q.-Q.M., A.S., and B.-Y.L.; project administration, H.-B.L.; resources, Q.-Q.M., A.S., and H.-B.L.; software, X.-Y.X., J.-M.M., and A.S.; supervision, R.-Y.G. and H.-B.L.; validation, X.-Y.X., and B.-Y.L.; visualization, X.-Y.X.; writing—original draft, X.-Y.X., and J.Z.; writing—review and editing, J.Z., R.-Y.G., X-.L.W., and H.-B.L.

Funding: This study was supported by the National Key R&D Program of China (No. 2018YFC1604405), the Fundamental Research Funds for the Central Universities (No. 19ykyjs24), the Agri-X Interdisciplinary Fund of Shanghai Jiao Tong University (No. Agri-X2017004), Shanghai Basic and Key Program (No. 18JC1410800), and the Key Project of Guangdong Provincial Science and Technology Program (No. 2014B020205002).

Conflicts of Interest: The authors declare no conflicts of interest.

References

1. Durazzo, A.; Lucarini, M.; Novellino, E.; Daliu, P.; Santini, A. Fruit-based juices: Focus on antioxidant properties—Study approach and update. *Phytother. Res.* **2019**, *33*, 1754–1769. [CrossRef] [PubMed]
2. Apak, R.; Ozyurek, M.; Guclu, K.; Capanoglu, E. Antioxidant Activity/Capacity measurement. 1. Classification, physicochemical principles, mechanisms, and electron transfer (ET)-Based assays. *J. Agric. Food Chem.* **2016**, *64*, 997–1027. [CrossRef] [PubMed]
3. Apak, R.; Ozyurek, M.; Guclu, K.; Capanoglu, E. Antioxidant Activity/Capacity measurement. 2. Hydrogen atom transfer (HAT)-Based, Mixed-Mode (Electron transfer (ET)/HAT), and lipid peroxidation assays. *J. Agric. Food Chem.* **2016**, *64*, 1028–1045. [CrossRef] [PubMed]
4. Apak, R.; Ozyurek, M.; Guclu, K.; Capanoglu, E. Antioxidant Activity/Capacity measurement. 3. Reactive oxygen and nitrogen species (ROS/RNS) scavenging assays, oxidative stress biomarkers, and Chromatographic/Chemometric assays. *J. Agric. Food Chem.* **2016**, *64*, 1046–1070. [CrossRef] [PubMed]
5. Niki, E. Antioxidant capacity of foods for scavenging reactive oxidants and inhibition of plasma lipid oxidation induced by multiple oxidants. *Food Funct.* **2016**, *7*, 2156–2168. [CrossRef] [PubMed]
6. Senevirathne, M.; Kim, S.H.; Siriwardhana, N.; Ha, J.H.; Lee, K.W.; Jeon, Y.J. Antioxidant potential of Ecklonia cava on reactive oxygen species scavenging, metal chelating, reducing power and lipid peroxidation inhibition. *Food Sci. Technol. Int.* **2006**, *12*, 27–38. [CrossRef]
7. Tang, G.Y.; Zhao, C.N.; Xu, X.Y.; Gan, R.Y.; Cao, S.Y.; Liu, Q.; Shang, A.; Mao, Q.Q.; Li, H.B. Phytochemical composition and antioxidant capacity of 30 Chinese teas. *Antioxidants* **2019**, *8*, 180. [CrossRef]
8. Huang, D.J.; Ou, B.X.; Prior, R.L. The chemistry behind antioxidant capacity assays. *J. Agric. Food Chem.* **2005**, *53*, 1841–1856. [CrossRef]
9. Gil, M.I.; Tomas-Barberan, F.A.; Hess-Pierce, B.; Holcroft, D.M.; Kader, A.A. Antioxidant activity of pomegranate juice and its relationship with phenolic composition and processing. *J. Agric. Food Chem.* **2000**, *48*, 4581–4589. [CrossRef]
10. Xu, D.P.; Li, Y.; Meng, X.; Zhou, T.; Zhou, Y.; Zheng, J.; Zhang, J.J.; Li, H.B. Natural antioxidants in foods and medicinal plants: Extraction, assessment and resources. *Int. J. Mol. Sci.* **2017**, *18*, 96. [CrossRef]
11. Li, A.N.; Li, S.; Zhang, Y.J.; Xu, X.R.; Chen, Y.M.; Li, H.B. Resources and biological activities of natural polyphenols. *Nutrients* **2014**, *6*, 6020–6047. [CrossRef] [PubMed]
12. Liu, Q.; Tang, G.; Zhao, C.; Feng, X.; Xu, X.; Cao, S.; Meng, X.; Li, S.; Gan, R.; Li, H. Comparison of antioxidant activities of different grape varieties. *Molecules* **2018**, *23*, 2432. [CrossRef] [PubMed]
13. Deng, G.; Lin, X.; Xu, X.; Gao, L.; Xie, J.; Li, H. Antioxidant capacities and total phenolic contents of 56 vegetables. *J. Funct. Foods* **2013**, *5*, 260–266. [CrossRef]
14. Kumagai, M.; Nishikawa, K.; Matsuura, H.; Umezawa, T.; Matsuda, F.; Okino, T. Antioxidants from the Brown Alga Dictyopteris Undulata. *Molecules* **2018**, *23*, 1214. [CrossRef]
15. Liu, X.; Yuan, W.; Sharma-Shivappa, R.; van Zanten, J. Antioxidant activity of phlorotannins from brown algae. *Int. J. Agric. Biol. Eng.* **2017**, *10*, 184–191. [CrossRef]
16. Zhao, C.N.; Tang, G.Y.; Cao, S.Y.; Xu, X.Y.; Gan, R.Y.; Liu, Q.; Mao, Q.Q.; Shang, A.; Li, H.B. Phenolic profiles and antioxidant activities of 30 tea infusions from green, black, oolong, white, yellow and dark teas. *Antioxidants* **2019**, *8*, 215. [CrossRef]
17. Hensley, K.; Robinson, K.A.; Gabbita, S.P.; Salsman, S.; Floyd, R.A. Reactive oxygen species, cell signaling, and cell injury. *Free Radic. Biol. Med.* **2000**, *28*, 1456–1462. [CrossRef]
18. Ray, P.D.; Huang, B.; Tsuji, Y. Reactive oxygen species (ROS) homeostasis and redox regulation in cellular signaling. *Cell Signal.* **2012**, *24*, 981–990. [CrossRef]

19. Inoguchi, T.; Li, P.; Umeda, F.; Yu, H.Y.; Kakimoto, M.; Imamura, M.; Aoki, T.; Etoh, T.; Hashimoto, T.; Naruse, M.; et al. High glucose level and free fatty acid stimulate reactive oxygen species production through protein kinase C-dependent activation of NAD(P)H oxidase in cultured vascular cells. *Diabetes* **2000**, *49*, 1939–1945. [CrossRef]
20. Zhang, Y.J.; Gan, R.Y.; Li, S.; Zhou, Y.; Li, A.N.; Xu, D.P.; Li, H.B. Antioxidant phytochemicals for the prevention and treatment of chronic diseases. *Molecules* **2015**, *20*, 21138–21156. [CrossRef]
21. Li, S.; Tan, H.; Wang, N.; Zhang, Z.; Lao, L.; Wong, C.; Feng, Y. The role of oxidative stress and antioxidants in liver diseases. *Int. J. Mol. Sci.* **2015**, *16*, 26087–26124. [CrossRef] [PubMed]
22. Leonard, S.S.; Xia, C.; Jiang, B.H.; Stinefelt, B.; Klandorf, H.; Harris, G.K.; Shi, X.L. Resveratrol scavenges reactive oxygen species and effects radical-induced cellular responses. *Biochem. Biophys. Res. Commun.* **2003**, *309*, 1017–1026. [CrossRef] [PubMed]
23. Paran, E.; Novack, V.; Engelhard, Y.N.; Hazan-Halevy, I. The effects of natural antioxidants from tomato extract in treated but uncontrolled hypertensive patients. *Cardiovasc. Drugs Ther.* **2009**, *23*, 145–151. [CrossRef]
24. Shang, A.; Cao, S.; Xu, X.; Gan, R.; Tang, G.; Corke, H.; Mavumengwana, V.; Li, H. Bioactive compounds and biological functions of garlic (*Allium sativum* L.). *Foods* **2019**, *8*, 246. [CrossRef] [PubMed]
25. Ishige, K.; Schubert, D.; Sagara, Y. Flavonoids protect neuronal cells from oxidative stress by three distinct mechanisms. *Free Radic. Biol. Med.* **2001**, *30*, 433–446. [CrossRef]
26. Yan, S.; Yang, H.; Lee, H.; Yin, M. Protective effects of maslinic acid against alcohol-induced acute liver injury in mice. *Food Chem. Toxicol.* **2014**, *74*, 149–155. [CrossRef]
27. Purohit, V.; Brenner, D.A. Mechanisms of alcohol-induced hepatic fibrosis: A summary of the Ron Thurman Symposium. *Hepatology* **2006**, *43*, 872–878. [CrossRef]
28. Zhao, J.; Chen, H.; Li, Y. Protective effect of bicyclol on acute alcohol-induced liver injury in mice. *Eur. J. Pharmacol.* **2008**, *586*, 322–331. [CrossRef]
29. Zhao, C.N.; Tang, G.Y.; Liu, Q.; Xu, X.Y.; Cao, S.Y.; Gan, R.Y.; Zhang, K.Y.; Meng, S.L.; Li, H.B. Five-Golden-Flowers tea: Green extraction and hepatoprotective effect against oxidative damage. *Molecules* **2018**, *23*, 2216. [CrossRef]
30. Zhao, H.; Li, H.; Lai, Q.; Yang, Q.; Dong, Y.; Liu, X.; Wang, W.; Zhang, J.; Jia, L. Antioxidant and hepatoprotective activities of modified polysaccharides from *Coprinus comatus* in mice with alcohol-induced liver injury. *Int. J. Biol. Macromol.* **2019**, *127*, 476–485. [CrossRef]
31. Xu, X.Y.; Zhao, C.N.; Cao, S.Y.; Tang, G.Y.; Gan, R.Y.; Li, H.B. Effects and mechanisms of tea for the prevention and management of cancers: An updated review. *Crit. Rev. Food Sci. Nutr.* **2019**. [CrossRef] [PubMed]
32. Gan, R.Y.; Li, H.B.; Sui, Z.Q.; Corke, H. Absorption, metabolism, anti-cancer effect and molecular targets of epigallocatechin gallate (EGCG): An updated review. *Crit. Rev. Food Sci. Nutr.* **2018**, *58*, 924–941. [CrossRef] [PubMed]
33. Cao, S.Y.; Zhao, C.N.; Gan, R.Y.; Xu, X.Y.; Wei, X.L.; Corke, H.; Atanasov, A.G.; Li, H.B. Effects and mechanisms of tea and its bioactive compounds for the prevention and treatment of cardiovascular diseases: An updated review. *Antioxidants* **2019**, *8*, 166. [CrossRef] [PubMed]
34. Park, H.J.; Lee, J.; Chung, M.; Park, Y.; Bower, A.M.; Koo, S.I.; Giardina, C.; Bruno, R.S. Green tea extract suppresses NF-kappa B activation and inflammatory responses in diet-induced obese rats with nonalcoholic steatohepatitis. *J. Nutr.* **2012**, *142*, 57–63. [CrossRef]
35. Levites, Y.; Weinreb, O.; Maor, G.; Youdim, M.; Mandel, S. Green tea polyphenol-epigallocatechin-3-gallate prevents N-methyl-4-phenyl-1,2,3,6-tetrahydropyridine-induced dopaminergic neurodegeneration. *J. Neurochem.* **2001**, *78*, 1073–1082. [CrossRef]
36. Aktas, O.; Prozorovski, T.; Smorodchenko, A.; Savaskan, N.E.; Lauster, R.; Kloetzel, P.M.; Infante-Duarte, C.; Brocke, S.; Zipp, F. Green tea epigallocatechin-3-gallate mediates T cellular NF-kappa B inhibition and exerts neuroprotection in autoimmune encephalomyelitis. *J. Immunol.* **2004**, *173*, 5794–5800. [CrossRef]
37. Marventano, S.; Salomone, F.; Godos, J.; Pluchinotta, F.; Del Rio, D.; Mistretta, A.; Grosso, G. Coffee and tea consumption in relation with non-alcoholic fatty liver and metabolic syndrome: A systematic review and meta-analysis of observational studies. *Clin. Nutr.* **2016**, *35*, 1269–1281. [CrossRef]
38. Wang, D.; Gao, Q.; Wang, T.; Zhao, G.; Qian, F.; Huang, J.; Wang, H.; Zhang, X.; Wang, Y. Green tea infusion protects against alcoholic liver injury by attenuating inflammation and regulating the PI3K/Akt/eNOS pathway in C57BL/6 mice. *Food Funct.* **2017**, *8*, 3165–3177. [CrossRef]

39. Hirsch, N.; Konstantinov, A.; Anavi, S.; Aronis, A.; Hagay, Z.; Madar, Z.; Tirosh, O. Prolonged feeding with green tea polyphenols exacerbates cholesterol-induced fatty liver disease in mice. *Mol. Nutr. Food Res.* **2016**, *60*, 2542–2553. [CrossRef]
40. Qin, G.Z.; Ning, Y.Y.; Lotlikar, P.D. Chemoprevention of aflatoxin B-1-initiated and carbon tetrachloride-promoted hepatocarcinogenesis in the rat by green tea. *Nutr. Cancer* **2000**, *38*, 215–222. [CrossRef]
41. Lu, Y.; Sun, J.; Petrova, K.; Yang, X.; Greenhaw, J.; Salminen, W.F.; Beger, R.D.; Schnackenberg, L.K. Metabolomics evaluation of the effects of green tea extract on acetaminophen-induced hepatotoxicity in mice. *Food Chem. Toxicol.* **2013**, *62*, 707–721. [CrossRef] [PubMed]
42. Del Rio, D.; Stewart, A.J.; Mullen, W.; Burns, J.; Lean, M.; Brighenti, F.; Crozier, A. HPLC-MSn analysis of phenolic compounds and purine alkaloids in green and black tea. *J. Agric. Food Chem.* **2004**, *52*, 2807–2815. [CrossRef] [PubMed]
43. Xiao, J.B.; Huo, J.L.; Jiang, H.X.; Yang, F. Chemical compositions and bioactivities of crude polysaccharides from tea leaves beyond their useful date. *Int. J. Biol. Macromol.* **2011**, *49*, 1143–1151. [CrossRef] [PubMed]
44. Kim, T.I.; Lee, Y.K.; Park, S.G.; Choi, I.S.; Ban, J.O.; Park, H.K.; Nam, S.Y.; Yun, Y.W.; Han, S.B.; Oh, K.W.; et al. L-Theanine, an amino acid in green tea, attenuates beta-amyloid-induced cognitive dysfunction and neurotoxicity: Reduction in oxidative damage and inactivation of ERK/p38 kinase and NF-kappa B pathways. *Free Radic. Bio. Med.* **2009**, *47*, 1601–1610. [CrossRef]
45. Higdon, J.V.; Frei, B. Tea catechins and polyphenols: Health effects, metabolism, and antioxidant functions. *Crit. Rev. Food Sci. Nutr.* **2003**, *43*, 89–143. [CrossRef]
46. Rusak, G.; Komes, D.; Likic, S.; Horzic, D.; Kovac, M. Phenolic content and antioxidative capacity of green and white tea extracts depending on extraction conditions and the solvent used. *Food Chem.* **2008**, *110*, 852–858. [CrossRef]
47. Zhao, Y.; Chen, P.; Lin, L.; Harnly, J.M.; Yu, L.L.; Li, Z. Tentative identification, quantitation, and principal component analysis of green pu-erh, green, and white teas using UPLC/DAD/MS. *Food Chem.* **2011**, *126*, 1269–1277. [CrossRef]
48. Galati, G.; Lin, A.; Sultan, A.M.; O'Brien, P.J. Cellular and in vivo hepatotoxicity caused by green tea phenolic acids and catechins. *Free Radic. Bio. Med.* **2006**, *40*, 570–580. [CrossRef]
49. Xu, H.; Luo, J.; Huang, J.; Wen, Q. Flavonoids intake and risk of type 2 diabetes mellitus: A meta-analysis of prospective cohort studies. *Medicine* **2018**, *97*, e0686. [CrossRef]
50. Godos, J.; Vitale, M.; Micek, A.; Ray, S.; Martini, D.; Del Rio, D.; Riccardi, G.; Galvano, F.; Grosso, G. Dietary polyphenol intake, blood pressure, and hypertension: A systematic review and Meta-Analysis of observational studies. *Antioxidants* **2019**, *8*, 152. [CrossRef]
51. Wang, X.; Ouyang, Y.Y.; Liu, J.; Zhao, G. Flavonoid intake and risk of CVD: A systematic review and meta-analysis of prospective cohort studies. *Br. J. Nutr.* **2014**, *111*, 1–11. [CrossRef] [PubMed]
52. Grosso, G.; Godos, J.; Lamuela-Raventos, R.; Ray, S.; Micek, A.; Pajak, A.; Sciacca, S.; D'Orazio, N.; Del Rio, D.; Galvano, F. A comprehensive meta-analysis on dietary flavonoid and lignan intake and cancer risk: Level of evidence and limitations. *Mol. Nutr. Food Res.* **2017**, *61*. [CrossRef] [PubMed]
53. Panza, V.P.; Brunetta, H.S.; de Oliveira, M.V.; Nunes, E.A.; Da Silva, E.L. Effect of mate tea (Ilex paraguariensis) on the expression of the leukocyte NADPH oxidase subunit p47(phox) and on circulating inflammatory cytokines in healthy men: A pilot study. *Int. J. Food Sci. Nutr.* **2019**, *70*, 212–221. [CrossRef] [PubMed]
54. Isomura, T.; Suzuki, S.; Origasa, H.; Hosono, A.; Suzuki, M.; Sawada, T.; Terao, S.; Muto, Y.; Koga, T. Liver-related safety assessment of green tea extracts in humans: A systematic review of randomized controlled trials. *Eur. J. Clin. Nutr.* **2016**, *70*, 1221–1229. [CrossRef]
55. Hu, J.; Webster, D.; Cao, J.; Shao, A. The safety of green tea and green tea extract consumption in adults - Results of a systematic review. *Regul. Toxicol. Pharmacol.* **2018**, *95*, 412–433. [CrossRef]
56. Baik, J.H.; Shin, K.S.; Park, Y.; Yu, K.W.; Suh, H.J.; Choi, H.S. Biotransformation of catechin and extraction of active polysaccharide from green tea leaves via simultaneous treatment with tannase and pectinase. *J. Sci. Food Agric.* **2015**, *95*, 2337–2344. [CrossRef]
57. Olempska-Beer, Z.S.; Merker, R.I.; Ditto, M.D.; DiNovi, M.J. Food-processing enzymes from recombinant microorganisms—A review. *Regul. Toxicol. Pharmacol.* **2006**, *45*, 144–158. [CrossRef]
58. DiCosimo, R.; McAuliffe, J.; Poulose, A.J.; Bohlmann, G. Industrial use of immobilized enzymes. *Chem. Soc. Rev.* **2013**, *42*, 6437–6474. [CrossRef]

59. Toushik, S.H.; Lee, K.T.; Lee, J.S.; Kim, K.S. Functional applications of lignocellulolytic enzymes in the fruit and vegetable processing industries. *J. Food Sci.* **2017**, *82*, 585–593. [CrossRef]
60. Rai, P.; Majumdar, G.C.; Dasgupta, S.; De, S. Optimizing pectinase usage in pretreatment of mosambi juice for clarification by response surface methodology. *J. Food Eng.* **2004**, *64*, 397–403. [CrossRef]
61. Pinelo, M.; Zeuner, B.; Meyer, A.S. Juice clarification by protease and pectinase treatments indicates new roles of pectin and protein in cherry juice turbidity. *Food Bioprod. Process.* **2010**, *88*, 259–265. [CrossRef]
62. Knorr, D.; Zenker, M.; Heinz, V.; Lee, D.U. Applications and ultrasonics in food potential of processing. *Trends Food Sci. Technol.* **2004**, *15*, 261–266. [CrossRef]
63. Mahapatra, K.; Nanda, R.K.; Bag, S.S.; Banerjee, R.; Pandey, A.; Szakacs, G. Purification, characterization and some studies on secondary structure of tannase from *Aspergillus awamori* nakazawa. *Process. Biochem.* **2005**, *40*, 3251–3254. [CrossRef]
64. Belmares, R.; Contreras-Esquivel, J.C.; Rodriguez-Herrera, R.; Coronel, A.R.; Aguilar, C.N. Microbial production of tannase: An enzyme with potential use in food industry. *LWT-Food Sci. Technol.* **2004**, *37*, 857–864. [CrossRef]
65. Khan, M.K.; Abert-Vian, M.; Fabiano-Tixier, A.; Dangles, O.; Chemat, F. Ultrasound-assisted extraction of polyphenols (flavanone glycosides) from orange (*Citrus sinensis* L.) peel. *Food Chem.* **2010**, *119*, 851–858. [CrossRef]
66. Chemat, F.; Rombaut, N.; Sicaire, A.; Meullemiestre, A.; Fabiano-Tixier, A.; Abert-Vian, M. Ultrasound assisted extraction of food and natural products. Mechanisms, techniques, combinations, protocols and applications. A review. *Ultrason. Sonochem.* **2017**, *34*, 540–560. [CrossRef] [PubMed]
67. Soria, A.C.; Villamiel, M. Effect of ultrasound on the technological properties and bioactivity of food: A review. *Trends Food Sci. Technol.* **2010**, *21*, 323–331. [CrossRef]
68. Awad, T.S.; Moharram, H.A.; Shaltout, O.E.; Asker, D.; Youssef, M.M. Applications of ultrasound in analysis, processing and quality control of food: A review. *Food Res. Int.* **2012**, *48*, 410–427. [CrossRef]
69. Soares, A.D.S.; Duarte Augusto, P.E.; de Castro Leite Junior, B.R.; Nogueira, C.A.; Rufino Vieira, E.N.; De Barros, F.A.R.; Stringheta, P.C.; Ramos, A.M. Ultrasound assisted enzymatic hydrolysis of sucrose catalyzed by invertase: Investigation on substrate, enzyme and kinetics parameters. *LWT-Food Sci. Technol.* **2019**, *107*, 164–170. [CrossRef]
70. Pingret, D.; Durand, G.; Fabiano-Tixier, A.; Rockenbauer, A.; Ginies, C.; Chemat, F. Degradation of edible oil during food processing by ultrasound: Electron paramagnetic resonance, physicochemical, and sensory appreciation. *J. Agric. Food Chem.* **2012**, *60*, 7761–7768. [CrossRef]
71. Xu, X.Y.; Meng, J.M.; Mao, Q.Q.; Shang, A.; Li, B.Y.; Zhao, C.N.; Tang, G.Y.; Cao, S.Y.; Wei, X.L.; Gan, R.Y.; et al. Effects of tannase and ultrasound treatment on the bioactive compounds and antioxidant activity of green tea extract. *Antioxidants* **2019**, *8*, 362. [CrossRef] [PubMed]
72. Wang, F.; Zhang, Y.J.; Zhou, Y.; Li, Y.; Zhou, T.; Zheng, J.; Zhang, J.J.; Li, S.; Xu, D.P.; Li, H.B. Effects of beverages on alcohol metabolism: Potential health benefits and harmful impacts. *Int. J. Mol. Sci.* **2016**, *17*, 354. [CrossRef] [PubMed]
73. Zhang, Y.J.; Wang, F.; Zhou, Y.; Li, Y.; Zhou, T.; Zheng, J.; Zhang, J.J.; Li, S.; Xu, D.P.; Li, H.B. Effects of 20 selected fruits on ethanol metabolism: Potential health benefits and harmful impacts. *Int. J. Environ. Res. Public Health* **2016**, *13*, 399. [CrossRef] [PubMed]
74. Hou, Z.; Qin, P.; Ren, G. Effect of anthocyanin-rich extract from black rice (*Oryza sativa* L. Japonica) on chronically alcohol-induced liver damage in rats. *J. Agric. Food Chem.* **2010**, *58*, 3191–3196. [CrossRef]
75. Zhang, J.; Xue, J.; Wang, H.; Zhang, Y.; Xie, M. Osthole improves Alcohol-Induced fatty liver in mice by reduction of hepatic oxidative stress. *Phytother. Res.* **2011**, *25*, 638–643. [CrossRef]
76. Zhang, S.; Zheng, L.; Dong, D.; Xu, L.; Yin, L.; Qi, Y.; Han, X.; Lin, Y.; Liu, K.; Peng, J. Effects of flavonoids from *Rosa laevigata* Michx fruit against high-fat diet-induced non-alcoholic fatty liver disease in rats. *Food Chem.* **2013**, *141*, 2108–2116. [CrossRef]
77. Kolankaya, D.; Selmanoglu, G.; Sorkun, K.; Salih, B. Protective effects of Turkish propolis on alcohol-induced serum lipid changes and liver injury in male rats. *Food Chem.* **2002**, *78*, 213–217. [CrossRef]
78. Zhao, L.; Jiang, Y.; Ni, Y.X.; Zhang, T.Z.; Duan, C.C.; Huang, C.; Zhao, Y.J.; Gao, L.; Li, S.Y. Protective effects of *Lactobacillus plantarum* C88 on chronic ethanol-induced liver injury in mice. *J. Funct. Foods* **2017**, *35*, 97–104. [CrossRef]

79. Xiao, C.Q.; Zhou, F.B.; Zhao, M.M.; Su, G.W.; Sun, B.G. Chicken breast muscle hydrolysates ameliorate acute alcohol-induced liver injury in mice through alcohol dehydrogenase (ADH) activation and oxidative stress reduction. *Food Funct.* **2018**, *9*, 774–784. [CrossRef]
80. Lu, Y.H.; Tian, C.R.; Gao, C.Y.; Wang, W.J.; Yang, W.Y.; Kong, X.; Chen, Y.X.; Liu, Z.Z. Protective effect of free phenolics from Lycopus lucidus Turcz. root on carbon tetrachloride-induced liver injury in vivo and in vitro. *Food Nutr. Res.* **2018**, *62*. [CrossRef]
81. Ajmo, J.M.; Liang, X.M.; Rogers, C.Q.; Pennock, B.; You, M. Resveratrol alleviates alcoholic fatty liver in mice. *Am. J. Physiol.-Gastroint. Liver Physiol.* **2008**, *295*, G833–G842. [CrossRef] [PubMed]

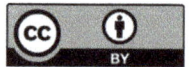

© 2019 by the authors. Licensee MDPI, Basel, Switzerland. This article is an open access article distributed under the terms and conditions of the Creative Commons Attribution (CC BY) license (http://creativecommons.org/licenses/by/4.0/).

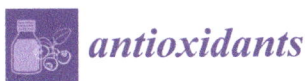

Article

Narrow-Leafed Lupin (*Lupinus angustifolius* L.) Seeds Gamma-Conglutin is an Anti-Inflammatory Protein Promoting Insulin Resistance Improvement and Oxidative Stress Amelioration in PANC-1 Pancreatic Cell-Line

Elena Lima-Cabello [1], Juan D. Alché [1], Sonia Morales-Santana [2], Alfonso Clemente [3] and Jose C. Jimenez-Lopez [1,4,*]

1. Department of Biochemistry, Cell & Molecular Biology of Plants, Estación Experimental del Zaidín, Spanish National Research Council (CSIC), Profesor Albareda 1, Granada E-18008, Spain; elena.lima@eez.csic.es (E.L.-C.); juandedios.alche@eez.csic.es (J.D.A.)
2. Proteomic Research Department, San Cecilio University Hospital, Biosanitary Research Institute of Granada (Ibs.GRANADA), Av. Dr. Olóriz 16, Granada E-18012, Spain; soniamoralessantana@hotmail.com
3. Department of Physiology and Biochemistry of Animal Nutrition, Estación Experimental del Zaidín, Spanish National Research Council (CSIC), Camino del Jueves, Granada E-18100, Spain; alfonso.clemente@eez.csic.es
4. The UWA Institute of Agriculture and School of Agriculture and Environment, The University of Western Australia, CRAWLEY Perth, WA 6019, Australia
* Correspondence: josecarlos.jimenez@eez.csic.es

Received: 3 November 2019; Accepted: 19 December 2019; Published: 23 December 2019

Abstract: (1) Background: Inflammation molecular cues and insulin resistance development are some of the main contributors for the development and advance of the pathogenesis of inflammatory-related diseases; (2) Methods: We isolated and purified γ-conglutin protein from narrow-leafed lupin (NLL or blue lupin) mature seeds using affinity-chromatography to evaluate its anti-inflammatory activities at molecular level using both, a bacterial lipopolysaccharide (LPS)-induced inflammation and an insulin resistance pancreatic cell models; (3) Results: NLL γ-conglutin achieved a plethora of functional effects as the strong reduction of cell oxidative stress induced by inflammation through decreasing proteins carbonylation, nitric oxide synthesis and inducible nitric oxide synthase (iNOS) transcriptional levels, and raising glutathione (GSH) levels and modulation of superoxide dismutase (SOD) and catalase enzymes activities. γ-conglutin induced up-regulated transcriptomic and protein levels of insulin signalling pathway IRS-1, Glut-4, and PI3K, improving glucose uptake, while decreasing pro-inflammatory mediators as iNOs, TNFα, IL-1β, INFγ, IL-6, IL-12, IL-17, and IL-27; (4) Conclusion: These results suggest a promising use of NLL γ-conglutin protein in functional foods, which could also be implemented in alternative diagnosis and therapeutic molecular tools helping to prevent and treat inflammatory-related diseases.

Keywords: 7S basic globulins; anti-inflammatory protein; antioxidant protein; cytokines; glutathione; iNOS; nitric oxide; oxidative stress; sweet lupins group

1. Introduction

The outcomes from epidemiological studies have revealed that an increasing number of health problems are affecting all societies around the globe as diabetes, insulin resistance, obesity, metabolic syndrome and cardiovascular diseases [1], where they have been associated to both scarce physical activity and the ingestion of high sugar–high lipid diets in metropolitan areas [2]. In this regard, there is an increasing demand of plant proteins highly beneficial for human health to be used for foodstuffs development and production and has prompted an increasing body of research covering diverse nutraceutical aspects in a number of crop plants. There is a strong interest focused in legumes, which are an economical important source of high-quality proteins compared to other plant foods [3].

Interestingly, lupin seeds, and particularly seeds from the species encompassing the "sweet lupin" group have been reported to exert beneficial effects in human health [4]. Thus, the dietary consumption of lupin seed proteins might provide preventive and protective effects (also complementing the current treatments for metabolic diseases) for different human inflammatory-related diseases such as metabolic syndrome, obesity, and high blood pressure (lowering capacity), type 2 diabetes mellitus (T2DM) development and triggered by uncontrolled glycemia throughout increasing insulin resistance, familial hypercholesterolemia and cardiovascular disease [5]. Different factors or stressors promote and stimulate immune-response-mediated inflammation leading to the molecular mechanisms underlying many of these diseases including defective insulin secretion and responses, and finally to the insulin resistance which has the pancreatic tissue as the key target for this disease evolution, progressing with an uncontrolled synthesis of pro-inflammatory mediators. Among them, interleukin 6 (IL-6), interleukin 1 (IL-1), interferon gamma (INFγ), tumor necrosis factor (TNF-α), chemokines (i.e., CCL2, CCL5), reactive oxygen species (ROS) as H_2O_2, peroxide and superoxide anion, nitric oxide (NO) overproduction, and nitrogen intermediate molecules, as well as adhesion molecules release (i.e., ICAM-1, VCAM-1) facilitating immune system cells attraction and movement through the tissues enhancing the inflammatory response [6]. The most frequently associated stressors are oxidative stress, alterations in gut microbiota that increase lipopolysaccharides (LPS) in blood, lipotoxicity, glucotoxicity and endoplasmic reticulum (ER) stress promoting misfolded proteins that may be deposited in the islets β-cells in form of amyloids [6]; these amyloid deposits enhance inflammatory response mediated by immune cells attracted to the pancreatic tissues [7].

Thus, lowering the synthesis and/or functional role of pro-inflammatory molecules has the advance of potentiate an anti-inflammatory reaction that may also help to the inflammatory-related diseases amelioration.

Searching for naturally-occurring compounds with the potential of anti-inflammatory responses has also increased parallel to the risen number of inflammation-related diseases. Only a few studies have described the anti-inflammatory properties of some seeds-derived bioactive hydrolysates of proteins; however, even more scarce are the studies concerning legume seed compounds with these potential functional activities. Interestingly, enzymatic hydrolysates of field pea seeds showed anti-inflammatory properties at molecular level by inhibiting several inflammation mediators' production, i.e., NO and TNFα [8]. Lunasin, a peptide derived of isolated 2S albumin that was found in soybean, as well in some cereal grains displayed great benefits related to cancer amelioration, cardiovascular disease improvement and lowering cholesterol [9]. In soybean, the anti-inflammatory properties of lunasin have been associated to its ability to suppress the NFκB functional pathway [10]. Seed protein hydrolysates from blue lupin were found to have the potential to inhibit phospholipase A2 and cyclooxygenase-2 enzymes that are involved in the inflammatory pathway [11]. Another further study showed the example of bioactive peptides with high homology with *Arabidopsis thaliana* 2S albumin and *Glycine max* lectin-like protein, which were associated with genes expression modulation of inflammatory molecules [12].

In this work, we have studied the anti-inflammatory properties of narrow-leafed lupin (NLL) γ-conglutin protein from mature seeds using in vitro human PANC-1 pancreatic cell-line in both, an induced inflammation model using bacteria lipopolysaccharide (LPS), and an induced insulin resistance (IR) cell model, with the aim of assessing the capability of NLL γ-conglutin to improve the oxidative stress homeostasis of cells, the inflammatory induced state and the IR improvement at molecular level by decreasing several pro-inflammatory mediators genes expression and proteins levels, as well as up-regulating of insulin signaling pathway gene expression.

2. Material and Methods

2.1. Isolation and Purification of γ-Conglutin from NLL Mature Seeds

The isolation and purification of γ-conglutin proteins from NLL was accomplished following the Czubiński et al. [13] method. Briefly, NLL seed proteins were extracted using Tris buffer pH 7.5 [20 mmol L^{-1}], having 0.5 mol L^{-1} NaCl/gr defatted seeds. After sample centrifugation at 20,000× g, 30 min at 4 °C, the supernatant was filtered using a 0.45 μm syringe filter of PVDF. Thus, the sample was ready to be introduced in a desalting column of Sephadex G-25 medium. The desalted crude protein sample was applied to a HiTrap Q HP column (GE Healthcare) previously equilibrated with Tris buffer pH 7.5 [20 mmol L^{-1}], where the proteins' separation was possible using a linear gradient [0 to 1 mol L^{-1}] of NaCl. Under these conditions, the γ-conglutin proteins were not retained on the media contained in the column. Thus, different fractions that contained γ-conglutin proteins were pooled and introduced on HiTrap SP HP column (GE Healthcare) previously equilibrated with Tris buffer pH 7.5 [20 mmol L^{-1}]. γ-conglutin proteins retained in this column were eluted with a linear gradient of NaCl [0 to 0.5 mol L^{-1}]. The γ-conglutin proteins were collected and directly used in the further SDS-PAGE analysis and fingerprinting characterization. The remaining protein was kept frozen at −80 °C.

2.2. Analysis of Purified γ-Conglutin Protein by Peptide Mass Fingerprinting

The identity proof of the purified γ-conglutin protein was achieved following peptide mass fingerprinting. Briefly, proteins (10 μg) were separated by SDS-PAGE using precast gels of 12% Bis-Tris (Invitrogen) under reduced conditions. Electrophoretic bands corresponding to γ-conglutin protein (bands 1 to 4, Supplementary Figure S1), were cut out from the gel and in-gel trypsin digested. These peptide fragments generated were subjected to desalt and concentration, to be afterward loaded onto the MALDI plate and analyzed. MALDI-MS spectra were generated in a 4700 Proteomics Analyzer (Applied Biosystems, Waltham, MA, USA), and these data were used for proteins ID validation (www.matrixscience.com).

2.3. SDS-PAGE and Immunoblotting

Analysis of protein extracts were made by mixing the samples sample buffer (6× concentrated) and heated during 5 min up to 95 °C. Proteins were separated by SDS-PAGE using gradient TGX gels of 4–20% acrylamide (Bio-Rad). To identify the molecular weight (MW) of separated proteins we used a MW marker for stained gels as Mark12 Unstained Standard (ThermoFisher Scientific), with a MW range between 2.5 to 200 kDa. The resolved protein bands were visualized in a Gel Doc™ EZ Imager (Bio-Rad, Berkeley, CA, USA). For immunoblotting, proteins were transferred to PVDF membranes, which afterward were blocked for 2 h at room temperature (RT) using 5% of non-fat dry milk dissolved in PBST (phosphate-buffered saline, 0.05% Tween-20). Different membranes were incubated with goat anti-TNFα (Abcam, ref. ab8348, Cambridge, UK) at 1:1000 dilution; anti-IL-1β (Abcam, ref. ab9722) at 1:500; anti-iNOS (Invitrogen, ref. PA1-036, Carlsbad, USA) at 1:1000; anti-IRS1 (Sigma-Aldrich, Ref. 06-248, Darmstadt, Germany) at 1:500; anti GLUT4 (Sigma-Aldrich, ref. 07-1401) at 1:1000; and anti-PI3K (Abcam, ref. 86714) at 1:500. All the incubations were made leaving the membranes overnight at 4 °C in constant movement. Next day, membranes were washed for 5 times with PBST, followed by incubation with horseradish peroxidase-conjugated anti-rabbit IgG (Sigma-Aldrich, ref. A9169) at 1:2500 dilution in 2% non-fat dry milk dissolved in PBST 24 for 2 h at RT. The membranes were then washed 5 times with PBST; signal development was achieved for each antibody by incubation with ECL Plus chemiluminescence following the manufacturer's instructions (Bio-Rad). The reactive bands in the membranes were detected by exposure to C-DiGit Blot Scanner (LI-COR).

2.4. Cell Culture and Treatment

The PANC-1 pancreatic cells were grown in poly-L-lysine-coated 75 cm^2 flasks (~2.5 × 10^6 cells/mL) in Dulbecco's modified Eagle's medium (DMEM) supplemented with heat-inactivated fetal bovine serum (10%) and 2 mM glutamine, all at final concentration, in a 5% CO_2/95% humidified atmosphere at 37 °C.

The pancreatic cells were maintained by serial passage in culture flasks and used in the experimental studies when the exponential phase was reached. Cells were grown to confluence and the monolayer culture was washed two times with phosphate-buffered solution (PBS, Sigma). The cells were then treated with trypsin-EDTA (Lonza) at 0.25% for 10 min. After 5 min centrifugation at 1000× g and two times PBS washing, PANC-1 cells were collected. Afterward, cells counting and viability assessment were achieved by using a Countess II FL Automated Cell Counter (Thermo Fisher) at both, the initial and final step of each experiment. Viability of cells was higher than 95%. Cell cultures were stablished at 80% of confluence and treated with LPS (1 µg/mL) for 24 h. PANC-1 cells were challenged with purified γ-conglutin protein for 24 h alone or in combination adding LPS. Aliquots of γ-conglutin protein stored at −20 °C in PBS were thawed just before use and dissolved in culture media to target concentrations and to be added to the cultures. After treatment, cells were harvested for further analyses.

2.5. MTT Assay for Cell Viability

Cell viability was evaluated using 3-(4,5-dimethylthiazol-2-yl)-2,5-diphenyltetrazolium bromide (MTT) following the manufacturer's instructions (Roche). Briefly, 96-well microtitre plates were inoculated at a density of 1×10^3 PANC-1 cells per well in 300 µL of growth media. Plates were incubated overnight under 5% CO_2 in humidified air to allow the cells to adhere to the wells. After incubation, cells were treated for 24 h with either LPS or γ-conglutin protein, and washed three times with PBS in order to prevent any interfering issue because of the phenolic compounds when making the MTT assay. A volume of 200 µL of free red-phenol DMEM containing 1 mg mL^{-1} of MTT was added to the cells, and these were incubated for 3 h. Metabolically active viable cells are able to convert MTT into formazan crystals (purple color), and the former compound was solubilized with 200 µL of DMSO to absorb at 570 nm (test) and 690 nm using a iMark microplate reader (Bio-Rad, USA).

2.6. Insulin Resistance PANC-1 Cell Model and Glucose Uptake

Culture PANC-1 control cells were seeded in DMEM supplemented with 10% (v/v) FBS, using 96-well microtiter plates under standard conditions (5% CO_2 and 37 °C in humidified air), and a density of 2×10^4 cells per mL in 200 mL. Optimal dose of insulin and treatment time as requisite to establish insulin-resistant IR_PANC-1 (IR-C) cells. Cells display reduced glucose uptake, and this is one of the main feature of the insulin resistance impaired glucose uptake since decreasing cells responses to glucose uptake to increasing levels of insulin. Thus, the cell culture was separated into two groups having six independent replicates per each group: (1) Cultured cells in 200 µL complete medium (control cells, group C); (2) Treated cells with insulin (10^{-5} to 10^{-9} nmol L^{-1}) when the cells became adherent (group IR-C). These PANC-1 cells were then cultured for 24, 48, and 72 h and the concentration of glucose in the media was measured using the glucose oxidase method (Abcam, UK). The concentration required to stablish IR-C PANC-1 cells was 10^{-7} nmol L^{-1} and cultured for 24 h. At this IR stage, it was evaluated whether cells were sensitive to insulin and to evaluate whether γ-conglutin protein can improve the insulin-dependent glucose uptake capacity of IR-C PANC-1 cells. Thus, these cells were separated in three groups, each one with six replicates: The control group (C), IR-C and the IR-C + γ-conglutin groups. After 24 h, 2 µL of culture supernatant was collected from each sample and glucose concentration was determined as described above. Cultures of IR-C cells were stablished to 80% confluence and challenged with γ-conglutin protein for 24 h. After the treatments, the cells were harvested for further analyses.

2.7. Quantitative Real-Time PCR

GLUT-4, IL-1β, iNOS, IRS-1, PI3K and TNFα mRNA expression were assayed by mean of Real-time quantitative PCR for each experimental group. Total RNA was isolated from group C using the RNeasy Tissue RNA isolation kit (Qiagen, Hilden, Germany). First strand cDNA was synthesized using a

High-Capacity cDNA Archive Kit (Applied Biosystems, Waltham, MA, USA). cDNA was prepared, diluted and subjected to real-time polymerase chain reaction (PCR), and amplified using TaqMan technology (LightCycler 480 quantitative PCR System, Roche, Basel, Switzerland) for gene expression assays. Primers and probes were used from the commercially available TaqMan Gene Expression Assays [IRS-1: Assay ID Hs00178563_m1, GLUT-4: Hs00168966_m1, PI3K: Hs00898511_m1, TNFα: Hs01555410_m1, IL-1β: Hs01075529_m1, iNOS: Hs00174128_m1, respectively]. Gene expression levels relative changes were assessed using the $2^{-\Delta\Delta Ct}$ method. The cycle number where the transcripts were detectable (CT) was normalized to the cycle number of β-actin detection as housekeeping gene (Assay ID: Hs99999903_m1, Applied Biosystems), and referred to as ΔCT, where the relative mRNA levels are presented as unit values of $2^{\wedge\,[CT\,(\beta\text{-actin})-CT\,(gene\,of\,interest)]}$, and displaying CT as the threshold cycle value. This parameter was defined as the fractional cycle number at which the target fluorescent signal passes a fixed threshold above baseline. PCR efficiency was assessed by TaqMan analysis on a standard curve for targets and endogenous control amplifications, which were highly similar.

2.8. ELISA Assays for INFγ and Cytokines Quantification

The cell cultured were prepared by cell counting and plated in six-well plates including 10^6 cells per well, and a duplicated well per group. After 24 h incubation, the media from treated culture was eliminated and cells were washed with PBS at 4 °C. To achieve proteins extraction, temperature of the plates was kept closely to 4 °C by placing these on ice, thus avoiding the denaturation of cytokines. One hundred microliters of buffer (150 mM sodium chloride, 1% NP-40, 50mM Tris pH 8) was added to each well and supplemented with 1 µL of protease inhibitor (Sigma) for 15 s. Scraped cells from the bottom of the wells were transferred to microcentrifuge tubes. These tubes were centrifuged at 12,500× g for 15 min at 4 °C. After this step, every supernatant was collected and diluted to a 1:4 ratio used for the ELISA quantification test of INFγ, IL-6, IL12p70, IL-17, and IL-27 (Diaclone). Data were statistically analyzed using the *t*-test.

2.9. Antioxidant Enzymatic Activity Assays

The cell cultures were prepared and after 24 h of incubation of the treated culture, growing media was removed, and cells washed with PBS at 4 °C. Cells from C, IR-C and IR-C cultures challenged with γ-conglutin protein were collected and used for the enzymatic activity assessment of SOD and catalase, as well as the GSH measurement (Canvax, Córdoba, Spain), following manufacturer's instructions. Data were analyzed by the statistical t-test.

2.10. Determination of Intracellular ROS and Nitric Oxide (NO)

C and IR-C cell cultures, challenged or not with γ-conglutin protein, were used for proteins extraction and following company instructions either for control or treatment samples (EMD Millipore, USA). A total proteins quantity of 25 µg was loaded onto polyacrylamide gels at 12% for proteins separation by SDS-PAGE. Achieved this step, proteins were transferred to PVDF membranes to be used for protein oxidation detection by using The OxyBlot™ Kit (EMD Millipore, Burlington, MA, USA) according to the manufacturer's instructions, This kit was used for the detection of carbonyl groups present into proteins because the proteins reaction with ROS. Measurements were developed at 485 nm and 530 nm excitation and emission wavelengths, respectively.

The total amount of NO, including nitrite/nitrate content, was measured using a commercial assay kit [ab65328, Abcam, Cambridge, UK] from C and IR-C culture cells before and after γ-conglutin protein challenges. Briefly, samples including every experimental group were deproteinized according to the manufacturer's instructions. An equal amount of sample (30 µL) and standards were loaded into 96-well microtiter plates. Nitrate reductase, enzyme cofactor and assay buffer were added following a 1 h of incubation at RT with Enhancer, Griess Reagent R1 and Griess Reagent R2. Just after incubation, samples were used to measure absorbance at 540 nm with an i-Mark microplate reader (Bio-Rad, USA).

The value of the blank control (medium without cells) was subtracted to the samples' values. Total nitrite/nitrate concentrations were calculated by using a standard curve.

2.11. Statistical Analysis

Data obtained from each experimental were expressed as means ± standard deviation (SD). Experimental assessment was developed at least three times. The one-way variance analysis was implemented using SPSS statistical software (SPSS Inc., Chicago, IL, USA). Statistical significance of differences ($p < 0.05$) in the analyzed data was evaluated with the use of SPSS software by analysis of variance and Dunnett analysis afterward.

3. Results and Discussion

3.1. Isolation and Purification of the NLL Anti-Inflammatory γ-Conglutin Protein

The γ-conglutin protein extraction, isolation and purification were accomplished following the methodology from Czubinski et al. [13] using mature NLL seeds as starting material. A representative SDS-PAGE is shown in supplementary Figure S1. The sample from γ-conglutin purification went to the electrophoretically separation under reduced conditions; several different electrophoretic bands were found for this protein. The most abundant forms were the separated α and β subunits, followed by the unreduced γ-conglutin (α + β subunits) and the uncleaved γ-conglutin precursor [14]. The γ-conglutin monomer is integrated by two subunits (α + β) linked by a single disulphide bridge, which is highly resistant to be broken under reducing conditions due to the structure of the monomeric protein [15].

The expected MW of the γ-conglutin monomer from these sequences is ~45 kDa. After reduction of the disulphide bridge, two electrophoretic bands of 30 kDa (α-subunit) and 17 kDa (β-subunit) were detected, in addition to a ~56.0 kDa band corresponding to the uncleaved γ-conglutin precursor (Supplementary Figure S1, Supplementary Table S1). The purity of this isolated protein assayed by SDS-PAGE under reducing conditions (Supplementary Figure S1) reached a 95%.

In order to identify the different bands showed in the SDS-PAGE gel corresponding to the isolated and purified γ-conglutin (Supplementary Figure S1), we performed an in-gel tryptic digestion of the cut bands, and these were subjected to separation of the peptides and MS-based analysis. The peptide mass data generated was searched against the MS protein sequence database enabled the unambiguous identification by mass peptide fingerprinting as γ-conglutin (NLL 7S-basic globulin) (Supplementary Table S1).

3.2. Cell Viability Assessment of the PANC-1 Cells Treated with γ-Conglutin Protein

In this study, we assessed the viability of PANC-1 cells under treatment of the γ-conglutin protein and the potential cytotoxicity of this protein. In order to evaluate whether inflammation inductor LPS and γ-conglutin produce cell cytotoxicity effects, the viability MTT assay was achieved on PANC-1 cells under separate treatments with LPS adding γ-conglutin, at increasing concentrations to complete the conditions of DMEM culture medium + FBS + antibiotic for 24 h. The LPS plus γ-conglutin had no significant ($p > 0.05$) effects on cell viability (Supplementary Table S2), when compared with the control (untreated) group. The cell cultures used as positive control lacked LPS and γ-conglutin protein. In order to complete the usefulness of the γ-conglutin protein study, trypan blue staining was also used for assessing PANC-1-pancreatic cells viability after treatment with LPS (1 µg/µL) and increasing concentrations (from 10 to 50 µg) of γ-conglutin for 24 h, finding significant differences ($p < 0.05$) in cell viability after 24 h of incubation only at 50 µg compared to the control (Supplementary Table S2).

Furthermore, a parallel study was made to assess the cell viability and cytotoxicity of increasing concentrations of insulin in order to know whether an insulin resistance model could be performed in PANC-1 pancreatic cells and to know the actual insulin concentration that should be used to stablish the model. An MTT assay was developed on PANC-1 cell finding that an important change in the percentage of viability was induced for insulin concentrations higher than 10^{-7} nmol L^{-1}

(Supplementary Table S3). Afterward, IR-C cells were assayed for viability using MTT kit when performed the addition of γ-conglutin protein for 24 h. No significant ($p > 0.05$) effect on cell viability (when treated with 25 μg of γ-conglutin protein) (Supplementary Table S4) was found after comparison with unchallenged IR-C group. When insulin was added alone (in the absence of γ-conglutin), these samples were used as a positive control. We also performed the cell viability assessment using trypan blue exclusion in IR-C pancreatic cells treated with increasing concentrations of this protein for a period of 24 h. No cell viability differences were found after 24 h of incubation in the presence of γ-conglutin.

These results suggest that γ-conglutin do not affect to the PANC-1 pancreatic cell integrity in both, the induced (LPS treatment) inflammation and the IR-C cell models.

3.3. Effect of γ-Conglutin Protein on the Inflammatory Process

Inflammatory-related illnesses as metabolic syndrome, T2DM, obesity and cardiovascular diseases are well known to be developed and chronically associated to a continuously sustained inflammatory state. Among different mechanisms hidden in the inflammatory-based diseases, different molecules namely stressors affect functional pancreatic tissues physiology, particularly β-islets, promoting the course of pathology, which also of course mainly depend of particular genetic backgrounds and environmental factors [16].

Nowadays, there is an increasing number of diabetes associated to obesity named "Diabesity epidemic", which is frequently coincidental with a pancreatic islet cells failure unable to generate enough amount of insulin and/or a developed decreasing sensitivity to insulin by tissues able to metabolize glucose. During the establishment of T2DM, sustained high levels of glucose may lead to organ damage, which is mediated by pancreatic β-cells tissue damage, and the enhancement of immune system inflammatory response because the synthesis and release of pro-inflammatory mediators as cytokines and chemokines (cells chemotactic factors). These processes create feed-forward progressive steps that further increases immune system cell content, promoting a chronic inflammatory state [17]. Thus, increasing levels of multiple factors as IL-1β, TNFα, and iNOS are important contributors for the development of inflammation since IL-1β-mediates β-cell dysfunction during the development of T2DM, while are able to activate the expression of iNOS with the result of an exacerbate synthesis of NO, promoting the up-regulation of pro-inflammatory genes [18]. In this regard, we evaluated the ability of γ-conglutin protein to modulate the mRNA levels of genes of pro-inflammatory mediators as potential anti-inflammatory targets (TNFα, IL-1β, and iNOS mRNA) in PANC-1 cells (Figure 1). Induced inflammatory state by LPS was significantly inhibited ($p < 0.05$) by γ-conglutin proteins at mRNA expression level in PANC-1 [−694, −2733, and −4208–fold, respectively, *versus* LPS treated culture cells] (Figure 1A). No statistically significant differences were observed in IL-1β cytokine, TNFα, and iNOS mRNA levels ($p > 0.05$) when challenges were performed with γ-conglutin + LPS as compared to the control group (Figure 1A). These results highlight the potential implications of γ-conglutin to decrease the pro-inflammatory capacity in PANC-1 cells by decreasing cytokines and iNOS genes expression levels, thus supporting the inflammatory process amelioration at molecular level. In this study, this lowering in the cellular pro-inflammatory capacity could be the result of the antioxidant capacity of γ-conglutin since changes in GSH levels, SOD and catalase activities was shown, helping to keep redox homeostasis in T2DM and other inflammatory-dependent diseases also affected by the oxidative stress [19]. On this line, the above results on PANC-1 pancreatic cells are in agreement with previous studies that shown a similar reduction in the expression levels of iNOS and IL-1β mRNA in T2DM blood culture [20].

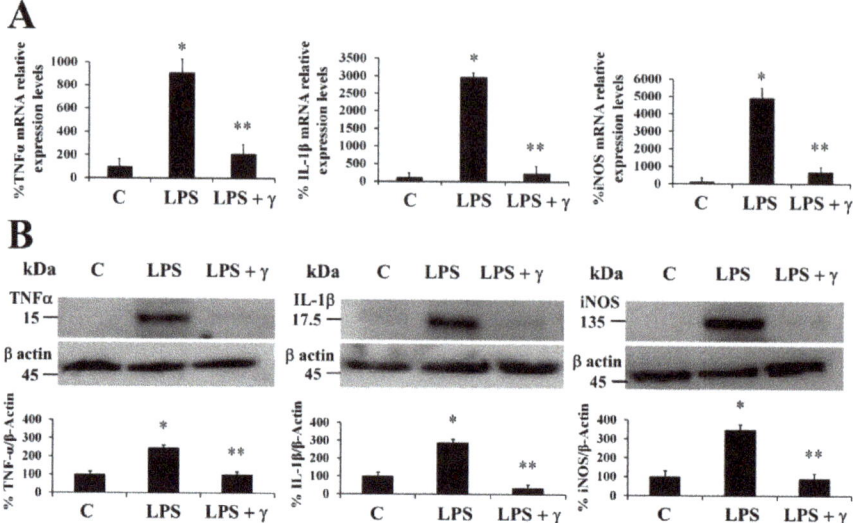

Figure 1. Narrow-leafed lupin (NLL) γ-conglutin decreases the mRNA expression and protein levels of TNFα, IL-1β, and iNOS on lipopolysaccharide (LPS)-induced inflammation pancreatic cells. PANC-1 cells were incubated for 24 h with LPS alone or γ-conglutin + LPS. (**A**) The bar graph shows mRNA levels determined by real-time RT-qPCR of TNFα, iNOS, and IL1β. (**B**) The bar graph shows protein levels determined by immunoblotting of TNFα, iNOS, and IL1β. Average value from triplicate experiments of each biomarker were relativized to the average value of their housekeeping actin protein in control samples. Then, average values from challenge experiments (calculated in the same way than controls) are relativized to these from their respective control values previously calculated. Data represent mean ± SD from three independent experiments. C: Untreated control culture cells; LPS: LPS-treated culture cells; LPS + γ: LPS + γ-conglutin challenge. $p < 0.05$ represents statistically significant differences associated with each figure. $p^* < 0.05$ LPS *versus* C; $p^{**} < 0.05$ LPS + γ-conglutin *versus* LPS. Challenges were made with LPS and/or γ-conglutin protein at 1 µg/mL and 25 µg, respectively.

It is well established that systemic production of IL-1β at local tissues plays a fundamental role in the progression of pancreatic dysfunction as β-cell apoptosis in T2DM. The advance of this disease is facilitated by a continued production of inflammatory molecular mediators that would have an initial development stage and further progression promoted by TNFα-/IL-1β-mediated iNOS synthesis and NO production [21]. We have also demonstrated that NLL γ-conglutin can reverse this state by decreasing the levels of TNFα, IL-1β and iNOS functional protein levels in PANC-1 [−158, −144, and −164-fold, respectively, *versus* LPS treated culture cells] (Figure 1B, Supplementary Table S5), while no statistically significant differences ($p > 0.05$) were observed in TNFα, IL-1β and iNOS protein levels when challenges were accomplished with γ-conglutin (LPS + γ) when compared to the control group (Figure 1B).

3.4. γ-Conglutin Protein Inhibits the Production of Different Cytokines and Pro-Inflammatory Mediators

Physiological circulating levels of cytokines have important implications in the functional regulation of pancreatic β-cells, although these produce different cytokines itself in response to physio-pathological states, playing also important roles in its own β-cells function [18]. When insulin resistance is stablished, increasing production of dangerous pro-inflammatory circulating mediators is also stablished. During the T2DM state progression, this non-physiological condition is characterized by an imbalance pro-inflammatory cytokines and mediators profile, led by the β-cell dysfunction and T2DM sustainable situation, which on the other hand, is based on the crosstalk among cytokines in pancreatic β-cells and immune tissues [22]. Thus, restoring the balance back to the increased levels of protective plasma circulating and β-cells cytokines could prevent and promote the treatment of this β-cell dysfunctional statement, and for extension the T2DM progression.

In this regard, we evaluated by ELISA method the potential anti-inflammatory effects of γ-conglutin protein through its capacity to modulate the amount of important pro-inflammatory mediator as INF-γ and cytokines (IL-6, IL-12p70, IL-17A, and IL-27) in both, an induced inflammation model (Figure 2, Supplementary Tables S5 and S6), and in an IR-C cell model (Supplementary Figure S2, Supplementary Tables S5 and S6) using PANC-1-pancreatic cells. Levels of INFγ and the above cytokines were assessed under basal conditions, after cell treatment with LPS, by challenging the cell culture with γ-conglutin protein after LPS and by adding LPS + γ-conglutin together, or alternatively with γ-conglutin after IR-C model is stablished (as explained in material and methods, Section 2.6). The protein levels of INF-γ and cytokines (IL-6, IL-12p70, IL-17A, and IL-27) significantly ($p < 0.05$) augmented (several-fold) after LPS challenges [LPS: +11335, +2979, +12127, +5632 and +5676-fold versus C, respectively] (Figure 2, Supplementary Table S6); and IR-C model [+8994, +1881, +11592, +5553, +5231-fold versus C, respectively] (Supplementary Figure S2, Supplementary Table S6) whereas the LPS + γ -conglutin protein challenges showed a significant reduction (several-folds) in protein levels [LPS: −256, −1849, −11786, −5339 and −6100-fold versus LPS treated cells, respectively], and IR-C model [−8644, −1839, −11409, −5659 and −5339-fold versus IR-C cells, respectively] (Supplementary Figure S2, Supplementary Table S5). These results are in agreement with these obtained from RT-qPCR, where reduced mRNA and proteins levels of the pro-inflammatory mediators TNFα, IL-1β, and iNOS were found in PANC-1-cells culture (Figure 1A, Figure 1B, Supplementary Tables S5 and S6). No statistically significant differences ($p > 0.05$) were observed in INF-γ and cytokines (IL-6, IL-12p70, IL-17A, and IL-27) protein levels when challenges were accomplished with γ-conglutin (LPS + γ) after comparison to the control group (Figure 2, Supplementary Figure S2).

Currently, scarce studies have showed results concerning the anti-inflammatory effects of plant peptides, usually promoted by the modulation of the balance regulation of pro-inflammatory interleukins, INFγ, TNFα and NO. In the case of studied soybean peptides, these inhibited mRNA iNOS expression levels and TNFα and NO production, while also reduced the pro-inflammatory enzymatic activity of COX-2 in LPS-induced macrophages [8]. Moreover, lunasin was shown to reduce the ROS production in macrophages induced by LPS while inhibiting the release of IL-6 and TNFα [11,12]. In this regard, we demonstrated that NLL γ-conglutin protein lowered the pro-inflammatory mediators' levels assayed. This anti-inflammatory capacity would be capable to manage the diseases developmental states promoting feed-forward process for the establishment of these chronic inflammatory-derived diseases as T2DM. Thus, lupin γ-conglutins may be capable to promote the improvement from the detrimental effects of several inflammatory molecular developments as follows:

(i) Lipotoxicity as a sustained high lipid diet induces the production of IL-1β, IL-6, which β-cells continued exposure induces exacerbate synthesis and release of ROS, while secretion of insulin is also inhibited. This combination promotes the apoptosis of the pancreatic β-cells [23]. Based in our research, challenging pancreatic β-cells with γ-conglutin decreased the mRNA expression of IL-1β, and protein levels of IL-1β and IL-6 in LPS-induced inflammation [LPS + γ: −2749; −146 and −1100-fold versus LPS treated cells, respectively] (Figure 1; Figure 2, Supplementary Table S5); and IR-C model [IR-C + γ: −177; −97 and −1849-fold versus IR-C cells, respectively] (Figure 3, Supplementary Figure S2, Supplementary Table S5).

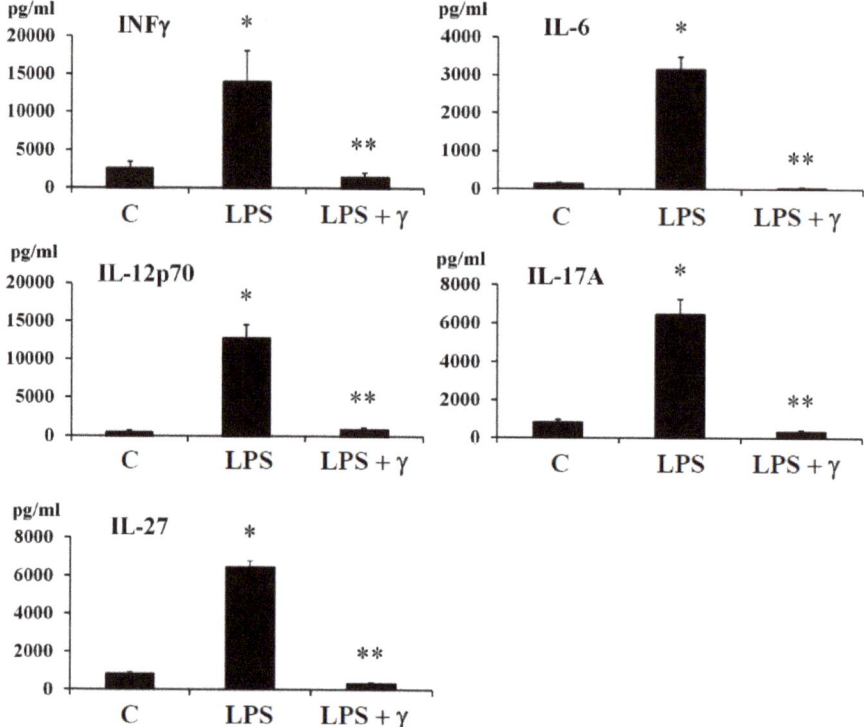

Figure 2. Effect of NLL γ-conglutin on the protein levels of pro-inflammatory cytokines. PANC-1 cells were incubated for 24 h with LPS alone, or γ-conglutin + LPS. The bar graph shows protein levels determined by ELISA of INFγ, IL-6, IL-12, IL-17, and IL-27. Data represent mean ± SD from three independent experiments. C: Untreated control culture cells; LPS: LPS-treated culture cells; LPS + γ: LPS + γ-conglutin challenge. $p < 0.05$ represents statistically significant differences associated with each figure. $p^* < 0.05$ LPS *versus* C; $p^{**} < 0.05$ LPS + γ-conglutin *versus* LPS. Challenges were made with LPS and/or γ-conglutin at 1 µg/mL and 25 µg, respectively.

(ii) Apoptosis of islets β-cells prompted by IL-1β and INFγ is stimulated by endoplasmic reticulum stress [24]. In this regard, β-cell apoptosis is also activated by the join action of INFγ and TNFα, together with the activation of Ca^{2+} channels. This situation induces the NO synthesis and consequently the endoplasmic reticulum stress pathway activation [25], leading to caspases activation and mitochondrial dysfunction [26]. In this concern, γ-conglutin may be able to prevent these mechanisms by suppressing the TNFα, IL-1β and INFγ mRNA and protein levels (Figures 1–3, Supplementary Figure S2, Supplementary Tables S5 and S6).

(iii) The synergistic action of IL-1β + INFγ, or even IL-1β + INFγ + TNFα cytokines in pancreatic tissues increases NO production as consequence of direct increasing of iNOS, resulting in islet β-cell destruction [27]. We have shown that mRNA expression levels of TNFα and IFNγ (apoptosis mediated molecules) were lowered after treatment with γ-conglutin (Figures 1–3, Supplementary Figure S2, Supplementary Tables S5 and S6), which may have a positive effect on the survival of islet β-cells [28].

(iv) IL-12 mRNA expression levels are increased by the effect of INFγ, while IL-12 promote signaling positive feed-back effect for raising levels of INFγ [29]. The γ-conglutin protein reduction effect of IL-12 mRNA levels (Figure 2, Supplementary Figure S2, Supplementary Tables S5 and S6) may decrease INFγ levels and its negative inflammatory effects.

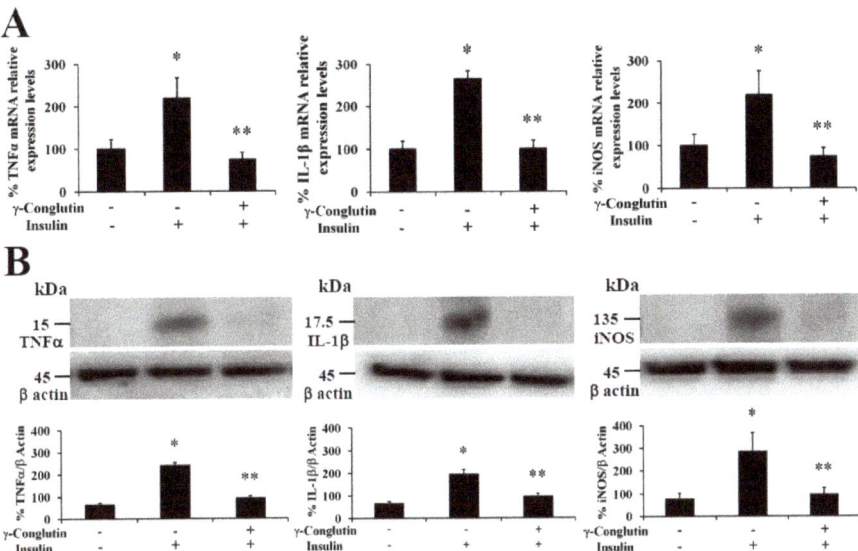

Figure 3. NLL γ-conglutin decreases the mRNA expression and protein levels of TNFα, IL-1β and iNOS on an insulin-resistance IR-C cell model. Control PANC-1 cells, and IR-C pancreatic cells were cultured for 24 h alone, or the former culture with γ-conglutin. (**A**) The bar graph shows mRNA levels determined by real-time RT-qPCR of TNFα, iNOS and IL1β. (**B**) The bar graph shows protein levels determined by immunoblotting of TNFα, iNOS and IL1β. Average value from triplicate experiments of each biomarker were relativized to the average value of their housekeeping actin protein in control samples. Then, average values from challenge experiments (calculated in the same way than controls) are relativized to these from their respective control values previously calculated. Data represent mean ± SD from three independent experiments. Control: Untreated control PANC-1 culture cells; IR-C: insulin resistant culture cells; IR-C + γ: IR-C + γ-conglutin challenge. $p < 0.05$ represents statistically significant differences associated with each figure. $p^* < 0.05$ IR-C *versus* control PANC-1 cells; $p^{**} < 0.05$ IR-C + γ-conglutin *versus* IR-C. Challenges were made with 25 µg of γ-conglutin.

(v) Important inflammatory cytokine, IL-17A, involved in the T2DM progressing, is able to induce ROS production, which also greatly affects to insulin resistance. A join action from IL-17 and INFγ acts as diabetes chronic state development [30]. Overall, IL-17A has pleiotropic functional effects comprising synthesis of IL-6 and TNFα, and chemokines (chemotaxis effect) on a diversity of cells [31]. Thus, the lowering of the IL-17 protein level (Figure 2, Supplementary Figure S2, Supplementary Tables S5 and S6) might reduce pro-inflammatory effects of IL-6 and TNFα (Figure 2, Supplementary Figure S2, Supplementary Tables S5 and S6), avoiding islet β-cell apoptosis and the recruitment of immune cells to local tissues, enhancing feed-forward mechanism of inflammation progression in islets [32] as preventive action for inflammation based T2DM progression.

3.5. γ-Conglutin Reverses the Insulin Resistance through Inflammation Amelioration while Improving Insulin Signalling Pathway in Pancreatic IR-C Cells

Insulin resistance is another consequence of a sustained inflammation, which has been observed in several pathophysiological processes, including metabolic disorders as hyperinsulinemia, hyperglycemia, and hypertriglyceridemia, being IR also an important cause of pre-diabetes establishment and T2DM development and obesity [33], affecting to different insulin target organs. Thus, amelioration of IR by NLL γ-conglutin may constitute a major approach to prevent and treat these metabolic disorders.

In this study, it was established an in vitro insulin-resistant (IR-C) cell model using PANC-1 cells to evaluate the insulin effects on glucose uptake and metabolism in IR-C cell. To evaluate glucose uptake, control cells were incubated with a range of insulin concentrations (between 10^{-5} to 10^{-9} nmol L^{-1}) for 24 h (Figure 4). Following an insulin concentration of 10^{-7} nmol L^{-1}, we found the most statistically significant reduction in the extracellular glucose depletion ($p < 0.05$) in comparison to control cells (without insulin treatment) (Figure 4A). The addition of 10^{-7} nmol L^{-1} of insulin promoted a time-dependent lowering ($p < 0.05$) of glucose consumption between 24–48 h when compared to control cells (Figure 4B). These results clearly showed the maintenance of the insulin resistance by IR-C cells for a period of 48 h after insulin treatment. Following 48 h, cells acquired a normal condition as control cells (C). These results are consistent with the increasing glucose uptake shown in Figure 3B after 72 h, while no statistically significant differences ($p > 0.05$) in glucose consumption was observed when compared to control cells without insulin treatment. Furthermore, the molecular mechanisms leading to glucose homeostasis and/or IR are still uncertain. However, NLL γ-conglutin might be able to contribute in this process of glucose homeostasis, as we have demonstrated in the current study that glucose uptake by IR-C cells is clearly induced by treatment with γ-conglutin protein, reaching higher glucose uptake levels after IR-C cells challenged with 25 μg of γ-conglutin protein, which glucose uptake increased more than 60% in comparison to IR-C cells ($p < 0.05$), which were assayed without γ-conglutin protein challenge (Figure 4C).

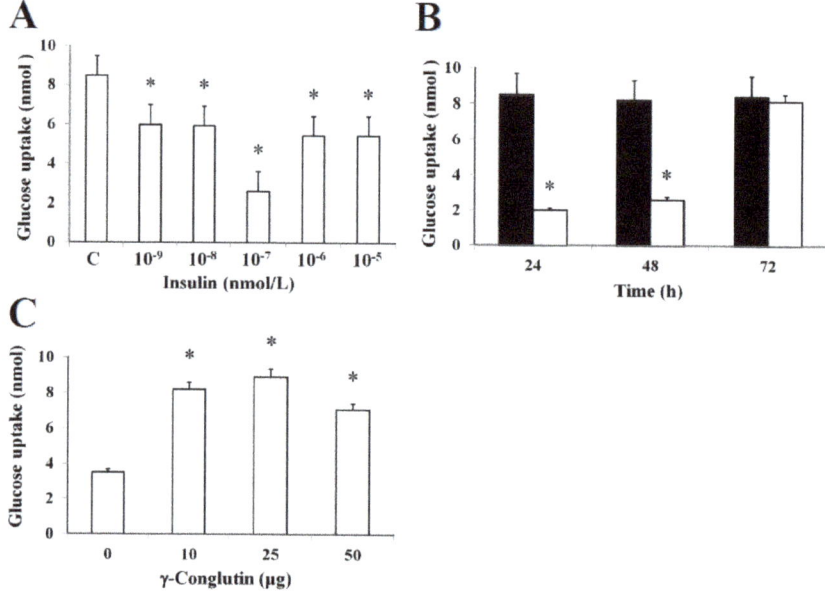

Figure 4. Insulin-resistant IR_PANC-1 cell model and glucose consumption promoted by γ-conglutin. (**A**) Increasing concentrations of insulin from 10^{-9} to 10^{-5} nmol/L showed that cell culture did uptake the lower level of glucose at 10^{-7} nmol/L in comparison to C cell culture, taking this concentration as the level of insulin where cells acquired the resistance state. (**B**) C cells were cultured for 24, 48 and 72 h, testing the glucose uptake of cultures including 10^{-7} nmol/L (white bars), in comparison to control C cells (black bars). In these assays were showed that insulin resistance state is preserved for 48 h. $p^* < 0.05$ IR-C *versus* C. (**C**) Glucose consumption by IR-C cells promoted by γ-conglutin at 0, 10, 25 and 50 μg was assayed after 24 h of culture. Values are shown as the mean ± SD from three independent experiments. $p < 0.05$ represents statistically significant differences associated with each figure. $p^* < 0.05$ treated cells (μg) *versus* control.

The treatment of pancreatic IR-C cells with γ-conglutin was also accomplished to determine whether this protein had effects on insulin resistance improvement throughout recovering the control-like associated mRNA expression levels of IRS-1, GLUT-4, and PI3K, key upstream and glucose transport mediators in the insulin signaling pathway [20], which would also be the reflect of a potential improvement in the glucose uptake and the inflammatory state on IR-C cells. The analysis of IRS-1, GLUT-4 and PI3K showed their up-regulation in their mRNA expression after γ-conglutin treatment in IR-C cells (Figure 5) [IRS-1: +70; GLUT-4: +97%; and PI3K: +90-fold, respectively], which differences were statistically significant compared to IR-C untreated cells ($p < 0.05$) (Figure 5A), as well as the mRNA expression level reduction of IRS-1, GLUT-4 and PI3K in IR-C cells [IRS-1: −93; GLUT-4: −84%; and PI3K: −89-fold, respectively] compared to control cells PANC-1 (Figure 5A).

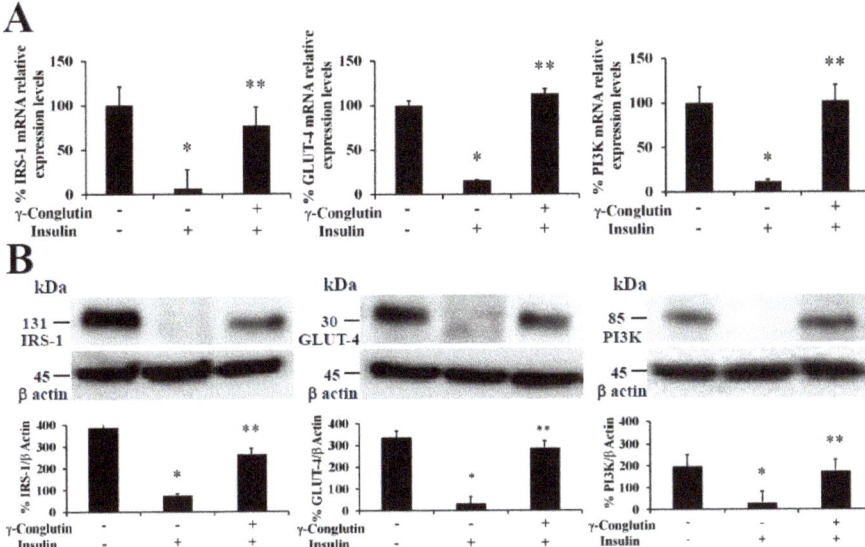

Figure 5. NLL γ-conglutin increases mRNA expression and protein levels of the insulin signaling pathway mediators IRS-1, PI3K and GLUT-4. PANC-1 cells or IR-C cell culture were incubated for 24 h alone, or the former culture with γ-conglutin. (**A**) The bar graph shows mRNA levels determined by real-time RT-qPCR of IRS-1, PI3K and GLUT-4. (**B**) The bar graph shows protein levels determined by immunoblotting of IRS-1, PI3K and GLUT-4. Average value from triplicate experiments of each biomarker were relativized to the average value of their housekeeping actin protein in control samples. Then, average values from challenge experiments (calculated in the same way than controls) are relativized to these from their respective control values previously calculated. Data represent mean ± SD from three independent experiments. Control: Untreated control PANC-1 culture cells; IR-C: insulin resistant culture cells; IR-C + γ: IR-C + γ-conglutin challenge. $p < 0.05$ represents statistically significant differences associated with each figure. $p^* < 0.05$ IR-C versus control PANC-1 cells; $p^{**} < 0.05$ IR-C + γ-conglutin versus IR-C. Challenges were made with 25 µg of γ-conglutin.

We have also demonstrated that NLL γ-conglutin can reverse this state by up-regulating the IRS-1, GLUT-4 and PI3K functional protein levels in IR-C cells [IRS-1: +266; GLUT-4: +185; and PI3K: +144-fold, respectively] (Figure 5B), after decreased proteins levels showed when PANC-1 control cells acquired the IR-C statement compared to the control group [IRS-1: −302; GLUT-4: −310; and PI3K: −166-fold, respectively] (Figure 5B). These results confirm that γ-conglutin protein would be capable to reduce significantly the blood glucose level by promoting glucose uptake by insulin sensitive tissues while ameliorating hyperglycemia via increasing GLUT-4 glucose transporter protein level and plasma membrane recruitment [34], and insulin signaling pathway upstream mediators IRS-1 and PI3K [20].

Furthermore, at the same time we also evaluated the capability of γ-conglutin protein to regulate the mRNA and protein levels of pro-inflammatory molecules as potential mechanism helping to reverse the IR-C cell statement. TNFα, IL-1β and iNOS were analyzed in IR-C culture (Figure 3). These pro-inflammatory mediators were significantly lowered in γ-conglutin protein treated IR-C cells, at the mRNA expression levels [TNFα: −158; IL-1β: −144; and iNOS: −164-fold, respectively, *versus* IR-C untreated cells] (Figure 3A), and at the protein levels [TNFα: −189; IL-1β: −146; and iNOS: −97-fold, respectively, *versus* IR-C untreated cells] (Figure 3B, Supplementary Table S6). No statistically significant differences ($p > 0.05$) were found for TNFα, IL-1β and iNOS levels in IR-C cells treated with γ-conglutin in comparison to the PANC-1 control group (Figure 3). These results highlight the potential implications of γ-conglutin to improve insulin resistance through inflammation amelioration at molecular level in PANC-1 pancreatic cells by decreasing cytokines and iNOS levels [20].

In this study, we have demonstrated for the first time that NLL γ-conglutin protein is able to help improving the insulin resistance state in PANC-1 cell line targeting two major molecular signaling cross-roads, restoring functional levels of insulin activation pathway mediators while decreasing several pro-inflammatory mediators' levels that worthwhile reinforces the first effect on PANC-1 cells. These outcomes are vital knowledge to be considered for successful anti-inflammatory insulin sensitizing new alternative therapies from natural plant sources.

3.6. Oxidative Stress Modulation by γ-Conglutin Protein as Anti-Inflammatory and Insulin Resistance Improvement Mechanism

Oxidative stress, understood as the cellular statement of excess reactive oxygen species (ROS) production, is a main factor in the T2DM development [35], through promoting IR development. Afterward, high amounts of blood glucose sustained long time causes damage on the enzymes superoxide dismutase (Cu/Zn-SOD), catalase (CAT), and glutathione molecule as the most important elements of the cell antioxidant defense system [36]. Thus, an excessive ROS production contributes to oxidative stress, a pro-inflammatory state, and mitochondrial dysfunction that in turn exacerbates IR [37]. It would be necessary a comprehensive knowledge about the relationship between oxidative stress and T2DM risk factors (inflammation and IR) in order to improve diabetes prevention and its associated complications. In this regard, signaling molecules as nitric oxide (NO) play a critical role of the inflammation pathogenesis acting as a pro-inflammatory molecule, together with cytokines and chemokines (e.g., TNFα, IL-6, IL-12), under oxidative stress situations because of the excessive NO and ROS production, i.e., IR [38], promoting islet β-cell apoptosis [39] and the progression of diseases concomitant with inflammation [40].

In the present study, we evaluated the oxidative homeostasis in inflammatory LPS-induced PANC-1 cells, as well as in IR-C cell model, after treatment with γ-conglutin protein. In both cases, we assessed the ROS production by measuring the levels of protein carbonylation, the covalent modifications of proteins induced by ROS, i.e., H_2O_2 or other derived molecules from the oxidative stress process by using an OxyBlot protein oxidation detection and immunoassay [41], and comparing them with control cells, LPS treated cells and IR-C cells, respectively, without any challenge with γ-conglutin. Very low levels of protein oxidation, generated through normal metabolic activity, were observed in untreated (control) cells with LPS (Supplementary Figure S3A), as well as in control PANC-1 cells before IR-C statement induction (Figure 6A). However, ROS production was significantly increased ($p < 0.05$) after LPS cells treatment (+677-fold, Supplementary Figure S3A), and in IR-C cells (+445-fold, Figure 6A), as significant ($p < 0.05$) increased levels of proteins carbonylation was detected. Treatments of these type of cells with γ-conglutin protein restored oxidative balance in both situations (LPS-induced cells: −423-fold, and IR-C cells: −445-fold, respectively; Supplementary Figure S3A, Figure 6A), in comparison to their respective inflammatory induced stages. These results suggest that γ-conglutin protein efficiently avoid at certain levels the ROS production (oxidative stress) in PANC-1 cells after inflammatory statement incensement, and that γ-conglutin exhibited strong anti-oxidant effect since this protein ameliorated the oxidative stress induced by LPS and in IR-C cell model. Interestingly, the present and future related studies would benefit from the comparative further analyses using other types of cell cultures, like primary islets and/or pancreatic β-cells and/or adipocyte cells to determine actions related to insulin secretion and islet inflammation.

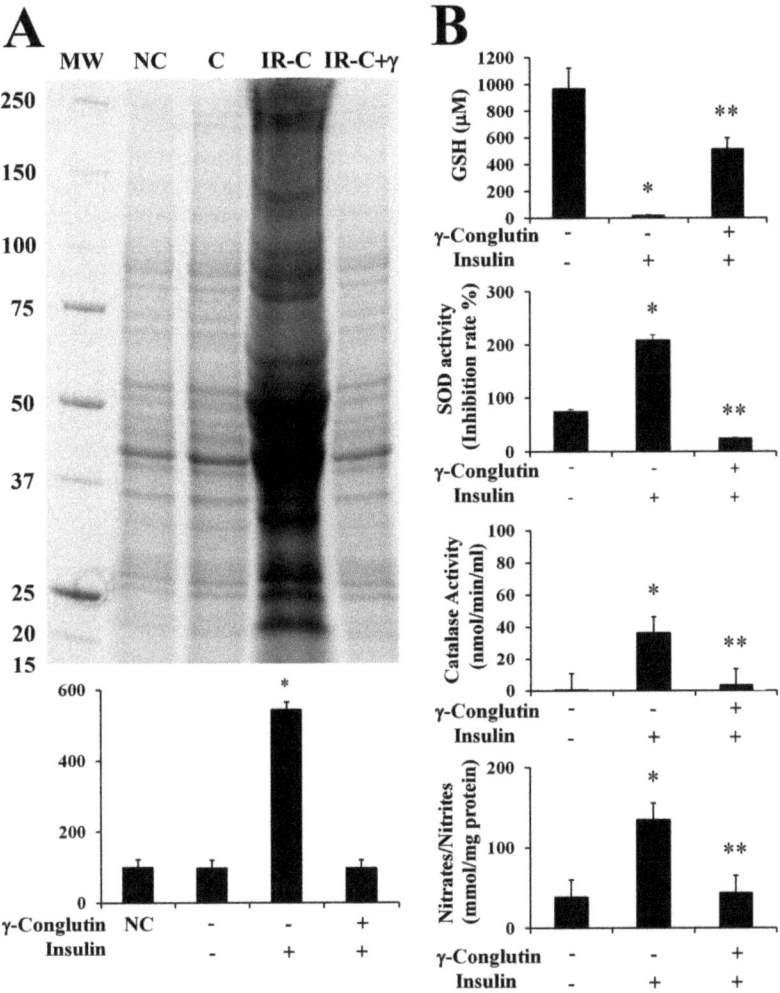

Figure 6. Effect of γ-conglutin on proteins oxidative modifications, antioxidant enzymatic activities and production of glutathione (GSH) and NO. (A) Changes in protein carbonyl formation were measured in IR-C cells after 24 h of incubation with γ-conglutin. Protein carbonyls were measured using an OxyBlot kit. Representative blots show basal carbonylation levels in C control PANC-1 cells, IR-C cells, and IR-C culture cells challenged with γ-conglutin. Graph y-axis represents arbitrary densitometry units. $p^* < 0.05$ IR-C cells *versus* C cells. (B) IR-C pancreatic cells were incubated for 24 h with γ-conglutin protein. GSH and NO production, as well as SOD and catalase activities were measured. Data represent mean ± SD from three independent experiments. $p < 0.05$ represents statistically significant differences associated with each figure. $p^* < 0.05$ IR-C *versus* control PANC-1 cells; $p^{**} < 0.05$ IR-C + γ-conglutin *versus* IR-C. Challenges were made with 25 µg of γ-conglutin.

Therefore, removal of free radicals is strongly dependent of enzymatic activities as superoxide dismutase (Cu/Zn-SOD), catalase (CAT) and glutathione (GSH) levels, representing crucial indicators of the cellular anti-oxidant capacity, and the oxidative stress cell state [35]. In the current study, we assessed the modulation of these antioxidant factors by γ-conglutin in the inflammatory LPS-induced PANC-1 cells, as well as in IR-C cell model, by measuring SOD and catalase activities, GSH levels and NO production, before and after the treatment with γ-conglutin (Supplementary Figure S3B, Figure 6B). We found a statistically significant ($p < 0.05$) decreased levels of GSH (LPS-induced inflammation cells: −660-fold; IR-C cells: −949-fold, respectively) (Supplementary Figure S3B, Figure 6B). Furthermore, the levels of SOD and catalase activity were strongly reduced after the same treatments with γ-conglutin protein in LPS-induced inflammatory statement (SOD: −677-fold; catalase: −142-fold, respectively) (Supplementary Figure S3B) and IR-C cells (SOD: −183-fold; catalase: −33-fold, respectively) (Figure 6B). These data showed that high GSH and low SOD levels and catalase activities might be regulated by γ-conglutin protein through direct or indirect marked effects in avoiding lipids and protein oxidative modifications, which is also supported by the concomitant large reduction of oxidative carbonylation (Supplementary Figure S3B, Figure 6B), and an overall oxidative stress balance improvement, translated also to an inflammation molecular cellular statement amelioration by γ-conglutin protein as an anti-oxidant protein.

Furthermore, we analyzed the NO production again in both induced inflammation cell models treated with γ-conglutin protein for 24 h. Statistically significant decreased levels of NO were found ($p < 0.05$) in the LPS-induced cells (−351-fold, Supplementary Figure S3B) and IR-C cells (−91-fold, Figure 6B), in comparison to inflammation induced cells without γ-conglutin protein treatment, showing again how γ-conglutin is able to ameliorate the inflammatory state of cells promoting lowering NO [42] and iNOS expression levels, showing potential uses in the improvement of T2DM and other inflammatory-based diseases.

These novel results clearly indicated that oxidative stress is a major point targeted by NLL γ-conglutin protein effects causing an improved stress balancing through reduced ROS-related pro-inflammatory mediators and increased anti-oxidative molecules. Indeed, such data can be helpful for the development of future antioxidant and new anti-inflammatory therapeutics avoiding the oxidative stress activation of inflammatory mediators involved in several chronic diseases, with the advantage of being a natural product from lupin seeds that can be implemented as a functional food.

4. Conclusions

In this study, treatment with NLL γ-conglutin protein to inflammation LPS-induced and IR-C in the PANC-1 pancreatic cell-line promoted: (i) Lowering expression of mRNA and proteins levels of key pro-inflammatory mediators as TNFα, IL-1β, and iNOS; ii) the up-regulation mRNA expression and increasing protein levels of IRS-1, and p85-PI3K, and GLUT-4 transporter, which are crucial biomarkers of the insulin signaling pathway activation. This up-regulation makes possible the recovery of the physiological condition of the cells as control cell-like situation from an induced inflammatory statement; (iii) glucose uptake in IR-C cells; (iv) a significant decrease ($p < 0.05$) in proteins levels of pro-inflammatory mediators INFγ, IL-6, IL-12, IL-17 and IL-27; (v) significant dropping oxidative stress in inflammation LPS-induced and IR-C pancreatic cells, as indicated by a reduced levels of protein carbonylation, improved glutathione (GSH) levels and lower SOD and catalase antioxidant enzymatic activities; (vi) reduction of NO production and down-regulation of iNOS in both, LPS-induced inflammation and IR-C pancreatic cells. This study is the first describing the anti-inflammatory effects at molecular level of the legume protein family 7S basic globulins or γ-conglutin, constituting strong evidences that NLL γ-conglutins play a crucial role in the development of novel functional foods and therapeutic options for the prevention and treatment of inflammatory-related diseases.

Supplementary Materials: The following are available online at http://www.mdpi.com/2076-3921/9/1/12/s1, Figure S1: Isolation and purification of NLL seed γ-conglutin protein; FigureS2: Effect of NLL γ-conglutin on the protein levels of pro-inflammatory cytokines; Figure S3: Effect of γ-conglutin on proteins oxidative modifications, antioxidant enzymatic activities and production of GSH and NO; Table S1: γ-conglutin peptides mass fingerprinting characterization; Table S2: Cell viability (%) and dose effects of NLL γ-conglutin protein; Table S3: Cell viability (%) on insulin resistance IR-C cell model; Table S4: Cell viability (%) and dose effects of purified NLL γ-conglutin protein on insulin resistance cell (IR-C) model; Table S5: Fold-change in protein levels of pro-inflammatory cytokines and iNOS; Table S6: Fold-change in protein levels of pro-inflammatory cytokines and iNOS.

Author Contributions: Conceptualization: J.C.J.-L. and E.L.-C.; Methodology: J.C.J.-L., E.L.-C., A.C.; Data Analysis: J.C.J.-L., E.L.-C., A.C.; Resources: J.C.J.-L., A.C., J.D.A.; Writing—Original Draft Preparation: J.C.J.-L.; Writing—Review and Editing: J.C.J.-L., A.C., J.D.A., S.M.-S.; Funding Acquisition: J.C.J.-L., A.C., J.D.A. All authors have read and agreed to the published version of the manuscript.

Funding: This research was partially funded by the European Research Program MARIE CURIE (FP7-PEOPLE-2011-IOF) grant ref. number PIOF-GA-2011-301550; The Spanish Ministry of Economy, Industry and Competitiveness for the grant ref. number RYC-2014-16536 (Ramon y Cajal Research Program); the grant ref. number BFU2016-77243-P; and the grant ref. number AGL2017-83772-R (AEI/FEDER, UE) funded by the Spanish Ministry of Science, Innovation and Universities" and "The APC was funded by the grant ref. number BFU2016-77243-P".

Acknowledgments: This study has been funded by the European Research Program MARIE CURIE (FP7-PEOPLE-2011-IOF) for through the grant ref. number PIOF-GA-2011-301550 to J.C.J.-L. and J.D.A.; The Spanish Ministry of Economy, Industry and Competitiveness for the grant ref. number RYC-2014-16536 (Ramon y Cajal Research Program) to J.C.J.-L.; the grant ref. number BFU2016-77243-P to J.D.A. and J.C.J.-L.; and the grant ref. number AGL2017-83772-R (AEI/FEDER, UE) funded by the Spanish Ministry of Science, Innovation and Universities to A.C.

Conflicts of Interest: The authors have declared that no competing interests exist.

References

1. Clark, M.; Hill, J.; Tilman, D. The Diet, health, and environment trilemma. *Ann. Rev. Environ. Res.* **2018**, *43*, 109–134. [CrossRef]
2. Dehghan, M.; Mente, A.; Zhang, X.; Swaminathan, S.; Li, W.; Mohan, V.; Lqbal, R.; Kumar, R.; Wentzel-Viljoen, E.; Rosengren, A.; et al. Associations of fats and carbohydrate intake with cardiovascular disease and mortality in 18 countries from five continents (PURE): A prospective cohort study. *Lancet* **2017**, *390*, 2050–2062. [CrossRef]
3. Robinson, G.H.J.; Balk, J.; Domoney, C. Improving pulse crops as a source of protein, starch and micronutrients. *Nutr. Bull.* **2019**, *44*, 202–215. [CrossRef] [PubMed]
4. Prusinski, J. White lupin (*Lupinus albus* L.)—Nutritional and health values in human nutrition—A Review. *Czech J. Food Sci.* **2017**, *35*, 95–105.
5. Delgado-Andrade, C.; Olías, R.; Jimenez-Lopez, J.C.; Clemente, A. Nutritional and beneficial effects of grain legumes on human health. *Arbor* **2016**, *313*, 192–779.
6. Turner, M.D.; Nedjai, B.; Hurst, T.; Pennington, D.J. Cytokines and chemokines: At the crossroads of cell signalling and inflammatory disease. *Biochim. Biophys. Acta* **2014**, *1843*, 2563–2582. [CrossRef] [PubMed]
7. Montane, J.; Cadavez, L.; Novials, A. Stress and the inflammatory process: A major cause of pancreatic cell death in type 2 diabetes. *Diabets Metab. Syndr. Obes.* **2014**, *7*, 25–34.
8. Ndiaye, F.; Vuong, T.; Duarte, J.; Aluko, R.E.; Matar, C. Anti-oxidant, anti-inflammatory and immunomodulating properties of an enzymatic protein hydrolysate from yellow field pea seeds. *Eur. J. Nutr.* **2012**, *51*, 29–37. [CrossRef]
9. Malaguti, M.; Dinelli, G.; Leoncini, E.; Bregola, V.; Bosi, S.; Cicero, A.F.; Hrelia, S. Bioactive peptides in cereals and legumes: Agronomical, biochemical and clinical aspects. *Int. J. Mol. Sci.* **2014**, *15*, 21120–21135. [CrossRef]
10. Cam, A.; de Mejia, E.G. RGD-peptide lunasin inhibits Akt-mediated NF-κB activation in human macrophages through interaction with the αVβ3 integrin. *Mol. Nutr. Food Res.* **2012**, *56*, 1569–1581. [CrossRef]
11. Millán-Linares, M.C.; Yust, M.M.; Alcaide-Hidalgo, J.M.; Millán, F.; Pedroche, J. Lupine protein hydrolysates inhibit enzymes involved in the inflammatory pathway. *Food Chem.* **2014**, *151*, 141–147. [CrossRef]
12. Millán-Linares, M.C.; Millán, F.; Pedroche, J.; Yust, M.M. GPETAFLR: A new anti-inflammatory peptide from *Lupinus angustifolius* L. protein hydrolysate. *J. Funct. Foods* **2015**, *18*, 358–367. [CrossRef]

13. Czubinski, J.; Barciszewski, J.; Gilski, M.; Szpotkowski, K.; Debski, J.; Lampart-Szczapa, E.; Jaskolski, M. Structure of γ-conglutin: Insight into the quaternary structure of 7S basic globulins from legumes. *Acta Crystallogr. D Biol. Crystallogr.* **2015**, *71*, 224–238. [CrossRef]
14. Terruzzi, I.; Senesi, P.; Magni, C.; Montesano, A.; Scarafoni, A.; Luzi, L.; Duranti, M. Insulin-mimetic action of conglutin-γ, a lupin seed protein, in mouse myoblasts. *Nutr. Metab. Cardiovasc. Dis.* **2011**, *21*, 197–205. [CrossRef]
15. Czubiński, J.; Montowska, M.; Fornal, E. Post-translational cleavage pattern of Lupinus angustifolius γ-conglutin. *J. Sci. Food Agric.* **2018**, *98*, 5212–5219. [CrossRef]
16. Halban, P.A.; Polonsky, K.S.; Bowden, D.W.; Hawkins, M.A.; Ling, C.; Mather, K.J.; Powers, A.C.; Rhodes, C.J.; Sussel, L.; Weir, G.C. β-cell failure in type 2 diabetes: Postulated mechanisms and prospects for prevention and treatment. *J. Clin. Endocriol. Metab.* **2014**, *99*, 1983–1992. [CrossRef]
17. Donath, M.Y.; Shoelson, S.E. Type 2 diabetes as an inflammatory disease. *Nat. Rev. Immunol.* **2011**, *11*, 98–107. [CrossRef]
18. Wang, C.; Guan, Y.; Yang, J. Cytokines in the progression of pancreatic β-cell dysfunction. *Int. J. Endocrinol.* **2010**, *2010*, 515136. [CrossRef]
19. Boudjou, S.; Oomah, B.D.; Zaidi, F.; Hosseinian, F. Phenolics content and antioxidant and anti-inflammatory activities of legume fractions. *Food Chem.* **2013**, *138*, 1543–1550. [CrossRef]
20. Lima-Cabello, E.; Alche, V.; Foley, R.C.; Andrikopoulos, S.; Morahan, G.; Singh, K.B.; Alché, J.D.; Jimenez-Lopez, J.C. Narrow-leafed lupin (*Lupinus angustifolius* L.) β-conglutin proteins modulate the insulin signalling pathway as potential type 2 diabetes treatment and inflammatory-related disease amelioration. *Mol. Nutr. Food Res.* **2017**, *61*, 1600819. [CrossRef]
21. Russell, M.A.; Morgan, N.G. The impact of anti-inflammatory cytokines on the pancreatic β-cell. *Islets* **2014**, *6*, 950547. [CrossRef]
22. Tanabe, K.; Amo-Shiinoki, K.; Hatanaka, M.; Tanizawa, Y. Interorgan crosstalk contributing to β-cell dysfunction. *J. Diabetes Res.* **2017**, *2017*, 3605178. [CrossRef]
23. Imai, Y.; Dobrian, A.D.; Morris, M.A.; Nadler, J.L. Islet inflammation: A unifying target for diabetes treatment? *Trends Endocrinol. Metab.* **2013**, *24*, 351–360. [CrossRef]
24. Gurzov, E.N.; Ortis, F.; Cunha, D.A.; Gosset, G.; Li, M.; Cardozo, A.K. Signaling by IL-1beta+IFN-gamma and ER stress converge on DP5/Hrk activation: A novel mechanism for pancreatic beta-cell apoptosis. *Cell Death Differ.* **2009**, *16*, 1539–1550. [CrossRef]
25. Ramadan, J.W.; Steiner, S.R.; Christina, M.; O'Neill, C.; Nunemaker, S. The central role of calcium in the effects of cytokines on beta-cell function: Implications for type 1 and type 2 diabetes. *Cell Calcium* **2011**, *50*, 481–490. [CrossRef]
26. Chang, I.; Cho, N.; Kim, S.; Kim, J.Y.; Kim, E.; Woo, J.E.; Nam, J.H.; Kim, S.J.; Lee, S.M. Role of calcium in pancreatic islet cell death by IFN/TNF. *J. Immunol.* **2004**, *1*, 7008–7014. [CrossRef]
27. Sekine, N.; Ishikawa, T.; Okazaki, T.; Hayashi, M.; Wollheim, C.B.; Fujita, T. Synergistic activation of NF-κB and inducible isoform of nitric oxide synthase induction by interferon-γ and tumor necrosis factor-α in INS-1 cells. *J. Cell. Physiol.* **2000**, *184*, 46–57. [CrossRef]
28. Salim, T.; Sershen, C.L.; May, E.E. Investigating the role of TNF-α and IFN-γ activation on the dynamics of iNOS gene expression in LPS stimulated macrophages. *PLoS ONE* **2016**, *11*, e0153289. [CrossRef]
29. Liu, J.; Cao, S.; Kim, S.; Chung, E.I.; Homma, Y.; Guan, X.; Violeta, J.; Ma, X.J. Interleukin-12: An update on its immunological activities, signalling and regulation of gene expression. *Curr. Immunol. Rev.* **2005**, *1*, 119–137. [CrossRef]
30. Marwaha, A.K.; Tan, S.; Dutz, J.P. Targeting the IL-17/IFN-γ axis as a potential new clinical therapy for type 1 diabetes. *Clin. Immunol.* **2014**, *154*, 84–89. [CrossRef]
31. Kawaguchi, M.; Adachi, M.; Oda, N.; Kokubu, F.; Huang, S.K. IL-17 cytokine family. *J. Allergy Clin. Immunol.* **2004**, *114*, 1265–1273. [CrossRef]
32. Vanbervliet, B.; Homey, B.; Durand, I.; Massacrier, C.; Aït-Yahia, S.; de Bouteiller, O.; Vicari, A.; Caux, C. Sequential involvement of CCR2 and CCR6 ligands for immature dendritic cell recruitment: Possible role at inflamed epithelial surfaces. *Eur. J. Immunol.* **2002**, *32*, 231–242. [CrossRef]
33. Chen, L.; Chen, R.; Wang, H.; Liang, F. Mechanisms linking inflammation to insulin resistance. *Int. J. Endocrinol.* **2015**, *2015*, 508409. [CrossRef]

34. Jaldin-Fincati, J.R.; Pavarotti, M.; Frendo-Cumbo, S.; Bilan, P.J.; Klip, A. Update on GLUT4 Vesicle Traffic: A Cornerstone of Insulin Action. *Trends Endocrinol. Metab.* **2017**, *28*, 597–611. [CrossRef]
35. Tangvarasittichai, S. Oxidative stress, insulin resistance, dyslipidemia and type 2 diabetes mellitus. *World J. Diabetes* **2015**, *6*, 456–480. [CrossRef]
36. Ighodaro, O.M.; Akinloy, O.A. First line defence antioxidants-superoxide dismutase (SOD), catalase (CAT) and glutathione peroxidase (GPX): Their fundamental role in the entire antioxidant defence grid. *Alex. J. Med.* **2018**, *54*, 287–293. [CrossRef]
37. Hurrle, S.; Hsu, W.H. The etiology of oxidative stress in insulin resistance. *Biomed. J.* **2017**, *40*, 257–262. [CrossRef]
38. Sharma, J.N.; Al-Omran, A.; Parvathy, S.S. Role of nitric oxide in inflammatory diseases. *Inflammopharmacology* **2007**, *15*, 252–259. [CrossRef]
39. McDaniel, M.L.; Kwon, G.; Hill, J.R.; Marshall, C.A.; Corbett, J.A. Cytokines and nitric oxide in islet inflammation and diabetes. *Proc. Soc. Exp. Biol. Med.* **1996**, *211*, 24–32. [CrossRef]
40. Fujimoto, M.; Shimizu, N.; Kunii, K.; Martyn, J.A.; Ueki, K.; Kaneki, M. A role for iNOS in fasting hyperglycemia and impaired insulin signalling in the liver of obese diabetic mice. *Diabetes* **2005**, *54*, 1340–1348. [CrossRef]
41. Dalle-Donne, I.; Rossi, R.; Giustarini, D.; Milzani, A.; Colombo, R. Protein carbonyl groups as biomarkers of oxidative stress. *Clin. Chim. Acta* **2003**, *329*, 23–38. [CrossRef]
42. Tripathi, P.; Tripathi, P.; Kashyap, L.; Singh, V. The role of nitric oxide in inflammatory reactions. *FEMS Immunol. Med. Microbiol.* **2007**, *51*, 443–452. [CrossRef] [PubMed]

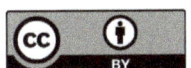

© 2019 by the authors. Licensee MDPI, Basel, Switzerland. This article is an open access article distributed under the terms and conditions of the Creative Commons Attribution (CC BY) license (http://creativecommons.org/licenses/by/4.0/).

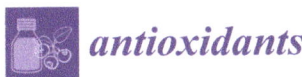

Article

In Vitro Antioxidant, Antiinflammation, and Anticancer Activities and Anthraquinone Content from *Rumex crispus* Root Extract and Fractions

Taekil Eom [1], Ekyune Kim [2,*] and Ju-Sung Kim [1,*]

[1] Majors in Plant Resource and Environment, College of Agriculture & Life Sciences, SARI, Jeju National University, Jeju 63243, Korea; taekil7@hanmail.net
[2] College of Pharmacy, Catholic University of Daegu, Gyeongsan 38430, Korea
* Correspondence: ekyune@cu.ac.kr (E.K.); aha2011@jejunu.ac.kr (J.-S.K.); Tel.: +82-53-850-3619 (E.K.); +82-64-754-3314 (J.-S.K.)

Received: 10 July 2020; Accepted: 7 August 2020; Published: 10 August 2020

Abstract: *Rumex crispus* is a perennial plant that grows in humid environments across Korea. Its roots are used in traditional Korean medicine to treat several diseases, including diseases of the spleen and skin and several inflammatory pathologies. In this study, different solvent fractions (*n*-hexane, dichloromethane, ethyl acetate, *n*-butanol, and aqueous fractions) from an ethanol extract of *R. crispus* roots were evaluated for the presence and composition of anthraquinone compounds and antioxidants by checking for such things as free radical scavenging activity, and electron and proton atom donating ability. In addition, anti-inflammatory activity was measured by NO scavenging activity and inflammatory cytokine production; furthermore, anti-cancer activity was measured by apoptosis-inducing ability. Polyphenolic and flavonoid compounds were shown to be abundant in the dichloromethane and ethyl acetate fractions, which also exhibited strong antioxidant activity, including free radical scavenging and positive results in FRAP, TEAC, and ORAC assays. HPLC analysis revealed that the dichloromethane fractions had higher anthraquinone contents than the other fractions; the major anthraquinone compounds included chrysophanol, emodin, and physcione. In addition, results of the anti-inflammatory assays showed that the ethyl acetate fraction showed appreciable reductions in the levels of nitric oxide and inflammatory cytokines (TNF-α, IL-1β, and IL-6) in Raw 264.7 cells. Furthermore, the anthraquinone-rich dichloromethane fraction displayed the highest anticancer activity when evaluated in a human hepatoma cancer cell line (HepG2), in which it induced increased apoptosis mediated by p53 and caspase activation.

Keywords: anthraquinone; free radical scavenging; inflammatory cytokines; apoptosis; *Rumex crispus*

1. Introduction

Reactive oxygen species (ROS), also known as oxygen-centered free radicals, are produced during normal metabolic processes and play an essential role in maintaining cellular homeostasis. ROS levels can increase as a result of exposure to chemical substances or other environmental stress resulting in oxidative stress [1]. When the intrinsic antioxidant system within an organism is damaged, it is not possible to remove these free radicals and the resulting oxidative stress can lead to various chronic diseases. A state of chronic oxidative stress can cause oxidative damage to various cellular components, including cell membranes, DNA, and proteins. It can also result in the activation of systemic chronic inflammatory responses via a number of different intracellular signaling pathways, ultimately exacerbating a variety of pathological conditions, including cardiovascular diseases, cancer, dementia, diabetes, autoimmune disorders, and aging [2]. One of the underlying signaling mechanisms triggered by excessive ROS generation is the activation of nuclear transcription factor κB (NF-κB), which acts as a transcriptional regulator of the innate immune system and can stimulate the release of a variety of pro-inflammatory cytokines from various tissues [3,4].

Inflammation is one of the self-defense responses used by organisms to defend against a wide range of external stimuli; however, excessive or prolonged inflammation can lead to the development of serious pathologies. The inflammatory response is characterized by the activation of macrophages and subsequent increases in the secretions of nitric oxide (NO), pro-inflammatory cytokines such as interleukin-1β (IL-1β), interleukin-6 (IL-6), and tumor necrosis factor-α (TNF-α), and cell adhesion molecules [5]. ROS-mediated chronic inflammatory responses can be inhibited by antioxidants. Various antioxidant compounds have been described in the literature with varying degrees of efficacy. The versatility of these compounds makes them ideal candidates for novel therapies. Various natural products have been shown to exhibit antioxidant properties and hence this is a growing field of interest. Plants have been identified as an especially rich source of antioxidant compounds, with most containing phenolic groups, which are known to play a crucial role in the removal of ROS. These phenolic compounds are generally secondary metabolites involved in stress responses and are known to perform various physiological functions, including antioxidant, anti-inflammatory, and anticancer functions [6,7]. The *Rumex* genus belongs to the Polygonaceae family and includes *R. crispus*, *R. acetosella*, *R. acetosa*, *R. aquatica*, *R. longifolius*, *R. gmelini*, *R. conglomeratus*, and *R. maritimus*. *R. crispus* is a perennial plant endemic to Korea which is found growing in humid environments. Its roots have been used as traditional medicinal materials in the treatment of several pathological conditions, including bladder infections, gallbladder disease, skin disease, and lymph node disorders. They have also been used as an adjuvant therapy in oriental medicine strategies used to treat cancer [8,9]. Several bioactive components of *R. crispus* have been identified and include saponins, tannins, flavonoids, essential oils, and anthraquinone derivatives such as chrysophanol and emodin [10–12]. This study was designed to evaluate the potential of new bioactive substances from *R. crispus* identified by analyzing their antioxidant, anti-inflammatory, and anticancer activities using root extracts and various extract fractions.

2. Materials and Methods

2.1. Materials

2,2-Diphenyl-1-picrylhydrazyl (DPPH), 2,2'-azobis(2-methylpropionamidine) dihydrochloride (AAPH), 2,2'-azino-bis(3-ethylbenzothiazoline-6-sulfonic acid) diammonium salt (ABTS), 2',7'-dichlorofluorescin (DCFH), trolox, Folin-Ciocalteu reagent, 2,4,6-tris (2-pyridyl)-s-triazine (TPTZ), gallic acid, quercetin, trichloroacetic acid (TCA), aluminum chloride hexahydrate (AlCl$_3$·6H$_2$O), phenazine methosulphate (PMS), β-nicotinamide adenine dinucleotide reduced disodium salt (NADH), nitro blue tetrazolium tablet (NBT), thiazolyl blue tetrazolium bromide (MTT), dimethyl sulfoxide (DMSO), and lipopolysaccharide (LPS) were purchased from Sigma-Aldrich (St. Louis, MO, USA). The human hepatoma cancer cell line HepG2 and mouse macrophage cell line Raw 264.7 were obtained from the American Type Culture Collection (Manassas, VA, USA). All western blot antibodies were obtained from Santa Cruz Biotechnology (Logan, UT, USA). All other chemicals used in this study were at least 99% pure.

2.2. Preparation of Extracts and Fractions

Dried *R. crispus* root powder was extracted three times using ten times its weight of ethanol and subjected to reflux for 12 h. After drying by evaporation in a vacuum rotary evaporator, the extract was suspended in water and fractionated with *n*-hexane (HF), dichloromethane (DCMF), ethyl acetate (EAF), *n*-butanol, (BF), and water (AF) three times, respectively. A total of five fractions were obtained after the solvents were removed.

2.3. Determination of Total Phenol and Flavonoid Contents

The total phenolic content was quantified using Folin–Ciocalteu reagent and a Gallic acid standard [13]. Briefly, 100 µL of each sample solution (1 mg/mL) was mixed in a test tube containing 3.5 mL distilled water and 500 µL 50% Folin–Ciocalteu reagent. The mixture was then allowed to react for 2 h, after which 500 µL of 20% Na_2CO_3 was added. The mixture was then placed in a dark room for 1 h, and the absorbance at 720 nm was recorded using a SpectraMax $M2^e$ microplate reader (Molecular Device, Sunnyvale, CA, USA). The total phenolic contents are expressed as gallic acid equivalents (mM GAE/g).

To analyze total flavonoid content of each sample, 500 µL of each sample (1 mg/mL) was mixed with 100 µL of 10% (w/v) aluminum chloride and 100 µL of 1.0 M potassium acetate. Then, 1.5 mL of ethanol and 2.8 mL of distilled water were added and mixed in. The mixture was then placed in a dark room for 1 h, and the absorbance at 415 nm was recorded using a SpectraMax $M2^e$ microplate reader [14]. The total flavonoid content is expressed as quercetin equivalents (mM QE/g).

2.4. HPLC Analysis of Anthraquinone Derivative

Anthraquinone derivatives in the R. crispus extracts and solvent fractions were analyzed using high performance liquid chromatography coupled with a PDA detection system (Shimadzu Prominence, Japan). The analysis was performed on a Triat C-18 column (250 mm × 4.6 mm, 5 µm) from YMC Co., Ltd. The column temperature was set to 40 °C and the detection wavelength was set to 450 nm. The mobile phase consisted of water containing 0.1% TFA (Trifluoro aceticacid) and 0.1% TFA containing methanol (B) with the gradient program set as follows: isocratic 20% B at 0–5 min, linear gradient 20–80% B at 5–15 min, linear gradient 80–90% B at 15–30 min, linear gradient 90–100% B at 30–35 min, isocratic 100% B at 35–40 min with flow rate of 1.0 mL/min.

2.5. DPPH Radical Scavenging Activity

The DPPH radical scavenging effect was evaluated using the published method with slight modifications [15]. Briefly, 160 µL of 1.5×10^{-4} M DPPH solution was mixed with 40 µL of a sample solution, incubated at room temperature for 30 min, and then absorbance at 540 nm was evaluated using a SpectraMax $M2^e$ microplate reader. The scavenging activity of the DPPH radicals was calculated as follows: ((Abs blank−Abs sample)/Abs blank) × 100. The radical scavenging activity was expressed as a concentration that inhibited the radicals by 50%.

2.6. Hydroxyl Radical Scavenging Activity

The hydroxyl radical scavenging activity was determined using the method described by Label and Bondy [16]. Briefly, the sample was mixed with 1 mM H_2O_2 and 0.2 mM $FeSO_4$, and incubated at 37 °C for 5 min. Esterase-treated 2 µM DCHF-DA was then added and the change in fluorescence was monitored on a SpectraMax $M2^e$ microplate reader, with excitation and emission wavelengths of 460 nm and 530 nm, respectively, for 30 min. The scavenging activity of the hydroxyl radicals was calculated as follows: ((FLU blank−FLU sample)/FLU blank) × 100. The radical scavenging activity was expressed as a concentration that inhibited the radicals by 50%.

2.7. Superoxide Radical Scavenging Activity

The superoxide radical scavenging effect was evaluated using the method reported by Liu et al. [17] with minor modifications. Briefly, the reagent mixture containing a 50 µL aliquot of a sample solution, 50 µL of 150 µM NBT, 50 µL of 468 µM NADH, and 50 µL of 60 µM phenazine methosulfate was incubated at room temperature for 5 min. The absorbance was measured at 560 nm and compared to the blank, and the superoxide anion radical scavenging activity was then calculated using the following equation: Scavenging effect, % = ((Abs sample − Abs blank)/Abs blank) × 100. The radical scavenging activity was expressed as a concentration that inhibited the radicals by 50%.

2.8. TEAC Assay

The TEAC method is based on the reaction of ABTS$^{•+}$ ions and was carried out according to the method described by Zulueta et al. [18] with minor modifications. An ABTS$^{•+}$ working solution was prepared daily by diluting the ABTS$^{•+}$ stock solution with distilled water to get an absorbance of 0.07 ± 0.02 at 734 nm. Briefly, 50 µL aliquots of the sample solutions were each mixed with 1.0 mL ABTS$^{•+}$ working solution. Each mixture was incubated at 25 °C in the dark for 5 min and absorbance was measured using a SpectraMax M2^e microplate reader at 734 nm. The sample extract activity was expressed as mM trolox/g dry sample and all determinations were carried out in triplicate.

2.9. ORAC Assay

ORAC measures the antioxidant inhibition of peroxyl-radical-induced oxidations and reflects radical chain-breaking antioxidant activity by H-atom transfer. This assay is based on the scavenging of peroxyl radicals generated by AAPH, which prevents the degradation of the fluorescein probe, and consequently, prevents the loss of fluorescence. For this study, we used the method described by Zulueta et al. [18]. A 75 mM phosphate buffer (pH 7.4) was used for all sample dilutions and reagent preparations. Aliquots of the sample extractions (50 µL) and the 150 µL 75 nM fluorescein solutions were placed in 96-black well microplates. The mixture was preincubated for 10 min at 37 °C. The reaction was initiated by adding 25 µL of 120 mM AAPH solution and the changes in the fluorescence were monitored using a SpectraMax M2^e microplate reader, with excitation and emission wavelengths of 460 nm and 530 nm, respectively, for 60 min. The sample extract activity was expressed as mM of trolox/g dry sample and all determinations were carried out in triplicate.

2.10. FRAP Assay

The FRAP value was determined using the method described by Benzie et al. [19] with slight modifications. Briefly, 50 µL aliquots of the sample extracts each were mixed with 1.5 mL FRAP working reagent prepared fresh daily. The FRAP working reagent consisted of 10 volumes of 300 mM acetate buffer (pH 3.6) mixed with 10 volumes of 20 mM FeCl$_3$. In addition, one volume of 10 mM TPTZ in 40 mM HCl, was also added to each sample and the final mixture was incubated at 37 °C in the dark for 30 min. Absorbance was measured after 30 min at 593 nm. The activities of each extract are expressed as mM of FeSO$_4$/g dry sample and all determinations were carried out in triplicate.

2.11. Cell Culture and Cell Viability Assays

HepG2 and Raw 264.7 cells were cultured in Dulbecco's modified Eagle's medium supplemented with 10% heated-inactivated fetal bovine serum, penicillin (100 U/mL), and streptomycin (100 µg/mL) at 37 °C in a humidified atmosphere of 95% air and 5% CO$_2$. The medium was changed every other day. Cell viability was measured using the MTT assay, which is based on the conversion of MTT to formazan crystals by mitochondrial dehydrogenases. Cells were cultured in 96-well plates (2.0×10^4 cells/well) with serum free media and treated with different concentrations of sample for 24 h. The R. crispus extracts and its solvent fractions were dissolved in 10% DMSO. The final concentration of DMSO in the culture medium never exceeded 0.1%. For the assay, 100 µL of MTT solution was added to each well and incubated for 4 h. Finally, 200 µL of DMSO was added to dissolve the formazan crystals and the absorbance was measured using a SpectraMax M2^e microplate reader at 540 nm.

2.12. NO Production

Raw 264.7 cells were cultured in 96-well plates using media without phenol red and pre-treated for 1 h with each of the test substrates. Cellular NO production was induced by adding 1 µg/mL LPS and incubating the mixture for 24 h. After incubation, 50 µL of conditioned media containing nitrite (primary stable oxidation product of NO) was mixed with the same volume of Griess reagent and incubated for 15 min. Absorbance of the mixture was measured using a SpectraMax M2^e microplate reader at 550 nm.

2.13. Cytokine Analysis

Production of IL-1β, IL-6, and TNF-α in Raw 264.7 cells was evaluated using Quantikine ELISA kits (R&D Systems, Minneapolis, MN, USA) as per the manufacturer's instructions. Cells were treated with different concentrations of test materials for 1 h and production of IL-1β, IL-6, and TNF-α was stimulated by adding 1 µg/mL LPS and incubating for a further 24 h. The supernatant was collected and the concentrations of IL-1β, IL-6, and TNF-α were quantified using the relevant kit protocol.

2.14. Annexin V-FITC/PI Analysis

To determine the magnitude of the apoptosis induced by DCMF, an Annexin V-fluorescein isothiocyanate (FITC) apoptosis detection kit (BD Pharmingen, San Diego, CA, USA) was used. Briefly, the cells were harvested, washed with PBS and binding buffer, and then stained with FITC-conjugated Annexin V and propidium iodide (PI) for 30 min in the dark. The mixture was then analyzed using an LSR Fortessa flow cytometer (Becton Dickinson, San Jose, CA, USA) according to the manufacturer's protocol.

2.15. Western Blot

HepG2 cells were cultured in DMEM at a density of 1×10^4 cells in 10 cm^2 cell culture dishes and incubated for 24 h. The cells were treated with different concentrations of DCMF for 24 h. The cells were lysed using RIPA buffer (Sigma-Aldrich, St. Louis, MO, USA) and supernatants were treated with a protease inhibitor cocktail and centrifuged at 2300× g for 10 min to remove the insoluble fraction. The protein concentrations of the supernatants were determined using a BCA protein assay kit (Thermo Science, Rockford, IL, USA).

The same amounts of cell lysates were analyzed on 10% SDS-PAGE and the proteins were blotted onto immuno-blot nitro-cellulose membranes and blocked with 5% BSA in TBS containing 0.1% Tween 20 (TBS-T) for 1 h. Then the primary monoclonal antibodies were added to the TBS-T (1:1000 dilutions) and incubated overnight. Antibody binding was detected using a horseradish peroxidase secondary antibody and enhanced using a chemi-luminescence ECL assay kit (Bio-Rad, Hercules, CA, USA) according to the manufacturer's instructions and imaged on a FUJIFILM LAS-4000 mini system (Tokyo, Japan). The basal levels of the proteins were normalized against β-actin or β-tubulin.

2.16. Statistical Analysis

Each experiment was performed at least three times and results are presented as means ± SDs (standard deviations). Statistical comparisons of the mean values were performed using one-way ANOVA followed by Duncan's multiple range test using Minitab 17 software (Minitab Inc., IL, USA, State College, PA, USA). Differences were considered significant at $p < 0.05$.

3. Results and Discussion

3.1. Analysis of Polyphenol, Flavonoid, and Anthraquinone Contents

Polyphenols are aromatic compounds containing more than two phenolic hydroxyl groups. They are classified into phenolic acids (e.g., caffeic acid and chlorogenic acid) and flavonoids (e.g., kaempferol and catechin) [20]. The total polyphenol and flavonoid contents for each of the extracts are described in Table 1. Analysis of the total polyphenol and flavonoid content in the *R. crispus* extracts and solvent fractions revealed that polyphenol content was highest in the ethyl acetate fraction (EAF), followed by the dichloromethane fraction (DCMF), ethanol extract (EE), aqueous fraction (AF), butanol fraction (BF), and finally, the hexane fraction (HF). The highest flavonoid content was detected in the DCMF, followed by HF, EAF, EE, AF, and BF. The antioxidant activity of polyphenolic compounds is attributed to their activities as electron donors and free radical scavengers. Therefore, the antioxidant effects of various plant extracts have been shown to be strongly linked with the relative phenolic content [21,22].

Table 1. Total phenolic and flavonoid contents of *Rumex crispus* L. root extracts and fractions [1].

Samples [2]	Total Phenols (mg GAE/g)	Total Flavonoids (mg QE/g)
EE	21.84 ± 1.15 [c]	14.58 ± 0.61 [d]
HF	10.68 ± 0.06 [e]	24.15 ± 0.47 [b]
DCMF	28.16 ± 1.42 [b]	30.67 ± 0.97 [a]
EAF	83.26 ± 2.49 [a]	21.31 ± 0.33 [c]
BF	19.03 ± 1.04 [c,d]	11.28 ± 0.40 [e]
AF	19.79 ± 0.32 [c,d]	11.52 ± 0.70 [e]

[1] Values are each expressed as a mean ± SD ($n = 3$). [2] EE: ethanol extracts. HF: *n*-hexane fractions. DCMF: dichloromethane fraction. EAF: ethyl acetate fraction. BF: *n*-buthanol fractions. AF: aqueous fraction. [a–e] Means with different superscripts in the same column are significantly different at $p < 0.05$.

An HPLC-DAD method was applied to identify the five anthraquinones, including aloeemodin, chrysophanol, emodin, physcion, and rhein, in *R. crispus* extracts and solvent fractions. Figure S1 shows the typical chromatograms of the standard solution containing the five anthraquinones and the *R. crispus* extracts and solvent fractions. The retention times of the aloeemodin, rhein, emodin, chrysophanol, and physcion were 22.2, 23.7, 27.3, 29.9, and 33.2 min, respectively (Figure S1). The concentrations of the major anthraquinones from *R. crispus* extracts and solvent fraction are summarized in Table 2. The major anthraquinones found in the samples analyzed in this study were chrysophanol, emodin, and physcion. The anthraquinone content was highest in the DCMF, followed by HF, EE, EAF, and BF. One gram of DCMF contained 66.96 mg chrysophanol, 160.43 mg emodin, and 34.90 mg physcion. One gram of HF contained 48.64 mg chrysophanol, 14.64 mg emodin, and 15.43 mg physcion. However, none of the anthraquinone compounds were detected in the AF. Anthraquinone derivatives are naturally occurring quinone compounds including naphthoquinones and benzoquinones, and are present in large quantities in plants such as Polygonaceae (*Rheum*, *Rumex*), Fabaceae (*Cassia*), Liliaceae (*Aloe*), Rhamnaceae (*Rhamnus*), and Rubiaceae (*Asperula*, *Coelospermum*, *Coprosma*, *Galium*, *Morinda*, and *Rubia*) [23]. Lim et al. [24] analyzed the anthraquinone contents of various *Rumex* species and found that emodin was highest in *R. crispus*. In addition, Smolarz et al. [25] investigated the anthraquinone contents of various *Rumex* species and found that the highest anthraquinone concentrations were found in the root extracts, with these extracts having substantially higher concentrations than those of the fruit extracts (70-fold) and the leaf extracts (10-fold). Most of these compounds are nonpolar with a 9,10-anthracenedione basic structure—a tricyclic aromatic organic compound with a formula of $C_{14}H_8O_2$, which is extracted by polar solvents like ethanol/water mixtures, ethanol, methanol, and acetone [26]. It has also been reported that these compounds are well dispersed in nonpolar solvents, such as hexane and dichloromethane [27].

Table 2. Anthraquinone derivative contents of *Rumex crispus* L. root extracts and fractions [1].

Samples [2]	Concentration (mg/g)					
	Aloeemodin	Chrysophanol	Emodin	Physcion	Rhein	Total
EE	0.141 ± 0.002 [c]	9.714 ± 0.02 [c]	8.779 ± 0.011 [d]	4.282 ± 0.006 [c]	0.057 ± 0.002 [d]	22.97 ± 0.026 [c]
HF	0.048 ± 0.006 [e]	48.644 ± 0.171 [b]	14.64 ± 0.037 [b]	15.433 ± 0.058 [b]	0.106 ± 0.001 [c]	79.095 ± 0.259 [b]
DCMF	0.595 ± 0.003 [a]	66.964 ± 0.244 [a]	160.434 ± 0.651 [a]	34.896 ± 0.109 [a]	0.466 ± 0.002 [a]	263.356 ± 0.666 [a]
EAF	0.218 ± 0.001 [b]	3.154 ± 0.009 [d]	13.627 ± 0.053 [c]	1.722 ± 0.006 [d]	0.151 ± 0.002 [b]	18.923 ± 0.062 [d]
BF	0.181 ± 0.007 [d]	0.083 ± 0.002 [e]	0.639 ± 0.004 [e]	0.054 ± 0.002 [e]	0.001>	0.856 ± 0.006 [e]
AF	-	-	-	-	-	-

[1] Values are each expressed as a mean ± SD ($n = 3$). [2] EE: ethanol extracts. HF: *n*-hexane fractions. DCMF: dichloromethane fraction. EAF: ethyl acetate fraction. BF: *n*-buthanol fractions. AF: aqueous fraction. [a–e] Means with different superscripts in the same column are significantly different at $p < 0.05$.

3.2. Radical Scavenging Activities of R. crispus Extracts and Fractions

The DPPH radical scavenging assay is used to assess the electron-donating ability of antioxidants to quench free radicals. In *R. crispus* root extracts and fractions, we observed that DPPH radical scavenging was the highest in the EAF, followed by the EE, BF, DCMF, and HF (Table 3). While the antioxidant activities of *R. crispus* leaf and fruit extracts have been extensively studied, there is limited information on these activities in its root extracts. Yildirim et al. [28] have reported that DPPH radical scavenging activity is higher in *R. crispus* fruit extracts with high polyphenol content than in leaf extracts. Consistent with the findings of this study, the radical scavenging ability of *R. japonica* extracts and fractions has also been found to be highest in extracts with high polyphenol content and low in extracts with low polyphenol content [29].

We measured the scavenging capacities of these extracts for hydroxyl radicals using the Fenton reaction assay, which is based on fluorescence emission after hydroxyl radicals generated by H_2O_2 and Fe^{2+} via the Fenton reaction with DCFH. The scavenging ability increased in all the extracts and fractions in a concentration-dependent manner. This is similar to the results for Trolox, a well-known antioxidant. Anusuya et al. [30] have reported that the hydroxyl radical scavenging abilities of *Rubus nepalensis* extracts are closely related to their polyphenol contents. Moreover, phenolic hydroxyl groups are known to rapidly quench hydroxyl radicals by donating hydrogen atoms or electrons, as evidenced by measuring the hydroxyl radical scavenging abilities of various phenolic acids [31]. This study also demonstrated that the EAF and DCMF which both had high polyphenol and flavonoid contents also had the highest hydroxyl scavenging abilities (Table 3).

Superoxide radicals have very low reactivity; however, within the body, they are rapidly transformed into H_2O_2, and then via the Fenton reaction, to highly reactive hydroxyl radicals, which interact with biomolecules, causing tissue damage. As with hydroxyl radical scavenging, the superoxide radical scavenging ability of *R. crispus* root extracts was strongest in the EAF and DCMF, followed by EE, BF, AF, and HF (Table 3). In a study of the antioxidant properties of *Rumex hastatus* extracts and fractions, superoxide radical scavenging ability has been linked to flavonoid content rather than phenolic content [32]. The present study showed that the EAF and DCMF fractions, with high flavonoid content, exhibited the highest superoxide radical scavenging ability.

Table 3. Free radical scavenging activity of *Rumex crispus* L. root extracts and fractions [1].

Samples [2]	EC_{50} [3]		
	DPPH Radical	Hydroxyl Radical	Superoxide Radical
EE	46.5 ± 2.6 [b]	19.65 ± 0.64 [c]	51.72 ± 2.00 [c]
HF	126.2 ± 1.3 [e]	62.47 ± 2.44 [f]	>200 [f]
DCMF	65.6 ± 1.2 [d]	0.54 ± 0.13 [a]	45.83 ± 2.00 [b]
EAF	11.9 ± 2.5 [a]	0.65 ± 0.06 [a]	4.45 ± 0.42 [a]
BF	55.1 ± 1.5 [c]	3.84 ± 0.35 [d]	61.00 ± 2.81 [d]
AF	44.2 ± 3.4 [b]	43.12 ± 0.00 [e]	71.29 ± 2.39 [e]

[1] Values are expressed as a mean ± SD ($n = 3$). [2] EE: ethanol extracts. HF: *n*-hexane fractions. DCMF: dichloromethane fraction. EAF: ethyl acetate fraction. BF: *n*-buthanol fractions. AF: aqueous fraction. [3] Effective concentration of substance that causes 50% inhibition. [a–e] Means with different superscripts in the same column are significantly different at $p < 0.05$.

3.3. Antioxidant Capacities of R. crispus Extracts and Fractions

The FRAP assay determines antioxidant activity by measuring electro transport. In this assay, the antioxidant activity was assessed by the reduction of Fe^{3+}-TPTZ to Fe^{2+}-TPTZ. The FRAP value of the extracts and fractions was the highest in the EAF, followed by the EE, AF, DCMF, BF, and HF (Table 4). The TEAC assay measures scavenging of $ABTS^+$ radicals by sulfur oxides through donation of hydrogen atoms or electrons, which are expressed as trolox equivalents. The highest electron-donating capacity was recorded for the EAF (5.65 mM TE/g), followed by the DCMF, EE, AF, BF, and HF

(Table 4). The ORAC assay is an experimental method recommended by the United States Department of Agriculture for the quantification of food antioxidant content based on electron transport capacity. Decomposition of AAPH produces peroxyl radicals, which react with fluorescein, leading to decreased fluorescence. Peroxyl radical scavenging measured as fluorescence reduction is then converted to trolox equivalents (TE). The ORAC value was highest in the EAF (4817 mM TE/g) and decreased in order from DCMF, to EE, then HF, then AF, and finally BF (Table 4).

The antioxidant capacities of R. crispus were highest in the EAF and DCMF, which is consistent with their total phenol and flavonoid contents. Similarly, the antioxidant activity of R. hastatus extracts has been reported to be highest in the EAF which has high total phenol and flavonoid concentrations [32]. Sahidi and Ambigaipalan [33] have reported that food antioxidant capacity is closely related to the total phenolic and flavonoid contents and have attributed it to the electron or H-atom-donating ability of phenolic hydroxyl groups. In this study, the antioxidant capacities were highest in the EAF and DCMF, which is consistent with their higher concentrations of phenolic and flavonoid compounds.

Table 4. FRAP, TEAC, and ORAC values of *Rumex crispus* L. root extracts and fractions [1].

Samples [2]	FRAP (mM FeSO$_4$/g)	TEAC (mM TE/g)	ORAC (mM TE/g)
EE	48.14 ± 0.47 [b]	2.46 ± 0.11 [c]	1396 ± 204 [b,c]
HF	13.66 ± 0.15 [e]	0.43 ± 0.06 [f]	983 ± 88 [c,d]
DCMF	37.74 ± 0.77 [c,d]	3.56 ± 0.11 [b]	1790 ± 246 [b]
EAF	135.58 ± 3.62 [a]	5.65 ± 0.00 [a]	4817 ± 331 [a]
BF	33.06 ± 0.80 [d]	1.97 ± 0.13 [d]	909 ± 121 [d]
AF	40.83 ± 0.16 [c]	2.30 ± 0.13 [c]	945 ± 87 [d]

[1] Values are expressed as a mean ± SD ($n = 3$). [2] EE: ethanol extracts. HF: *n*-hexane fractions. DCMF: dichloromethane fraction. EAF: ethyl acetate fraction. BF: *n*-buthanol fractions. AF: aqueous fraction. [a–e] Means with different superscripts in the same column are significantly different at $p < 0.05$.

3.4. Anti-Inflammation Activities of R. crispus Extracts and Fractions

To assess the anti-inflammatory activities of R. crispus extracts and fractions, we measured their cytotoxicities in mouse leukemic monocyte macrophage cells (Raw 264.7). Raw 264.7 cells were treated with 25–400 μg/mL of R. crispus extracts and fractions, and cell survival was measured after 24 h using the WST-1 assay. Cell viabilities of R. crispus extracts and fractions are summarized in Figure 1A. The EE, BF, and AF did not show cytotoxicity within the indicated concentration range. The EE and HF were not cytotoxic at a concentration of 25–200 μg/mL, but at 400 μg/mL cell survival decreased to 75.24% and 60.94%, respectively. The EAF showed the highest cytotoxicity, decreasing cell survival to 60.20%, 2.62%, and 17.33% at 100, 200, and 400 μg/mL, respectively (Figure 1A).

Excessive NO production from L-arginine due to an overexpression of inducible NO synthase (iNOS) during acute or chronic inflammation is known to accelerate inflammatory responses [34]. We assessed the inhibition of NO production induced by LPS at non-cytotoxic concentrations (25 and 50 μg/mL) for each of the extract fractions. Consistent with the results of the antioxidant assays the EAF and DCMF showed the highest inhibitions of NO production, while other fractions did not exhibit any inhibitory effects (Figure 1B). Previous studies on the anti-inflammatory activities of R. crispus leaf extracts and fractions have also reported high levels of inflammatory activity in the DCMF and EAF, which agrees with the findings of this study [35]. Based on the results of the NO inhibition assay, we used the EAF for further cell-based experiments.

Cytokines play a pivotal role in inflammatory responses by directly affecting the proliferation and activity of immune cells [36]. Among the pro-inflammatory cytokines, TNF-α is an essential mediator in the development of systemic inflammatory responses, and its synthesis is increased by NO generated by LPS-stimulated macrophages. TNF-α increases the expressions of chemokines and cell adhesion molecules, thereby accelerating pro-inflammatory responses [37]. IL-1β and IL-6 are multifunctional cytokines secreted by macrophages activated by various pro-inflammatory stimuli; these cytokines are also implicated in the induction of autoimmune diseases, and they act by accelerating inflammatory responses through autocrine signaling [38]. Figure 2 shows the inhibition of IL-1β, IL-6, and TNF-α secretion following EAF treatment using the enzyme-linked immunosorbent assay (ELISA). The secretion of pro-inflammatory cytokines by Raw 264.7 cells was sharply increased following LPS stimulation and decreased after treatment with EAF in a concentration-dependent manner. IL-1β, IL-6, and TNF-α were suppressed by 28%, 65%, and 68%, respectively, when treated with 50 µg/mL EAF.

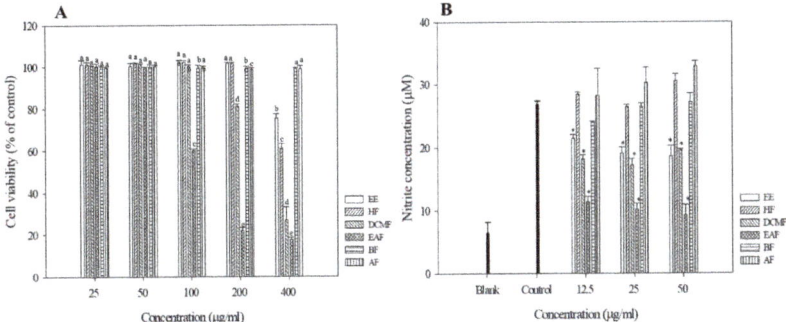

Figure 1. Cell viabilities of *R crispus* extracts and solvent fractions. (**A**) NO production (**B**) in Raw 264.7 cells. RAW 264.7 cells were treated with various concentrations (25, 50, 100, 200, 400 µg/mL) of *R. crispus* extracts and fractions for 24 h. Cell viability was measured by MTT assay. RAW 264.7 cells were pre-incubated with 12.5, 25, and 50 µg/mL of extracts and fractions for 1 h and then treated with 1 µg/mL of LPS for 24 h. The NO production was measured by the Griess reagent system. Data are represented as means ± SEMs. The different superscripts are significantly different at $p < 0.05$. * Statistical significance of the difference between LPS and LPS + sample treatment groups: * $p < 0.05$.

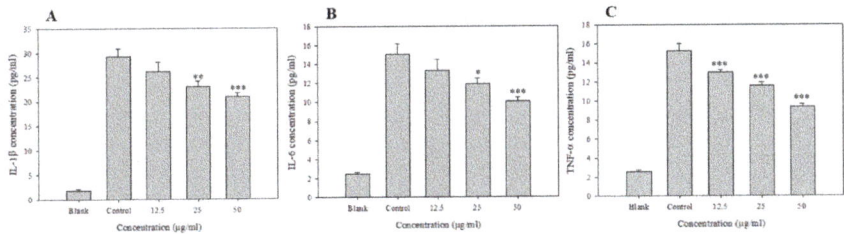

Figure 2. Inhibition of LPS induced IL-1b, IL-6 and TNF-a in the EAF. RAW 264.7 cells were preincubated with 12.5 or 25 µg/mL of EAF for 1 h and then treated with 1 µg/mL of LPS for 24 h. The IL-1β, IL-6, and TNF-α production was measured by ELISA, as described in Materials and Methods. Data are represented as means ± SEMs. * Statistical significance of the difference between LPS and LPS + sample treatment groups: * $p < 0.05$, ** $p < 0.01$, *** $p < 0.001$.

In a study of the anti-inflammatory activity in *R. crispus* leaf extracts and fractions, Im et al. [35] found that the EAF displayed higher concentration-dependent activity than the extracts in inhibiting the expression of COX-2 and iNOS involved in the production of PGE_2 and NO. In this study, the anti-inflammatory effects were verified by the reduced expression of all the pro-inflammatory cytokines apart from TNF-α [39].

3.5. Anticancer Activities of R. crispus Extracts and Fractions

We measured the cytotoxic activities of the fractions against the HepG2 human hepatoma cancer cell line. Among the extracts and fractions, anthraquinone-rich fractions HF and DCMF appeared to be the most potent inhibitors of HepG2 cell proliferation, but the other fractions showed no cytotoxicity. The DCMF inhibited cell growth in a dose-dependent manner. Treatment with HF for 24 h inhibited cell viability with rates of approximately 97%, 90%, 70%, 55%, and 35% at concentrations of 25, 50, 100, 200, and 400 μg/mL, respectively. Treatment with DCMF for 24 h resulted in inhibition of cell viability with rates of approximately 95%, 82%, 61%, 53%, and 27% at concentrations of 25, 50, 100, 200, and 400 μg/mL, respectively (Figure 3A).

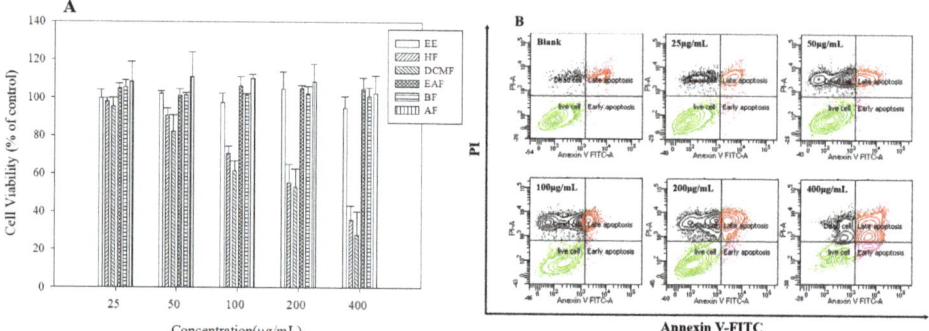

Figure 3. Cell viability of *R crispus* extracts and solvent fractions. (**A**) apoptosis induced (**B**) in HepG2 cells. HepG2 cells were treated with various concentrations (25, 50, 100, 200, 400 μg/mL) of *R. crispus* extracts and fractions for 24 h. Cell viability was measured by MTT assay. Flow cytometry analysis of apoptosis after exposure to various concentrations (25, 50, 100, 200, 400 μg/mL) of DCMF for 24 h, using annexin V-FITC/PI. The lower right indicates the percentage of early apoptotic cells; the upper right indicates the percentage of necrotic and late apoptotic cells.

A previous study has shown that anticancer activities of *Rumex* species are closely related to their anthraquinone contents [8,40]. In this study, anticancer activity was highest in the HF and DCMF, which is consistent with their anthraquinone content. Based on these results we used the DCMF for further cell-based experiments. As a decrease in cell proliferation may result from the induction of apoptosis, we investigated whether treatment with the DCMF induced apoptosis in HepG2 cells. HepG2 cells were treated with DCMF at various concentrations; then Annexin V-FITC and PI fluorescence was determined by flow cytometry (Figure 3B). After treatment with 50, 100, 150, and 200 μg/mL DCMF for 48 h, the percentages of apoptotic cells were 13.3%, 15.9%, 25.6%, and 71.3%, respectively. These results suggest that the DCMF inhibited the proliferation of HepG2 cells by inducing apoptosis in a concentration-dependent manner.

3.6. Modulation of Apoptotic Regulation

Bcl-2 proteins play a complex regulatory role in apoptosis [41]. Treatment with DCMF resulted in decreased Bcl-2 expression, while Bax protein expression was increased in a dose dependent manner. DCMF showed increased p53 tumor suppressor protein expression in HepG2 cells (Figure 4A). These results indicate that part of the DCMF-mediated inhibition of HepG2 cells is related to apoptosis through its effects of p53 and Bcl-2 protein expression. In order to determine whether this inhibition is related to the induction of apoptosis, HepG2 cells were exposed to DCMF and their caspase activity was evaluated. DCMF treatment resulted in increased levels of cleaved caspase-3, -8, and -9. This result was confirmed by the progressive proteolytic cleavage of the poly (ADP-ribose) polymerase (PARP), a downstream target of activated caspase, in HepG2 cells treated with DCMF (Figure 4B). These data agree with the other experiments that suggest that DCMF treatment induces apoptosis in HepG2 cells.

DCMF-induced apoptosis in HepG2 cell was confirmed by the characteristic pattern of Annexin V/PI staining, activation of caspases (-3, -8, and -9), and cleavage of PARP. Activated caspases regulate the execution-phases of cell apoptosis by degrading specific structural, regulatory, and DNA repair proteins within the cell [42]. Activated caspase-9 then initiates the proteolytic activity of other downstream caspases, such as caspase-3. The activation of caspase-3 results in the cleavage of key cellular proteins, such as PARP [43]. Tumor suppressor protein p53 also plays key roles in cell fate, cell growth, and death, via the regulation of the cell cycle proteins [44] and apoptosis induced proteins (Apaf1, Bad, Bax, and Fas) [45]. Treatment with DCMF decreased anti-apoptotic Bcl-2 protein and increased pro-apoptotic Bax protein expression. In addition, DCMF treatment increased p53 tumor suppressor protein levels. These results demonstrate that DCMF-induced apoptosis in HepG2 human hepatoma cancer cells is affected via the induction of p53, activation of Bax, inhibition of Bcl-2, processing of caspases, and cleavage of PARP.

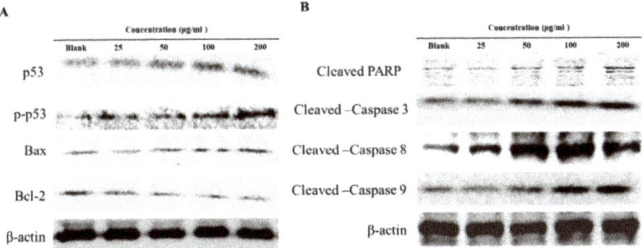

Figure 4. Effects of DCMF on the Bcl-2 family and p53 (**A**) and caspase family (**B**) protein expression in HepG2 cells. HepG2 were treated with the indicated concentrations of DCMF for 24 h. The equal amounts of cellular proteins were probed with the indicated antibodies, and the proteins were visualized using an ECL detection system. Actin was used as an internal control.

4. Conclusions

Several studies have demonstrated that natural polyphenol-containing products reduce ROS which are risk factors for age-related diseases. This study examined whether *R. crispus* extracts and fractions could exert any inhibitory effects on oxidative stress-related reactions and inflammation in vitro. The ethanol extracts of *R. crispus* were separated into hexane, dichloromethane, ethyl acetate, butanol, and aqueous fractions based on polarity. Antioxidant activity was evaluated using various assays and was shown to be highest in the DCMF and EAF, corresponding to their high polyphenol and flavonoid contents. In addition, the anti-inflammatory tests revealed that high antioxidant activity correlated with inhibitory effects on NO production, and that the EAF also reduced the secretion of pro-inflammatory cytokines in a concentration-dependent manner. In addition, DCMF was shown to inhibit HepG2 human hepatoma cancer cell growth and induce cellular apoptosis. DCMF-induced apoptosis is facilitated by p53 tumor suppressor protein-mediated Bcl-2 family protein regulation and caspase family protein activation. The results of this study suggest that *R. crispus* could be used as a natural alternative to synthetic antioxidants and anti-inflammatory agents.

Supplementary Materials: The following are available online at http://www.mdpi.com/2076-3921/9/8/726/s1, Figure S1: Chromatogram of *Rumex crispus* root extract and fractions at 420 nm. a: Aloe-emodin, b: Rhein, c: Emodin, d: Chrysophanol. e: Physcion (EE).

Author Contributions: Conceptualization, T.E. and J.-S.K.; formal analysis, J.-S.K.; investigation, E.K.; methodology, T.E. and E.K.; project administration, J.-S.K. and E.K.; writing—original draft, T.E. All authors have read and agreed to this version of the manuscript.

Funding: This research was supported as a Basic Science Research Program through the National Research Foundation of Korea (NRF) funded by the Ministry of Education (grant number 2013R1A1A2065215).

Conflicts of Interest: The authors have no conflicts of interest to declare.

References

1. Finkel, T. Signal transduction by reactive oxygen species. *J. Cell Biol.* **2011**, *194*, 7–15. [CrossRef] [PubMed]
2. Valko, M.; Leibfritz, D.; Moncol, J.; Cronin, M.T.; Mazur, M.; Telser, J. Free radicals and antioxidants in normal physiological functions and human disease. *Int. J. Biochem. Cell Biol.* **2007**, *39*, 44–84. [CrossRef] [PubMed]

3. Morgan, M.J.; Liu, Z.G. Crosstalk of reactive oxygen species and NF-kappaB signaling. *Cell Res.* **2011**, *21*, 103–115. [CrossRef] [PubMed]
4. Mittal, M.; Siddiqui, M.R.; Tran, K.; Reddy, S.P.; Malik, A.B. Reactive oxygen species in inflammation and tissue injury. *Antioxid. Redox Signal.* **2014**, *20*, 1126–1167. [CrossRef] [PubMed]
5. Grivennikov, S.I.; Greten, F.R.; Karin, M. Immunity, inflammation, and cancer. *Cell* **2010**, *140*, 883–899. [CrossRef] [PubMed]
6. Rahman, I.; Biswas, S.K.; Kirkham, P.A. Regulation of inflammation and redox signaling by dietary polyphenols. *Biochem. Pharmacol.* **2006**, *72*, 1439–1452. [CrossRef] [PubMed]
7. Haslam, E. Natural polyphenols (vegetable tannins) as drugs: Possible modes of action. *J. Nat. Prod.* **1996**, *59*, 205–215. [CrossRef]
8. Vasaa, A.; Orban-Gyapai, O.; Hohmann, J. The *Geneus Rumex*: Review of traditional uses, phytochemistry and pharmacoly. *J. Ethnopharmacol.* **2015**, *175*, 198–228. [CrossRef]
9. Bello, O.M.; Fasinu, P.S.; Bello, O.E.; Ogbesejana, A.B.; Adetunji, C.O.; Dada, A.O.; Ibitoye, O.S.; Aloko, S.; Oguntoye, O.S. Wild vegetable *Rumex acetosa* Linn.: Its ethonobotany, pharmacology and phytochemistry—A review. *S. Afr. J. Bot.* **2019**, *125*, 149–160. [CrossRef]
10. Yang, J.Y.; Wang, Z.Z.; Mao, X.J.; Xu, Q.L.; Lin, R.C.; Dai, Z. Determination of free and total anthraquinones in 3 kinds of *Rumex* by HPLC: A comparative study. *Chin. J. Pharm. Anal.* **2017**, *37*, 615–623.
11. Jang, S.J.; Kuk, Y.I. Effects of different fractions of *Rheum palmatum* root extract and anthraquinone compounds on fungicidal, insecticidal, and herbicidal activities. *J. Plant. Dis Protect.* **2018**, *125*, 451–460. [CrossRef]
12. Prateeksha; Yusuf, M.A.; Singh, B.N.; Sudheer, S.; Kharwar, R.N.; Siddiqui, S.; Abdel-Azeem, A.M.; Fraceto, L.F.; Dashora, K.; Gupta, V.K. Chrysophanol: A natural anthraquinone with multifaceted biotherapeutic potential. *Biomolecules* **2019**, *9*, 68. [CrossRef] [PubMed]
13. Singleton, V.L.; Orthofer, R.; Lamuela-Raventos, R.M. Analysis of total phenols and other oxidation substrates and antioxidants by means of Folin-Ciocalteu reagent. *Method Enzymol.* **1999**, *299*, 152–178.
14. Pekal, A.; Pyrzynska, K. Evaluation of aluminium complexation reaction for flavonoid content assay. *Food Anal. Method* **2014**, *7*, 1776–1782. [CrossRef]
15. Eom, T.K.; Senevirathne, M.; Kim, S.K. Synthesis of phenolic acid conjugated chitooligosaccharides and evaluation of their antioxidant activity. *Environ. Toxicol. Pharm.* **2012**, *34*, 519–527. [CrossRef]
16. Lebel, C.P.; Bondy, S.C. Sensitive and rapid quantitation of oxygen reactive species formation in rat synaptosomes. *Neurochem. Int.* **1990**, *17*, 435–440. [CrossRef]
17. Liu, F.; Ooi, V.E.C.; Chang, S.T. Free radical scavenging activities of mushroom polysaccharide extracts. *Life Sci.* **1997**, *60*, 763–771. [CrossRef]
18. Zulueta, A.; Esteve, M.J.; Frigola, A. ORAC and TEAC assays comparison to measure the antioxidant capacity of food products. *Food Chem.* **2009**, *114*, 310–316. [CrossRef]
19. Benzie, I.F.F.; Strain, J.J. Ferric reducing antioxidant power assay: Direct measure of total antioxidant activity of biological fluids and modified version for simultaneous measurement of total antioxidant power and ascorbic acid concentration. *Method Enzymol.* **1999**, *299*, 15–27.
20. Manach, C.; Scalbert, A.; Morand, C.; Remesy, C.; Jimenez, L. Polyphenols: Food sources and bioavailability. *Am. J. Clin. Nutr.* **2004**, *79*, 727–747. [CrossRef]
21. Kaur, C.; Kapoor, H.C. Anti-oxidant activity and total phenolic content of some Asian vegetables. *Int. J. Food Sci. Tech.* **2002**, *37*, 153–161. [CrossRef]
22. Maisuthisakul, P.; Suttajit, M.; Pongsawatmanit, R. Assessment of phenolic content and free radical-scavenging capacity of some Thai indigenous plants. *Food Chem.* **2007**, *100*, 1409–1418. [CrossRef]
23. Malik, E.M.; Muller, C.E. Anthraquinones as pharmacological tools and drugs. *Med. Res. Rev.* **2016**, *36*, 705–748. [CrossRef] [PubMed]
24. Lim, J.P.; Park, Y.S.; Hong, M.W.; Kim, D.K. Qunatotative analysis of anthraquinones from the roots of Korean natural *Rumex* spcies plant. *Kor. J. Pharm.* **2011**, *42*, 297–301.
25. Wegiera, M.; Smolarz, H.D.; Wianowska, D.; Dawidowicz, A.L. Anthracene derivatives in some species of *Rumex*, L. genus. *Acta Soc. Bot. Pol.* **2007**, *76*, 103–108.
26. Duval, J.; Pecher, V.; Poujol, M.; Lesellier, E. Research advances for the extraction, analysis and uses of anthraquinones: A review. *Ind. Crop. Prod.* **2016**, *94*, 812–833. [CrossRef]
27. Lee, N.J.; Choi, J.H.; Koo, B.S.; Ryu, S.Y.; Han, Y.H.; Lee, S.I.; Lee, D.U. Antimutagenicity and cytotoxicity of the constituents from the aerial parts of *Rumex acetosa*. *Biol. Pharm. Bull.* **2005**, *28*, 2158–2161. [CrossRef]

28. Yildirim, A.; Mavi, A.; Kara, A.A. Determination of antioxidant and antimicrobial activities of *Rumex crispus* L. extracts. *J. Agric. Food Chem.* **2001**, *49*, 4083–4089. [CrossRef]
29. Elzaawely, A.A.; Xuan, T.D.; Tawata, S. Antioxidant and antibacterial activities of *Rumex japonicus* HOUTT. Aerial parts. *Biol. Pharm. Bull.* **2005**, *28*, 2225–2230. [CrossRef]
30. Ansuya, N.; Gomathi, R.; Manian, S.; Sivaram, V.; Menon, A. Evalution of *Basella rubra* L., *Rumex nepalensis* spreng. and *Commelina benghalensis* L. for antioxidant activity. *Int. J. Pharm. Pharm. Sci.* **2012**, *4*, 714–720.
31. RiceEvans, C.A.; Miller, N.J.; Paganga, G. Structure-antioxidant activity relationships of flavonoids and phenolic acids. *Free Radic. Biol. Med.* **1996**, *20*, 933–956. [CrossRef]
32. Sahreen, S.; Khan, M.R.; Khan, R.A. Phenolic compounds and antioxidant activities of *Rumex hastatus* D. Don. leaves. *J. Med. Plants Res.* **2011**, *5*, 2755–2765.
33. Shahidi, F.; Ambigaipalan, P. Phenolics and polyphenolics in foods, beverages and spices: Antioxidant activity and health effects—A review. *J. Funct. Foods* **2015**, *18*, 820–897. [CrossRef]
34. Aktan, F. iNOS-mediated nitric oxide production and its regulation. *Life Sci.* **2004**, *75*, 639–653. [CrossRef] [PubMed]
35. Im, N.K.; Jung, Y.S.; Choi, J.H.; Yu, M.H.; Jeong, G.S. Inhibitoy effect of leaves of *Rumex crispus* L. on LPS-induced nitric oxide production and the expression of iNOS and COX-2 in macrophage. *Nat. Prod. Sci.* **2014**, *20*, 51–57.
36. Ng, S.; Galipeau, J. Concise review: Engineering the fusion of Cytokines for the modulation of immune cellular responses in cancer and autoimmune disorders. *Stem Cell Transl. Med.* **2015**, *4*, 66–73. [CrossRef] [PubMed]
37. Bradley, J.R. TNF-mediated inflammatory disease. *J. Pathol.* **2008**, *214*, 149–160. [CrossRef]
38. Dinarello, C.A. Immunological and inflammatory functions of the interleukin-1 family. *Annu. Rev. Immunol.* **2009**, *27*, 519–550. [CrossRef]
39. Ishihara, K.; Hirano, T. IL-6 in autoimmune disease and chronic inflammatory proliferative disease. *Cytokine Growth F R* **2002**, *13*, 357–368. [CrossRef]
40. Xie, Q.C.; Yang, Y.P. Anti-proliferative of physcion 8-O-beta-glucopyranoside isolated from *Rumex japonicus* Houtt. on A549 cell lines via inducing apoptosis and cell cycle arrest. *BMC Complement. Altern. Med.* **2014**, *14*, 377. [CrossRef]
41. Borner, C. The Bcl-2 protein family: Sensors and checkpoints for life-or-death decisions. *Mol. Immunol.* **2003**, *39*, 615–647. [CrossRef]
42. Casciolarosen, L.A.; Miller, D.K.; Anhalt, G.J.; Rosen, A. Specific cleavage of the 70-Kda protein-component of the U1 small nuclear ribonucleoprotein is a characteristic biochemical feature of apoptotic cell-death. *J. Biol. Chem.* **1994**, *269*, 30757–30760.
43. Li, P.; Nijhawan, D.; Budihardjo, I.; Srinivasula, S.M.; Ahmad, M.; Alnemri, E.S.; Wang, X.D. Cytochrome c and dATP-dependent formation of Apaf-1/caspase-9 complex initiates an apoptotic protease cascade. *Cell* **1997**, *91*, 479–489. [CrossRef]
44. Issaeva, N. p53 signaling in cancers. *Cancers* **2019**, *11*, 332. [CrossRef] [PubMed]
45. Chipuk, J.E.; Green, D.R. Dissecting p53-dependent apoptosis. *Cell Death Differ.* **2006**, *13*, 994–1002. [CrossRef] [PubMed]

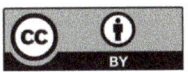

© 2020 by the authors. Licensee MDPI, Basel, Switzerland. This article is an open access article distributed under the terms and conditions of the Creative Commons Attribution (CC BY) license (http://creativecommons.org/licenses/by/4.0/).

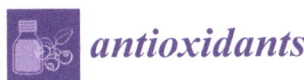

Article

Phytochemical Characterization of *Dillenia indica* L. Bark by Paper Spray Ionization-Mass Spectrometry and Evaluation of Its Antioxidant Potential Against t-BHP-Induced Oxidative Stress in RAW 264.7 Cells

Md Badrul Alam [1,2,†], Arif Ahmed [3,†], Syful Islam [3], Hee-Jeong Choi [1], Md Abdul Motin [4], Sunghwan Kim [3,5,*] and Sang-Han Lee [1,2,6,*]

1. Department of Food Science and Biotechnology, Graduate School, Kyungpook National University, Daegu 41566, Korea; mbalam@knu.ac.kr (M.B.A.); choi930302@gmail.com (H.-J.C.)
2. Food and Bio-Industry Research Institute, Inner Beauty/Antiaging Center, Kyungpook National University, Daegu 41566, Korea
3. Department of Chemistry, Kyungpook National University, Daegu 41566, Korea; arifahmed83@gmail.com (A.A.); msi412@yahoo.com (S.I.)
4. Department of Chemistry, University of California, Riverside, CA 92521, USA; mdabdulm@ucr.edu
5. Mass Spectrometry Converging Research Center and Green-Nano Materials Research Center, Daegu 41566, Korea
6. knu BnC, Daegu 41566, Korea
* Correspondence: sunghwank@knu.ac.kr (S.K.); sang@knu.ac.kr (S.-H.L.); Tel.: +82-053-950-7754 (S.K. & S.-H.L.); +82-010-2537-7659 (S.-H.L.); Fax: +82-053-950-6772 (S.K. & S.-H.L.)
† These authors have an equal contribution.

Received: 6 October 2020; Accepted: 5 November 2020; Published: 9 November 2020

Abstract: The antioxidant effects of the ethyl acetate fraction of *Dillenia indica* bark (DIBEt) and the underlying mechanisms were investigated in *tert*-butyl hydroperoxide (t-BHP)-stimulated oxidative stress in RAW 264.7 cells. Paper spray ionization-mass spectroscopy with positive-ion mode tentatively revealed 27 secondary metabolites in *D. indica* bark extract; predominant among them were alkaloids, phenolic acids, and flavonoids. A new triterpenoid (nutriacholic acid) was confirmed in DIBEt for the first time. DIBEt had strong free radical-scavenging capabilities and was also able to reduce t-BHP-induced cellular reactive oxygen species (ROS) generation in RAW 264.7 cells. DIBEt was found to prevent oxidative stress by boosting the levels of heme oxygenase-1 (HO-1) through the up-regulation of nuclear factor erythroid 2-related factor 2 (Nrf2) via the regulation of extracellular signal-regulated kinase (ERK) phosphorylation in RAW 264.7 cells. These results support the potential of DIBEt for defense against oxidative stress-stimulated diseases.

Keywords: antioxidant; *Dillenia indica*; heme oxygenase 1 (HO-1); nuclear factor erythroid 2-related factor 2 (Nrf2); RAW 264.7 cells

1. Introduction

Among the various signaling molecules, reactive oxygen species (ROS) and reactive nitrogen species (RNS) play critical roles in maintaining cellular homeostasis. Redox imbalance precisely participates in the pathogenesis and pathophysiology of numerous chronic diseases [1]. However, macrophage cells serve as the first line of defense in infected cells, and activated macrophages are a major source of ROS and RNS triggers epigenetic modifications, leading to the pathogenesis of chronic diseases [2]. Thus, activated macrophage models can identify the active components for functional diet development through a multiple-target strategy [2]. Natural medicinal products have been exploited in medical practice for centuries. Phytochemicals with inherent antioxidant potential orchestrate innumerable cellular defensive signaling cascades directly or indirectly and might have remedial applications for oxidative stress-induced disorders [3]. Thus, it is essential to understand and validate the bioactivities of natural compounds and their molecular mechanisms to form concrete scientific evidence for their clinical use and effectiveness and to meet regulatory challenges.

Nuclear factor erythroid 2-related factor 2 (Nrf2) activation triggers the induction of various detoxifying and antioxidant enzymes, such as heme oxygenase-1 (HO-1) and NAD(P)H quinone oxidoreductase 1 (NQO1) [4]. In the resting state, cytosolic Kelch-like ECH-associated protein 1 (Keap1) causes the degradation of Nrf2 through the ubiquitin-proteasome system. During stress conditions or xenobiotic challenge, the reactive cysteine residue of Keap1 is modified, causing the conformational change of Keap1 structure that prevents Nrf2 degradation, which is then free to translocate to the nucleus and bind to antioxidant-related elements (AREs) in the promoter regions of antioxidant and cytoprotective genes [4]. Furthermore, the activation of mitogen-activated protein kinase (MAPK), phosphatidylinositol 3-kinase/Akt (PI3K/AKT), and protein kinase C (PKC) also boosts Nrf2 nuclear translocation [5].

Instrumental analytical techniques, such as high-performance liquid chromatography (HPLC) and gas chromatography (GC) coupled with mass spectrometry (MS), have been applied to qualitatively and quantitatively explore the secondary metabolites of medicinal plants or foods. Although these techniques are very accurate and precise, they are very time-consuming and require laborious sample preparation and high costs. In contrast, paper spray ionization-MS (PSI-MS) requires minimal sample preparation time, boosts the ionization of compounds under mild experimental conditions, and furnishes ultrafast examinations of complex matrices at low cost [6]. Thus, PSI-MS has been widely accepted in resveratrol evaluation in red wine [7], chemical composition and fraud verification of whiskey and beer [8], medicines, pesticide analysis in fruits and vegetables, and food additives and their byproducts [9].

Dillenia indica (family Dilleniaecae) is commonly known as elephant apple. The pulp of the fruit is applied on the scalp to cure dandruff and hair loss, and the sepal has been used to treat stomach disorders since ancient times [10]. Evidence suggested that *D. indica* possesses various medicinal properties, such as anticancer [11], antimicrobial, antioxidant [12], analgesic, anti-inflammatory [13], and antidiabetic and its associated complications, such as hyperlipidemia [14], diabetic nephropathy, and neuropathy. However, little information is available on the chemical composition of *D. indica* bark (DIB). Therefore, this study aimed to provide further information on the chemical composition of the ethyl acetate fraction of DIB (DIBEt) through the determination of total phenolic and total flavonoid contents and in-vitro antioxidant capacity. The bioactive components of DIBEt were screened using PSI-MS. Furthermore, the focus was on the regulatory role of DIBEt on the expression of antioxidant enzymes in RAW 264.7 cells and the underlying mechanisms.

2. Materials and Methods

2.1. Plant Materials and Extraction

DIB was collected from Jahangirnagar University, Bangladesh, in August 2018 and taxonomically identified by the National Herbarium of Bangladesh (voucher specimen no. 49403) and retained in the laboratory for future reference. Dried and coarsely powdered barks (100 g) were extracted by shaking with ethanol at 60 °C for 12 h (three times) and dried in a rotary vacuum evaporator. The ethanolic extract (DIBE; 18.21 g) was suspended in 200 mL deionized water and partitioned sequentially with n-hexane, chloroform, and ethyl acetate using separating funnels in a stepwise manner. After vacuum filtration, the solutions were concentrated in a rotary vacuum evaporator. The n-hexane fraction (DIBH; 1.70 g), chloroform extract (DIBC; 2.44 g), ethyl acetate fraction (DIBEt; 8.55 g), and aqueous fraction (DIBW; 5.18 g) were dissolved in deionized water at 30 mg/mL concentration.

DIBEt was dissolved in deionized water and then diluted with HPLC-grade ethanol at 10 mg/mL concentration for PSI-tandem MS (MS/MS). The sample solution was vortexed for 1 min and sonicated for 5 min in a Powersonic 410 sonication bath (Hwashin Technology Co., Gyeonggi, Korea) for a homogeneous mixture.

2.2. PSI-MS

A 2 µL stock solution (10 mg/mL) was loaded using a disposable glass Pasteur pipette (Volac; Poulten & Graf Ltd., Barking, UK) onto the center of a chromatographic paper tip (Whatman 1 Chr., Kent, UK). The positive-ion mode of the Q-Exactive orbitrap MS (Thermo Fisher Scientific, Inc., Rockford, IL, USA) was used to collect the data over the range of m/z 50–600. To make a sharp tip, the chromatographic paper was cut into dimensions of 6 mm base and 14 mm height. A syringe pump (Fusion 100T; Chemyx, Stafford, TX, USA) was used to load the ethanol solvent onto the sample-loaded paper at a flow rate of 15 µL/min. A spray voltage of 4.5 kV was directly applied to the paper tip for the ionization of the sample. The other parameters for the PSI experiment were as follows: capillary temperature 300, S-lens RF level 50, mass resolution 140,000 (full-width at half-maximum), and maximum injection time 150 ms. The automatic gain control was set to 1×10^6.

To perform the MS/MS experiments, three different stepped normalized collision energies (10, 30, and 50) were used with the same instrument. The instrument was operated in the positive-ion mode. The other operative parameters for the MS/MS experiments were as follows: sheath and auxiliary gas flow rate 10 and 0 (arbitrary units), respectively; spray voltage 3.60 kV; capillary temperature 300; and S-lens RF level 50.

2.3. Data Processing

Mass spectral data obtained from the orbitrap MS were processed using Xcalibur 3.1 with Foundation 3.1 (Thermo Fisher Scientific). Compounds were tentatively identified by matching their exact (calculated) masses of protonated (M + H) adducts with measured m/z values and PSI-MS/MS fragmentation patterns from the in-house MS/MS database, and online databases such as the Human Metabolome Database [15] and METLIN [16], and the literature. The compound structures were drawn using ChemDraw Professional 15.0 (PerkinElmer, Waltham, MA, USA).

2.4. Radical-Scavenging Activity Assays

DPPH, ABTS, superoxide, and hydroxyl radical-scavenging assays were conducted to evaluate the free radical-scavenging potential of DIB extract following the procedures outlined by Alam et al. [3]. Ascorbic acid and quercetin were used as positive controls for DPPH and ABTS and superoxide and hydroxyl radical-scavenging assays, respectively. The following equation was adapted to calculate the percent inhibition:

$$\text{Radical-scavenging activity (\% inhibition)} = \left(\frac{\text{Abs}_{\text{control}} - \text{Abs}_{\text{sample}}}{\text{Abs}_{\text{control}}} \right) \times 100$$

where $\text{Abs}_{\text{control}}$ is the absorbance of the control sample and $\text{Abs}_{\text{sample}}$ is the absorbance of the experimental sample. All samples were analyzed in triplicate.

To determine the reducing power potential, ferric reducing antioxidant power (FRAP) and cupric reducing antioxidant capacity (CUPRAC) assays were performed according to the method described by Alam et al. [17]. The reducing power potential was expressed as the ascorbic acid-equivalent antioxidant value (µM) calculated from the standard curve of ascorbic acid. The oxygen radical absorbance capacity (ORAC) assay [18] was performed using Trolox, a water-soluble analog of vitamin E, as a positive control. The antioxidant potentiality was calculated as the Trolox-equivalent antioxidant value (µM).

2.5. Cell Culture and Cell Viability Assay

RAW 264.7 cells (American Type Culture Collection, Rockville, MD, USA) were maintained in Dulbecco's modified Eagle medium (DMEM) supplemented with 10% fetal bovine serum (FBS) and streptomycin-penicillin (100 µg/mL each; Hyclone, Logan, UT, USA) at 37 °C and 5% CO_2. The cells were seeded in 96-well plates (5×10^5 cells/mL) for 24 h and subsequently treated with DIBEt (1–100 µg/mL) for the next 24 h. Cell viability was measured using the 3-(4,5-dimethylthiazol-2-yl)-2,5-diphenyltetrazolium bromide (MTT) assay, as described previously [19].

2.6. Measurement of Intracellular ROS

The generation of *tert*-butyl hydroperoxide (t-BHP)-induced ROS as a cellular oxidative stress biomarker was determined by the 2',7'-dichlorofluorescein diacetate (DCFH-DA) method [3].

2.7. Reverse Transcription-Polymerase Chain Reaction (RT-PCR)

Total RNA was isolated using TRIzol (Invitrogen, Carlsbad, CA, USA). RT & Go Mastermix (MP Biomedicals, Seoul, Korea) was used to prepare cDNA by implementing the manufacturer's protocols. As described in Supplementary Table S1, various primers were used to perform RT-PCR using a PCR Thermal Cycler Dice TP600 (Takara Bio, Inc., Otsu, Japan) [17].

2.8. Western Blot Analysis

Cells were lysed and harvested using radioimmunoprecipitation assay buffer. Nuclear and cytosolic proteins were extracted by applying the nuclear and cytoplasmic extraction kit (Sigma-Aldrich, St. Louis, MO, USA). The bicinchoninic acid protein assay kit (Pierce, Rockford, IL, USA) was used to confirm the protein content. An adequate amount of protein (30 µg) was subjected to Western blot analysis, as described in a previous report using various antibodies (Supplementary Table S2) [20].

2.9. Statistical Analysis

Statistical analysis was performed using SigmaPlot version 12.5 (Systat Software, Inc., Chicago, IL, USA). Data were expressed as mean ± standard deviation (SD; $n = 3$). One-way analysis of variance (ANOVA) followed by Dunnett's multiple comparison test was performed to determine the significance of the differentiation and fusion indices. $p < 0.05$ was considered significant.

3. Results and Discussion

3.1. Identification of Secondary Metabolites of DIBEt

The identification and characterization of the related compounds from DIBEt were performed in two steps. In the first step, PSI-MS was used to identify the major *m/z* peaks with a full-scan MS, and then characterized using PSI-MS/MS to obtain the MS/MS fragment of the obtained *m/z* from the first step. Figure 1 corresponds to the total ion chromatogram of DIBEt in PSI-MS in positive-ion mode, revealing 27 secondary metabolites presented with their molecular formula, monoisotopic mass of experimental ions, and calculated ions in positive modes (Table 1). All compounds identified in DIBEt were classified into nitrogen compounds, phenolic acids, flavonoids, amino acids, triterpenoids, and others.

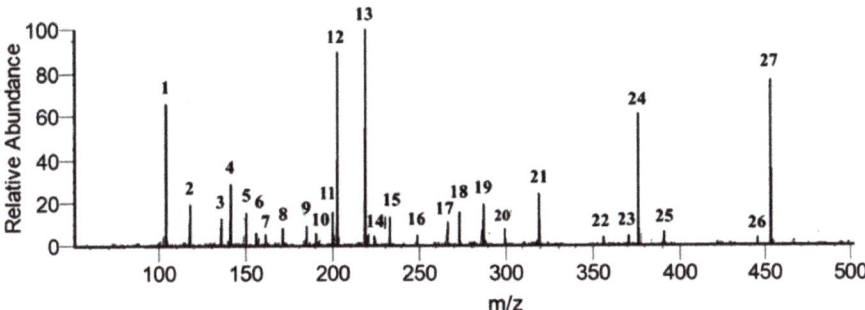

Figure 1. PSI-MS parent ion peak of the identified compounds of DIBEt.

Three phenolic acids (3,4-dihydroxy-5-methoxybenzoic acid, 2-caffeoylisocitric acid, and 2-O-caffeoylhydroxycitric acid) and seven flavonoids (naringenin, kaempferol, 5,7-dimethoxyapigenin, 6,7,3′-trihydroxy-2′,4′-dimethoxyisoflavan (bryaflavan), formononetin 7-glucoronide, amoradinin, and mallotus B (isoallorottlerin), along with the Na and K adducts of glucose) were identified. Twelve nitrogen compounds [γ-aminobutyric acid (GABA), N-isopropylhydrazinecarboxamide, hydroxymethylserine, triethanolamine, 5-acetyl-2,4-dimethylthiazole, dialanine, 4-methylthiazole-5-propionic acid, L-α-aminosuberic acid, 1,3-bis(carbamoylcarbamoyl)urea (carbonyldibiuret), linamarin, 2-(glucosyloxy)isobutyraldoxime, and N-acetyl-3,5,11,18-tetrahydroxyoctadecyl-2-amine] were also confirmed. One fatty acid (11-dodecenoic acid) and one triterpenoid (nutriacholic acid) were confirmed for the first time in this genus (Figure 2). Peaks 1–3, 5–8, 10, 14–16, and 23 were characterized as nitrogen compounds, such as GABA, N-isopropylhydrazinecarboxamide, hydroxymethylserine, triethanolamine, 5-acetyl-2,4-dimethylthiazole, dialanine, 4-methylthiazole-5-propionic acid, L-α-aminosuberic acid, 1,3-bis(carbamoylcarbamoyl)urea, linamarin, 2-(glucosyloxy)isobutyraldoxime, and N-acetyl-3,5,11,18-tetrahydroxyoctadecyl-2-amine, with the parent ion peak at m/z 104.1075, 118.0866, 136.0619, 150.1131, 156.0428, 161.0966, 172.0434, 190.1081, 233.0633, 248.1138, 266.1233, and 376.2597, respectively [21]. The detailed fragmentation patterns are given in Supplementary Figure S1. Seven flavonoids [naringenin (17), kaempferol (18), 5,7-dimethoxyapigenin (19), 6,7,3′-trihydroxy-2′,4′-dimethoxyisoflavan (20), formononetin 7-glucoronide (25), amoradinin (26), and mallotus B (27)] were also confirmed. Naringenin and kaempferol yielded a major fragment ion at m/z 153.01 and 119.05 and/or 121.02 due to $^{1,3}A$ and $^{0,2}B$ fragmentation, respectively. Polyphenolics also produced at m/z (M + H-44 u) and (M + H-18 u) by losing CO_2 and water molecules, respectively, in positive-ion mode due to the abundance of carboxyl or hydroxyl groups. The detailed fragmentation patterns are given in Supplementary Figure S2. Furthermore, peaks 9, 21, and 22 were confirmed as 3,5-dihydroxy-4-methoxybenzoic acid, 2-caffeoylisocitric acid, and 2-O-caffeoylhydroxycitric acid with the parent ion peak at m/z 185.0445, 355.0697, and 371.0754, respectively (fragmentation patterns in Supplementary Figure S3). Peak 24 was suggested as nutriacholic acid [m/z 391.2841 (M + H)] and yielded a major fragmentation ion at m/z 207.14 due to the cleavage of C_8–C_{14} and C_9–C_{11} followed by water loss at m/z 189.13 (Supplementary Figure S4) [22].

Table 1. Characterization of the secondary metabolites of DIBEt by PSI-MS/MS.

No.	Compound Name	MW	MM	EF	(M + H) m/z [a]	(M + H) m/z [b]	PSI-MS/MS (Positive Ionization)
1	γ-Aminobutyric acid (GABA)	103.121	103.063	$C_4H_9NO_2$	104.108	104.071	87.04, 60.02, 58.07
2	N-Isopropylhydrazinecarboxamide	117.152	117.09	$C_4H_{11}N_3O$	118.087	118.098	101.06, 59.07, 58.06
3	Hydroxymethylserine	135.119	135.053	$C_4H_9NO_4$	136.062	136.061	119.035
4	Ethyl maltol	140.138	140.047	$C_7H_8O_3$	141.055	141.055	140.06, 126.03, 123.04, 113.06, 108.02, 81.04
5	Triethanolamine	149.188	149.105	$C_6H_{15}NO_3$	150.113	150.113	132.10, 120.10, 103.06, 88.07
6	5-Acetyl-2,4-dimethylthiazole	155.22	155.04	$C_7H_{10}NOS$	156.043	155.048	140.03, 122.07, 81.04
7	Dialanine	160.171	160.085	$C_6H_{12}N_2O_3$	161.097	161.092	145.06, 144.07, 131.06, 118.05, 101.07, 88.04, 72.04
8	4-Methylthiazole-5-propionic acid	171.214	171.035	$C_7H_9NO_2S$	172.043	172.043	156.06, 141.08, 128.07, 113.07
9	3,5-Dihydroxy-4-methoxybenzoic acid	184.157	184.037	$C_8H_8O_5$	185.045	185.045	170.02, 155.03, 126.02, 109.03, 95.05, 91.02, 77.04
10	L-α-Aminosuberic acid	189.211	189.1	$C_8H_{15}NO_4$	190.108	190.108	173.08, 130.09, 128.07, 113.06, 101.06, 70.01
11	11-Dodecenoic acid	198.306	198.162	$C_{12}H_{22}O_2$	199.169	199.169	181.16, 127.08, 95.09, 85.03
12	Glucose Na adduct				203.053	203.052	
13	Glucose K adduct				219.027	219.026	
14	1,3-Bis(carbamoylcarbamoyl)urea (Carbonyldibiuret)	232.156	232.056	$C_5H_8N_6O_5$	233.063	233.063	216.08, 188.09, 145.03, 119.01, 102.05
15	Linamarin	247.247	247.106	$C_{10}H_{17}NO_6$	248.114	248.113	230.10, 182.08, 128.07, 115.04, 98.04
16	2-(Glucosyloxy) isobutyraldoxime	265.262	265.112	$C_{10}H_{19}NO_7$	266.123	266.123	248.11, 230.10, 182.08, 128.07, 115.04, 98.04
17	Naringenin	272.256	272.068	$C_{15}H_{12}O_5$	273.076	273.076	153.01, 147.04, 119.05
18	Kaempferol	286.239	286.048	$C_{15}H_{10}O_6$	287.056	287.055	269.04, 141.05, 213.05, 165.02, 153.02, 137.02, 121.02
19	5,7-Dimethoxyapigenin	298.29	298.084	$C_{17}H_{14}O_5$	299.056	299.091	271.10, 253.09, 179.03, 137.06, 123.04
20	6,7,3′-Trihydroxy-2′,4′-dimethoxyisoflavan (Bryaflavan)	318.325	318.11	$C_{17}H_{18}O_6$	319.116	319.11	301.11, 245.08, 195.10, 167.07, 153.05, 149.05, 137.02
21	2-Caffeoylisocitric acid	354.267	354.059	$C_{15}H_{14}O_{10}$	355.07	355.066	310.07, 121.03, 203.02, 192.03, 177.04
22	2-O-caffeoylhydroxycitric acid	370.26	370.053	$C_{15}H_{14}O_{11}$	371.075	371.061	311.04, 279.05, 267.05, 237.04
23	N-Acetyl-3,5,11,18-tetrahydroxyoctadecyl-2-amine	375.52	375.295	$C_{20}H_{41}NO_5$	376.26	376.303	358.30, 340.28, 226.18, 161.15, 147.14, 137.06, 123.04, 109.10
24	Nutriacholic acid	390.62	390.277	$C_{24}H_{38}O_4$	391.284	391.284	361.27, 207.14, 189.13, 161.13, 149.13
25	Formononetin 7-glucoronide	444.38	444.105	$C_{22}H_{20}O_{10}$	445.12	445.113	413.12, 251.07, 137.02, 123.04
26	Amoradinin	452.521	452.219	$C_{27}H_{32}O_6$	453.231	453.231	391.15, 373.14, 361.14, 207.07, 191.07
27	Mallotus B (Isoallorottlerin)	518.554	518.194	$C_{30}H_{30}O_8$	519.205	519.202	339.17, 237.11

[a] Observed parent ion m/z (M + H); [b] Calculated parent ion m/z (M + H). MW, average molecular weight (g/mol); MM, monoisotopic molecular mass (g/mol); EF, elemental formula.

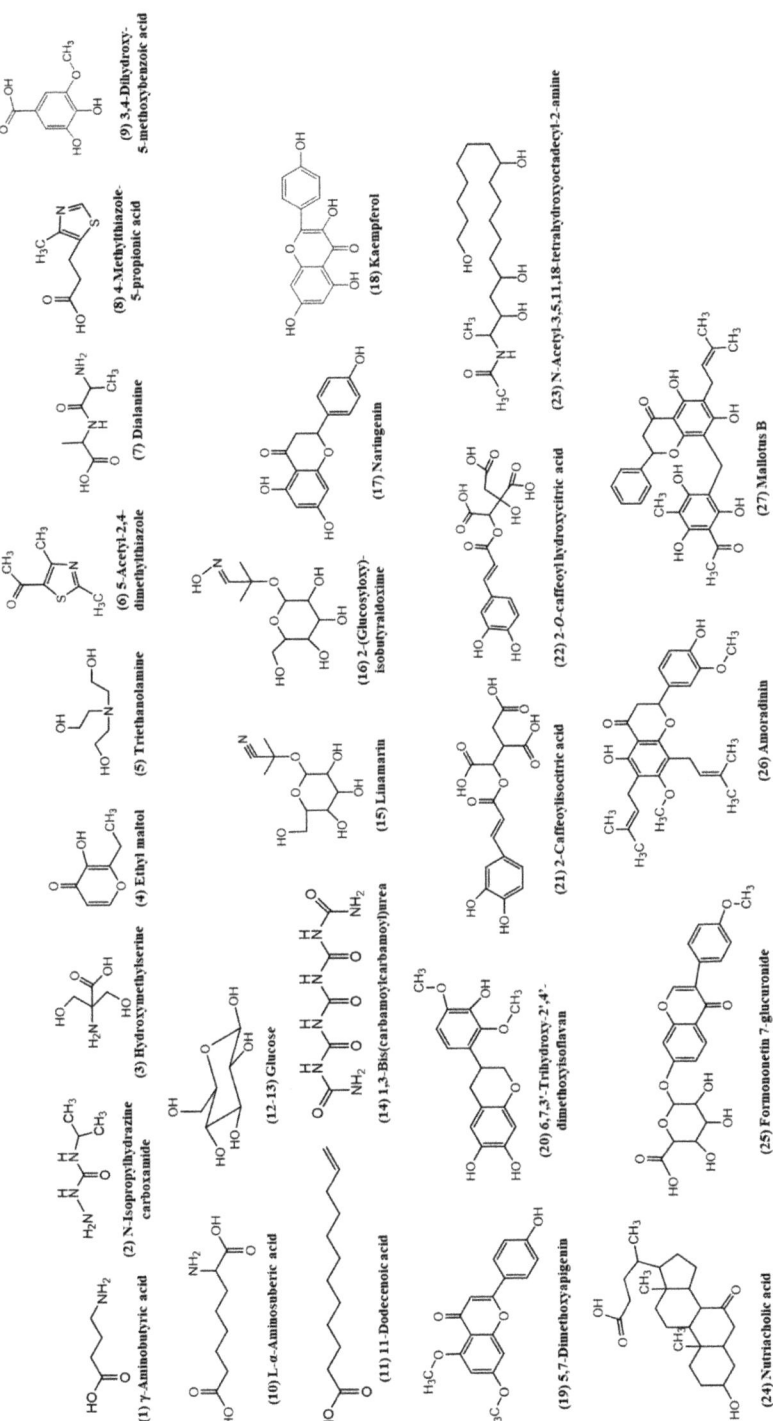

Figure 2. Chemical structures of the identified compounds of DIBEt by PSI-MS/MS.

3.2. Radical-Scavenging Activities of DIB Extracts

Various molecular mechanisms and/or the synergism between them may cause the attribution of antioxidant activity of the secondary metabolites present in plants. Thus, the evaluation of the antioxidant activity of plant extracts should be performed via several methods. DPPH, ABTS, superoxide and hydroxyl radical-scavenging assays, and FRAP, CUPRAC, and ORAC assays were performed to assess the antioxidant potential of various organic and aqueous DIB extracts. All organic and aqueous DIB extracts significantly scavenged DPPH and ABTS radicals in a dose-dependent manner (Figure 3A; Supplementary Figure S5). DIBEt showed 7.34- and 3.81-fold higher DPPH and ABTS radical-scavenging activities, respectively, than ascorbic acid used as a positive control, with IC_{50} of 1.87 ± 0.13 and 7.58 ± 0.10 µg/mL for DIBEt and 13.79 ± 0.87 and 28.90 ± 0.16 µg/mL for ascorbic acid, respectively. Other extracts showed DPPH and ABTS radical-scavenging activities in the following order: DIBE (IC_{50}, 5.12 ± 0.68 µg/mL) > DIBW (IC_{50}, 5.82 ± 0.18 µg/mL) > DIBC (IC_{50}, 50.13 ± 1.08 µg/mL) > DIBH (IC_{50}, 63.79 ± 2.19 µg/mL) and DIBE (IC_{50}, 9.95 ± 0.05 µg/mL) > DIBW (IC_{50}, 17.54 ± 1.15 µg/mL) > DIBC (IC_{50}, 91.00 ± 0.86 µg/mL) > DIBH (IC_{50}, >100 µg/mL), respectively. Previous studies revealed that the methanolic extracts of *D. indica* fruits showed strong DPPH radical-scavenging activity followed by petroleum ether, ethyl acetate, and water extract with IC_{50} of 31.25, 65.77, 97.25, and 106.95 µg/mL, respectively [12,23]. Compared to previous studies, this study revealed that DIB is more powerful to scavenge DPPH radicals. The superoxide and hydroxyl radical-scavenging abilities of DIB extracts were evaluated by the PMS-NADH superoxide-generating system and Fenton reaction in a dose-dependent manner, respectively (Figure 3B; Supplementary Figure S6). DIBEt had 5.70- and 7.10-fold higher superoxide and hydroxyl radical-scavenging potential than quercetin, with IC_{50} of 2.47 ± 0.05 and 1.58 ± 0.06 µg/mL for DIBEt and 14.12 ± 0.77 and 11.21 ± 1.06 µg/mL for quercetin, respectively. Other extracts had superoxide and hydroxyl radical-scavenging activities in the following order: DIBE (IC_{50}, 14.78 ± 1.15 µg/mL) > DIBW (IC_{50}, 14.48 ± 0.17 µg/mL) > DIBC (IC_{50}, >100 µg/mL) > DIBH (IC_{50}, >100 µg/mL) and DIBE (IC_{50}, 7.85 ± 0.02 µg/mL) > DIBW (IC_{50}, 9.54 ± 0.09 µg/mL) > DIBC (IC_{50}, 22.41 ± 2.17 µg/mL) > DIBH (IC_{50}, 23.85 ± 0.47 µg/mL), respectively. Das et al. [23] reported that the methanolic extract of *D. indica* fruits had powerful superoxide and hydroxyl radical-scavenging activities with IC_{50} of 51.49 and 51.82 µg/mL, respectively. In contrast, this study showed that various organic and aqueous DIB extracts are more powerful to scavenge superoxide and hydroxyl radicals.

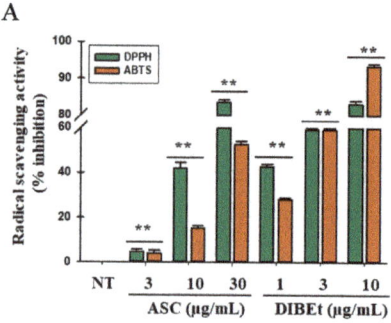
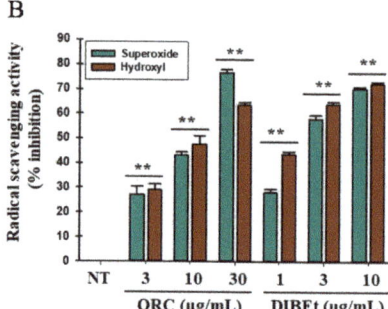

Figure 3. Cont.

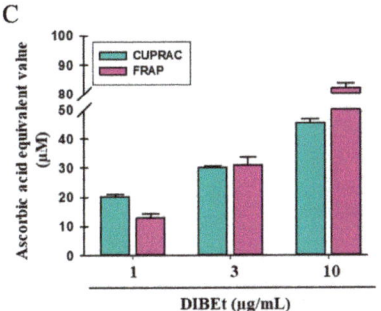
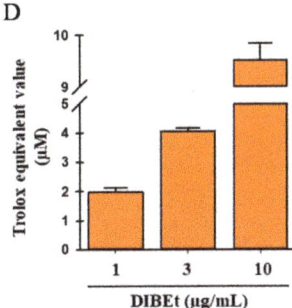

Figure 3. Radical-scavenging effects of DIBEt. DPPH and ABTS (**A**) and superoxide and hydroxyl (**B**) radical-scavenging activities of DIBEt. Ascorbic acid (ASC) and quercetin (QRC) were considered as standard antioxidant molecules. The reducing power of DIBEt was examined by CUPRAC, FRAP, and ORAC assays (**C**). The ascorbic acid-equivalent antioxidant capacity was calculated for CUPRAC and FRAP assays, and (**D**) the ORAC activity was expressed as the Trolox-equivalent antioxidant capacity. Mean ± SD ($n = 3$). ** $p < 0.01$.

CUPRAC, FRAP, and ORAC assays were performed to determine whether DIBEt is capable to donate electrons and establish that DIBEt has a strong reducing power potential in a dose-dependent manner (Figure 3C; Supplementary Figure S7). At 10 µg/mL, DIBEt showed 34.52 ± 0.37 and 81.37 ± 0.57 µM ascorbic acid-equivalent reducing power for CUPRAC and FRAP assays, respectively. Other extracts showed ascorbic acid-equivalent reducing power activities in the following order: DIBE (30.64 ± 0.58 µM) > DIBW (24.51 ± 1.13 µM) > DIBC (11.85 ± 2.03 µM) > DIBH (4.22 ± 0.28 µM) and DIBE (21.08 ± 1.25 µM) > DIBW (19.72 ± 0.80 µM) > DIBC (6.80 ± 0.89 µM) > DIBH (3.30 ± 1.57 µM) for CUPRAC and FRAP assays, respectively. DIBEt showed 9.43 ± 1.97 µM Trolox-equivalent antioxidant capacity at 10 µg/mL in the ORAC assay. Other extracts showed Trolox-equivalent antioxidant capacity in the following order: DIBE (7.87 ± 0.04 µM) > DIBW (5.55 ± 0.27 µM) > DIBC (3.10 ± 0.20 µM) > DIBH (2.74 ± 0.13 µM). Based on these interpretations, DIBEt has a very strong potential to donate/transfer hydrogen/electrons to oxidants to neutralize them.

Studies revealed that phenolic compounds, such as phenol and flavonoids, have strong redox properties capable of quenching singlet and triplet oxygen, adsorbing and neutralizing free radicals, and/or decomposing peroxides, resulting in superior antioxidant potential [17,24,25]. Thus, total phenolic and flavonoid contents were found in the plant chosen for the study (Supplementary data S8). In addition, Pearson coefficient (ρ) and linear regression analyses were performed to correlate the polyphenol, flavonoid, and antioxidant activities of DIB extracts. The results showed substantial correlation for DPPH, ABTS, and hydroxyl radical-scavenging activities ($\rho = -0.939$, -0.918, and -0.853, respectively) and moderate correlation for superoxide radical-scavenging activity ($\rho = -0.622$). A negative ρ-value (-1) stands for a perfect positive correlation, as a correlation between polyphenol and free radical-scavenging abilities was found using IC_{50}. The data were also supported by previous studies describing that the antioxidant activity is highly influenced by the presence of total phenol content, and has a linear correlation between phenolic content and antioxidant activity, but the total flavonoid content provided a mixed function [3,26].

The radical-scavenging and reducing power activities of the identified constituents of DIBEt were also tested. The identified compounds showed a strong radical-scavenging activity (IC_{50}) in the order of naringenin > kaempferol > 3,4-dihydroxy-5-methoxybenzoic acid > ethyl maltol > dialanine > GABA ≅ linamarin. Naringenin also showed the highest reducing power activity, with an ascorbic acid-equivalent of 33.32 ± 0.31 and 54.34 ± 0.29 µM for CUPRAC and FRAP assays, respectively, followed by kaempferol > 3,4-dihydroxy-5-methoxybenzoic acid > ethyl maltol > dialanine > GABA ≅ linamarin (Table 2).

Table 2. Antioxidant activities of commercially available identified compounds from DIBEt.

	Compound Name	DPPH [a]	ABTS [a]	CUPRAC [b]	FRAP [b]
1	GABA	>100	>100	0.12 ± 1.51	0.91 ± 1.25
2	Ethyl maltol	29.42 ± 0.85	34.52 ± 0.35	21.05 ± 1.15	28.52 ± 0.55
3	Dialanine	85.69 ± 0.25	92.57 ± 0.53	09.55 ± 0.25	11.02 ± 1.52
4	3,4-Dihydroxy-5-methoxybenzoic acid	18.25 ± 1.52	12.05 ± 0.45	25.15 ± 0.85	35.25 ± 0.89
5	Linamarin	>100	>100	0.32 ± 0.94	0.71 ± 0.65
6	Naringenin	4.52 ± 0.12	3.98 ± 0.78	33.32 ± 0.31	54.34 ± 0.29
7	Kaempferol	10.32 ± 0.54	5.21 ± 0.45	31.02 ± 0.57	45.53 ± 0.92

[a] Radical-scavenging activities as IC_{50} (μg/mL). [b] Ascorbic acid-equivalent reducing power (μM). GABA, ethyl maltol, dialanine, 3,4-dihydroxy-5-methoxybenzoic acid, naringenin, and kaempferol were purchased from Sigma-Aldrich (catalog nos. A2129, W348708, A9502, CDS003720, N5893, and 60010, respectively). Linamarin was purchased from Cayman Chemical (Ann Arbor, MI, USA). All standards of purity were >98%.

Studies revealed that 3,4-dihydroxy-5-methoxybenzoic acid and 2-*O*-caffeoylhydroxycitric acid have strong free radical-scavenging activities, with IC_{50} of 10.69 and 6.05 μg/mL and 10.23 and 4.32 μg/mL for DPPH and ABTS assays, respectively [27,28]. Flavonoids, such as naringenin, kaempferol, and 6,7,3′-trihydroxy-2′,4′-dimethoxyisoflavan, also have very strong free radical-scavenging activities as reported by previous studies [29,30]. Triethanolamine, dialanine, and linamarin have also been studied for their antioxidant properties [31,32]. GABA- and mallotus B-containing plant extracts also showed excellent antioxidant properties and protect RIN-m5F pancreatic cells from hydrogen peroxide-induced oxidative stress [33,34].

3.3. DIBEt Attenuates t-BHP-Induced Cellular Oxidative Stress

Among all extracts, DIBEt has the highest antioxidant potential triggered to evaluate the potential of DIBEt to scavenge oxidative stress-induced cellular ROS generation with cellular toxicity. t-BHP, a short-chain analog of lipid peroxide, is widely accepted as a model substance to induce oxidative stress in cells and tissues and evaluate the molecular mechanisms of cellular alterations caused by oxidative stress [35]. More than 95% of cell viability was noted at DIBEt concentrations up to 50 μg/mL (Figure 4A; Supplementary Figure S9). In addition, Figure 4B demonstrates that DIBEt has an immense potential to attenuate oxidative stress-induced cellular ROS generation in a concentration-dependent manner with that of gallic acid (30 μg/mL) without showing cellular toxicity. Excessive ROS formation triggers oxidative stress, leading to cell death. Detailed research has revealed that antioxidants mitigated the deleterious effects of ROS and retard many effects that cause cellular death [3,36,37].

3.4. Effects of DIBEt on Antioxidant Enzyme Expression in RAW 264.7 Cells

The first-line antioxidant defense system, including superoxide dismutase, catalase, glutathione peroxidase (GPx), and glutathione, critically maintains cellular redox homeostasis [37]. Various stimuli can induce HO-1 expression, conferring cell protection from oxidative stress by maintaining antioxidant/oxidant homeostasis [38]. In Figure 4C,D, the mRNA expression and protein levels of the first-line antioxidant enzymes SOD1, catalase, and GPx-1 and the phase II enzyme HO-1 were extremely extenuated in t-BHP-treated cells, respectively, but DIBEt treatment dose-dependently reversed this trend. Naringenin also enhanced the mRNA expression and protein levels of first-line antioxidant enzymes in the t-BHP model. These data suggest that increased mRNA and protein levels of antioxidant enzymes by DIBEt plays a critical role in cellular homeostasis and protects against oxidative stress-induced cell death.

Studies revealed that medicinal plants or foods possess abundant polyphenolic compounds that boost SOD1, CAT, and GPx activities, decreasing oxidative stress [39,40]. Evidence showed that polyphenolic acids, such as naringenin, kaempferol, apigenin, and formononetin aglycone, and their glycosidic form and caffeoylisocitric acid have a potential to boost first-line antioxidant proteins, leading to cell protection against oxidative stress [41–45]. Therefore, the presence of phenolic acids and flavonoids in DIBEt may play a major role in boosting the expression of first-line antioxidant enzymes/proteins as the principal mechanism accounting for protecting DIBEt against oxidative stress.

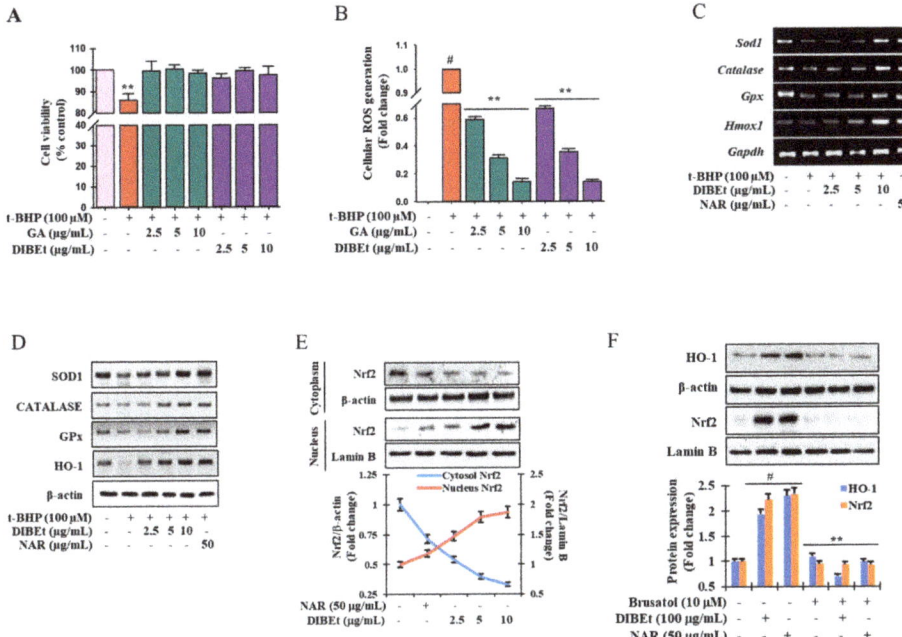

Figure 4. Protective effects of DIBEt against t-BHP-induced cell toxicity and intracellular ROS generation through the up-regulation of antioxidant enzymes via Nrf2 activation. Cells were treated with DIBEt and gallic acid (GA) at the indicated concentrations for 12 h and then exposed to 100 μM t-BHP for 6 h. Cell viability percentage (**A**) and intracellular ROS (**B**) were determined by MTT assay and the DCFH-DA method, respectively. Mean ± SD (n = 3). # $p < 0.001$, compared to no treatment; ** $p < 0.05$, compared to t-BHP treatment. SOD1, catalase, GPx, and phase II antioxidant enzyme (such as HO-1) mRNA (**C**) and protein expression (**D**) were analyzed by RT-PCR and Western blot, respectively. Nrf2 protein expression (**E**) was measured by Western blot. Cells were treated with an Nrf2 inhibitor (brusatol) with and without DIBEt and naringenin (NAR). Nrf2 and HO-1 protein levels were analyzed by Western blot (**F**). Mean ± SD (n = 3). # $p < 0.001$, compared to no treatment; ** $p < 0.05$, compared to sample treatment. (+): presence; (-): absence.

3.5. Effects of DIBEt on Phase II Enzymes Mediated by Nrf2 Nuclear Translocation in RAW 264.7 Cells

An important transcription factor, Nrf2, binds to the ARE in the promoter regions of cytoprotective genes and acts as a master regulator of antioxidative responses [46]. Thus, immunoblotting was performed to evaluate the role of DIBEt on Nrf2 regulation. In Figure 4E, the nuclear Nrf2 content was markedly increased in association with decreased cyto-Nrf2 levels after DIBEt treatment. Furthermore, brusatol, a pharmacological inhibitor of Nrf2, was used to confirm the role of DIBEt on the activation of phase II detoxifying enzymes through Nrf2 regulation. Nrf2 protein levels were greatly diminished by brusatol treatment, which was not reestablished despite the application of DIBEt and naringenin (Figure 4F). Furthermore, DIBEt and naringenin treatment was also unable to restore the basal HO-1 protein levels in brusatol-treated cells (Figure 4F). This observation conferred that DIBEt might disrupt the proteasomal degradation of Nrf2 in the cytoplasm by Keap1 and facilitate Nrf2 nuclear translocation, resulting in the up-regulation of HO-1 expression. Studies revealed that extracts from various medicinal plants or foods, such as *Nymphaea nouchali* flowers, *Lannea coromandelica* bark, and *Ginkgo biloba* bark, can activate Nrf2-mediated phase II enzyme expression in RAW 264.7, Hepa-1c1c7, and Hep G2 cells [3,17,47]. Furthermore, naringenin, kaempferol, apigenin, and formononetin aglycone and their glycosidic form can modulate the Nrf2/ARE/HO-1 signaling cascade, leading to the attenuation of oxidative stress-mediated melanocytes and kidney and neuronal death [43–45].

3.6. DIBEt Regulates Nrf2 Translocation Via Activation of MAPK to Lessen Oxidative Stress

MAPKs act as a downstream effector in antioxidant responses. The activation of MAPKs can manifest the activation of Nrf2. In-vitro and in-vivo studies have revealed that extracellular signal-regulated kinase (ERK), JNK, and p38 MAPK positively regulate ARE-containing reporter or detoxifying genes via Nrf2-dependent mechanisms [48,49]. In Figure 5A, ERK1/2 was phosphorylated from 15 to 180 min and peaked at 30 min after DIBEt exposure, whereas p38 and JNK phosphorylation was absent in DIBEt-treated cells. Furthermore, to confirm the role of ERK1/2 phosphorylation in Nrf2 translocation to the nucleus and induction of HO-1 expression, U0126, a specific inhibitor of ERK1/2, was used in DIBEt-treated cells. As expected, in Figure 5B, Nrf2 nuclear translocation and subsequently HO-1 expression were successfully enhanced in DIBEt-treated cells, which were strongly mitigated in U0126-treated cells, suggesting that ERK activation plays a critical role in DIBEt-induced Nrf2 translocation into the nucleus and subsequent boost of HO-1 expression in RAW 264.7 cells. Moreover, according to previous reports, dietary antioxidants can cause MAPK activation accountable for cell protection against oxidative stress [50].

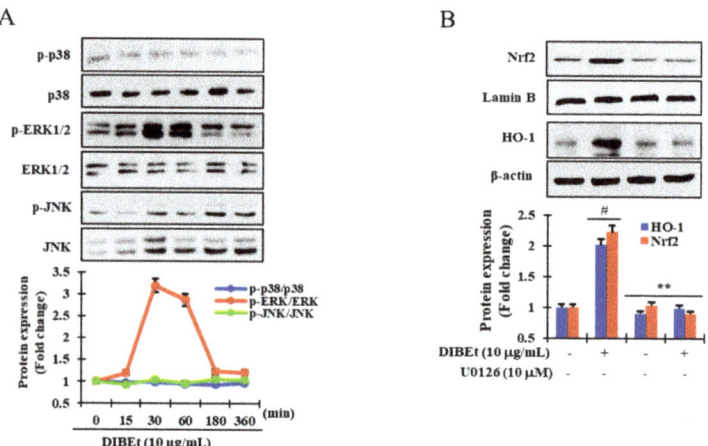

Figure 5. DIBEt facilitates Nrf2 translocation by activating ERK1/2. RAW 264.7 cells were pretreated with DIBEt (10 µg/mL) at the indicated times. Immunoblotting was performed to evaluate kinase activity (**A**). Cells were treated with DIBEt in the presence and absence of the specific inhibitor U0126. The protein levels of Nrf2 and HO-1 were analyzed by Western blot (**B**). Mean ± SD ($n = 3$). # $p < 0.001$; ** $p < 0.05$, compared to no treatment. Statistical analysis was performed using one-way ANOVA.

4. Conclusions

Oxidative stress is a major causative condition for the development and progression of numerous acute and chronic clinical disorders. Thus, antioxidants may cause health benefits as prophylactic agents. In this study, DIBEt contained various polyphenolic compounds as confirmed by PSI-MS/MS and showed superior antioxidant activity in cell-free and cellular levels. DIBEt treatment successfully lessened oxidative stress and cell death, most likely by (i) reducing ROS generation and (ii) boosting the expression of endogenous antioxidant enzymes and/or Nrf2-mediated HO-1 expression. DIBEt pretreatment may cause the activation of ERK1/2 signaling pathways involved in the cytoprotective effects of DIBEt. The findings provide new insights into the cytoprotective effects and mechanisms of DIB against oxidative stress, which may be used as treatment for oxidative stress-induced disorders.

Supplementary Materials: The following are available online at http://www.mdpi.com/2076-3921/9/11/1099/s1, Figure S1: Mass fragmentation of nitrogen compounds in DIB extracts. Figure S2: Mass fragmentation of flavonoids in DIB extracts. Figure S3: Mass fragmentation of phenolic acids in DIB extracts. Figure S4: Mass fragmentation of ethyl maltol, 11-dodecenoic acid, and the triterpenoid nutriacholic acid in DIB extracts. Figure S5: DPPH and ABTS radical-scavenging activities of various organic and aqueous DIB extracts. Figure S6: Superoxide and hydroxyl radical-scavenging activities of various organic and aqueous DIB extracts. Figure S7: CUPRAC and FRAP activities of various organic and aqueous DIB extracts. Figure S8: Total phenol (A) and flavonoid (B) content of various organic and aqueous DIB extracts. Figure S9: Cell viability of DIBEt. Table S1: List of primer sequences used in this study. Table S2: List of antibodies used in this study.

Author Contributions: M.B.A., A.A., S.I. and H.-J.C. performed the research. M.B.A., A.A., M.A.M., S.K. and S.-H.L. designed the research study and analyzed the data. M.B.A., A.A., S.K. and S.-H.L. wrote the paper. M.B.A. and S.-H.L. revised the paper. All authors have read and agreed to the published version of the manuscript.

Funding: This study was supported by a National Research Foundation of Korea grant funded by the Ministry of Science and ICT (2020R1A2C2011495).

Acknowledgments: M.B.A. and H.-J.C. were supported by the BK21Plus Creative Innovative Group for Leading Future Functional Food Industry, Kyungpook National University.

Conflicts of Interest: The authors declare no conflict of interest.

References

1. Banerjee, J.; Das, A.; Sinha, M.; Saha, S. Biological efficacy of medicinal plant extracts in preventing oxidative damage. *Oxidative Med. Cell. Longev.* **2018**, *2018*, 7904349. [CrossRef] [PubMed]
2. Castaneda, O.A.; Lee, S.C.; Ho, C.T.; Huang, T.C. Macrophages in oxidative stress and models to evaluate the antioxidant function of dietary natural compounds. *J. Food Drug Anal.* **2017**, *25*, 111–118. [CrossRef] [PubMed]
3. Alam, M.B.; Ju, M.K.; Lee, S.H. DNA protecting activities of *Nymphaea nouchali* (Burm. f) flower extract attenuate t-BHP-induced oxidative stress cell death through Nrf2-mediated induction of heme oxygenase-1 expression by activating MAP-kinases. *Int. J. Mol. Sci.* **2017**, *18*, 2069. [CrossRef] [PubMed]
4. Taguchi, K.; Motohashi, H.; Yamamoto, M. Molecular mechanisms of the Keap1-Nrf2 pathway in stress response and cancer evolution. *Genes Cells* **2011**, *16*, 123–140. [CrossRef] [PubMed]
5. Baird, L.; Dinkova-Kostova, A.T. The cytoprotective role of the Keap1-Nrf2 pathway. *Arch. Toxicol.* **2011**, *85*, 241–272. [CrossRef] [PubMed]
6. Wang, H.; Liu, J.; Cooks, R.G.; Ouyang, Z. Paper spray for direct analysis of complex mixtures using mass spectrometry. *Angew. Chem. (Int. Ed. Engl.)* **2010**, *49*, 877–880. [CrossRef] [PubMed]
7. Di Donna, L.; Taverna, D.; Indelicato, S.; Napoli, A.; Sindona, G.; Mazzotti, F. Rapid assay of resveratrol in red wine by paper spray tandem mass spectrometry and isotope dilution. *Food Chem.* **2017**, *229*, 354–357. [CrossRef] [PubMed]
8. Teodoro, J.A.R.; Pereira, H.V.; Sena, M.M.; Piccin, E.; Zacca, J.J.; Augusti, R. Paper spray mass spectrometry and chemometric tools for a fast and reliable identification of counterfeit blended Scottish whiskies. *Food Chem.* **2017**, *237*, 1058–1064. [CrossRef] [PubMed]
9. Li, A.; Wei, P.; Hsu, H.C.; Cooks, R.G. Direct analysis of 4-methylimidazole in foods using paper spray mass spectrometry. *Analyst* **2013**, *138*, 4624–4630. [CrossRef] [PubMed]
10. Saiful Yazan, L.; Armania, N. Dillenia species: A review of the traditional uses, active constituents and pharmacological properties from pre-clinical studies. *Pharm. Biol.* **2014**, *52*, 890–897. [CrossRef]
11. Kumar, D.; Mallick, S.; Vedasiromoni, J.R.; Pal, B.C. Anti-leukemic activity of *Dillenia indica* L. fruit extract and quantification of betulinic acid by HPLC. *Phytomed. Int. J. Phytother. Phytopharmacol.* **2010**, *17*, 431–435. [CrossRef]
12. Abdille, M.H.; Singh, R.; Jayaprakasha, G.; Jena, B. Antioxidant activity of the extracts from *Dillenia indica* fruits. *Food Chem.* **2005**, *90*, 891–896. [CrossRef]
13. Deraedt, R.; Jouquey, S.; Delevallee, F.; Flahaut, M. Release of prostaglandins E and F in an algogenic reaction and its inhibition. *Eur. J. Pharmacol.* **1980**, *61*, 17–24. [CrossRef]
14. Grover, J.K.; Yadav, S.; Vats, V. Medicinal plants of India with anti-diabetic potential. *J. Ethnopharmacol.* **2002**, *81*, 81–100. [CrossRef]

15. Wishart, D.S.; Feunang, Y.D.; Marcu, A.; Guo, A.C.; Liang, K.; Vazquez-Fresno, R.; Sajed, T.; Johnson, D.; Li, C.; Karu, N.; et al. HMDB 4.0: The human metabolome database for 2018. *Nucleic Acids Res.* **2018**, *46*, D608–D617. [CrossRef] [PubMed]
16. Guijas, C.; Montenegro-Burke, J.R.; Domingo-Almenara, X.; Palermo, A.; Warth, B.; Hermann, G.; Koellensperger, G.; Huan, T.; Uritboonthai, W.; Aisporna, A.E.; et al. METLIN: A technology platform for identifying knowns and unknowns. *Anal. Chem.* **2018**, *90*, 3156–3164. [CrossRef] [PubMed]
17. Alam, M.B.; Kwon, K.R.; Lee, S.H.; Lee, S.H. *Lannea coromandelica* (Houtt.) Merr. induces heme oxygenase 1 (HO-1) expression and reduces oxidative stress via the p38/c-Jun N-terminal kinase-nuclear factor erythroid 2-related factor 2 (p38/JNK-NRF2)-mediated antioxidant pathway. *Int. J. Mol. Sci.* **2017**, *18*, 266. [CrossRef] [PubMed]
18. Ou, B.; Huang, D.; Hampsch-Woodill, M.; Flanagan, J.A.; Deemer, E.K. Analysis of antioxidant activities of common vegetables employing oxygen radical absorbance capacity (ORAC) and ferric reducing antioxidant power (FRAP) assays: A comparative study. *J. Agric. Food Chem.* **2002**, *50*, 3122–3128. [CrossRef] [PubMed]
19. Alam, M.B.; Ju, M.K.; Kwon, Y.G.; Lee, S.H. Protopine attenuates inflammation stimulated by carrageenan and LPS via the MAPK/NF-kappaB pathway. *Food Chem. Toxicol.* **2019**, *131*, 110583. [CrossRef]
20. Rahman, M.S.; Hee Choi, Y.; Seok Choi, Y.; Alam, M.B.; Han Lee, S.; Cheol Yoo, J. A novel antioxidant peptide, purified from *Bacillus amyloliquefaciens*, showed strong antioxidant potential via Nrf-2 mediated heme oxygenase-1 expression. *Food Chem.* **2018**, *239*, 502–510. [CrossRef]
21. Piraud, M.; Vianey-Saban, C.; Petritis, K.; Elfakir, C.; Steghens, J.P.; Morla, A.; Bouchu, D. ESI-MS/MS analysis of underivatised amino acids: A new tool for the diagnosis of inherited disorders of amino acid metabolism. Fragmentation study of 79 molecules of biological interest in positive and negative ionisation mode. *Rapid Commun. Mass Spectr. RCM* **2003**, *17*, 1297–1311. [CrossRef] [PubMed]
22. Shiojima, K.; Arai, Y.; Masuda, K.; Takase, Y.; Ageta, T.; Ageta, H. Mass spectra of pentacyclic triterpenoids. *Chem. Pharmaceut. Bull.* **1992**, *40*, 1683–1690. [CrossRef]
23. Das, M.; Sarma, B.P.; Ahmed, G.; Nirmala, C.B.; Choudhury, M.K. In vitro anti oxidant activity total phenolic content of *Dillenia indica Garcinia penducalata*, commonly used fruits in Assamese cuisine. *Free Radic. Antioxid.* **2012**, *2*, 30–36. [CrossRef]
24. Kumaran, A.; Karunakaran, R.J. In vitro antioxidant activities of methanol extracts of five *Phyllanthus* species from India. *LWT-Food Sci. Technol.* **2007**, *40*, 344–352. [CrossRef]
25. Astley, S.B. Dietary antioxidants—Past, present and future? *Trends Food Sci. Technol.* **2003**, *14*, 93–98. [CrossRef]
26. Holasova, M.; Fiedlerova, V.; Smrcinova, H.; Orsak, M.; Lachman, J.; Vavreinova, S. Buckwheat—The source of antioxidant activity in functional foods. *Food Res. Int.* **2002**, *35*, 207–211. [CrossRef]
27. Huyut, Z.; Beydemir, Ş.; Gülçin, İ. Antioxidant and antiradical properties of selected flavonoids and phenolic compounds. *Biochem. Res. Int.* **2017**, *2017*, 7616791. [CrossRef]
28. Kapepula, P.M.; Kabamba Ngombe, N.; Tshisekedi Tshibangu, P.; Tsumbu, C.; Franck, T.; Mouithys-Mickalad, A.; Mumba, D.; Tshala-Katumbay, D.; Serteyn, D.; Tits, M.; et al. Comparison of metabolic profiles and bioactivities of the leaves of three edible Congolese *Hibiscus* species. *Nat. Prod. Res.* **2017**, *31*, 2885–2892. [CrossRef]
29. Cavia-Saiz, M.; Busto, M.D.; Pilar-Izquierdo, M.C.; Ortega, N.; Perez-Mateos, M.; Muñiz, P. Antioxidant properties, radical scavenging activity and biomolecule protection capacity of flavonoid naringenin and its glycoside naringin: A comparative study. *J. Sci. Food Agric.* **2010**, *90*, 1238–1244. [CrossRef] [PubMed]
30. Wang, J.; Fang, X.; Ge, L.; Cao, F.; Zhao, L.; Wang, Z.; Xiao, W. Antitumor, antioxidant and anti-inflammatory activities of kaempferol and its corresponding glycosides and the enzymatic preparation of kaempferol. *PLoS ONE* **2018**, *13*, e0197563. [CrossRef]
31. Canabady-Rochelle, L.L.; Harscoat-Schiavo, C.; Kessler, V.; Aymes, A.; Fournier, F.; Girardet, J.M. Determination of reducing power and metal chelating ability of antioxidant peptides: Revisited methods. *Food Chem.* **2015**, *183*, 129–135. [CrossRef]
32. Baran, M.Y.; Emecen, G.; Simon, A.; Tóth, G.; Kuruuzum-Uz, A. Assessment of the antioxidant activity and genotoxicity of the extracts and isolated glycosides with a new flavonoid from *Lotus aegaeus* (Gris.) Boiss. *Ind. Crops Prod.* **2020**, *153*, 112590. [CrossRef]
33. Gangwar, M.; Goel, R.K.; Nath, G. *Mallotus philippinensis* Muell. Arg (Euphorbiaceae): Ethnopharmacology and phytochemistry review. *Biomed. Res. Int.* **2014**, *2014*, 213973. [CrossRef] [PubMed]
34. Tang, X.; Yu, R.; Zhou, Q.; Jiang, S.; Le, G. Protective effects of γ-aminobutyric acid against H_2O_2-induced oxidative stress in RIN-m5F pancreatic cells. *Nutr. Metab.* **2018**, *15*, 60. [CrossRef] [PubMed]

35. Zou, X.; Gao, J.; Zheng, Y.; Wang, X.; Chen, C.; Cao, K.; Xu, J.; Li, Y.; Lu, W.; Liu, J. Zeaxanthin induces Nrf2-mediated phase II enzymes in protection of cell death. *Cell Death Dis.* **2014**, *5*, e1218. [CrossRef]
36. Poljsak, B.; Šuput, D.; Milisav, I. Achieving the balance between ROS and antioxidants: When to use the synthetic antioxidants. *Oxidative Med. Cell. Longev.* **2013**, *2013*, 956792. [CrossRef] [PubMed]
37. He, L.; He, T.; Farrar, S.; Ji, L.; Liu, T.; Ma, X. Antioxidants maintain cellular redox homeostasis by elimination of reactive oxygen species. *Cell. Physiol. Biochem.* **2017**, *44*, 532–553. [CrossRef]
38. Araujo, J.A.; Zhang, M.; Yin, F. Heme oxygenase-1, oxidation, inflammation, and atherosclerosis. *Front. Pharmacol.* **2012**, *3*, 119. [CrossRef]
39. Fernández-Pachón, M.S.; Berná, G.; Otaolaurruchi, E.; Troncoso, A.M.; Martín, F.; García-Parrilla, M.C. Changes in antioxidant endogenous enzymes (activity and gene expression levels) after repeated red wine intake. *J. Agric. Food Chem.* **2009**, *57*, 6578–6583. [CrossRef]
40. Crespo, I.; García-Mediavilla, M.V.; Almar, M.; González, P.; Tuñón, M.J.; Sánchez-Campos, S.; González-Gallego, J. Differential effects of dietary flavonoids on reactive oxygen and nitrogen species generation and changes in antioxidant enzyme expression induced by proinflammatory cytokines in Chang liver cells. *Food Chem. Toxicol.* **2008**, *46*, 1555–1569. [CrossRef] [PubMed]
41. Schröter, D.; Neugart, S.; Schreiner, M.; Grune, T.; Rohn, S.; Ott, C. Amaranth's 2-caffeoylisocitric acid—An anti-inflammatory caffeic acid derivative that impairs NF-κB signaling in LPS-challenged RAW 264.7 macrophages. *Nutrients* **2019**, *11*, 571. [CrossRef] [PubMed]
42. Du, W.; An, Y.; He, X.; Zhang, D.; He, W. Protection of kaempferol on oxidative stress-induced retinal pigment epithelial cell damage. *Oxidative Med. Cell. Longev.* **2018**, *2018*, 1610751. [CrossRef]
43. Wang, K.; Chen, Z.; Huang, L.; Meng, B.; Zhou, X.; Wen, X.; Ren, D. Naringenin reduces oxidative stress and improves mitochondrial dysfunction via activation of the Nrf2/ARE signaling pathway in neurons. *Int. J. Mol. Med.* **2017**, *40*, 1582–1590. [CrossRef]
44. Aladaileh, S.H.; Hussein, O.E.; Abukhalil, M.H.; Saghir, S.A.M.; Bin-Jumah, M.; Alfwuaires, M.A.; Germoush, M.O.; Almaiman, A.A.; Mahmoud, A.M. Formononetin upregulates Nrf2/HO-1 signaling and prevents oxidative stress, inflammation, and kidney injury in methotrexate-induced rats. *Antioxidants (Basel Switz.)* **2019**, *8*, 430. [CrossRef]
45. Zhang, B.; Wang, J.; Zhao, G.; Lin, M.; Lang, Y.; Zhang, D.; Feng, D.; Tu, C. Apigenin protects human melanocytes against oxidative damage by activation of the Nrf2 pathway. *Cell Stress Chaperones* **2020**, *25*, 277–285. [CrossRef]
46. Vomund, S.; Schäfer, A.; Parnham, M.J.; Brüne, B.; von Knethen, A. Nrf2, the master regulator of anti-oxidative responses. *Int. J. Mol. Sci.* **2017**, *18*, 2772. [CrossRef]
47. Liu, X.-P.; Goldring, C.E.; Copple, I.M.; Wang, H.-Y.; Wei, W.; Kitteringham, N.R.; Park, B.K. Extract of *Ginkgo biloba* induces phase 2 genes through Keap1-Nrf2-ARE signaling pathway. *Life Sci.* **2007**, *80*, 1586–1591. [CrossRef]
48. Shen, G.; Hebbar, V.; Nair, S.; Xu, C.; Li, W.; Lin, W.; Keum, Y.S.; Han, J.; Gallo, M.A.; Kong, A.N. Regulation of Nrf2 transactivation domain activity. The differential effects of mitogen-activated protein kinase cascades and synergistic stimulatory effect of Raf and CREB-binding protein. *J. Biol. Chem.* **2004**, *279*, 23052–23060. [CrossRef] [PubMed]
49. Bellezza, I.; Giambanco, I.; Minelli, A.; Donato, R. Nrf2-Keap1 signaling in oxidative and reductive stress. *Biochim. Biophys. Acta Mol. Cell Res.* **2018**, *1865*, 721–733. [CrossRef]
50. Yoon, J.; Ham, H.; Sung, J.; Kim, Y.; Choi, Y.; Lee, J.-S.; Jeong, H.-S.; Lee, J.; Kim, D. Black rice extract protected HepG2 cells from oxidative stress-induced cell death via ERK1/2 and Akt activation. *Nutr. Res. Pract.* **2014**, *8*, 125–131. [CrossRef]

Publisher's Note: MDPI stays neutral with regard to jurisdictional claims in published maps and institutional affiliations.

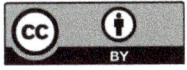

© 2020 by the authors. Licensee MDPI, Basel, Switzerland. This article is an open access article distributed under the terms and conditions of the Creative Commons Attribution (CC BY) license (http://creativecommons.org/licenses/by/4.0/).

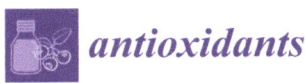

Article

Colon Bioaccessibility under In Vitro Gastrointestinal Digestion of a Red Cabbage Extract Chemically Profiled through UHPLC-Q-Orbitrap HRMS

Luana Izzo [1,*], Yelko Rodríguez-Carrasco [2], Severina Pacifico [3], Luigi Castaldo [1], Alfonso Narváez [1] and Alberto Ritieni [1,4]

1. Department of Pharmacy, University of Naples "Federico II", Via Domenico Montesano 49, 80131 Naples, Italy; luigi.castaldo2@unina.it (L.C.); alfonso.narvaezsimon@unina.it (A.N.); alberto.ritieni@unina.it (A.R.)
2. Laboratory of Food Chemistry and Toxicology, Faculty of Pharmacy, University of Valencia, Av. Vicent Andrés Estellés s/n, 46100 Burjassot, Valencia, Spain; yelko.rodriguez@uv.es
3. Department of Environmental, Biological and Pharmaceutical Sciences and Technologies, University of Campania "Luigi Vanvitelli", Via Vivaldi 43, 81100 Caserta, Italy; severina.pacifico@unicampania.it
4. Health Education and Sustainable Development, Federico II University, 80131 Naples, Italy
* Correspondence: luana.izzo@unina.it; Tel.: +39-081-678116

Received: 4 September 2020; Accepted: 2 October 2020; Published: 6 October 2020

Abstract: Red cabbage is a native vegetable of the Mediterranean region that represents one of the major sources of anthocyanins. The aim of this research is to evaluate the antioxidant capability and total polyphenol content (TPC) of a red cabbage extract and to compare acquired data with those from the same extract encapsulated in an acid-resistant capsule. The extract, which was qualitatively and quantitatively profiled by UHPLC-Q-Orbitrap HRMS analysis, contained a high content of anthocyanins and phenolic acids, whereas non-anthocyanin flavonoids were the less abundant compounds. An in vitro gastrointestinal digestion system was utilized to follow the extract's metabolism in humans and to evaluate its colon bioaccessibility. Data obtained showed that during gastrointestinal digestion, the total polyphenol content of the extract digested in the acid-resistant capsule in the Pronase E stage resulted in a higher concentration value compared to the extract digested without the capsule. Reasonably, these results could be attributed to the metabolization process by human colonic microflora and to the genesis of metabolites with greater bioactivity and more beneficial effects. The use of red cabbage extract encapsulated in an acid-resistant capsule could improve the polyphenols' bioaccessibility and be proposed as a red cabbage-based nutraceutical formulation for counteracting stress oxidative diseases.

Keywords: red cabbage; in vitro gastrointestinal digestion; antioxidants; acid-resistant capsule; bioaccessibility; UHPLC-Q-Orbitrap HRMS

1. Introduction

Red cabbage (*Purple Brassica oleracea* L. var. *capitata F. rubra*) is a native vegetable of the Mediterranean region that originated in Europe in the 16th century and nowadays is largely consumed worldwide. Among different vegetables in the human diet, it represents one of the major sources of polyphenolic compounds, especially anthocyanins [1]. Anthocyanins are natural glycoside compounds belonging to the flavonoids group, and they are mainly responsible for the colors of fruits, vegetables, and flowers. The flavylium (2-phenylchromenylium) ion represents the basic molecular skeleton of anthocyanins, whose sugar-free components are anthocyanidin aglycones. Among naturally anthocyanidins known until now, merely six principal types are common in fruit and vegetables, which mainly differ in the oxygenation degree of the flavonoid B-ring (e.g., hydroxyl and/or methoxyl groups). Thus, anthocyanins variability in plants is mainly due to the sugar moieties identity and number as well as to the diversity in acylated substituents [both aromatic (largely hydroxycinnamic acids, and/or simple C_6C_1 acids) or aliphatic acids (e.g., malonic acid)], which could be linked to the anthocyanin core or directly to the anthocyanidin nucleus. Particularly, the red cabbage matrix contains cyanidin 3-diglucoside-5-glucoside derivatives highly conjugated with sugars such as glucose and xylose and acyl groups including caffeoyl, p-coumaroyl, feruloyl, p-hydroxybenzoyl, sinapoyl, and oxaloyl [2,3].

The overproduction of reactive oxygen and nitrogen species (ROS/RNS) could occur in living organisms at an uncontrolled rate, defining oxidative stress condition onset, which is correlated with various forms of health damage including chronic age-related diseases, atherosclerosis, carcinogenesis, and neurodegenerative disorders. A healthy nutrition, mainly based on fruits and vegetables, is suggested to delay or positively modulate the dynamic balance between oxidants and antioxidants, thanks to plant foods diversity in bioactive compounds, such as polyphenols. Polyphenols are exogenous antioxidant compounds that are able to prevent and/or inhibit the genesis of pathophysiological perturbations in redox circuitry. According to Sies et al. [4], the oxidative stress represents "a disturbance in the pro-oxidant–antioxidant balance in favor of the former, leading to potential damage". Anthocyanins are known to have a wide range of health-promoting properties for human health including cytoprotective activity, which might be due to the ability of anthocyanins to decrease cell death, lactate dehydrogenase (LDH) release, caspase 3 activation, and DNA damages [5]. Moreover, scientific reports support an increase in the cytoprotective effect as a result of the anthocyanin-rich diet [6].

To fully preserve or augment polyphenols bioactivity and achieve an efficient therapeutic activity, these compounds often need to be formulated into bioavailable dosage nutraceutical forms [7,8]. Indeed, new formulations by using polyphenols from dietary plants are continuously investigated also for safeguarding polyphenol chemical features that could be compromised during their metabolism fates in humans. This is particularly true for anthocyanins and anthocyanidin compounds, which are highly instable and very sensitive to degradation by oxygen, temperature, light, enzymes, and pH, and whose availability after gastrointestinal digestion could limit their beneficial effect on health.

The correlation of the anthocyanins' consumption and beneficial effects on human health has been reported by many scientific studies and includes sundry protective effects on human health such as antioxidant, anti-inflammatory, anticancer activity, and effects on the cardiovascular, neurodegenerative, and metabolic systems [9–11]. To confer beneficial health effects, bioactive compounds need to be bioavailable and reach, after gastrointestinal (GI) digestion, target tissues in the human body. Although fruits and vegetables are an abundant source of polyphenols and other bioactive compounds, the available amount of these substances after small intestine digestion is significantly reduced [12].

Anthocyanins are stable in the acid conditions existing in the stomach, whereas their stability decreases with the increase in the pH value in the small intestine. Therefore, the bioavailability of these compounds is affected [13]. In particular, it was observed that at pH > 7, anthocyanidins undergo degradation, and that the presence of sugar moieties in anthocyanins favors an increase in terms of stability at neutral pH in respect to their aglycones [14]. Thus, diglycosides are more stable than monoglycosides, which is explained by the hindrance from sugar parts that prevent the degradation into phenolic acids and aldehydes [2]. Accordingly, it is important to define the effect of such polyphenols and their stability during the digestion process and consequentially, their bioaccessibility and their possible beneficial effects. Until now, limited information describing the in vivo effects of the GI process on dietary polyphenols has been reported [15–17].

Thus, the aim of this scientific research is as follows: (i) to prepare red-cabbage extracts based on different extracting mixtures, evaluated for their total polyphenol content (TPC) and the antiradical and reducing properties; (ii) to compare the antioxidant activity of red cabbage extract showing the highest TPC value with data from the same extract encapsulated in an acid-resistant capsule, and (iii) to assess the bioaccessibility of the extract, such as it is, and its encapsulated formula through an in vitro gastrointestinal digestion, with a view to propose the use of the red-cabbage nutraceutical formulation in slowing down or delaying oxidative stress onset.

The polyphenolic profile of the prepared red cabbage extract was ascertained through ultra-high-performance liquid chromatography coupled to a high-resolution Orbitrap mass spectrometry.

2. Materials and Methods

2.1. Reagents and Materials

Methanol (MeOH), ethanol (EtOH), acetic acid (AcOH), formic acid (FA), and acetonitrile (AcN) HPLC grade were purchased from Merck (Darmstadt, Germany). Deionized water (<18 MΩ x cm resistivity) was obtained from a Milli-Q water purification system (Millipore, Bedford, MA, USA).

Potassium chloride (KCl), potassium thiocyanate (KSCN), monosodium phosphate (NaH_2PO_4), sodium sulfate (Na_2SO_4), potassium persulphate ($K_2S_2O_8$), sodium chloride (NaCl), sodium bicarbonate ($NaHCO_3$), sodium carbonate (Na_2CO_3), hydrochloric acid (HCl), pepsin (250 U/mg solid) from porcine gastric mucosa, pancreatin (4 USP) from porcine pancreas, protease from *Streptomyces griseus*, also named Pronase E (3.5 U/mg solid), and Viscozyme L were purchased from Sigma Aldrich (Milan, Italy).

The compound of 2,2-azinobis (3-ethylbenzothiazoline-6-sulphonic acid) diammonium salt (ABTS), ferrous chloride ($FeCl_2$), 1,1-Diphenyl-2-picrylhydrazyl (DPPH), 2,4,6-tris(2-pyridyl)-1,3,5-triazine (TPTZ), Folin–Ciocalteu reagent, (±)-6-Hydroxy-2,5,7,8-tetramethylchromane-2-carboxylic acid commonly called Trolox ($C_{14}H_{18}O_4$), and gallic acid ($C_7H_6O_5$) were acquired from Sigma Aldrich (Milan, Italy). All other chemicals and reagents were of analytical grade.

2.2. Sampling

Red cabbage (*Brassica oleracea* L. var. *capitata* F. *rubra*) plants were grown in different fields located in Campania, South of Italy. All bulbs (n = 10) were harvested in September 2019. After the samples arrived in the laboratory, the cabbage samples with mechanical damage and visible spoilage were separated. Red cabbage samples were rapidly washed under running tap water and chopped into small pieces before being frozen and freeze-dried (Lyovapor™ L-200, Buchi srl, Milan, Italy). After lyophilization, the dry weight of the samples obtained was recorded; then, they were milled into powder (particle size 200 μm) using a laboratory mill. The powders were stored at −80 °C until analysis. All the analyses were performed in triplicate, the replicates were independents and results expressed as mean ± SD. Dry matter content of red cabbage corresponded to 12%.

2.3. Red Cabbage Polyphenolic Extraction

Polyphenols were extracted according to the procedure reported by Grace et al. [18] with some modifications. Briefly, 2.5 g of freeze-dried red cabbage was introduced into a 50-mL Falcon tube (Conical Polypropylene Centrifuge Tube; Thermo Fisher Scientific, Milan, Italy) and extracted with 30 mL of five different mixtures: (1) MeOH:H_2O (60:40) 0.1% FA; (2) MeOH:H_2O (70:30) 0.1% AcOH; (3) MeOH:H_2O (80:20) 0.1% FA; (4) H_2O 0.1% FA; (5) EtOH:H_2O (70:30) 0.1% AcOH. The samples were vortexed (ZX3; VEPL Scientific, Usmate, Italy) for 2 min and sonicated (LBS 1; Zetalab srl, Padua, Italy) for 30 min (vortexed at 10-min intervals). Then, the mixture was centrifuged for 10 min at 4000 rpm at 20 °C. The supernatant was collected and filtrated through a 0.22 μm filter. A portion of the extracts was kept in refrigeration conditions until further analysis.

Moreover, another part of the red cabbage polyphenol extract obtained with mixture 1 after lyophilization was employed for the capsules' formulation. In particular, the capsules contained 1000 mg of red cabbage polyphenolic extract. The capsules used were acid-resistant (hydroxypropyl cellulose E464, gellan gum E418, titanium dioxide E171).

2.4. Determination of Total Phenolic Content (TPC)

The Folin–Ciocalteu method was used for determining the total phenolic content in accordance with the procedure reported by Izzo et al. [19]. Briefly, 500 µL of deionized water and 125 µL of the Folin–Ciocalteu reagent 2 N were added to 125 µL of red cabbage extract. The tube was mixed and incubated for 6 min in dark conditions. Then, 1.25 mL of 7.5% of sodium carbonate solution and 1 mL of deionized water were added. The reaction mixture was maintained in dark for 90 min. Finally, the absorbance at 760 nm was measured through a spectrophotometer system. Results were expressed as mg of gallic acid equivalents (GAE)/g of dry weight sample.

2.5. UHPLC-Q-Orbitrap HRMS Analysis

The qualitative and quantitative profile of bioactive compounds were performed by Ultra High-Pressure Liquid Chromatograph (UHPLC, Dionex UltiMate 3000, Thermo Fisher Scientific, Waltham, MA, USA) equipped with a degassing system, a Quaternary UHPLC pump working at 1250 bar, and an autosampler device. Chromatographic separation was carried out with a thermostated (T = 25 °C) Kinetex 1.7 µm F5 (50 × 2.1 mm, Phenomenex, Torrance, CA, USA) column. The mobile phase consisted of 0.1% FA in water (A) and 0.1% FA in methanol (B). The injection volume was 1 µL. The gradient elution program was as follows: an initial 0% B, increased to 40% B in 1 min, to 80% B in 1 min, and to 100% B in 3 min. The gradient was held for 4 min at 100% B, reduced to 0% B in 2 min, and another 2 min for column re-equilibration at 0%. The total run time was 13 min, and the flow rate was 0.5 mL/min.

The mass spectrometer was operated in both negative and positive ion mode by setting 2 scan events: full ion MS and all ion fragmentation (AIF). The following settings were used in full MS mode: resolution power of 70,000 Full Width at Half Maximum (FWHM) (defined for m/z 200), scan range 80–1200 m/z, automatic gain control (AGC) target 1×10^6, injection time set to 200 ms and scan rate set at 2 scan/s. The ion source parameters were as follows: spray voltage 3.5 kV; capillary temperature 320 °C; S-lens RF level 60, sheath gas pressure 18, auxiliary gas 3, and auxiliary gas heater temperature 350 °C.

For the scan event of AIF, the parameters in the positive and negative mode were set as follows: mass resolving power = 17,500 FWHM; maximum injection time = 200 ms; scan time = 0.10 s; ACG target = 1×10^5; scan range = 80–120 m/z; isolation window to 5.0 m/z; and retention time to 30 s. The collision energy was varied in the range of 10 to 60 eV to obtain representative product ion spectra.

For accurate mass measurement, identification and confirmation were performed at a mass tolerance of 5 ppm for the molecular ion and for both fragments. Data analysis and processing were performed using Xcalibur software, v. 3.1.66.10 (Xcalibur, Thermo Fisher Scientific, Waltham, MA, USA).

2.6. Antioxidant Activity

2.6.1. ABTS Radical Cation Scavenging Assay

Free radical-scavenging activity was measured by using the method reported by Luz et al., [20]. Briefly, 9.6 mg of 2,2-azinobis (3-ethylbenzothiazoline-6-sulphonic acid) diammonium salt was solubilized in 2.5 mL of deionized water (7 mM) and 44 µL of solution of potassium persulfate ($K_2S_2O_8$; 2.45 mM) were added. The solution was kept in dark conditions at room temperature for 16 h prior to use. Afterward, ABTS$^{•+}$ solution was diluted with ethanol to reach an absorbance value of 0.70 (±0.02) at 734 nm. Then, to 1 mL of ABTS$^{•+}$ solution with an absorbance of 0.700 ± 0.050, 0.1 mL of opportunely diluted sample was added. After 2.5 min wait, the absorbance was immediately measured at 734 nm. Results were expressed as millimoles of Trolox Equivalents (TE)/kg of dry weight sample.

2.6.2. DPPH Free Radical-Scavenging Assay

The total free radical-scavenging activity of the analyzed samples was determined using the method suggested by Brand-Williams et al. [21] with modifications. Briefly, 1,1-diphenyl-2-picrylhydrazyl (4.0 mg) was solubilized in 10 mL of methanol and then diluted to reach a value of 0.90 (±0.02) at 517 nm. This solution was used to perform the assay, and 200 µL of sample extract was added to 1 mL of working solution. Results were expressed as mmol Trolox Equivalents (TE)/kg of dry weight sample.

2.6.3. Ferric Reducing Antioxidant Power

The antioxidant capacity of red cabbage samples was estimated spectrophotometrically following the procedure of Benzie and Strain [22]. The ferric reducing/antioxidant power (FRAP) reagent was prepared by mixing acetate buffer (0.3 M; pH 3.6), TPTZ solution (10 mM), and ferric chloride solution (20 mM) in the proportion of 10:1:1 (*v/v/v*). Freshly prepared working FRAP reagent was used to perform the assay. Briefly, 0.150 mL of the appropriately diluted sample was added to 2850 mL of FRAP reagent. The value of absorbance was recorded after 4 min at 593 nm.

The method is based on the reduction of Fe^{3+} TPTZ complex (colorless complex) to Fe^{2+}-tripyridyltriazine (intense blue color complex) formed by the action of electron-donating antioxidants at low pH. Results were expressed as mmol Trolox Equivalents (TE)/kg of dry weight sample. All the determinations were performed in triplicate.

2.7. In Vitro Simulated Gastrointestinal Digestion

The in vitro gastrointestinal digestion, composed by oral, gastric, and intestinal phases (both duodenal and colon phases), was performed according to the standardized in vitro digestion model (INFOGEST method) [23] with some modifications (Figure 1). The simulated salivary, gastric, and intestinal fluid was prepared in accordance with the proportion salts reported by Castaldo et al. in Table 8 of the materials and methods section.

In the oral phase, 1 g of extract and one capsule contained 1 g of extract were mixed with 3.5 mL of warmed simulated salivary fluid (SSF). Then, 0.5 mL of α-amylase enzyme (50 mg of 250 U/mg solid), 25 µL of 0.3 M $CaCl_2$ $(H_2O)_2$, and 975 µL of water were added and thoroughly mixed. Afterward, the pH of the mixture was adjusted to 7 with HCl 1 M, and the sample was incubated for 2 min at 37 °C at 150 rpm in an orbital shaker (KS130 Basic IKA, Argo Lab, Milan, Italy).

In order to simulate the gastric phase, 7.5 mL of simulated gastric fluid (SGF), 1.6 mL of pepsin (59.2 mg of 4 USP), 5 µL of 0.3 M $CaCl_2$ $(H_2O)_2$, and 695 µL of water were added and thoroughly mixed. The pH value was adjusted to 3 using HCl 6 M. The sample was incubated for 120 min at 37 °C at 150 rpm in an orbital shaker (KS130 Basic IKA, Argo Lab, Milan, Italy).

In the intestinal phase, 11 mL of simulated intestinal fluid (SIF), 5 mL of pancreatin (20 mg of 4 USP), 2.5 mL of bile salts (150 mg), 40 µL of 0.3 M $CaCl_2$ $(H_2O)_2$, and 1300 µL of water were added and thoroughly mixed. The pH value was adjusted to 7 using NaOH 6 M. The sample was incubated for 120 min at 37 °C at 150 rpm in an orbital shaker (KS130 Basic IKA, Argo Lab, Milan, Italy).

To the end of the intestinal phase, the tube was centrifuged at 5000 rpm for 10 min. To simulate the colon digestion process, the supernatant was collected, while 5 mL of Pronase E (1 mg/mL water solution) was added to the pellet. In this step, the pH value was adjusted to 8 using NaOH 1M and incubated for 60 min at 37 °C. Afterward, the supernatant was collected, lyophilized, and stored. The residue pellet was mixed with 150 µL of Viscozyme L, and the pH value was adjusted to 4 and incubated for 16 h at 37 °C. Finally, the supernatant was collected, stored, and lyophilized whereas the pellet was eliminated. All the supernatants collected during the different in vitro digestion phases were freeze-dried and then dissolved in MeOH:H_2O (6:4, *v/v*) containing 0.1% FA for the evaluation of antioxidant activity and total polyphenols content.

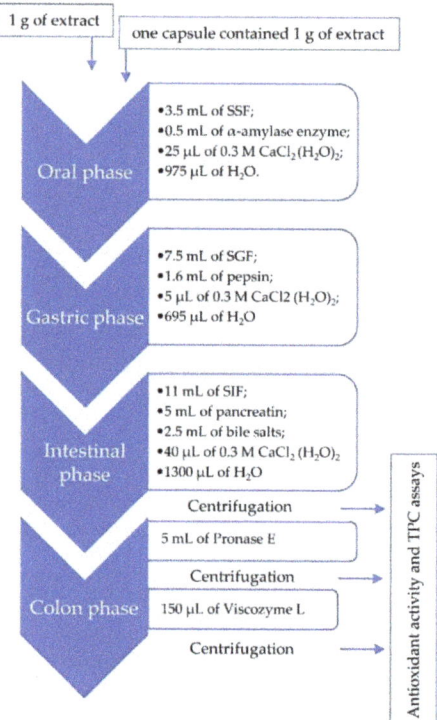

Figure 1. Overview and flow diagram of a simulated in vitro digestion method. SSF: simulated salivary fluid; SGF: simulated gastric fluid; SIF: simulated intestinal fluid.

2.8. Statistical Analysis

Statistical analysis of data was performed by two-way ANOVA analysis (SPSS 13.0) followed by the Tukey–Kramer multiple comparison test to evaluate significant differences; p-values ≤ 0.05 were considered as significant. All the determinations were performed in triplicate, and results were expressed as mean ± standard deviation (SD).

3. Results and Discussion

In this context, considering the diversity in polyphenol compounds of red cabbage, herein, the total polyphenol content and the antioxidant capability of red cabbage extracts obtained by using five different extracting mixtures were firstly evaluated. The red cabbage extract from the hydroalcoholic solution MeOH:H_2O (6:4, v/v), acidified with 0.1% FA, appeared to be the most active. Thus, this extract, which was chemically profiled by UHPLC-Q-Orbitrap HRMS, underwent an in vitro gastrointestinal digestion simulation, together with its encapsulated form. Accordingly, the effects of the GI process on the extract as it is and that formulated in an acid-resistant capsule were compared.

3.1. Red Cabbage Extract Bioactivity

In the first approach, efficient extraction mixtures to maximize polyphenol recovery, mainly in its anthocyanin component, were explored. The choice of the solvent represents an important step in the extraction process because of its impact on the yield of bioactive compounds and consequently on human system effects. As reported by Lapornik et al. [24], who studied the solvent effect on the extraction of anthocyanins and other polyphenols from grape and red currant, ethanol and methanol extracts resulted in a major amount of bioactive compounds than water extracts. Methanol exhibits slightly better characteristics than ethanol as an extracting solvent. Since methanol and ethanol are less polar than water, they are more effective in degrading cell walls (due to their apolar feature), favoring anthocyanins and polyphenols releasing from cells. However, it must be considered that ethanol is more suitable than methanol for a safe application in the food sector [25,26]. Taking into account these previous observations, in the current scientific research, total polyphenol content (TPC) and antioxidant activity of red cabbage extracts obtained by using five different mixtures of extraction solvents are evaluated and reported in Table 1. TPC data ranged from 15.798 to 19.986 mg GAE/g. Acidified water is less suitable for the extraction of phenolic compounds from red cabbage, followed by acidified ethanol/water mixture, which showed a 2.95% increase in extraction efficiency in respect to water extract. Hydroalcoholic solution based on methanol as an alcoholic component also differed in their TPC content, and the MeOH:H_2O (6:4) solution acidified with 0.1% formic acid appeared to elicit the best extracting properties. Indeed, beyond the ratio of alcohol to water, the type of acid component also could affect extraction overall. In fact, considering a variation of the MeOH/water ratio from 7:3 (v/v) to 8:2 (v/v) leads to a comparable TPC yield where acetic acid is used instead of formic acid. Moreover, the phenol recovery was estimated, taking account of the relative TPC value, and it showed a percentage increase of 26.5% in MeOH:H_2O (6:4) plus 0.1% FA with respect to acidified water extract. A similar trend was observed also assessing antioxidant activity through ABTS and DPPH antiradical tests, as well as by the ferric reducing/antioxidant power assay. Data acquired are in the range of 45.128–50.849, 23.498–36.242, and 67.759–87.095 mmol Trolox®/kg for ABTS, DPPH, and FRAP, respectively. It appears clear that the potential antioxidant capacity of red cabbage extract could be affected by the typology and polarity of the extraction mixture used or methodology applied [26], and a great variability could be verified when the total phenolics content from previous scientific studies in the literature was consulted.

Table 1. Total polyphenol content and antioxidant data of red cabbage extracts obtained using five different extractants. Values are reported as mean ± SD of independent experiments performed in triplicate. Statistic significance was calculated with two-way ANOVA analysis.

Red Cabbage Extract	TPC * (mg GAE/g)	ABTS *	DPPH * (mmol Trolox/kg)	FRAP *
MeOH:H_2O (6:4) 0.1% FA	19.986 ± 0.132 [a]	50.849 ± 2.955 [d]	36.242 ± 0.068 [f]	87.095 ± 0.699 [h]
MeOH:H_2O (7:3) 0.1% AcOH	17.591 ± 0.721 [b]	49.978 ± 1.408 [d]	34.466 ± 0.168 [f]	85.379 ± 0.349 [h]
MeOH:H_2O (8:2) 0.1% FA	17.541 ± 0.304 [b]	45.128 ± 1.065 [e]	24.003 ± 0.056 [g]	68.759 ± 0.349 [i]
H_2O 0.1% FA	15.798 ± 0.566 [c]	47.906 ± 1.411 [d]	23.498 ± 0.345 [g]	67.833 ± 1.325 [i]
EtOH:H_2O (7:3) 0.1% AcOH	16.262 ± 0.528 [c]	49.324 ± 0.761 [d]	24.701 ± 0.166 [g]	81.884 ± 1.277 [h]

* results are referred to dry weight (dw). [a–h] Mean values with different superscript letters are significantly different by Tukey–Kramer multiple comparison test.

Antioxidant activity data measured through the three spectrophotometrical assays (ABTS, DPPH, and FRAP test) are in line with those from other studies [27,28]. The Relative Antioxidant Capacity Index (RACI) was determined in accordance with the method previously reported by Pacifico et al. [29]. The standard score was calculated as the average of the standard scores obtained from the raw data for the various antioxidant methods. The TPC value highlights that MeOH:H_2O (6:4, v/v) 0.1% FA extract was more active than the others (Figure 2) and that an increase in methanol amount corresponds to a gradual decrease in antioxidant capacity. As shown in Table 2, a wide variability in the TPC of different red cabbage extracts was found in the literature. The concentration ranged between 0.10 and 116.00 mg/kg dry weight (dw). Presumably, the mixture MeOH:H_2O (6:4, v/v) results were a good compromise applicable to the extraction of red cabbage bioactive compounds. By increasing the percentage of methanol, the TPC content decreases. This effect could be due to the major solubility of anthocyanins, which are contained in high quantity in red cabbage, in a high percentage of acidified water, whereas polyphenols are more soluble in methanol.

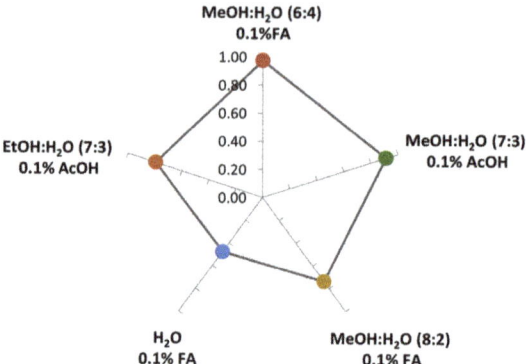

Figure 2. Relative Antioxidant Capacity Index (RACI) was used to integrate the antioxidant capacity values generated from the different applied methods.

Table 2. Recent surveys reporting the total phenolic content (mg GAE/g) in red cabbage extract. GAE: gallic acid equivalents.

References	TPC (mg GAE/g) dw *	Extraction Solvent	Sample Origin
Leja et al., 2010 [30]	3.90–31.11	80% MeOH	Poland
Upadhyay et al., 2016 [31]	28.25	80% MeOH	India
Fusari et al., 2020 [32]	0.099	Ultrapure H_2O	Argentina
Erken et al., 2017 [33]	313.73	EtOH/acetone	Turkey
Murador et al., 2016 [27]	3.56	0.5% HCl in MeOH	Brazil
Podsędek et al., 2017 [34]	10.1–19.6	70% MeOH	Poland
Podsędek et al., 2006 [35]	16.8–21.42	70% MeOH	Poland
Oroian et al., 2017 [36]	84.75	MeOH	Romania
Tanongkankit et al., 2010 [37]	496.92–739.24	acetone–H_2O (1:1, v/v)	Thailand
Jaiswal et al., 2012 [38]	18.45	70% MeOH	Ireland
Kusznierewicz et al., 2007 [39]	2.4–4.9	0.1% HCl (1 N) in MeOH	Poland/Belgium Germany/England
Tabart et al., 2018 [28]	18.51	acetone/H_2O/AcOH, (70:28:2, $v/v/v$)	Belgium
Cruz et al., 2016 [40]	89.33–116	70% MeOH/ H_2O boiled	Brazil
Caramês et al., 2020 [41]	48.37–87.12	MeOH/H_2O/AcOH (0.58:0.38:0.04, $v/v/v$)	Brazil

* results are adjusted and expressed in the same measurement unit as mg GAE/g dry weight.

Cruz et al. [40] reported higher TPC content in red cabbage extract (up to 116.00 mg/g) obtained with a hydromethanolic mixture (7:3, MeOH:H_2O, $v:v$), whereas in the here analyzed samples, all extracts were obtained by different mixtures acidified with AcOH or FA.

Murador et al. [27] evaluated the effects of different home cooking techniques on kale and red cabbage and demonstrated that these procedures seemed to have no significant effect on TPC in red cabbage. On the contrary, the cooking process facilitated the extraction of bioactive compounds due to the capability to soften the vegetable tissues, ameliorating the activity. Moreover, Wiczkowski et al. [42] determined the antioxidant activity of red cabbage varieties (Langedijker Dauer 2, Kissendrup, Koda, Kalibos, and Langedijker Polona) in two diversified lengths of the vegetation period (year 2008, 2009). The result of antioxidant activity measured through ABTS assay ranged between 87.99 and 168.76 and from 101.06 to 169.46 mmol Trolox/kg dry weight (dw) for two diversified lengths of the vegetation period, respectively. The varieties of red cabbage obtained in 2009 were characterized by a higher ability to radical scavenge than that grown in 2008, indicating that the differences in antioxidant capacity of red cabbage occurred in a variety-dependent manner. Nevertheless, amongst *Brassica* vegetables, red cabbage, brussels sprouts, and broccoli possess the highest antioxidant capacity and the contribution to health improvement can be related to their capacity [43].

3.2. In Vitro Bioaccessibility of Red Cabbage Polyphenols

The bioaccessibility of total phenolic compounds, which was calculated using the Folin–Ciocalteu method, and antioxidant activity determined by DPPH, ABTS, and FRAP tests during the in vitro gastrointestinal digestion are presented in Tables 3 and 4. The in vitro gastrointestinal digestion was evaluated according to the INFOGEST procedure until the duodenal stage. Subsequently, to reproduce the microbiota occurring in the colon phase, the combined action of Pronase E and Viscozyme L. was utilized [44,45].

Table 3. Total polyphenol content of red cabbage extract compared to that of the same extract encapsulated in an acid-resistant capsule. Values are reported as mean ± SD of independent experiments performed in triplicate. Statistic significance was calculated with two-way ANOVA analysis.

Red Cabbage In Vitro GI Digestion		TPC (mg GAE/g)	
	Phase	Extract	Capsule *
1	Intestinal phase	22.287 ± 0.295 [a]	22.738 ± 0.339 [a]
2	Pronase E	0.124 ± 0.003 [b]	4.434 ± 0.069 [c]
3	Viscozyme L	0.994 ± 0.060 [d]	0.102 ± 0.022 [e]

* results are referred to dry weight (dw) of extract; red cabbage extract was encapsulated in polyethylene capsule and used in in vitro digestion process. [a–e] Mean values with different superscript letters are significantly different by Tukey–Kramer multiple comparison test.

Table 4. Antioxidant data by means of 2,2-azinobis (3-ethylbenzothiazoline-6-sulphonic acid) diammonium salt (ABTS), 1,1-diphenyl-2-picrylhydrazyl (DPPH), and ferric reducing/antioxidant power (FRAP) methods of red cabbage extract compared to that of the same extract encapsulated in an acid-resistant capsule. Values are reported as mean ± SD of independent experiments performed in triplicate.

		Red Cabbage In Vitro GI Phase		
		1 Intestinal phase	2 Pronase E	3 Viscozyme L
ABTS (mmol Trolox/kg)	Capsule	76.755 ± 1.483 [a]	0.682 ± 0.044 [b]	2.600 ± 0.220 [d]
	Extract	78.513 ± 1.783 [a]	12.820 ± 0.949 [c]	2.626 ± 0.067 [d]
DPPH (mmol Trolox/kg)	Capsule	44.985 ± 2.547 [e]	0.150 ± 0.003 [f]	4.074 ± 0.126 [h]
	Extract	45.762 ± 1.773 [e]	7.268 ± 1.095 [g]	0.008 ± 0.001 [i]
FRAP (mmol Trolox/kg)	Capsule	90.778 ± 2.128 [j]	2.055 ± 0.355 [k]	28.954 ± 1.793 [m]
	Extract	91.958 ± 1.502 [j]	132.931 ± 0.939 [l]	0.528 ± 0.074 [b]

* Results are referred to dry weight (dw) of extract; [a–m] Mean values with different superscript letters are significantly different by Tukey–Kramer multiple comparison test.

An improvement of bioactivity was observed for the extract digested in an acid-resistant capsule after the colonic stage compared to the extract digested without capsule. In fact, the total polyphenols content of extract digested in an acid-resistant capsule in the Pronase E resulted in a significantly higher concentration than the extract digested without capsule: 4.434 and 0.124 mg GAE/g, respectively. A similar trend was also observed by evaluating the antioxidant activity (Table 4); encapsulation appeared to favor an increase in antiradical and reducing capability mainly at the Viscozyme L stage. In GI digestion, polyphenols may interact with food constituents and be subjected to further degradation or metabolization that could affect their uptake. The presence of dietary fiber in fruits and vegetables is able to influence and modulate the phytochemicals bioaccessibility [46]. In this context, Podsędek et al. [47] have evaluated the stability of red cabbage antioxidant compounds, principally anthocyanins, during GI, concluding that the latter are affected by cabbage composition and vegetable constituents, including dietary fiber. During intestinal digestion, anthocyanins' stability is hard dependent on food matrices. Notwithstanding, compared to other matrices, red cabbage has demonstrated a greater stability [43].

Some studies showed that anthocyanins have low absorption and high metabolism, and their bioavailability is lower compared with other subclasses of polyphenols [48,49]. Despite the reduced bioavailability, Sodagari et al. [50] reported that up to 70% of anthocyanins derived by foods could reach the colon. Hence, a regular intake of foods rich in anthocyanins could result in beneficial effects on human health.

Chemical modifications occurring during gastrointestinal digestion including the activity of gut microbiota lead to a releasing of smaller compounds, the principal responsible for the increased antioxidant activity. Although polyphenols were poorly absorbed in the duodenum, they can exert their antioxidant activities in the lower gut, which is able to metabolize these compounds, generating metabolites with greater activity [43]. It is speculated that bioactive compounds could be metabolized by human colonic microflora, generating metabolites with greater bioactivity and more beneficial effects. Specifically, anthocyanins, forming the majority of the polyphenols of red cabbage, are metabolized by glycosidase from gut microflora through cleavage of the C-ring to produce easily absorbed phenolic acids. Glycosidase, in the ileum, supports metabolism and the absorption of glycosides [51]. Moreover, Chen et al. [52] demonstrated that mulberry's anthocyanins were metabolized to phenolic acids such as chlorogenic, protocatechuic, caffeic, and ferulic acids by the action of intestinal microflora in a percentage of 46.17%.

Several studies have also demonstrated that polyphenols from foods could have dissimilar bioaccessibilities. Most of the polyphenols are stable in the acidic gastric environment and degraded due to the neutral conditions encountered in the small intestine, which contribute to a reduced uptake into blood [12]. The in vitro GI digestion represents a valid tool to understand the behavior of compounds and the amounts that are effectively subjected to mucosal absorption. By using oral administration, macromolecules derived by food need firstly to be digestive and reduced in small bioactive compounds, and after withstanding to the pH in the GI tract, they could reach the absorption site in the small intestine [53]. Polyphenols metabolized by the combined action of Viscozyme and Pronase lead to the release of smaller compounds, the principal being responsible for the increased antioxidant activity [45]. Foods, including fruits and vegetables, represent an important source of bioactive compounds having numerous beneficial health effects such as antioxidant capacity [54]. As proved by scientific studies, GI digestion plays an important role in the antioxidant capacity, because the availability of bioactive compounds is influenced by the digestion process [55]. It seems that digestion could modify the antioxidant properties of foods, but there are contrasting opinions [56,57]. The antioxidant activity of dietary supplements commonly ingested as a source of antioxidant polyphenols was investigated by Henning et al. [58]. In addition, in this latest case, the stability was evaluated by determining the total phenolic content by Folin–Ciocalteu assay, and the antioxidant capacity was assessed by using DPPH, FRAP, and ABTS tests. Although polyphenols provide the major antioxidant potency, their results highlight that digestion may alter antioxidant properties depending on polyphenol content.

Naturally, the behavior of different classes of molecules during digestion is no overall standard. This finding was broadly demonstrated by Chen et al. [54], who evaluated the total phenolic content (TPC) and antioxidant activity before and after the in vitro digestion of thirty-three fruits, deriving large variations in the results. A significant improvement in TPC after gastric step was observed for eight fruits, but for the other twenty-five, it resulted in an increase after the duodenal phase. The same trend was observed by the antioxidant activity performed through DPPH, ABTS, and FRAP tests; the values significantly increased for some fruits but decreased for others.

It is demonstrated that some classes of polyphenols are able to increase their concentration after the gastric phase, justifying their high sensitivity to alkaline conditions. In fact, the majority of antioxidant compounds are degraded by alkaline pH, causing a substantial loss in the activity after the intestinal stage [57].

Unfortunately, polyphenols had not demonstrated high long-term stability and are characterized by sensitivity to heat and light. Moreover, polyphenols present a poor bioavailability because of low water solubility [59]. Finally, some of these compounds possess a bitter and astringent taste that limits their use in food or in oral medications. To circumvent these drawbacks, some processes that are able to enhance polyphenol bioavailability have been reported [60–62]. The use of an acid-resistant capsule in the digestion process acted as a protective agent and allowed us to avoid the consequence of gastric ambient on the bioactive molecules. In particular, acid-resistant capsules protect bioactive compounds from degradation or alteration of their chemical structure caused by changes in pH or the action of digestive enzymes. The acid-resistant capsules represent a useful strategy to conduct bioactive molecules until the intestinal district, where the bioactive compounds are favorably absorbed and exert their activity.

3.3. Identification and Quantification of Red Cabbage Bioactive Compounds Analyzed through UHPLC-Q-Orbitrap HRMS

Bioactive compounds of red cabbage MeOH:H_2O (6:4, *v/v*) extract were profiled through UHPLC-Q-Orbitrap HRMS. A total of 40 different polyphenolic compounds including phenolic acids, flavonoids and anthocyanins were tentatively identified by combining MS and MS/MS spectra (Tables S1 and S2 in Supplementary Material). Experiments were carried out both in ESI⁻ and ESI⁺ mode. Phenolic acids and flavonoids exhibited better fragmentation patterns producing the deprotonated molecular ion [M-H]⁻, whereas anthocyanins were investigated in positive ESI mode. Unambiguous identification of some compounds is carried out by comparison to their relative reference pure standards. The quantitative determination of target analytes was carried out using calibration curves at eight concentration levels. Each calibration curve was prepared in triplicate. Regression coefficients >0.990 were obtained. The quantification of compounds that had no standard to generate a curve was based on a representative standard of the same group. This is the case of cyanidin derivatives, which are quantified by using the calibration curve of cyanidin 3,5-diglucoside.

Screening in full scan mass chromatograms enables the identification of untargeted compounds and retrospective data analysis. The confirmation of the structural characterization of untargeted analytes was based on the accurate mass measurement, elemental composition assignment, retention time, and MS/MS fragmentation. Sensitivity was assessed by the limit of detection (LOD) and limit of quantification (LOQ). LOD is defined as the minimum concentration that enables the analyte identification with a mass error below 5 ppm. LOQ is the lowest analyte concentration that allows the analyte quantitated at defined levels for imprecision and accuracy <20%.

Red cabbage has its own characteristic anthocyanin pattern that includes acylated anthocyanins, which affect the antioxidant activity. In particular, anthocyanins with cyanidin-3-diglucoside-5-glucoside core, non-acylated, mono-acylated, or diacylated with *p*-coumaric, caffeic, ferulic, and sinapic acids were found to be the predominant compounds, which was in accordance with data reported by several scientific studies [63–65]. Indeed, according to Charron et al. [66], the dominant form of anthocyanins in the investigated red cabbage extract was cyanidin-3-diglucoside-5-glucoside, which appeared as the first main peak of the investigated extract. The compound showed the [M]$^+$ ion at m/z 773.21057 and the main MS^2 fragment ions at m/z 611.06012 [M-Glc]$^+$, 449.16882 [M-2Glc]$^+$, and 287.05219 [M-3Glc]$^+$ (Table S1). It constituted 39.5% of the anthocyanin fraction, which represented 26% of the investigated extract. Three abundant sinapoyl derivatives of the previous compound were also tentatively identified (Table 5). In particular, cyanidin-3-(sin)-diglucoside-5-glucoside and cyanidin-3-(sin)sophoroside-5-glucoside shared the molecular formula $C_{44}H_{51}O_{25}$ and the neutral loss of a sinapic acid-H_2O moiety, whereas cyanidin-3(sin)(sin)sophoroside-5-glucoside showed the [M]$^+$ ion at m/z 1185.32959 (Table S1). Cyanidin-3-(caf)(sin)soph-5-glucoside showed the [M]$^+$ ion at m/z 1141.30261, and cyanidin 3(sin)triglucoside-5-glucoside ([M]$^+$ ion at m/z 1141.32544) was also identified. The latter compound and cyanidin 3(caf)(fer)sophorosyl-5-glucoside, along with seven other acylated anthocyanidins (cyan-3(caf)(sin)soph-5-glu; cyan-3(p-coum)triglu-5-glu; cyan-3(p-coum)soph-5-(suc)glu; cyan-3(glucop-sin)(p-coum)soph-5-glu; cyan-3(glucop-sin)(fer)soph-5-glu; cyan-3(glucop-sin)(sin)soph-5-glu; cyan-3(fer)soph-5-(sin)glu)) were identified for the first time by Arapitsas et al. [64], who analyzed the red cabbage anthocyanin profile using HPLC/DAD-ESI/Qtrap MS.

Mizgier et al. [67] analyzed the phenolic compounds and antioxidant capacity of red cabbage extract, confirming that more than 80% was constituted from acylated compounds. The total anthocyanin content of the red cabbage extracts was reported to be equal to 175.1 mg/g dry weight, which was expressed as cyanidin-3-glucoside equivalents.

Wiczkowski et al. [63] studied the red cabbage anthocyanins profile and analyzed the correlation of antioxidant activity and acylated compounds, demonstrating that cyanidin 3-diglucoside-5-glucoside diacylated with sinapic acid had the highest radical-scavenging activities. Acylated cyanidin glycosides showed higher antioxidant capacity than the non-acylated form of cyanidin glycosides. In this case, the total content of anthocyanins in red cabbage was 2.32 mg/g on dry weight, which was calculated based on cyanidin equivalents [63]. Dominant forms of anthocyanins in this red cabbage were non-acylated compounds, which comprised 27.6% of the total red cabbage anthocyanins, whereas mono-acylated and diacylated anthocyanins covered 38.4% and 34.1%, respectively.

Other reports evidenced that red cabbage is an excellent vegetable containing a high content of anthocyanins, which were in the range from 40 to 188 mg Cy 3-glcE/100 g fresh weight [68,69].

Voća et al. [70], who analyzed the difference in chemical composition between cabbage cultivars, reported the highest content of anthocyanins in red cabbage extract (until 750.71 mg/kg fresh weight). In red cabbage cultivars, even 3.9 times higher antioxidant capacity was reported compared to the other cultivars. Another report estimated the total anthocyanins content of the red cabbage extract equal to 4984.13 ± 101.62 µg/g dry weight [71]. In addition, the flavonoids composition was analyzed by Voća et al. as well [70]; red cabbage contains, besides anthocyanins, other phenolic compounds also. In particular, the most abundant part of the extract (73.7%) consisted in C_6C_3 phenolic acids as sinapic acid (6325.025 ± 3.568 µg/g dry weight), ferulic acid (2768.48 ± 29.18 µg/g dry weight), and p-coumaric acid (4518.52 ± 15.83 µg/g dry weight), beyond C_6C_1 phenolic acids such as vanillic acid (5961.13 ± 29.08 µg/g dry weight) and protocatechuic acid (2881.17 ± 15.59 µg/g dry weight). Thus, sinapic acid covered 37.5% of phenolic acids.

Finally, non-anthocyanin flavonoids were found in a negligible portion, as they constituted only 0.38% of the extract. In particular, among flavonols, kaempferol appeared to mostly contain 17.371 ± 0.23 µg/g dry weight, followed by rutin and its aglycone quercetin, whose relative contents were estimated to be equal to 15.302 ± 0.96 and 4.359 ± 0.33 µg/g dry weight. The flavanol epigallocatechin constituted 23.965 ± 0.16 µg per g of dry extract.

Table 5. Quantitation of the main anthocyanin compounds in the investigated red cabbage extract, as well as of the most abundant non-anthocyanin flavonoids and phenolic acids. Results are expressed as mean ± SD from three independent determinations.

Compound	Red Cabbage Content (mg/kg)	SD
Anthocyanins		
Cyanidin 3-diglucoside-5-glucoside	2344.684	9.198
Cyanidin 3-soph-5-xyloside	24.660	5.115
Cyanidin 3,5-diglucoside	306.750	12.450
Cyanidin 3-galactoside	7.000	1.170
Cyanidin 3-(sin)soph-5-glucoside	514.153	11.001
Cyanidin 3-(sin)triglucoside-5-glucoside	131.554	4.225
Cyanidin 3-(glucofer)-diglucoside-5-glucoside	10.549	0.617
Cyanidin 3-(p-coum)-glucoside-5-glucoside	13.395	3.542
Cyanidin 3-(caf)-diglucoside-5-glucoside	22.115	2.892
Cyanidin 3-(fer)-glucoside-5-glucoside	28.009	2.759
Cyanidin 3-(sin)glucoside-5-glucoside	153.803	11.370
Cyanidin 3-(p-coum)-diglucoside-5-glucoside	340.812	8.372
Cyanidin 3-(fer)soph-5-glucoside	268.096	9.925
Cyanidin	112.793	2.745
Cyanidin 3-(sin)-diglucoside-5-glucoside	727.842	13.723
Cyanidin 3-(caf)(p-coum)-diglucoside-5-glucoside	5.680	0.056
Cyanidin 3-(caf)(sin)soph-5-glucoside	31.820	8.544
Cyanidin 3-(sin)(p-coum)soph-5-glucoside	186.841	11.523
Cyanidin 3-(sin)(fer)soph-5-glucoside	195.990	11.289
Cyanidin 3-(sin)(sin)soph-5-glucoside	506.567	8.600
Other flavonoids		
Epicatechin	1.544	0.232
Epigallocatechin	23.965	0.161
Rutin	15.302	0.963
Kaempferol	17.371	0.228
Quercetin	4.359	0.326
Genistein	24.122	1.471
Phenolic acids		
Caffeic acid	39.356	1.250
Chlorogenic acid	55.316	5.581
p-Coumaric acid	3689.235	2.356
Ferulic acid	2533.965	3.161
Protocatechuic acid	2056.230	2.102
Sinapic acid	6325.025	3.568
Syringic acid	17.069	0.532
Vanillic acid	2136.250	3.256

* Results are referred to dry weight (dw) of extract; sin = sinapoyl; soph = sophoroside; fer = feruloyl; p-coum = p-coumaroyl; caf = caffeoyl; glucofer = glucoferoyl.

4. Conclusions

Red cabbage is a rich source of phenolic acids and flavonoids. Among the latter, anthocyanins represent the most abundant class. Indeed, the full exploitation of the beneficial antioxidant efficacy of these compounds requires their extraction optimization. In this context, extractive procedures on red cabbage provided an extract rich in cyanidin-3-diglucoside-5-glucoside and its acylated compounds. In particular, UHPLC-Q-Orbitrap HRMS analysis highlighted the diversity in sinapoyl derivatives, and sinapic acid was also the most representative phenolic acid in the extract. The chemically profiled extract was screened for its antiradical and reducing capabilities, whereas its stability and bioaccesibility were proved to be preserved in an acid-resistant capsule. Indeed, based on the data acquired, improvements for all the evaluated bioactivities (TPC and antioxidant activity) were observed during the Pronase E and/or Viscozyme L phases of the in vitro gastrointestinal digestion of the red cabbage extract in an acid-resistant capsule. An increase in the colonic phase in TPC was also observed, as well as a similar trend for the other evaluated antioxidant activities. During gastrointestinal digestion, bioactive compounds could be metabolized by human colonic microflora, generating metabolites with greater bioactivity and more beneficial effects. Thus, the use of an acid-resistant capsule in the digestion process could protect bioactive compounds, ameliorating their bioaccessibility. In this context, red cabbage extract encapsulated in an acid-resistant capsule could be a valid alternative to produce a new nutraceutical formulation useful for preventing or slowing down oxidative stress-related diseases onset.

Supplementary Materials: The following are available online at http://www.mdpi.com/2076-3921/9/10/955/s1, Table S1: Chromatographic and spectrometric parameters including retention time, adduct ion, theoretical and measured mass (*m/z*), accuracy and sensibility for anthocyanins (n = 20) in the investigated red cabbage extract. RT = Retention Time, Table S2: Chromatographic and spectrometric parameters including retention time, adduct ion, theoretical and measured mass (*m/z*), accuracy and sensibility for phenolic acids and flavonoids (n = 20) in the investigated red cabbage extract. RT = Retention Time.

Author Contributions: Conceptualization, L.I. and A.R.; methodology, L.I.; formal analysis, L.I.; investigation, L.I., L.C. and A.N.; resources, A.R.; writing, original draft preparation, L.I.; writing, review and editing, Y.R.-C., S.P.; supervision, A.R and S.P.; project administration, A.R.; funding acquisition, A.R. All authors have read and agreed to the published version of the manuscript.

Funding: This research received no external funding.

Conflicts of Interest: The authors declare no conflict of interest

References

1. Shankar, S.; Segaran, G.; Sundar, R.D.V.; Settu, S.; Sathiavelu, M. Brassicaceae-A Classical Review on Its Pharmacological Activities. *Int. J. Pharm. Sci. Rev. Res.* **2019**, *55*, 107–113.
2. Araceli, C.; MadeLourdes, P.-H.; Maelena, P.; JoseA, R.; Carlosandrés, G. Chemical studies of anthocyanins: A review. *Food Chem.* **2009**, *113*, 859–871. [CrossRef]
3. Saigo, T.; Wang, T.; Watanabe, M.; Tohge, T. Diversity of anthocyanin and proanthocyanin biosynthesis in land plants. *Curr. Opin. Plant. Biol.* **2020**, *55*, 93–99. [CrossRef] [PubMed]
4. Seis, H. Oxidative stress:from basic research to clinical application. *Am. J. Med.* **1991**, *91*, S31–S38. [CrossRef]
5. Bellocco, E.; Barreca, D.; Laganà, G.; Calderaro, A.; El Lekhlifi, Z.; Chebaibi, S.; Smeriglio, A.; Trombetta, D. Cyanidin-3-O-galactoside in ripe pistachio (Pistachia vera L. variety Bronte) hulls: Identification and evaluation of its antioxidant and cytoprotective activities. *J. Funct. Foods* **2016**, *27*, 376–385. [CrossRef]
6. Zhu, F. Anthocyanins in cereals: Composition and health effects. *Food Res. Int.* **2018**, *109*, 232–249. [CrossRef] [PubMed]
7. Poljsak, B. Strategies for reducing or preventing the generation of oxidative stress. *Oxidative Med. Cell. Longev.* **2011**, *2011*. [CrossRef]
8. Nita, M.; Grzybowski, A. The role of the reactive oxygen species and oxidative stress in the pathomechanism of the age-related ocular diseases and other pathologies of the anterior and posterior eye segments in adults. *Oxidative Med. Cell. Longev.* **2016**, *2016*. [CrossRef]
9. Kong, J.-M.; Chia, L.-S.; Goh, N.-K.; Chia, T.-F.; Brouillard, R. Analysis and biological activities of anthocyanins. *Phytochemistry* **2003**, *64*, 923–933. [CrossRef]
10. Pojer, E.; Mattivi, F.; Johnson, D.; Stockley, C.S. The case for anthocyanin consumption to promote human health: A review. *Compr. Rev. Food Sci. Food Saf.* **2013**, *12*, 483–508. [CrossRef]
11. Sandoval-Ramírez, B.A.E.; Catalán, U.R.; Fernández-Castillejo, S.; Rubió, L.; Macià, A.; Solà, R. Anthocyanin tissue bioavailability in animals: Possible implications for human health. A systematic review. *J. Agric. Food Chem.* **2018**, *66*, 11531–11543. [CrossRef] [PubMed]
12. Hu, B.; Liu, X.; Zhang, C.; Zeng, X. Food macromolecule based nanodelivery systems for enhancing the bioavailability of polyphenols. *J. Food Drug Anal.* **2017**, *25*, 3–15. [CrossRef] [PubMed]
13. Liu, Y.; Tikunov, Y.; Schouten, R.E.; Marcelis, L.F.; Visser, R.G.; Bovy, A. Anthocyanin biosynthesis and degradation mechanisms in Solanaceous vegetables: A review. *Front. Chem.* **2018**, *6*, 52. [CrossRef] [PubMed]
14. Wahyuningsih, S.; Wulandari, L.; Wartono, M.; Munawaroh, H.; Ramelan, A. *The Effect of pH and Color Stability of Anthocyanin on Food Colorant*; IOP Conference Series: Materials Science and Engineering; IOP Publishing: Bristol, UK, 2017; p. 012047. [CrossRef]

15. Wootton-Beard, P.C.; Moran, A.; Ryan, L. Stability of the total antioxidant capacity and total polyphenol content of 23 commercially available vegetable juices before and after in vitro digestion measured by FRAP, DPPH, ABTS and Folin–Ciocalteu methods. *Food Res. Int.* **2011**, *44*, 217–224. [CrossRef]
16. Bouayed, J.; Deußer, H.; Hoffmann, L.; Bohn, T. Bioaccessible and dialysable polyphenols in selected apple varieties following in vitro digestion vs. their native patterns. *Food Chem.* **2012**, *131*, 1466–1472. [CrossRef]
17. Lorenzo, J.M.; Estévez, M.; Barba, F.J.; Thirumdas, R.; Franco, D.; Munekata PE, S. Polyphenols: Bioaccessibility and bioavailability of bioactive components. In *Innovative Thermal and Non-Thermal Processing, Bioaccessibility and Bioavailability of Nutrients and Bioactive Compounds*; Elsevier: Amsterdam, The Netherlands, 2019; pp. 309–332. [CrossRef]
18. Grace, M.H.; Esposito, D.; Dunlap, K.L.; Lila, M.A. Comparative analysis of phenolic content and profile, antioxidant capacity, and anti-inflammatory bioactivity in wild Alaskan and commercial *Vaccinium* berries. *J. Agric. Food Chem.* **2014**, *62*, 4007–4017. [CrossRef]
19. Izzo, L.; Castaldo, L.; Narváez, A.; Graziani, G.; Gaspari, A.; Rodríguez-Carrasco, Y.; Ritieni, A. Analysis of Phenolic Compounds in Commercial *Cannabis sativa* L. Inflorescences Using UHPLC-Q-Orbitrap HRMS. *Molecules* **2020**, *25*, 631. [CrossRef]
20. Luz, C.; Izzo, L.; Graziani, G.; Gaspari, A.; Ritieni, A.; Mañes, J.; Meca, G. Evaluation of biological and antimicrobial properties of freeze-dried whey fermented by different strains of *Lactobacillus plantarum*. *Food Funct.* **2018**, *9*, 3688–3697. [CrossRef]
21. Brand-Williams, W.; Cuvelier, M.-E.; Berset, C. Use of a free radical method to evaluate antioxidant activity. *Lwt Food Sci. Technol.* **1995**, *28*, 25–30. [CrossRef]
22. Benzie, I.F.; Strain, J.J. The ferric reducing ability of plasma (FRAP) as a measure of "antioxidant power": The FRAP assay. *Anal. Biochem.* **1996**, *239*, 70–76. [CrossRef]
23. Minekus, M.; Alminger, M.; Alvito, P.; Ballance, S.; Bohn, T.; Bourlieu, C.; Carriere, F.; Boutrou, R.; Corredig, M.; Dupont, D. A standardised static in vitro digestion method suitable for food—An international consensus. *Food Funct.* **2014**, *5*, 1113–1124. [CrossRef] [PubMed]
24. Lapornik, B.; Prošek, M.; Wondra, A.G. Comparison of extracts prepared from plant by-products using different solvents and extraction time. *J. Food Eng.* **2005**, *71*, 214–222. [CrossRef]
25. Ignat, I.; Volf, I.; Popa, V.I. A critical review of methods for characterisation of polyphenolic compounds in fruits and vegetables. *Food Chem.* **2011**, *126*, 1821–1835. [CrossRef] [PubMed]
26. Khoddami, A.; Wilkes, M.A.; Roberts, T.H. Techniques for analysis of plant phenolic compounds. *Molecules* **2013**, *18*, 2328–2375. [CrossRef]
27. Murador, D.C.; Mercadante, A.Z.; de Rosso, V.V. Cooking techniques improve the levels of bioactive compounds and antioxidant activity in kale and red cabbage. *Food Chem.* **2016**, *196*, 1101–1107. [CrossRef]
28. Tabart, J.; Pincemail, J.; Kevers, C.; Defraigne, J.-O.; Dommes, J. Processing effects on antioxidant, glucosinolate, and sulforaphane contents in broccoli and red cabbage. *Eur. Food Res. Technol.* **2018**, *244*, 2085–2094. [CrossRef]
29. Pacifico, S.; Galasso, S.; Piccolella, S.; Kretschmer, N.; Pan, S.P.; Marciano, S.; Monaco, P. Seasonal variation in phenolic composition and antioxidant and anti-inflammatory activities of *Calamintha nepeta* (L.) Savi. *Food Res. Int.* **2015**, *69*, 121–132. [CrossRef]
30. Leja, M.; Kamińska, I.; Kołton, A. Phenolic compounds as the major antioxidants in red cabbage. *Folia Hortic.* **2010**, *22*, 19–24. [CrossRef]
31. Upadhyay, R.; Sehwag, S.; Singh, S.P. Antioxidant activity and polyphenol content of *Brassica oleracea* varieties. *Int. J. Veg. Sci.* **2016**, *22*, 353–363. [CrossRef]
32. Fusari, C.M.; Nazareno, M.A.; Locatelli, D.A.; Fontana, A.; Beretta, V.; Camargo, A.B. Phytochemical profile and functionality of *Brassicaceae* species. *Food Biosci.* **2020**, 100606. [CrossRef]
33. Erken, O.; Kaya, S. Free radical scavenging activity, phenolic. *Fresenius Environ. Bull.* **2017**, *26*, 4383–4389.
34. Podsędek, A.; Majewska, I.; Kucharska, A.Z. Inhibitory potential of red cabbage against digestive enzymes linked to obesity and type 2 diabetes. *J. Agric. Food Chem.* **2017**, *65*, 7192–7199. [CrossRef] [PubMed]
35. Podsedek, A.; Sosnowska, D.; Redzynia, M.; Anders, B. Antioxidant capacity and content of Brassica oleracea dietary antioxidants. *Int. J. Food Sci. Technol.* **2006**, *41*, 49–58. [CrossRef]
36. Oroian, M.; Leahu, A.; Dutuc, A.; Dabija, A. Optimization of Total Monomeric Anthocyanin (TMA) and Total Phenolic Content (TPC) Extractions from Red Cabbage (*Brassica oleracea* varcapitata f. rubra): Response Surface Methodology versus Artificial Neural Network. *Int. J. Food Eng.* **2017**, *13*, 1–11. [CrossRef]

37. Tanongkankit, Y.; Chiewchan, N.; Devahastin, S. Effect of processing on antioxidants and their activity in dietary fiber powder from cabbage outer leaves. *Dry. Technol.* **2010**, *28*, 1063–1071. [CrossRef]
38. Jaiswal, A.K.; Gupta, S.; Abu-Ghannam, N. Kinetic evaluation of colour, texture, polyphenols and antioxidant capacity of Irish York cabbage after blanching treatment. *Food Chem.* **2012**, *131*, 63–72. [CrossRef]
39. Kusznierewicz, B.; Bartoszek, A.; Wolska, L.; Drzewiecki, J.; Gorinstein, S.; Namieśnik, J. Partial characterization of white cabbages (*Brassica oleracea* varcapitata f. alba) from different regions by glucosinolates, bioactive compounds, total antioxidant activities and proteins. *Lwt Food Sci. Technol.* **2008**, *41*, 1–9. [CrossRef]
40. Cruz, A.B.; Pitz, H.D.S.; Veber, B.; Bini, L.A.; Maraschin, M.; Zeni, A.L.B. Assessment of bioactive metabolites and hypolipidemic effect of polyphenolic-rich red cabbage extract. *Pharm. Biol.* **2016**, *54*, 3033–3039. [CrossRef]
41. Caramês, E.T.; Alamar, P.D.; Pallone, J.A.L. Bioactive Compounds and Antioxidant Capacity in Freeze-Dried Red Cabbage by FT-NIR and MIR Spectroscopy and Chemometric Tools. *Food Anal. Methods* **2020**, *13*, 78–85. [CrossRef]
42. Wiczkowski, W.; Topolska, J.; Honke, J. Anthocyanins profile and antioxidant capacity of red cabbages are influenced by genotype and vegetation period. *J. Funct. Foods* **2014**, *7*, 201–211. [CrossRef]
43. Shahidi, F.; Ambigaipalan, P. Phenolics and polyphenolics in foods, beverages and spices: Antioxidant activity and health effects–A review. *J. Funct. Foods* **2015**, *18*, 820–897. [CrossRef]
44. Castaldo, L.; Narváez, A.; Izzo, L.; Graziani, G.; Ritieni, A. In Vitro Bioaccessibility and Antioxidant Activity of Coffee Silverskin Polyphenolic Extract and Characterization of Bioactive Compounds Using UHPLC-Q-Orbitrap HRMS. *Molecules* **2020**, *25*, 2132. [CrossRef] [PubMed]
45. Annunziata, G.; Maisto, M.; Schisano, C.; Ciampaglia, R.; Daliu, P.; Narciso, V.; Tenore, G.C.; Novellino, E. Colon bioaccessibility and antioxidant activity of white, green and black tea polyphenols extract after in vitro simulated gastrointestinal digestion. *Nutrients* **2018**, *10*, 1711. [CrossRef] [PubMed]
46. Lucas-González, R.; Viuda-Martos, M.; Álvarez JA, P.; Fernández-López, J. Changes in bioaccessibility, polyphenol profile and antioxidant potential of flours obtained from persimmon fruit (*Diospyros kaki*) co-products during in vitro gastrointestinal digestion. *Food Chem.* **2018**, *256*, 252–258. [CrossRef]
47. Podsędek, A.; Redzynia, M.; Klewicka, E.; Koziołkiewicz, M. Matrix effects on the stability and antioxidant activity of red cabbage anthocyanins under simulated gastrointestinal digestion. *Biomed. Res. Int.* **2014**, *2014*. [CrossRef]
48. Han, F.; Yang, P.; Wang, H.; Fernandes, I.; Mateus, N.; Liu, Y. Digestion and absorption of red grape and wine anthocyanins through the gastrointestinal tract. *Trends Food Sci. Technol.* **2019**, *83*, 211–224. [CrossRef]
49. Tian, L.; Tan, Y.; Chen, G.; Wang, G.; Sun, J.; Ou, S.; Chen, W.; Bai, W. Metabolism of anthocyanins and consequent effects on the gut microbiota. *Crit. Rev. Food Sci. Nutr.* **2019**, *59*, 982–991. [CrossRef]
50. Sodagari, H.R.; Farzaei, M.H.; Bahramsoltani, R.; Abdolghaffari, A.H.; Mahmoudi, M.; Rezaei, N. Dietary anthocyanins as a complementary medicinal approach for management of inflammatory bowel disease. *Expert Rev. Gastroenterol. Hepatol.* **2015**, *9*, 807–820. [CrossRef]
51. Khalifa, I.; Zhu, W.; Li, K.-K.; Li, C.-M. Polyphenols of mulberry fruits as multifaceted compounds: Compositions, metabolism, health benefits, and stability—A structural review. *J. Funct. Foods* **2018**, *40*, 28–43. [CrossRef]
52. Chen, H.; Chen, J.; Yang, H.; Chen, W.; Gao, H.; Lu, W. Variation in total anthocyanin, phenolic contents, antioxidant enzyme and antioxidant capacity among different mulberry (*Morus* sp.) cultivars in China. *Sci. Hortic.* **2016**, *213*, 186–192. [CrossRef]
53. Rein, M.J.; Renouf, M.; Cruz-Hernandez, C.; Actis-Goretta, L.; Thakkar, S.K.; da Silva Pinto, M. Bioavailability of bioactive food compounds: A challenging journey to bioefficacy. *Br. J. Clin. Pharmacol.* **2013**, *75*, 588–602. [CrossRef] [PubMed]
54. Chen, H.; Sang, S. Biotransformation of tea polyphenols by gut microbiota. *J. Funct. Foods* **2014**, *7*, 26–42. [CrossRef]
55. Palafox-Carlos, H.; Ayala-Zavala, J.F.; González-Aguilar, G.A. The role of dietary fiber in the bioaccessibility and bioavailability of fruit and vegetable antioxidants. *J. Food Sci.* **2011**, *76*, R6–R15. [CrossRef] [PubMed]
56. Tagliazucchi, D.; Verzelloni, E.; Conte, A. The first tract of alimentary canal as an extractor. Release of phytochemicals from solid food matrices during simulated digestion. *J. Food Biochem.* **2012**, *36*, 555–568. [CrossRef]

57. Bermúdez-Soto, M.-J.; Tomás-Barberán, F.-A.; García-Conesa, M.-T. Stability of polyphenols in chokeberry (*Aronia melanocarpa*) subjected to in vitro gastric and pancreatic digestion. *Food Chem.* **2007**, *102*, 865–874. [CrossRef]
58. Henning, S.M.; Zhang, Y.; Rontoyanni, V.G.; Huang, J.; Lee, R.-P.; Trang, A.; Nuernberger, G.; Heber, D. Variability in the antioxidant activity of dietary supplements from pomegranate, milk thistle, green tea, grape seed, goji, and acai: Effects of in vitro digestion. *J. Agric. Food Chem.* **2014**, *62*, 4313–4321. [CrossRef]
59. Parisi, O.I.; Puoci, F.; Restuccia, D.; Farina, G.; Iemma, F.; Picci, N. Polyphenols and their formulations: Different strategies to overcome the drawbacks associated with their poor stability and bioavailability. In *Polyphenols in Human Health and Disease*; Academic Press: London, UK, 2014; pp. 29–45. [CrossRef]
60. Munin, A.; Edwards-Lévy, F. Encapsulation of natural polyphenolic compounds; a review. *Pharmaceutics* **2011**, *3*, 793–829. [CrossRef]
61. Esfanjani, A.F.; Assadpour, E.; Jafari, S. M Improving the bioavailability of phenolic compounds by loading them within lipid-based nanocarriers. *Trends Food Sci. Technol.* **2018**, *76*, 56–66. [CrossRef]
62. Ribas-Agustí, A.; Martín-Belloso, O.; Soliva-Fortuny, R.; Elez-Martínez, P. Food processing strategies to enhance phenolic compounds bioaccessibility and bioavailability in plant-based foods. *Crit. Rev. Food Sci. Nutr.* **2018**, *58*, 2531–2548. [CrossRef]
63. Wiczkowski, W.; Szawara-Nowak, D.; Topolska, J. Red cabbage anthocyanins: Profile, isolation, identification, and antioxidant activity. *Food Res. Int.* **2013**, *51*, 303–309. [CrossRef]
64. Arapitsas, P.; Sjöberg, P.J.; Turner, C. Characterisation of anthocyanins in red cabbage using high resolution liquid chromatography coupled with photodiode array detection and electrospray ionization-linear ion trap mass spectrometry. *Food Chem.* **2008**, *109*, 219–226. [CrossRef] [PubMed]
65. Wu, X.; Prior, R.L. Identification and characterization of anthocyanins by high-performance liquid chromatography–electrospray ionization–tandem mass spectrometry in common foods in the United States: Vegetables, nuts, and grains. *J. Agric. Food Chem.* **2005**, *53*, 3101–3113. [CrossRef] [PubMed]
66. Charron, C.S.; Kurilich, A.C.; Clevidence, B.A.; Simon, P.W.; Harrison, D.J.; Britz, S.J.; Baer, D.J.; Novotny, J.A. Bioavailability of anthocyanins from purple carrot juice: Effects of acylation and plant matrix. *J. Agric. Food Chem.* **2009**, *57*, 1226–1230. [CrossRef] [PubMed]
67. Mizgier, P.; Kucharska, A.Z.; Sokół-Łętowska, A.; Kolniak-Ostek, J.; Kidoń, M.; Fecka, I. Characterization of phenolic compounds and antioxidant and anti-inflammatory properties of red cabbage and purple carrot extracts. *J. Funct. Foods* **2016**, *21*, 133–146. [CrossRef]
68. Ahmadiani, N.; Robbins, R.J.; Collins, T.M.; Giusti, M.M. Anthocyanins contents, profiles, and color characteristics of red cabbage extracts from different cultivars and maturity stages. *J. Agric. Food Chem.* **2014**, *62*, 7524–7531. [CrossRef]
69. Podsędek, A. Natural antioxidants and antioxidant capacity of *Brassica* vegetables: A review. *Lwt Food Sci. Technol.* **2007**, *40*, 1–11. [CrossRef]
70. Voća, S.; Šic Žlabur, J.; Dobričević, N.; Benko, B.; Pliestić, S.; Filipović, M.; Galić, A. Bioactive compounds, pigment content and antioxidant capacity of selected cabbage cultivars. *J. Cent. Eur. Agric.* **2018**, *19*, 593–606. [CrossRef]
71. Koss-Mikołajczyk, I.; Kusznierewicz, B.; Wiczkowski, W.; Płatosz, N.; Bartoszek, A. Phytochemical composition and biological activities of differently pigmented cabbage (*Brassica oleracea* varcapitata) and cauliflower (*Brassica oleracea* var. botrytis) varieties. *J. Sci. Food Agric.* **2019**, *99*, 5499–5507. [CrossRef]

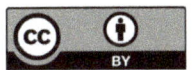

© 2020 by the authors. Licensee MDPI, Basel, Switzerland. This article is an open access article distributed under the terms and conditions of the Creative Commons Attribution (CC BY) license (http://creativecommons.org/licenses/by/4.0/).

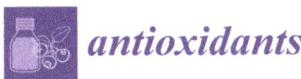

Article

Improvement of Health-Promoting Functionality of Rye Bread by Fortification with Free and Microencapsulated Powders from *Amelanchier alnifolia* Nutt

Sabina Lachowicz [1],*, Michał Świeca [2] and Ewa Pejcz [1]

1. Department of Fermentation and Cereals Technology, Wrocław University of Environmental and Life Science, Chełmońskiego 37 Street, 51-630 Wroclaw, Poland; ewa.pejcz@upwr.edu.pl
2. Department of Biochemistry and Food Chemistry, Agricultural University, Skromna 8, 20-704 Lublin, Poland; michal.swieca@up.lublin.pl
* Correspondence: sabina.lachowicz@up.wroc.pl

Received: 10 June 2020; Accepted: 10 July 2020; Published: 13 July 2020

Abstract: This study established the appropriate amounts of a functional Saskatoon berry fruit powder in fortified rye bread acceptable to consumers and determined the potential relative bioaccesibility of bioactive compounds exhibiting antioxidant activity, and enzymatic in vitro inhibitory activity against lipoxygenase, cyclooxigenase-1, cyclooxigenase-2, acetylcholinesterase, pancreatic lipase α-glucosidase, and α-amylase, as well as the relative digestibility of nutrients. The content of polyphenolic compounds and antioxidant capability were strongly, positively correlated with the content of the functional additive. The highest phenolics content and antioxidant activity were determined in the products enriched with the powders microencapsulated with maltodextrin (an increase by 91% and 53%, respectively, compared with the control). The highest overall acceptability was shown for the products with 3% addition of the functional additive, regardless of its type. The simulated in vitro digestion released phenols (with the highest bioaccessibility shown for anthocyanins) and enhanced the antioxidant activity of rye bread. In turn, the microencapsulation contributed to the improvement in the relative bioaccesibility of antioxidant compounds. Bread fortification led to an increased inhibitory activity against α-amylase, α-glucosidase, and lipoxygenase. Furthermore, the additive microencapsulated with maltodextrin and inulin improved the capacity to inhibit the activities of pancreatic lipase and cyclooxygenase-2. The results presented allowed concluding that the powders from Saskatoon berry fruits, especially microencapsulated ones, may be a promising functional additive dedicated for the enrichment of rye bread.

Keywords: rye bread; microencapsulation; phenolics; in vitro relative bioaccessibility; lipoxygenase; cyclooxygenase; acetylcholinesterase; biological activity

1. Introduction

Rye bread is an integral element of a man's diet as a good source of nutrients, including compounds that exhibit a broad spectrum of antioxidant activity. These properties are mainly ascribed to the phenolic compounds of cereal grains [1], which also exhibit anti-carcinogenic and anti-inflammatory activities and are recommended in the prevention of many degenerative diseases [1–3]. The consumption of rye bread has increased over the last years also owing to the nutritive value and higher bioaccessibility of its grain components, as well as a lower gluten content [2,3].

The production process of rye bread involves fermentation with sourdough, which positively affects the finished products by acidifying the dough, inhibiting α-amylase activity, developing flavor values, increasing the solubility of pentosans, and also by increasing their nutritive value and antioxidant potential [1,2]. In addition, this technology extends the shelf life of bread by preventing crumb sticking and mold appearance [2].

Worthy of attention is the recent development of the sector of functional food products, which offer increased nutritive and health values that may help prevent many diseases [2,4]. Considering their high intake, food products such as bread can serve as an excellent carrier of functional ingredients that can be introduced at any stage of the technological process. However, when designing fortified/supplemented foods, attention should be paid to their biological value as well as to their sensory profile, including in particular their acceptability by consumers [5]. Investigations conducted so far have demonstrated the fortification of rye bread with grape and tomato pomace to have a positive effect on its nutritive value and its flavor values [4,6]. Considering the properties and composition of Saskatoon berry, a worthwhile alternative to common bread types can be offered by rye bread with the addition of powder from its fruits. Saskatoon berry fruits exhibit a high antioxidant activity that is strongly correlated with the contents of phenolic compounds, vitamins, minerals, free and bound amino acids, and organic acids [7–9]. Furthermore, Saskatoon berry fruits exhibit strong antibacterial activity against *Escherichia coli* (VTT E-94564), *Enterococcus hirae* (ATCC 10542), and *Staphylococcus aureus* (VTT E-70045). Their components also exhibit inhibiting activities of α-amylase and α-glucosidase [9–11]. The study conducted by Zhao et al. [12] demonstrated that powders from *Amelanchier alnifolia* Nutt. could alleviate hyperlipidemia, hyperglycemia, and blood vessel inflammation induced by high-saccharose and high-fat diet. According to Juricova et al. [7], the Saskatoon berry fruit is additionally responsible for the anti-inflammatory and chemo-protective potency. The sweet taste of the Saskatoon berry fruit can also contribute to the improvement of taste values of sourdough bread by masking its sour taste. On the other hand, establishing the optimal amount of the additive is important as well, because a too high amount of fruit powder can decrease the taste value and cause the appearance of bitterness resulting from a high content of polymerized procyanidins [9].

Another critical issue is the protection of thermolabile bioactive compounds during bread baking at high temperatures. A solution to this problem can be offered by entrapping functional additives in carriers in the microencapsulation process, which allows minimizing losses of health-promoting compounds valuable for a human body. This solution will be worth considering while designing food products with functional characteristics, where not only their production technology, but also their nutritional aspects need to be strongly considered. The effectiveness of microencapsulation has been confirmed in studies into the use of curcumin or Garcinia fruits as functional additives to wheat bread, which demonstrated a higher content of polyphenolic compounds in final products compared with the crude additives [13,14]. The cited authors demonstrated the microencapsulated additive not to affect the complexity of the production process or quality traits of bread, but to contribute to the greater stability of bioactive compounds. According to recent literature, the protection of compounds ensured by the carriers can also contribute to the mitigation of the adverse effects of polyphenolic compounds on sensory properties of the finished products [15] including, for example, the appearance of a bitter and an astringent taste [13]. What is more, the use of microencapsulated food additives has been reported to positively affect the quality traits of bakery products, including bread, by improving their color, dough yield, or even texture [16].

Other important aspects that need to be considered while designing fortified food products include the potential in vitro bioaccesibility of compounds identified in functional additives that are often neglected in the assessment of the real value of such products, as well as the effect their additive has on the nutritive value. As reported by Gawlik-Dziki et al. [17], the quality and quantity of extracted nutrients and their potential health-promoting value determined after simulated in vitro digestion can differ from those obtained for the chemical extracts only. What is more, the bioaccesibility of components of the functional additive will also depend on its interactions (antagonistic or synergistic) with food components or on of its behavior in the digestive system [14]. Therefore, the determination of the potential relative bioaccesibility and biological value of functional food products is essential for the assessment of the effectiveness and safety of the fortification process.

This study examined the effectiveness of rye bread fortification with pure and microencapsulated powders from Saskatoon berry fruits. The study of quality and health-promoting properties was extended with the analysis of potential relative bioaccesibility that indicates the real value of fortified functional food. Furthermore, it aimed to establish the appropriate amounts of a functional additive from Saskatoon berry fruits acceptable by consumers and to determine the antioxidant activity and enzymatic in vitro inhibitory activity against lipoxygenase, cyclooxigenase-1, cyclooxigenase-2, acetylcholinesterase, pancreatic lipase, α-glucosidase, and α-amylase, as well as the relative digestibility of nutrients of fortified rye bread.

2. Materials and Methods

2.1. Reagents

Acetonitrile, formic acid, methanol, ABTS (2,2′-azinobis(3-ethylbenzothiazoline-6-sulfonic acid), 6-hydroxy-2,5,7,8-tetramethylchroman-2-carboxylic acid (Trolox), 2,4,6-tri(2-pyridyl)-s-triazine (TPTZ), 2,2-Di(4-tert-octylphenyl)-1-picrylhydrazyl (DPPH), methanol, acetic acid, phosphate buffered saline (pH 7.4), LOX Activity Assay kit, AChE Assay kit, α-amylase from porcine pancreas, α-glucoamylase from Rhizopus sp., lipase from porcine pancreas, trini-trobenzenesulfonic acid, NaH_2PO_4, and 3,5-dini-trosalicylic acid were purchased from Sigma-Aldrich (Steinheim, Germany). COX Inhibitor Screening Assay Kit was purchased from Cayman (No. 560131; Ann Arbor, MI, USA). (−)-Epicatechin, (+)-catechin, chlorogenic acid, neochlorogenic acid, cryptochlorogenic acid, dicaffeic acid, procyanidin A2, procyanidin B2, p-coumaric acid, caffeic acid, 4-caffeoylquinic, kampferol-3-O-galactoside, quercetin-3-O-rutinoside, quercetin-3-O-galactoside, quercetin-3-O-glucoside, cyanidin-3-O-arabinoside, cyanidin-3-O-xyloside, cyanidin-3-O-galactoside, and cyanidin-3-O-glucoside were purchased from Extrasynthese (Lyon, France). Acetonitrile for ultra-performance liquid chromatography (UPLC; gradient grade) and ascorbic acid were from Merck (Darmstadt, Germany). The carriers (30%) applied to produce powders were maltodextrin DE (20–40) and inulin (Beneo-Orafti, Belgium).

2.2. Materials

Fruits—"Smoky" cultivar of Saskatoon berry and rye flour type 720—were used in this work. Saskatoon berry was collected in the year 2019 from BIOGRIM company (Wojciechow, Lublin, Poland), and the rye flour was from Good Mills Poland company (Stradunia, Poland). The freeze drying pure fruit powder (FP) as additives was prepared as described previously by Lachowicz et al. [18]. Meanwhile, the freeze drying encapsulated fruit powder with maltodextrin (FPM) and inulin (FPI) as additives was prepared as described previously by Lachowicz et al. [19]. The resulting Saskatoon berry fruit was ground in Thermomix (Wuppertal, Vorkwek, Germany) at 40 °C for 10 min. For encapsulation fruit, 70% of grounded fruit (w/w) and 30% of carrier (maltodextrin or inulin) were mixed. Furth, grounded fruit and encapsulated fruit were frozen at −80 °C. Next, the freeze drying method of FP and FPM as well as FPI (≈200 g of each sample) was carried out in a freeze dryer (Christ Alpha 1–4 LSC; Germany) for 24 h at a reduced pressure of 65 Pa. The temperature in the drying chamber was −60 °C, while the heating plate reached 30 °C.

2.3. Rye Bread Preparation

The rye doughs were made according to a previously description by Pejcz et al. [3]. Dough samples were made using double-phase type. Yeasts (1%), salt (0.5%), and sourdough (50% of rye flour) were used to make rye flour. The rye dough was fermented by LV2 starter cultures. The next step was placing the dough in a baking tin (at 30 °C for last fermentation). Different rye breads were using different content of fruit powder: 1, 2, 3, 4, 5, and 6%. Breads were baked in a laboratory oven (Brabender, Duisburg, Germany) for 35 min/230 °C. Whole baking experiments were performed twice. Each sample of bread after 24 h was freeze-dried and milled for analysis. The rye bread sample without addition was considered to be the control sample. Symbols of samples: rye bread without additives (BRC) and with fruit powder from 1% (BR1) to 6% (BR6); rye bread with fruit powder encapsulated with maltodextrin from 1% (BRM1) to 6% (BRM6); and rye bread with fruit powder encapsulated with inulin from 1% (BRI1) to 6% (BRI6). The amount of encapsulated fruit powders with maltodextrin (FPM) and encapsulated fruit powders with inulin (FPI) added to bread was calculated per the amount of crude fruit powder (FP).

2.4. Sensory Attributes and Colour Parameters

The sensory properties of the obtained rye bread with supplementation were determined using a ten-degree hedonic scale: 1—"I do not like it extremely" to 10—"I like it extremely". The assessment included the following quality attributes such as aroma, taste, crumb, crust colour, texture, and consistency. It was conducted by a group of 22 panelists (11 men and 11 women in the age group of 20–70). Coded samples were provided to the panelists for the evaluation at 20 °C in a plastic plate.

Colour properties such as L*, a*, and b* of control and enriched rye bread were determined with a Konika Minolta CR-400 colorimeter (Wroclaw Poland). Bread samples were analysed against a white ceramic reference plate (L* = 93.92; a* = 1.03; b* = 0.52), and colour parameters L* (lightness or brightness: black = 0, white = 100), a* (greenness = −a*, redness = +a*), and b* (blueness = −b*, yellowness = +b*) values were recorded. Total change in colour of rye bread samples (ΔE^*) was calculated as follows:

$$\Delta E* = \sqrt{(L_0^* - L^*)^2 + (a_0^* - a^*)^2 + (b_0^* - b^*)^2}$$

2.5. Extraction Procedures

2.5.1. Digestion In Vitro

In vitro simulated digestion was made on the basis of the method described by Minekus et al. [20]. For gastrointestinal digestion, the freeze-dried rye bread (250 mg) was mixed with PBS buffer (phosphate-buffered saline) (0.5 mL; pH 7.4) and simulated salivary fluid (1 mL). After that, the sample was shaken (10 min/37 °C). Next, the pH of the mixture was changed to pH 3 using 6 M HCl, and the samples were shaken for 120 min at 37 °C. After that, pH of digests was changed to 7 using 1 M NaOH. The samples underwent intestinal digestion in vitro for 120 min. After that, the activity of enzymes was stopped using methanol (1:1 ratio). The samples were centrifuged (at 19,000× g/10 min) and used for the test.

2.5.2. Chemical Extraction

Freeze-dried rye bread samples (1 g) were mixed with 30% of UPLC-grade methanol (10 mL) with 1% of acetic acid. After that, the extract was sonicated for 20 min (Sonic 6D, Polsonic, Warsaw, Poland) and centrifuged (at 19,000× g/10 min). Finally, the extract was filtered by hydrophilic PTFE (politetrafluoroetylen) 0.20 μm membrane (Millex Samplicity Filter, Darmstadt, Germany) and used for testing—chemical extract (CE).

2.5.3. Buffer Extraction

Freeze-dried rye bread (~1 g) was mixed with 20 mL of PBS buffer (pH 7.4), and extracted for 1 h. After the extraction, the extracts were centrifuged (6900× g/15 min) and the samples were used for analysis—buffer extracts (BE).

2.6. Identyfication and Quantyfication of Polyphenolic Compounds

Determination of polyphenolic compounds of freeze-dried rye bread sample was carried out using an ACQUITY ultra performance liquid chromatography system equipped with a photodiode array detector with a binary solvent manager (Waters Corporation, Milford, MA, USA) series with a mass detector G2 Q/Tof Micro mass spectrometer (Waters, Manchester, U.K.) equipped with an electrospray ionization (ESI) source operating in negative and positive modes [21]. Separations of polyphenolic compounds were carried out using a UPLC BEH C18 column (1.7 µm, 2.1 × 100 mm, Waters Corporation, Milford, MA, USA) at 30 °C. The extracts (10 µL) were injected, and the elution was completed in 15 min with a sequence of linear gradients and isocratic flow rates of 0.45 mL min^{-1}. The mobile phase consisted of solvent A (2.0% formic acid, v/v) and solvent B (100% acetonitrile). The program began with isocratic elution with 99% solvent A (0–1 min), and then a linear gradient was used until 12 min, lowering solvent A to 0%; from 12.5 to 13.5 min, the gradient returned to the initial composition (99% A), and then it was held constant to re-equilibrate the column. The analysis was carried out using full-scan, data-dependent MS scanning from m/z 100 to 1500. Leucine enkephalin was used as the reference compound at a concentration of 500 pg/µL, at a flow rate of 2 µL/min, and the [M − H]$^-$ ion at 554.2615 Da was detected. The [M − H]$^-$ ion was detected during 15 min analysis performed within ESI–MS accurate mass experiments, which were permanently introduced via the LockSpray channel using a Hamilton pump. The lock mass correction was ±1.000 for the mass window. The mass spectrometer was operated in negative- and positive-ion mode, set to the base peak intensity (BPI) chromatograms, and scaled to 12,400 counts per second (cps) (100%). The optimized MS conditions were as follows: capillary voltage of 2500 V, cone voltage of 30 V, source temperature of 100 °C, desolvation temperature of 300 °C, and desolvation gas (nitrogen) flow rate of 300 L/h. Collision-induced fragmentation experiments were performed using argon as the collision gas, with voltage ramping cycles from 0.3 to 2 V. Characterization of the single components was carried out via the retention time and the accurate molecular masses. Each compound was optimized to its estimated molecular mass [M − H]$^-$/[M + H]$^+$ in the negative and positive mode before and after fragmentation. The data obtained from UPLC–MS were subsequently entered into the MassLynx 4.0 ChromaLynx Application Manager software (Waters Corporation, Milford, MA, USA). On the basis of these data, the software is able to scan different samples for the characterized substances. The runs were monitored at the following wavelength: flavonol glycosides at 360 nm. The PDA spectra were measured over the wavelength range of 200–800 nm in steps of 2 nm [21]. The results were as mg per 100 g of dry substances (d.s.).

2.7. Health-Promoting Properties

2.7.1. Antiradical Capacity

Rye bread (1 g) was mixed with 80% of methanol and water (10 mL) + 1% hydrochloric acid, and incubated for 20 min under sonication (Sonic 6D, Polsonic, Warsaw, Poland). Next, the slurry was centrifuged at 19,000× g for 10 min, and the supernatant was filtered through a hydrophilic PTFE 0.20 µm membrane (Merck, Darmstadt, Germany) and used for analysis.

The ABTS method was performed according to the method described by Re et al. [22]. ABTS$^{•+}$ was generated by oxidation of ABTS with potassiumpersulphate. The ABTS$^{•+}$ solution was diluted to an absorbance of 0.7 ± 0.05 at 734 nm. Then, 0.03 mL of extract was mixed with 2.97 mL of ABTS$^{•+}$ solution and left for 6 min at 25 °C. Next, the absorbance was measured at 734 nm using the UV-2401 PC spectrophotometer (Shimadzu, Kyoto, Japan). The results of antiradical capacity were expressed as Trolox equivalents in µmol per g d.s.

The DPPH method was carried out with the method described by Yen and Chen [23]. Then, 0.50 mL of extract was mixed with ethanol (1.5 mL) and DPPH$^{•+}$ solution (0.5 mL), and left for 10 min at 25 °C. Next, the absorbance was measured at 517 nm using the UV-2401 PC spectrophotometer (Shimadzu, Kyoto, Japan). The results of antiradical activity were expressed as Trolox equivalents in µmol per g d.s.

2.7.2. Reducing Potential

The FRAP test was made on the basis of the method described by Benzie and Strain [24]. First, 0.1 mL of extract was prepared with 0.9 mL of clean H_2O with 3 mL of ferric complex. Next, after 10 min, the absorbance was checked at 593 nm using the UV-2401 PC spectrophotometer (Shimadzu, Kyoto, Japan). The results of reducing activity were expressed as Trolox equivalents in µmol per g d.s.

2.7.3. Ability to Inhibit the Activity of COX 1 and COX-2

The effect of the bread extract on COX-1 and COX-2 (cyclooxygenase-1 and cyclooxygenase-2) activities was tested using COX Inhibitor Screening Assay Kit (Cayman, No. 560131). One unit of inhibitor activity (IU) was defined as the activity inhibiting 1 unit of enzyme activity. The results were expressed in kIU per g of d.s.

2.7.4. Ability to Inhibit the Activity of Lipoxygenase (LOX)

The LOX inhibitory assay was made on the basis of the method described by Axelroad et al. [25] with modifications. LOX activity was tested by BioTek Microplate Readers in absorbance at 234 nm. The reaction mixture contained 0.245 mL 1/15 mol/L phosphate buffer, 0.002 mL of lipoxygenase solution (167 U/mL), and 0.005 mL of inhibitor solution. After preincubation of the mixture at 30 °C for 10 min, the reaction was initiated by adding 0.008 mL 2.5 mmol/L linoleic acid. One unit of LOX activity was defined as the activity oxidizing 0.12 µmole of linoleic acid per 1 min at reaction conditions. One unit of inhibitor activity (IU) was defined as the activity inhibiting 1 unit of enzyme activity. The results were expressed in kIU per g of d.s.

2.7.5. Ability for Inhibit Acetylcholinesterase Activity (AChE)

The effect of the bread extract on AChE was tested by AChE Assay Kit (Sigma-Aldrich, No. CS0003). One unit of inhibitor activity (IU) was defined as the activity inhibiting 1 unit of enzyme activity. The results were expressed in kIU per g of d.s.

2.7.6. Activity of α-Amylase Inhibitors

α-Amylase inhibitor (αA) activity was made on the basis of the method described by Jakubczyk et al. [26]. α-Amylase from hog pancreas (50 U/mg) was dissolved in the 100 mM phosphate buffer (containing 6 mM NaCl, pH 7.0). To measure the α-amylase inhibitory activity, a mixture of 25 µL of α-amylase solution and 25 µL of sample was firstly incubated at 40 °C for 5 min. Then, 50 µL of 1% (w/v) soluble starch (dissolved in 100 mM phosphate buffer containing 6 mM NaCl, pH 7) was added. After 10 min, the reaction was stopped by adding 100 µL of 3,5-dinitrosalicylic acid (DNS) and was heated for 10 min. The mixture was then made up to 300 µL with double distilled water and absorbance 540 nm was measured using BioTek Microplate Readers. One αA inhibitory unit (AIU) was as the activity of αA that inhibited one unit of enzyme. αA was as AIU/mg of sample.

2.7.7. Activity of α-Glucoamyalse Inhibitors

α-Glucoamyalse inhibitor (αG) activity was made on the basis of the method described by Jakubczyk et al. [26]. Firstly, 10 µL of α-glucosidase (1 U/mL) and 20 µL 1% saccharose were added to 0.5 mL of 0.1 mol/L phosphor buffer, pH 6.8. The reaction was incubated at 37 °C for 5 min, stopped by adding 100 µL of 3,5-dinitrosalicylic acid (DNS), and heated for 10 min. The mixture was then made up to 300 µL with double distilled water and absorbance 540 nm was measured. For the αGIA measurement, 10 µL of α-glucosidase (1 U/mL) and 50 µL of the sample were added to 0.45 mL of 0.1 mol/L phosphor buffer pH 6.8. After the incubation at 37 °C for 5 min, 20 µL of 1% saccharose was added. The reaction was incubated at 37 °C for 50 min, stopped by adding 100 µL of 3,5-dinitrosalicylic acid (DNS), and heated for 10 min. The absorbance was tested at 540 nm using BioTek Microplate

Readers (Bad Friedrichshall, Germany). One αG inhibitory unit (αGAU) was as the activity of αG that inhibited one unit of enzyme. αGA was as AIU/mg of sample.

2.7.8. Activity of Lipase Inhibitors

Lipase inhibitory (LP) activity was made on the basis of the method described by Jakubczyk et al. [26]. First, 2 µL, 100 mg mL^{-1} was added to 5 µL of the sample and 142 µL of 100 mM potassium phosphate buffer, pH 7.5. After preincubation at 30 °C for 3 min, the reaction was initiated by mixing the reaction mixture with 1 µL of a 100 mM pNPA solution in dimethyl sulfoxide (DMSO). The absorbance was tested at 405 nm using BioTek Microplate Readers. Lipase One LP inhibitory unit (AIU) was as the activity of inhibitor that inhibited one unit of enzyme. LP was as IU/mg of sample.

2.7.9. Theoretical Approach

For a clear picture of the relationships between the activity of sample and bioaccessibility of their phenols, as well as pro-healthy properties, the following parameters were described by Gawlik-Dziki et al. [17].

Phenolics bioaccessibility index (ACP), which is an indication of the bioaccessibility of phenolic compounds [15]:

$$ACP = C_D/C_R$$

where C_D = amount of components after simulated gastrointestinal digestion and C_R = amount of components after chemical extraction (raw extract).

The biological bioaccessibility index (BAC), which is an indication of the bioaccessibility of antioxidative compounds [15]:

$$BAC = A_R/A_D$$

where A_D = extract after simulated gastrointestinal digestion and A_R = raw extract.

2.8. Relative Digestibility (RD)

2.8.1. Relative Digestibility Proteins

The RD of proteins was expressed as the differences in the content of free amino groups (FAGs) evaluated for the samples after the in vitro digestion [27]. The amount of FAG was evaluated using the TNBS method [28]. Rye bread (20 µL) was prepared with 0.2 M NaH$_2$PO$_4$ buffer (0.980 mL; pH 8.0) and 0.1% TNBS (0.5 mL). After 30 min, the absorbance was tested at 340 nm and the amount of FAG was as L-leucine standard (µg per mL).

2.8.2. Relative Digestibility Starch

The RD of starch was as the difference in the content of reducing sugars (RS) evaluated for the samples after the in vitro digestion [27]. The amount of RS was evaluated by DNSA. Bread (0.2 mL) was prepared with H$_2$O (0.3 mL) and DNSA reagent (0.5 mL). Next, the substance was incubated at 100 °C/10 min. After that, the absorbance was tested at 540 nm. The amount of RS was as maltose standard (µg per mL).

2.9. Statistical Analysis

All experimental results were mean ± SD of two parallel experiments ($N = 18$ for bioactive compounds, enzymatic activity, and relative digestibility; $N = 20$ for colour parameters). Extractions were repeated three times for all analyzed samples. One and multi-way analysis of variance (ANOVA), Duncan's multiple range, as well as median test were analyzed by Statistica 12.5 (Kraków, Poland).

3. Results and Discussion

3.1. Sensory Evaluation and Colour Parameters

The sensory assessment of rye breads demonstrated that the use of pure fruit powder (FP), encapsulated fruit powders with maltodextrin (FPM), and encapsulated fruit powders with inulin (FPI) had an insignificant effect on loaf appearance (Figure 1)—the highest scores were given to BRP3, BRM3, and BRI3, as well as to BRM4 and BRI4 breads, whereas the lowest ones were given to the breads with 6% content of the functional additive. In turn, statistically significant differences were noted in terms of aroma and taste, mainly in the breads with 5% and 6% contents of FP, FPM, and FPI compared with the breads with 1% and 4% contents of the functional additive. This happened probably because this content of the additive contributed to the bitter aftertaste and fruity aroma that merged with the acid flavor of rye bread. Deterioration of the sensory traits of breads with berry fruit can also result from a high content of procyanidin polymers that may cause a bitter and astringent aftertaste [13,29]. The highest scores were given by panelists to the breads with 3% and 4% contents of the powders, which were the most effective in making the rye bread taste intensity milder. Considering crumb porosity and elasticity, no statistically significant differences were noted, except for the breads with fruit powder levels of 5% and 6%, in which the values of these parameters slightly decreased. Summing up, the highest score in the overall acceptability assessment was given by the panelists to the bread with 3% content of the functional additive, regardless of functional additive type, as well as to the product with 4% content of the microencapsulated additive. The panelists evaluated this product as more desirable than the control bread. For this reason, the test can be successfully used for the production of sourdough rye breads. In turn, the microencapsulation of the functional additives allowed increasing its content in bread to 4%. This was also confirmed in a study that demonstrated that breads with the addition of a microencapsulated extract from *Garcinia cowa* fruit were scored higher by panelists than the crude fruit extract [13]. Rye breads could also be successfully supplemented with 5% of tomato pomace additive, which improved their taste values [4]. Other investigations have confirmed the feasibility of fortifying rye breads with saffron at levels of 0.08% and 0.12% [30] as well as with grape pomace at the level up to 6% [6], with both additives ensuring product acceptability by consumers.

Saskatoon berry fruit added as a supplement to rye bread (pure powder (FP) and powders encapsulated with maltodextrin (FPM), and inulin (FPI)) significantly diversified the colour of the crumb and crust of rye bread (Table 1). After preparation of rye bread, it was observed that, with the higher amount of FP, FPM, and FPI in rye product production, the L* parameter was lower, which indicates that the enriched rye breads were darker. Thus, BRC was brighter compared with breads with functional additives. In addition, the higher the fruit powder used, the higher the value of the a* parameter and the lower the value of the b* parameter. In turn, the use of encapsulated powder masked the red colour of the fruit powder used. Similar observations of colour were noted by Ezhilarasi et al. [13] for wheat bread supplemented with a fruit powder made from *Garcinia cowa*. The ΔE parameter was calculated for rye bread enriched with additives from pure FP and encapsulated FPM, as well as FPI, and the higher the proportion of additives, the higher the ΔE parameter value. The values of ΔE parameter for crumb bread with 1% and 2% of additives were <5 units, which indicates no difference to distinguish the colours of the two products. Meanwhile, the highest saturation of crust colour was noted in the sample with 6% of additives. Similar observations of change of colour were obtained by Bajerska et al. [30] through the use of saffron to make rye bread. In the case of pure and encapsulate fruit powder, no significant difference in color was noted.

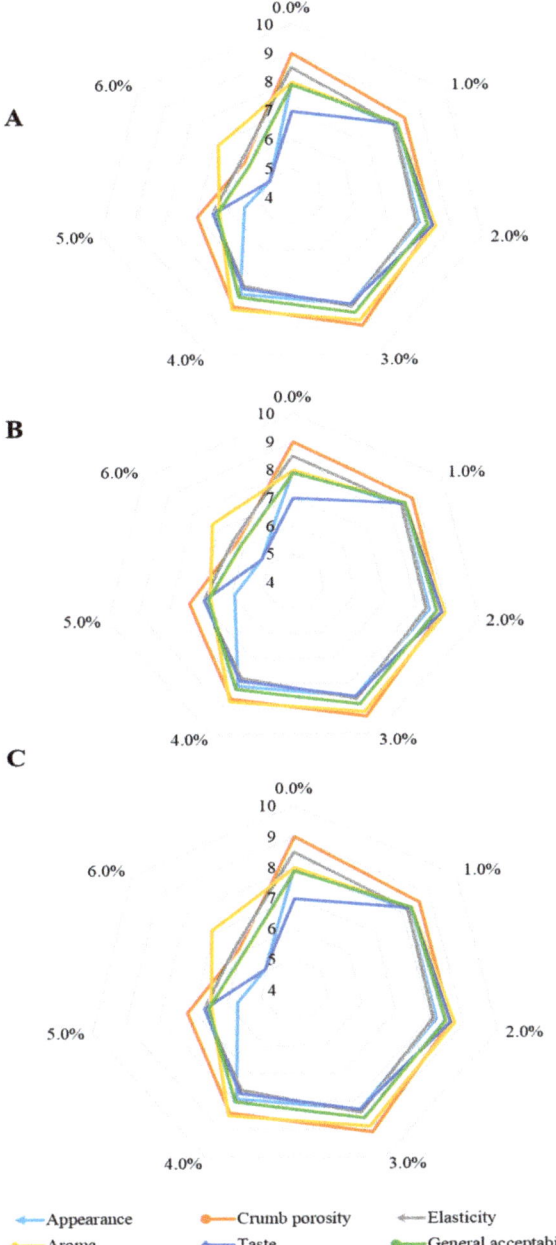

Figure 1. Sensory evaluation of rye bread fortified with fruit powder (**A**), fruit powders covered with maltodextrin (**B**), and fruit powder covered with inulin (**C**).

Table 1. The colour parameter of enriched rye bread. FP, pure fruit powder; FPM, encapsulated fruit powders with maltodextrin; FPI, encapsulated fruit powders with inulin.

	Shares [%]	Rye Bread Enriched with FP				Rye Bread Enriched with FPM				Rye Bread Enriched with FPI			
		L*	a*	b*	ΔE	L*	a*	b*	ΔE	L*	a*	b*	ΔE
Bread crust/dried fruit	BC	52.3 ± 1.0a [1]	2.8 ± 0.1e	17.0 ± 0.3a	-	-	-	-	-	-	-	-	-
	B1	49.3 ± 1.0b	3.9 ± 0.1d	14.1 ± 0.3b	4.4 ± 0.1f	50.2 ± 1.0a	3.2 ± 0.1e	14.3 ± 0.3a	3.5 ± 0.1f	49.7 ± 1.0a	3.4 ± 0.1e	14.5 ± 0.3a	3.7 ± 0.1e
	B2	48.1 ± 1.0c	4.0 ± 0.1d	12.0 ± 0.2c	6.6 ± 0.1e	49.4 ± 1.0b	3.7 ± 0.1d	13.5 ± 0.3b	4.7 ± 0.1e	49.1 ± 1.0a	3.8 ± 0.1d	13.9 ± 0.3b	4.6 ± 0.1d
	B3	46.2 ± 0.9d	4.9 ± 0.1c	11.2 ± 0.2d	8.7 ± 0.2d	47.4 ± 0.9d	4.5 ± 0.1c	12.6 ± 0.3c	6.8 ± 0.1c	47.1 ± 0.9b	4.6 ± 0.1b	13.0 ± 0.3c	6.8 ± 0.1b
	B4	44.9 ± 0.9e	5.8 ± 0.1b	9.2 ± 0.2e	11.2 ± 0.2c	48.4 ± 1.0c	4.3 ± 0.1c	13.0 ± 0.3b	5.8 ± 0.1d	47.7 ± 1.0b	4.2 ± 0.1c	12.9 ± 0.3c	6.4 ± 0.1c
	B5	42.8 ± 0.9f	6.6 ± 0.1b	8.2 ± 0.2f	13.5 ± 0.3b	45.5 ± 0.9e	4.8 ± 0.1b	11.4 ± 0.2d	9.0 ± 0.2b	47.5 ± 1.0b	4.7 ± 0.1b	12.6 ± 0.3c	6.8 ± 0.1b
	B6	40.5 ± 0.8g	7.3 ± 0.1a	6.2 ± 0.1g	16.6 ± 0.3a	43.1 ± 0.9f	5.2 ± 0.1a	8.6 ± 0.2e	12.7 ± 0.3a	44.9 ± 0.9c	5.2 ± 0.1a	9.5 ± 0.2d	10.8 ± 0.2a
Bread crumb/dried fruit	BCC	40.5 ± 0.8a	7.5 ± 0.2a	9.1 ± 0.2a	-	-	-	-	-	-	-	-	-
	B1C	39.9 ± 0.8b	6.4 ± 0.1b	7.8 ± 0.2b	1.8 ± 0.1c	40.7 ± 0.8a	5.3 ± 0.1b	7.9 ± 0.2b	2.5 ± 0.1e	40.3 ± 0.8a	5.7 ± 0.1b	8.0 ± 0.2b	2.1 ± 0.1e
	B2C	39.8 ± 0.8b	6.3 ± 0.1b	7.8 ± 0.2b	1.9 ± 0.1c	40.8 ± 0.8a	5.8 ± 0.1a	8.7 ± 0.2a	1.8 ± 0.1f	40.6 ± 0.8a	6.0 ± 0.1a	9.0 ± 0.2a	1.6 ± 0.1f
	B3C	38.4 ± 0.8b	5.7 ± 0.1c	5.7 ± 0.1c	4.4 ± 0.1b	39.3 ± 0.8b	5.2 ± 0.1b	6.4 ± 0.1c	3.7 ± 0.1d	39.1 ± 0.8b	5.4 ± 0.1b	6.6 ± 0.1d	3.6 ± 0.1d
	B4C	38.7 ± 0.8b	5.2 ± 0.1c	5.6 ± 0.1c	4.6 ± 0.1b	41.7 ± 0.8a	3.8 ± 0.1c	7.9 ± 0.2b	4.1 ± 0.1c	41.0 ± 0.8a	3.7 ± 0.1c	7.8 ± 0.2c	4.1 ± 0.1c
	B5C	36.6 ± 0.7c	3.4 ± 0.1e	2.8 ± 0.1e	8.4 ± 0.2a	39.0 ± 0.8b	2.5 ± 0.1d	3.9 ± 0.1e	7.4 ± 0.1a	40.6 ± 0.8a	2.4 ± 0.1e	4.3 ± 0.1e	7.0 ± 0.1b
	B6C	35.9 ± 0.7c	4.8 ± 0.1d	3.2 ± 0.1d	7.9 ± 0.2a	38.2 ± 0.8c	3.5 ± 0.1c	4.5 ± 0.1d	6.5 ± 0.1b	39.8 ± 0.8b	3.4 ± 0.1d	4.9 ± 0.1e	5.9 ± 0.1a

[1] Values are expressed as the mean (n = 20) ± standard deviation. Mean values bearing different letters in the same row denote statistical difference (a > b > c ... etc.).

3.2. Phenolic Compounds and Their Relative Bioaccesibility

The available literature provides sparse reports on rye bread enrichment with plant material [4–6,29]. The effect of rye bread fortification through the addition of pure fruit powder (FP), encapsulated fruit powders with maltodextrin (FPM), and encapsulated fruit powders with inulin (FPI) on the profile and content of polyphenolic compounds is presented in Table 2. Protective effects of carriers on polyphenolic compounds were demonstrated. The content of polyphenolic compounds in powders additionally protected by carriers after freeze-drying was two times higher compared with pure powders (Table S1) [18,19]. Additionally, enriched products in microencapsulated powders after bread baking contained on average a 1.8 times higher content of polyphenolic compounds than breads enriched with pure powder compared with the content of these compounds before baking [18,19]. The total content of polyphenols in BRC reached 127.2 mg/100 g d.s. Already at 1% FP, the mean content of polyphenols was three times higher compared with the control bread, while the 6% addition of crude FP caused a 13-fold increase. In the breads enriched with microencapsulated FPM and FPI, the content of phenols was by ca. 10% and 12% higher than in the breads with crude FP. This could be owing to the protection of these compounds during bread baking. Many authors have confirmed that carriers used in the microencapsulation process protected bioactive compounds from degradation [7,31,32], while the high temperature used during bread baking could contribute to the degradation of phenols in the breads with crude FP. Compared with the breads fortified with crude FP, greater protection of compounds was noted in the group of anthocyanins and in the group of phenolic acids, which reached 11% and 8% as well as 8% and 15% in the breads with FPM and FPI, respectively. These compounds are particularly unstable at high temperatures [18,31,33] and require additional protection that can be ensured by the microencapsulation process. In addition, our observations concerning bread fortification were consistent with earlier reports addressing rye bread enrichment with saffron [30], tomato pomace [4], green tea [5], and grape pomace [6], which demonstrated that the supplementation of rye breads contributed to an increase in the content of polyphenolic compounds.

Table 2. The content of polyphenols in rye bread [mg/100 g d.s.].

Compounds				Bread Sample					
				BR1	BR2	BR3	BR4	BR5	BR6
Anthocyanins	cyanidin-3-O-galactoside	ND	FP FPM FPI	18.7 ± 0.2m [1] 60.8 ± 0.5k 65.9 ± 0.6j	38.3 ± 0.3l 69.9 ± 0.6j 75.8 ± 0.7i	88.2 ± 0.8i 107 ± 1h 108 ± 1h	135 ± 1g 130 ± 1g 136 ± 1g	195 ± 1f 230 ± 2d 213 ± 1e	281 ± 2c 322 ± 2a 298 ± 2b
	cyanidin-3-O-glucoside	ND	FP FPM FPI	2.5 ± 0.1j 6.2 ± 0.1i 6.4 ± 0.1i	6.8 ± 0.1i 7.1 ± 0.1h 7.4 ± 0.1h	8.7 ± 0.1g 10.3 ± 0.1f 8.8 ± 0.1g	18.1 ± 0.2c 11.0 ± 0.1e 10.9 ± 0.1e	30.0 ± 0.3b 12.2 ± 0.1e 11.7 ± 0.1e	41.8 ± 0.4a 14.6 ± 0.1d 14.0 ± 0.1d
	cyanidin-3-O-arabinoside	ND	FP FPM FPI	ND 3.2 ± 0.1f 3.4 ± 0.1f	2.3 ± 0.1g 3.6 ± 0.1f 3.9 ± 0.1f	3.6 ± 0.1f 4.1 ± 0.1e 4.2 ± 0.1e	5.5 ± 0.1c 4.2 ± 0.1e 4.4 ± 0.1e	7.5 ± 0.1b 5.0 ± 0.1d 4.7 ± 0.1e	11.1 ± 0.1a 6.0 ± 0.1c 5.6 ± 0.1c
	cyanidin-3-O-xyloside	ND	FP FPM FPI	ND 3.3 ± 0.1g 3.1 ± 0.1g	3.8 ± 0.1f 3.6 ± 0.1f	4.1 ± 0.1e 4.1 ± 0.1e 3.7 ± 0.1f	5.0 ± 0.1c 4.6 ± 0.1d 3.6 ± 0.1f	7.2 ± 0.1b 4.4 ± 0.1d 4.5 ± 0.1d	10.1 ± 0.1a 5.2 ± 0.1c 5.4 ± 0.1c
	SUM	ND	FP FPM FPI	21.2 ± 0.9n 73.5 ± 2.8l 78.8 ± 3.1l	47.4 ± 1.8m 84.5 ± 3.3k 90.6 ± 3.5j	104 ± 4i 125 ± 5h 124 ± 5h	163 ± 6f 150 ± 6g 155 ± 6g	240 ± 9e 252 ± 11d 234 ± 10e	344 ± 13b 348 ± 15a 323 ± 14c
Flavan-3-ols	B-type procjanidin dimer	10.1 ± 0.1o	FP FPM FPI	11.0 ± 0.2n 20.6 ± 0.4k 19.1 ± 0.4l	11.5 ± 0.2m 23.7 ± 0.5j 22.0 ± 0.4j	30.2 ± 0.6g 39.4 ± 0.8e 27.7 ± 0.6i	37.1 ± 0.7f 49.6 ± 1.0d 29.6 ± 0.6g	36.3 ± 0.7f 55.5 ± 1.1c 49.9 ± 1.0d	38.8 ± 0.8e 66.6 ± 1.3a 59.9 ± 1.2b
	Epigallocatechin x	12.3 ± 0.1k	FP FPM FPI	25.1 ± 0.5j 23.7 ± 0.5j 30.4 ± 0.6h	32.2 ± 0.6g 27.2 ± 0.5i 36.2 ± 0.7f	37.6 ± 0.8e 39.5 ± 0.8d 44.6 ± 0.9b	39.9 ± 0.8d 46.6 ± 0.9b 44.4 ± 0.9b	43.4 ± 0.9c 43.8 ± 0.9c 45.1 ± 0.9b	44.9 ± 0.9b 54.5 ± 1.1a 55.8 ± 1.1a
	B-type procjanidin dimer	16.0 ± 0.2o	FP FPM FPI	31.8 ± 0.6g 14.9 ± 0.3n 21.2 ± 0.4l	30.6 ± 0.6g 17.1 ± 0.3m 23.2 ± 0.5k	41.7 ± 0.8d 29.5 ± 0.6h 26.5 ± 0.5j	49.7 ± 1.0c 29.7 ± 0.6h 28.0 ± 0.6i	55.8 ± 1.1b 31.4 ± 0.6g 29.3 ± 0.6h	53.8 ± 1.1a 35.7 ± 0.7e 33.6 ± 0.7f
	(+)-Catechin	4.0 ± 0.1m	FP FPM FPI	12.0 ± 0.2l 17.3 ± 0.3k 19.8 ± 0.4j	31.4 ± 0.6h 19.9 ± 0.4j 22.8 ± 0.5i	36.1 ± 0.7f 37.1 ± 0.7f 34.2 ± 0.7g	48.5 ± 1.0d 42.0 ± 0.8e 42.7 ± 0.9e	52.9 ± 1.1c 48.6 ± 1.0d 52.8 ± 1.1c	59.3 ± 1.2b 58.3 ± 1.2b 63.3 ± 1.3a
	(−)-Epicatechin	9.4 ± 0.3k	FP FPM FPI	11.3 ± 0.2j 13.9 ± 0.3i 13.3 ± 0.3i	14.7 ± 0.3h 15.9 ± 0.3 15.3 ± 0.3	15.3 ± 0.3g 18.4 ± 0.4e 17.7 ± 0.4f	19.9 ± 0.4d 18.1 ± 0.4e 18.3 ± 0.4e	21.5 ± 0.4c 24.8 ± 0.5b 16.4 ± 0.3	28.0 ± 0.6a 27.8 ± 0.6a 19.7 ± 0.4d
	SUM	51.8 ± 1.0n	FP FPM FPI	91.3 ± 9.6m 90.3 ± 4.1m 104 ± 6l	120 ± 10k 104 ± 5l 120 ± 8k	161 ± 10i 164 ± 9h 151 ± 10j	195 ± 12f 186 ± 13g 163 ± 11h	210 ± 14d 204 ± 13e 194 ± 15f	225 ± 12c 243 ± 16a 232 ± 19b

Table 2. Cont.

	Compounds			Bread Sample					
				BR1	BR2	BR3	BR4	BR5	BR6
Phenolic acids	protokatechumic acid	0.9 ± 0.1j	FP	3.1 ± 0.1h	4.9 ± 0.1g	6.2 ± 0.1e	8.3 ± 0.1c	9.5 ± 0.1b	10.5 ± 0.1a
			FPM	0.9 ± 0.1j	1.1 ± 0.1i	4.8 ± 0.0g	0.7 ± 0.0j	1.0 ± 0.1i	1.2 ± 0.1i
			FPI	6.9 ± 0.1e	7.9 ± 0.1c	5.8 ± 0.1f	5.5 ± 0.1f	5.6 ± 0.1f	6.8 ± 0.1d
	vanilic acid	2.5 ± 0.1d	FP	3.5 ± 0.1b	3.3 ± 0.1b	3.6 ± 0.1a	3.8 ± 0.1a	3.3 ± 0.1b	3.6 ± 0.1a
			FPM	2.0 ± 0.1d	2.3 ± 0.1d	2.1 ± 0.0d	2.0 ± 0.0d	2.1 ± 0.1d	2.5 ± 0.1c
			FPI	1.9 ± 0.1d	2.1 ± 0.1d	2.3 ± 0.1d	2.3 ± 0.1d	2.3 ± 0.1d	2.7 ± 0.1c
	caffeic acid	0.9 ± 0.1g	FP	3.1 ± 0.1f	3.5 ± 0.1f	4.2 ± 0.1e	4.6 ± 0.1e	5.2 ± 0.1d	5.7 ± 0.1d
			FPM	3.1 ± 0.1f	3.6 ± 0.1f	7.3 ± 0.1b	7.3 ± 0.1b	6.9 ± 0.1c	8.3 ± 0.1a
			FPI	5.1 ± 0.1d	5.9 ± 0.1d	7.2 ± 0.1b	7.3 ± 0.1b	7.2 ± 0.1b	8.6 ± 0.1a
	3-O-caffequinic acid	0.2 ± 0.1m	FP	60.1 ± 1.0g	72.2 ± 1.0g	86.6 ± 1.1e	103 ± 1d	106 ± 1c	110 ± 1a
			FPM	72.7 ± 0.7l	83.6 ± 0.8k	103 ± 1i	109 ± 1g	116 ± 0e	140 ± 3b
			FPI	89.1 ± 0.8j	102 ± 1i	106 ± 1h	110 ± 0g	114 ± 0f	137 ± 1c
	ferulic acid	5.0 ± 0.1b	FP	5.2 ± 0.1b	5.2 ± 0.1b	5.7 ± 0.1b	6.1 ± 0.1a	5.4 ± 0.1.0b	5.9 ± 0.1a
			FPM	3.1 ± 0.1f	3.6 ± 0.1d	3.6 ± 0.0d	3.5 ± 0.0e	3.7 ± 0.1d	4.4 ± 0.1c
			FPI	3.1 ± 0.1f	3.4 ± 0.1e	3.4 ± 0.1e	3.5 ± 0.1e	3.3 ± 0.1e	3.9 ± 0.1d
	5-O-caffequinic acid	0.4 ± 0.1	FP	43.3 ± 0.4k	49.5 ± 0.4j	76.6 ± 0.7g	102 ± 1e	115 ± 1c	127 ± 1b
			FPM	58.4 ± 0.5i	67.2 ± 0.6h	102 ± 1e	104 ± 1e	115 ± 1c	138 ± 1a
			FPI	75.2 ± 0.7g	86.5 ± 0.8f	104 ± 1e	107 ± 1d	113 ± 1c	136 ± 1a
	3-p-coumaroylquinic acid	0.8 ± 0.1h	FP	3.4 ± 0.1g	4.0 ± 0.1g	6.6 ± 0.1g	17.3 ± 0.2e	39.2 ± 0.4b	43.2 ± 0.4a
			FPM	15.4 ± 0.1f	17.7 ± 0.2e	23.0 ± 0.2d	23.2 ± 0.2d	23.6 ± 0.2d	28.3 ± 0.3c
			FPI	17.4 ± 0.2e	20.0 ± 0.2d	21.6 ± 0.2d	23.5 ± 0.2d	25.2 ± 0.2d	30.2 ± 0.3c
	4-O-caffequinic acid	0.2 ± 0.1j	FP	2.2 ± 0.1i	4.9 ± 0.1g	7.3 ± 0.1e	12.1 ± 0.1b	14.1 ± 0.1a	15.4 ± 0.1a
			FPM	3.5 ± 0.1i	4.0 ± 0.1g	5.8 ± 0.1f	7.2 ± 0.1e	8.3 ± 0.1d	10.0 ± 0.1c
			FPI	3.3 ± 0.1i	3.8 ± 0.1h	7.7 ± 0.1e	8.1 ± 0.1d	8.4 ± 0.1d	10.1 ± 0.1c
	SUM	10.9 ± 0.2l	FP	124 ± 2o	148 ± 3n	197 ± 4k	259 ± 5g	298 ± 6c	322 ± 6b
			FPM	159 ± 3m	183 ± 4l	253 ± 5h	257 ± 5g	277 ± 6e	333 ± 7a
			FPI	202 ± 4j	232 ± 5i	259 ± 5g	268 ± 5f	280 ± 6d	336 ± 7a
Flavonols	Kaempferol-3-O-galactoside	3.1 ± 0.1j	FP	3.3 ± 0.1j	7.3 ± 0.1h	12.6 ± 0.3f	21.5 ± 0.4c	26.3 ± 0.5b	31.5 ± 0.6a
			FPM	6.5 ± 0.1i	7.4 ± 0.1h	10.9 ± 0.2g	14.0 ± 0.3f	16.3 ± 0.3e	19.2 ± 0.4d
			FPI	7.5 ± 0.1h	8.4 ± 0.2h	10.3 ± 0.2g	13.3 ± 0.3f	13.9 ± 0.3f	16.7 ± 0.3e
	Quercetin-3-O-arabinoglucoside	4.2 ± 0.1j	FP	1.8 ± 0.1f	2.3 ± 0.1e	2.6 ± 0.1d	2.9 ± 0.1d	3.6 ± 0.1b	4.0 ± 0.0a
			FPM	2.5 ± 0.1e	2.9 ± 0.1d	3.4 ± 0.1c	3.4 ± 0.1c	3.7 ± 0.1b	4.2 ± 0.1a
			FPI	2.5 ± 0.1e	2.9 ± 0.1d	3.3 ± 0.1c	3.3 ± 0.1c	3.7 ± 0.1b	4.1 ± 0.0a
	Kaempferol-3-O-glucoside	32.0 ± 0.3g	FP	34.0 ± 0.7f	36.0 ± 0.7e	37.9 ± 0.8d	42.6 ± 0.9c	48.1 ± 1.1b	51.0 ± 1.1b
			FPM	34.3 ± 0.7f	39.1 ± 0.8d	40.8 ± 0.8c	48.1 ± 1.0b	49.0 ± 1.0b	53.0 ± 1.1a
			FPI	33.5 ± 0.7f	35.3 ± 0.7e	37.1 ± 0.7d	41.8 ± 0.8c	41.9 ± 0.8c	50.3 ± 1.0b
	Quercetin-3-O-rutinoside	3.1 ± 0.1h	FP	3.3 ± 0.1g	7.3 ± 0.1f	10.6 ± 0.1d	11.5 ± 0.1c	12.3 ± 0.1b	15.2 ± 0.1a
			FPM	6.0 ± 0.1e	7.1 ± 0.1d	9.7 ± 0.1b	9.4 ± 0.1c	12.2 ± 0.1a	13.6 ± 0.1a
			FPI	6.0 ± 0.1e	6.9 ± 0.1d	9.5 ± 0.1c	11.8 ± 0.1a	12.0 ± 0.1a	13.4 ± 0.1a

Table 2. Cont.

	Compounds		BC		Bread Sample					
					BR1	BR2	BR3	BR4	BR5	BR6
Flavonols	Quercetin-3-O-robinobioside		1.1 ± 0.1j	FP	2.5 ± 0.1i	3.5 ± 0.1g	3.7 ± 0.1g	8.1 ± 0.1d	10.0 ± 0.1b	11.3 ± 0.1a
				FPM	3.1 ± 0.1h	3.6 ± 0.1g	6.1 ± 0.1f	6.1 ± 0.1f	8.4 ± 0.1d	9.4 ± 0.1c
				FPI	3.0 ± 0.1h	3.5 ± 0.1g	6.1 ± 0.1f	5.9 ± 0.1f	7.4 ± 0.1e	8.3 ± 0.1d
	Quercetin-3-O-galactoside		4.2 ± 0.1h	FP	16.3 ± 0.1i	23.8 ± 0.2h	29.1 ± 0.3g	41.4 ± 0.4e	50.7 ± 0.5b	54.6 ± 0.6a
				FPM	29.7 ± 0.3g	34.1 ± 0.3f	34.3 ± 0.3f	41.6 ± 0.4e	50.8 ± 0.5d	56.8 ± 0.5c
				FPI	31.0 ± 0.3f	35.6 ± 0.3f	34.4 ± 0.3f	51.7 ± 0.5d	59.9 ± 0.5b	67.1 ± 0.6a
	Quercetin-3-O-glucoside		ND	FP	4.1 ± 0.1j	4.7 ± 0.1i	6.1 ± 0.1g	7.0 ± 0.1e	7.8 ± 0.1d	8.9 ± 0.1b
				FPM	3.6 ± 0.1k	4.1 ± 0.1j	5.5 ± 0.1h	6.7 ± 0.1f	7.6 ± 0.1d	8.6 ± 0.1b
				FPI	4.1 ± 0.1j	4.7 ± 0.1i	6.6 ± 0.1f	7.9 ± 0.1d	8.1 ± 0.1c	9.1 ± 0.1a
	Quercetin-3-O-arabinoside		1.8 ± 0.01g	FP	1.7 ± 0.01g	2.2 ± 0.01f	3.4 ± 0.1d	3.8 ± 0.1c	4.3 ± 0.1b	5.6 ± 0.1a
				FPM	1.9 ± 0.01g	2.1 ± 0.01f	2.2 ± 0.01f	2.6 ± 0.1e	2.7 ± 0.1e	2.9 ± 0.1e
				FPI	1.8 ± 0.01g	1.9 ± 0.01g	2.0 ± 0.01f	2.3 ± 0.1f	2.3 ± 0.1f	2.8 ± 0.1e
	Quercetin-3-O-xyloside		ND	FP	2.4 ± 0.1i	3.8 ± 0.1h	4.6 ± 0.1f	5.5 ± 0.1d	6.8 ± 0.1b	7.0 ± 0.a
				FPM	3.9 ± 0.1h	4.5 ± 0.1g	4.8 ± 0.1f	5.2 ± 0.1e	6.1 ± 0.1c	6.9 ± 0.1b
				FPI	4.4 ± 0.1g	5.1 ± 0.1e	5.2 ± 0.1e	5.5 ± 0.1d	5.9 ± 0.1c	6.6 ± 0.1b
	Quercetin-deoxyhexo-hexoside		ND	FP	0.5 ± 0.1c	0.5 ± 0.1c	0.6 ± 0.1b	0.8 ± 0.1a	0.9 ± 0.1a	1.0 ± 0.0a
				FPM	0.3 ± 0.1d	0.3 ± 0.1d	0.4 ± 0.1c	0.5 ± 0.1c	0.8 ± 0.1a	0.9 ± 0.1a
				FPI	0.4 ± 0.1d	0.4 ± 0.1d	0.5 ± 0.1kc	0.7 ± 0.1b	0.7 ± 0.1b	0.8 ± 0.0a
	SUM		43.5 ± 1.3o	FP	69.9 ± 1.4n	88.2 ± 1.8m	106 ± 2	133 ± 3h	155 ± 3e	171 ± 3c
				FPM	91.9 ± 1.8l	105 ± 2k	118 ± 2i	138 ± 3g	158 ± 3d	176 ± 4b
				FPI	94.2 ± 1.9l	105 ± 2k	115 ± 2j	144 ± 3f	156 ± 3e	179 ± 4a
	Sum of phenols		106 ± 3o	FP	306 ± 14n	404 ± 18m	568 ± 25j	751 ± 34f	904 ± 43c	1062 ± 56a
				FPM	415 ± 20m	477 ± 23l	661 ± 3 2h	731 ± 35g	891 ± 49d	1100 ± 66b
				FPI	479 ± 23l	547 ± 27k	649 ± 32i	730 ± 36g	863 ± 47e	1071 ± 62a

[1] Values are expressed as the mean (n = 18) ± standard deviation. Mean values bearing different letters in the same row denote statistical difference (a > b > c …. etc.). ND—not detected; BC—control rye bread; BR1–BR5—breads with fruit powders (1–6%); FP—additives fruit powders; FPM—additives of encapsulated fruit powders with maltodextrin; FPI—additives of encapsulated fruit powders with inulin.

The use of the functional additive, especially in the form of FPM and FPI, significantly improved the content of polyphenolic compounds in the products examined; however, relative bioaccesibility assessment in the simulated digestive system in vitro was conducted for better identification of the fortification effect in the products with the highest level of the additive (3%) acceptable by consumers (Table 3). Compared with the chemical extracts, the results obtained after simulated in vitro digestion demonstrated that the control sample had a 1.4-fold higher content of phenolic compounds, including a 1.3-fold higher content of flavan-3-ols, as well as a 3.4-fold higher content of phenolic acids, and a 1.2-fold lower content of flavonols. The relative bioaccessibility index computed for BRC showed that phenolic acids were more bioaccessible than the other groups of polyphenolic compounds. In turn, compared with the chemical extracts, the samples of bread enriched with FP obtained after in vitro digestion had a 1.3-fold higher content of polyphenolic compounds, including 5.5-fold and 1.2-fold higher contents of anthocyanins and flavonols, as well as 1.7-fold and 1.2-fold lower contents of phenolic acids and flavan-3-ols, respectively. Analogously, the breads fortified with FPM contained 2-fold higher amount of polyphenols, including 6.1, 1.1, 1.4, and 1.3 times more anthocyanins, flavan-3-ols, phenolic acids, and flavonols, respectively, compared with the chemical extracts. In turn, the breads supplemented with FPI were also characterized by a 2-fold higher content of phenols, including 6.4-fold, 1.2-fold, and 1.3-fold higher contents of anthocyanins, flavan-3-ols, and phenolic acids, respectively, as well as by a 1.2 times lower content of flavonols. The relative bioaccessibility index estimated for the enriched rye bread demonstrated that anthocyanins were highly bioaccessible, and that flavan-3-ols and phenolics were poorly bioaccessible upon the use of FP. The highest relative bioaccessibility index was computed for the breads with FPM addition followed by those with FPI addition, which may indicate that these carriers, and maltodextrin in particular, contributed to greater release of the compounds tested during in vitro digestion. This observation can be explained by better protection of these compounds during bread baking. Besides, it has been described earlier that the digestion process itself can enhance the release of phenolic compounds [34,35], while the low relative bioaccessibility of the compounds could suggest interactions with bread matrix components, which had earlier been reported for the wheat bread enriched with green coffee grains or with broccoli sprouts [17]. The results obtained may also suggest that the use of the powdered functional additive increased the content of phenols, which affected a higher relative bioaccessibility of the rye bread examined, which is indicative of the additive's effectiveness. In contrast, the microencapsulated functional additive was more effective than the additive without the carrier in increasing the potential relative bioaccessibility of the compounds tested. This was also confirmed by Vitaglione et al. [14], who demonstrated that the fortification of wheat bread with microencapsulated curcumin contributed to greater relative bioaccessibility of bioactive compounds compared with the non-microencapsulated material. According to the authors above, this could be owing to the impaired interactions between the compounds tested and bread matrix. However, the mechanisms of action of the microencapsulated functional additives during simulated in vitro digestion of rye bread require further extensive research. Such attempts will be undertaken in the future.

Table 3. Potentially bioaccessible phenolic compounds in the control and enriched rye bread.

	Compounds	Bread Sample				Relative Accessibility Index			
		BRC	BRP3	BRM3	BRI3	BRC	BRP3	BRM3	BRI3
Anthocyanins	ANT1	-	503 ± 2c [1]	662 ± 2b	695 ± 2a	-	5.7	6.2	6.4
	ANT2	-	34.8 ± 0.1b	45.8 ± 0.2a	48.1 ± 0.2a	-	4.0	4.4	5.4
	ANT3	-	17.3 ± 0.1b	22.7 ± 0.1a	23.8 ± 0.1a	-	4.8	5.6	5.7
	ANT4	-	23.0 ± 0.1b	30.3 ± 0.1a	31.8 ± 0.1a	-	5.7	7.4	8.5
	SUM	-	578 ± 239c	761 ± 315b	799 ± 202a	-	5.5	6.1	6.4
Flavan-3-ols	F3O1	16.7 ± 0.3d	27.2 ± 0.5c	40.2 ± 0.8a	36.6 ± 0.7b	1.7	0.9	1.0	1.3
	F3O2	14.2 ± 0.8c	30.5 ± 0.6b	42.7 ± 0.8a	43.3 ± 0.8a	1.1	0.8	1.1	1.0
	F3O3	13.1 ± 0.6d	5.4 ± 0.1c	30.1 ± 0.6a	23.4 ± 0.7b	0.1	0.1	1.0	0.9
	F3O4	4.3 ± 0.2d	14.4 ± 0.2c	37.8 ± 0.7b	44.2 ± 0.8a	1.7	0.8	1.0	1.0
	F3O5	10.2 ± 0.2c	6.1 ± 0.1d	18.7 ± 0.3b	22.8 ± 0.4a	1.1	0.4	1.0	1.3
	SUM	58.5 ± 1.1c	83.7 ± 1.2b	169 ± 3a	170 ± 3a	1.2	0.6	1.0	1.2
Phenolic acid	PA1	2.5 ± 0.1a	1.6 ± 0.1b	2.5 ± 0.1a	2.7 ± 0.1a	2.8	0.3	0.5	0.5
	PA2	5.1 ± 0.1a	0.9 ± 0.1b	1.5 ± 0.1b	1.6 ± 0.1b	2.0	0.3	0.7	0.7
	PA3	12.3 ± 0.1a	5.5 ± 0.1d	8.8 ± 0.1c	9.2 ± 0.1b	15.0	0.8	0.4	0.4
	PA4	5.5 ± 0.1a	2.7 ± 0.1c	4.3 ± 0.1b	4.6 ± 0.1b	5.9	0.7	0.6	0.6
	PA5	2.7 ± 0.1c	121 ± 1b	221 ± 1a	219 ± 1a	17.0	1.0	2.1	2.1
	PA6	5.5 ± 0.1a	2.7 ± 0.1c	4.3 ± 0.1b	4.5 ± 0.1b	1.1	0.5	1.2	1.3
	PA7	0.7 ± 0.1c	63.2 ± 0.3b	99.8 ± 0.4a	95.7 ± 0.4a	1.7	0.8	1.0	0.9
	PA8	1.4 ± 0.1c	6.1 ± 0.1b	9.7 ± 0.1a	10.1 ± 0.1a	7.5	0.8	1.7	1.3
	SUM	35.8 ± 3.7d	204 ± 21c	352 ± 47a	347 ± 39b	3.3	0.9	1.4	1.3
Flavonols	FL1	4.1 ± 0.1b	22.5 ± 0.1a	24.7 ± 0.1a	23.6 ± 0.1a	1.3	1.8	2.3	2.3
	FL2	5.1 ± 0.1b	2.3 ± 0.2a	3.1 ± 0.2a	3.2 ± 0.2a	1.2	0.9	0.9	1.0
	FL3	28.7 ± 0.1c	38.8 ± 0.2b	52.7 ± 0.2a	40.7 ± 0.2b	0.9	1.0	1.3	1.1
	FL4	7.0 ± 0.1b	9.6 ± 0.1a	10.5 ± 0.1a	10.1 ± 0.1a	2.3	0.9	1.1	1.1
	FL5	5.1 ± 0.1b	5.2 ± 0.1a	5.7 ± 0.1a	5.4 ± 0.1a	4.4	1.4	0.9	0.9
	FL6	-	40.3 ± 0.2a	44.3 ± 0.2a	42.3 ± 0.2a	-	1.4	1.3	1.2
	FL7	-	8.1 ± 0.1a	8.9 ± 0.1a	8.5 ± 0.1a	-	1.3	1.6	1.3
	FL8	4.9 ± 0.1d	9.2 ± 0.1a	6.4 ± 0.1b	5.1 ± 0.1c	2.7	2.7	2.9	2.6
	FL9	-	12.6 ± 0.1a	13.8 ± 0.1a	13.2 ± 0.1a	-	2.7	2.9	2.6
	FL10	-	5.4 ± 0.1a	5.9 ± 0.1a	5.6 ± 0.1a	-	2.1	2.5	2.3
	SUM	54.9 ± 9.1d	153 ± 15c	176 ± 18a	157 ± 15b	1.2	1.4	1.5	1.4
Sum of polyphenols		144 ± 25d	1047 ± 217c	1492 ± 270b	1506 ± 292a	1.4	1.6	1.9	2.1

[1] Values are expressed as the mean (n = 18) ± standard deviation. Mean values bearing different letters in the same row denote statistical difference (a > b > c … etc.). BRC—rye bread control; BRP3—rye bread with 3% of fruit powder; BRM3—rye bread with 3% of fruit powders with maltodextrin; BRI3—rye bread with 3% of fruit powders with inulin; FP—additives fruit powders; FPM—additives of encapsulated fruit powders with maltodextrin; FPI—additives of encapsulated fruit powders with inulin; PC—sum of phenolic compounds; ANT—sum of anthocyanins; FL—sum of flavonols; PA—sum of phenolic acid; F3O—sum of flavan-3-ols (monomers and oligomers); F3O1—B-type procyjanidin dimer; F3O2—epigallocatechin; F3O3—B-type procyanidin dimer; F3O4—(−)-Epicatechin; F3O5—(+)-Catechin; FL1—kampferol-3-O-galactoside; FL2—kampferol-3-O-glucoside; FL3—quercetin-3-O-arabinoglucoside; FL4—quercetin-3-O-rutinoside; FL5—quercetin-3-O-robinobioside; FL6—quercetin-3-O-galactoside; FL7—quercetin-3-O-glucoside; FL8—quercetin-3-O-arabinoside; FL9—quercetin-3-O-xyloside; FL10—quercetin-3-O-deoxy-hexoside; ANT1—cyanidin-3-O-galactoside; ANT2—cyanidin-3-O-glucoside; ANT3—cyanidin-3-O-arabinoside; ANT4—cyanidin-3-O-xyloside; PA1—protocatechuic acid; PA2—vanilic acid; PA3—caffeic acid; PA4—3-O-caffequinic acid; PA5—ferulic acid; PA6—5-O-p-coumaroylquinic acid; PA7, 3-O-p-coumaroylquinic acid; PA8—4-O-p-coumaroylquinic acid.

3.3. Pro-Healthy Potency and Their Bioaccesibility

The antioxidant activity of BRC analyzed in ABTS, DPPH, and FRAP tests reached 13.09, 3.04, and 21.00 µmol Trolox/g d.s., respectively (Table 4), and was consistent with the literature data [3]. The addition of Saskatoon berry fruit powder improved the antioxidant potential of the fortified breads compared with BRC. Even the 1% addition of FP, FPM, and FPI to rye bread increased its antiradical activity and reducing properties by 5%, 7.5%, and 6%; 6%, 7%, and 6.5%; as well as by 6%, 8%, and 6.2%, respectively. In turn, the 6% addition of FP, FPM, and FPI increased both the reducing (FRAP) and antiradical potential (ABTS and DPPH) by 39%, 46%, and 46.5%; 39%, 46%, and 47%; as well as by 40%, 47.5%, and 48%, respectively. The increased antioxidant potential of the supplemented rye breads could be owing to sourdough fermentation, because—as reported by Banu et al. [2]—it can increase the extractability of polyphenols from both the additive and rye flour. The baking process of rye bread can also contribute to an increase of its antioxidant potential owing to the appearance of Maillard reaction products [36]. Compared with the use of crude FP, rye bread fortification with microencapsulated FPM and FPI contributed to the greater protection of compounds exhibiting antioxidant potential by 9% and 8% on average in the FRAP assay, by 8% and 7% on average in the ABTS assay, and by 13% and 8% on average in the DPPH assay, respectively. However, there were no statistically significant differences between the microencapsulated additives. Earlier studies have demonstrated rye bread supplementation with grape pomace at the level of 10% to cause a 10-fold increase in its reducing potential [6]. In turn, rye bread fortification with 0.16% of saffron resulted in a 1.6-fold increase in its antiradical activity [30]. A green tea extract added at the level of 1.1% caused a 13-fold increase in the antioxidant activity of rye bread compared with the control sample [5]. As in the study by Mildner-Szkudlarz et al. [6], the higher value of the antioxidant potential was strongly correlated with the amount of polyphenolic compounds, that is, $r^2 = 0.801$ in the FRAP test and 0.837 in the ABTS test. A similar observation was noted in this work where strong Pearson correlation between polyphenols and antioxidant activity was $r^2 = 0.928$ for FRAP assay, $r^2 = 0.929$ for ABTS assay, and $r^2 = 0.892$ for DPPH assay. In addition, in accordance with the findings reported by Ezhilarasi et al. [13], the microencapsulated functional additives from Garcinia fruits ensured 2-fold greater protection of the antioxidant activity in wheat bread compared with the non-microencapsulated ones. The use of microencapsulated red grape seeds also caused a two times higher antioxidant potential of wheat cookies compared with the product containing a crude additive from grape seeds [37]. The higher antiradical and reducing properties can be owing to the greater protection of bioactive compounds during high-temperature baking [13,37].

However, the antioxidant potential of the bioaccessible fraction of the breads with 3% content of the additive was significantly higher compared with that of the chemical extracts, that is, by 20%, 23%, and 50% in the case of BRP3; by 63%, 27%, and 64% in the case of BRM3; and by 54%, 26%, and 53% in the case of BRI3, while measured with the FRAP, ABTS, and DPPH tests, respectively (Table 5). The analyses demonstrated that in vitro digestion could affect the release of polyphenols from a bread matrix, thereby leading to an increase in their antioxidant activity [33]. Similar results were obtained upon wheat bread enrichment with flaxseed hulls [38] and green coffee extracts [35]. The value of the relative bioaccesibility index computed for the antioxidant activity pointed to high in vitro relative bioaccesibility of these breads. In the FRAP test, the highest value of the relative bioaccesibility index was demonstrated for BRI3 (2.36), whereas the lowest one was for BRC (0.71), while in the ABTS and DPPH test, the highest value of this index was shown for the products containing the functional additive microencapsulated with maltodextrin (3.15 and 2.78). In turn, earlier studies have shown that interactions of bioactive compounds with the matrix of food products can reduce their antioxidant potential [27], which was noted in the case of BRC in our study. In turn, the highest relative bioaccesibility of the microencapsulated functional additives can be owing to the better release of compounds with the antioxidant activity during in vitro digestion or to the protective effect on the formation of complexes with rye bread components. Similar observations were made for the wheat bread enriched with microencapsulated curcumin [14].

Table 4. The antioxidant activity of rye bread fortification with functional additives without and with carriers.

Antioxidant Activity [μmol TE/g ds.]	BRC	Form of Supplement	BR1	BR2	BR3	BR4	BR5	BR6
FRAP	21.0 ± 0.42g [1]	FP	22.30 ± 0.45f	22.60 ± 0.37d	24.40 ± 0.45e	26.70 ± 0.53c	29.50 ± 0.59b	34.80 ± 0.70a
		FPM	22.70 ± 0.45e	22.90 ± 0.46e	26.50 ± 0.53d	30.20 ± 0.60c	32.30 ± 0.65b	39.00 ± 0.78a
		FPI	22.32 ± 0.33f	23.06 ± 0.40e	25.48 ± 0.45d	28.76 ± 0.58c	32.60 ± 0.65b	39.22 ± 0.78a
ABTS	13.09 ± 0.26g	FP	13.93 ± 0.27f	14.14 ± 0.49c	15.24 ± 0.40e	16.68 ± 0.43d	18.43 ± 0.79b	21.73 ± 0.80a
		FPM	14.19 ± 0.46d	14.32 ± 0.32f	16.58 ± 0.34e	18.84 ± 0.68c	20.27 ± 0.73b	24.39 ± 0.87a
		FPI	13.95 ± 0.35d	14.41 ± 0.35d	15.93 ± 0.33e	17.98 ± 0.63c	20.40 ± 0.73b	24.50 ± 0.87a
DPPH	3.04 ± 0.02k	FP	3.34 ± 0.12j	3.58 ± 0.05i	3.62 ± 0.09i	4.27 ± 0.17g	4.50 ± 0.20f	5.46 ± 0.17d
		FPM	3.70 ± 0.09i	3.66 ± 0.07i	6.94 ± 0.21b	4.51 ± 0.12f	5.14 ± 0.13e	8.51 ± 0.12a
		FPI	3.57 ± 0.15i	3.62 ± 0.17i	4.04 ± 0.08h	4.60 ± 0.19f	5.12 ± 0.09e	5.98 ± 0.10c

[1] Values are expressed as the mean (n = 18) ± standard deviation. Mean values bearing different letters in the same row denote statistical difference (a > b > c … etc.). BC—control rye bread; BR1–BR6—breads with fruit powders (1–6%); FP—additives fruit powders; FPM—additives of encapsulated fruit powders with maltodextrin; FPI—additives of encapsulated fruit powders with inulin; ABTS—2,2′-azinobis(3-ethylbenzothiazoline-6-sulfonic acid; DPPH—2,2-Di(4-tert-octylphenyl)-1-picrylhydrazyl.

Table 5. Ability to inhibit the activity of enzymes related to metabolic syndrome.

In Vitro Potency		Extract	Bread Sample				Relative Accessibility Index			
			BRC	BRP3	BRM3	BRI3	BRC	BRP3	BRM3	BRI3
Antioxidant activity [μmol TE/g d. s.]	ABTS	EBD	13.09 ± 0.26c [1]	15.24 ± 0.40a	16.58 ± 0.34b	15.93 ± 0.33b	2.20	2.48	3.15	2.72
		PBE	28.78 ± 0.24c	37.44 ± 0.31a	52.24 ± 0.24b	43.37 ± 0.25b				
	DPPH	EBD	3.04 ± 0.02d	3.62 ± 0.09c	6.94 ± 0.21a	4.04 ± 0.08b	1.70	2.00	2.78	2.13
		PBE	5.17 ± 0.39d	7.23 ± 0.21c	19.29 ± 0.72a	8.60 ± 0.28b				
	FRAP	EBD	21.00 ± 0.42c	24.39 ± 0.37d	26.53 ± 0.53a	25.48 ± 0.45b	0.71	1.25	1.84	2.36
		PBE	15.00 ± 0.71d	30.48 ± 0.41c	48.70 ± 0.51b	52.99 ± 0.39a				
Pro-health potency	Inhibition of LOX activity [kIU/g ds]	EBD	1257 ± 30b	1549 ± 2a	121 ± 2c	1116 ± 2d	0.56	2.04	1.25	1.37
		PBF	70.00 ± 0.14c	3168 ± 5d	147 ± 2b	1530 ± 3a				
	Inhibition of COX-1 activity [kIU/g ds]	EBD	4.22 ± 0.84b	8.32 ± 0.66a	-	-	0.37	-	-	-
		PBF	1.56 ± 0.11a	-	-	-				
	Inhibition of COX-2 activity [kIU/g ds]	EBD	7.75 ± 0.55d	10.71 ± 1.14c	19.33 ± 0.39a	15.96 ± 0.32b	0.91	0.36	0.43	0.54
		PBF	7.06 ± 1.41c	3.85 ± 0.77d	8.29 ± 0.66b	8.57 ± 0.71a				
	Inhibition of AChE activity [IU/g ds]	EBD	23.54 ± 0.47b	20.73 ± 0.41d	21.90 ± 0.44c	24.50 ± 0.49a	-	-	-	-
		PBF	-	-	-	-				

[1] Values are expressed as the mean (n = 18) ± standard deviation. Mean values bearing different letters in the same row denote statistical difference (a > b > c … etc.). EBD—extracts buffer digestion; PBE—potentially bioaccessible fraction; BRC—rye bread control; BRP3—rye bread with 3% of fruit powder; BRM3—rye bread with 3% addition of fruit powder microcapsulated with maltodextrin; BRI3—rye bread with 3% addition of fruit powder microcapsulated inulin; LOX—lipoxygenase; COX—cyclooxygenases.

Many of the previous studies have demonstrated the in vitro digestion to act as an extractor of compounds with potential relative bioaccessibility and capable of inhibiting enzymes responsible for the induction of inflammatory conditions, including the activity of lipoxygenase (LOX) [17,39]. The effect of in vitro digestion on the selected activities of bread with the optimal content of the functional additive (3%) is presented in Table 5. The highest ability to inhibit LOX activity in the buffered extracts was determined in BRP3 samples, and it was 1.2 times higher compared with BRC. There were no statistically significant differences in the capability for LOX activity inhibition between various forms of the additive (BRC, BRM3, and BRI3). The in vitro digestion caused an increase in the ability to inhibit LOX activity by ca. 29%, with the highest increase noted for BRP3 (over 50%). The relative bioaccessibility index pointed to a high relative bioaccessibility of the supplemented breads, that is,

2.04 (BRP3) 1.25 (BRM3), and 1.37 (BRI3), whereas poor relative bioaccesibility was demonstrated for BRC (0.56). It can be hypothesized that the breads fortified with the fruit powder can suppress the generation of reaction oxygen species (ROS) at the lipoxygenase pathways, thus leading to the inhibition of inflammatory conditions in the body, particularly in the gastrointestinal tract wherein the ROS can lead to the development of carcinogenic lesions [40].

In addition, the breads with the functional additives were determined for their capability to inhibit cyclooxygenases (COX), compared with BRC. The addition of crude FP to bread caused a 2-fold increase in the ability to inhibit COX-1 activity, whereas no such activity was demonstrated in BRM3 and BRI3 products (Table 5). The in vitro digestion caused a 2.5-fold suppression in COX-1 inhibiting activity of BRC, whereas no such activity was observed in the breads fortified with functional additives. In turn, the anti-inflammatory activity analyzed against the inhibition of COX-2 activity in the fortified breads BRP3, BRI3, and BRM3 was 1.3-fold, 2.1-fold, and 2.5-fold higher, respectively, compared with BRC. In the potentially bioaccessible fraction, the best COX-2 inhibiting effect was achieved for BRM3 and BRI3. The potential to inhibit the activity of COX-2 is significant as it is activated in the event of the inflammatory reaction of the body [41] and is responsible for the synthesis of prostaglandin E2, which promotes the development of carcinogenic lesions [42]. The high anti-inflammatory activity against COX-2 can be owing to a higher content of polyphenolic compounds in the products. It was confirmed in the study conducted by Moschon et al. [43], who noted that the microencapsulated products characterized by a higher content of phenols had a higher biological value, including the anti-inflammatory activity.

The use of Saskatoon berry fruits microencapsulated with inulin had only a negligible effect on AChE activity inhibition (an increase by 5%) compared with BRC, whereas no AChE inhibition was noted in the breads with 3% addition of FP and FPM. In turn, the negligibly higher ability to inhibit the activity of this enzyme determined in the products with FPI addition can be owing to the health-promoting properties of inulin [44]. Unfortunately, this activity was not detected in the fractions obtained after in vitro digestion.

Investigations conducted so far have proved that polyphenolic compounds can inhibit the activities of digestive hydrolases, including the activity of pancreatic lipase, being responsible for dietary fat absorption, as well as activities of α-glucosidase (αG) and α-amylase (αA) responsible for the hydrolysis of carbohydrates [10,12]. All additives used for bread fortification were able to inhibit αA activity. The highest inhibition was demonstrated for BRP3 and BRM3, and it was 2.8 and 2.6 times higher compared with BRI3, and 5.3 and 5.6 times higher compared with BRC (Table 6). The control bread exhibited a marginal ability to inhibit αG. This activity was a dozen times higher in BRP3, BRM3, and BRI3. In turn, the ability to inhibit the activity of pancreatic lipase was demonstrated for BRM3 and BRI3, and it was 1.3 and 1.2 times higher compared with BRC, and 1.3 and 1.4 times higher compared with BRP3. It can be concluded that the use of functional additive had a positive effect on the breads' ability to inhibit activities of αA and αG. In contrast, only the microencapsulated additives inhibited the activity of pancreatic lipase. The high inhibition of digestive enzymes can be owing to the presence of polyphenolic compounds in the additives. This was confirmed by Zhang et al. [45], who noted a strong correlation between the amount of polyphenols and the anti-diabetic activity of lentil. However, an undesirable effect was observed in the rye breads fortified with the microencapsulated powder, which involved the reduction of the potential to inhibit activities of αG and αA compared with FP. It is likely that the carrier can be responsible for masking enzyme inhibitors (polyphenols) and inhibiting their interactions. Considering the phenolic profile of the analyzed breads, it can be speculated that they effectively influence the inhibition of hyperglycemia and obesity, likewise in the study conducted by Zhao et al. [12], who demonstrated that powders from *Amelanchier alnifolia* Nutt. could alleviate hyperlipidemia, hyperglycemia, and blood vessel inflammation induced by high-saccharose and high-fat diet. In addition, the research carried out by Bajerska et al. [30] proved that rye bread enrichment with saffron could lead to the enhanced secretion of insulin and reduced blood levels of glucose and triglycerides. Furthermore, as shown by the literature data [46], the sourdough rye bread itself displays high anti-diabetic and anti-obesity potentials and, according to results of our study, these effects can be enhanced by rye bread fortification. Nevertheless, these metabolic effects need to be further explored in future research.

Table 6. Enzymatic in vitro inhibition activity of enriched rye bread.

Sample	Inhibition of α-Amylase Activity [U/g]	Inhibition of α-Glucosidase Activity [U/g]	Inhibition of Pancreatic Lipase Activity [U/g]
BRC	4.58 ± 0.09d [1]	0.04 ± 0.01d	1.20 ± 0.02c
BRP3	46.62 ± 0.93a	4.04 ± 0.08a	1.03 ± 0.02d
BRM3	41.58 ± 0.83b	2.32 ± 0.05b	1.27 ± 0.03b
BRI3	16.09 ± 0.32c	2.04 ± 0.04c	1.43 ± 0.03a

[1] Values are expressed as the mean (n = 18) ± standard deviation. Mean values bearing different letters in the same row denote statistical difference (a > b > c ... etc.). BRP3—rye bread with 3% of fruit powder; BRM3—rye bread with 3% of fruit powders with maltodextrin; BRI3—rye bread with 3% of fruit powders with inulin.

3.4. Relative Digestibility of Starches and Proteins

Functional additives with a high content of polyphenols usually reduce the relative bioaccesibility of nutrients. Considering the above, analyses were conducted to determine the effect of the functional additives on the relative digestibility of starch and proteins (Table 7). In the case of starch digestibility, it was found to decrease upon rye bread enrichment with FP, FPM, and FPI, with the most significant decrease determined in BRP3 (ca. 25%) and BRM3 (ca. 21%). Similar observations were made upon wheat bread enrichment with green coffee powder [35]. The fortification of wheat bread with sorghum flour also led to a ca. 40% decrease in the relative digestibility of starch [47]. Investigations conducted so far have shown that the reduced digestibility of starch and protein can be attributed to polyphenolic compounds present in the plant material, chlorogenic acid in particular [48]. In turn, the fruit powder with the addition of maltodextrin and inulin only slightly decreased protein digestibility (by ca. 16% and 14%, respectively), whereas the use of FP increased it by 27%. Reduced digestibility of protein and starch was also reported upon pasta enrichment with carob flour [27]. In turn, the decreased digestibility of proteins in the in vitro analyses can be owing to the interactions between bioactive compounds of plant origin and components of the bread matrix, leading to the formation of complexes that can be either completely excreted with digested products or inhibit activities of digestive enzymes in the gastrointestinal tract [27]. In addition, the reduction in the relative digestibility of protein can be owing to the fact that rye bread may be a better substrate for digestive enzymes [2].

Table 7. Relative digestibility of starch and proteins.

Bread	Free Reducing Sugars [mg/g]	Released Sugar [mg/g]	Relative Digestibility of Starch	Free Amino Acids and Peptides [mg/g]	Released Amino Acids and Peptides [mg/g]	Relative Digestibility of Proteins
BRC	54.7 ± 1.1d [1]	473 ± 9a	100 ± 2a	4.4 ± 0.1c	82.3 ± 1.6b	100 ± 2a
BRP3	248 ± 5a	354 ± 7d	75.0 ± 1.5d	6.9 ± 0.1a	105 ± 2a	127 ± 2b
BRM3	158 ± 3b	371 ± 7c	78.4 ± 1.6c	4.2 ± 0.1d	68.5 ± 1.4d	83.3 ± 1.7d
BRI3	100 ± 2c	442 ± 8b	93.4 ± 1.9b	4.8 ± 0.1b	70.8 ± 1.4c	86.0 ± 1.7c

[1] Values are expressed as the mean (n = 18) ± standard deviation. Mean values bearing different letters in the same row denote statistical difference (a > b > c ... etc.). BRC—rye bread control; BRP3—rye bread with 3% of fruit powder; BRM3—rye bread with 3% addition of fruit powder microcapsulated with maltodextrin; BRI3—rye bread with 3% addition of fruit powder microcapsulated inulin.

4. Conclusions

The enrichment of rye breads with fruits offers an effective method for the improvement of their biological value. The addition of Saskatoon berry fruit powders to rye bread caused a significant increase in the content of their polyphenols and their antioxidant activity, compared with the control products. The higher the content of the functional additive, the higher the content of antioxidant compounds and their particular groups. Bread supplemented with 3% of the fruit powder, regardless of its form, was acceptable in terms of its sensory attributes and colour. The simulated in vitro digestion showed that anthocyanins of the supplemented rye bread were highly bioaccessible compounds, whereas the least bioaccessible turned out to be flavan-3-ols. Among the functional additives studied, the highest value of the antioxidant potential and the highest relative bioaccesibility of flavonols, flavan-3-ols, and phenolic acids were achieved in BRM3. The addition of fruits caused an insignificant reduction in the relative digestibility of starch and proteins. Bread fortification led to the enhanced capability for the inhibition of α-glucosidase and α-amylase activities, whereas in the case of BRM3 and BRI3 analyses, it additionally showed the ability to inhibit the activity of pancreatic lipase and cyclooxigenase-2 as well as a low inhibitor activity against acetylcholinesterase. On the basis of the above results, it can be concluded that the Saskatoon berry fruit powders, especially these subjected to the microencapsulation process, are valuable and prospective functional additives that increase the attractiveness and nutritive value of rye bread.

Supplementary Materials: The following are available online at http://www.mdpi.com/2076-3921/9/7/614/s1, Table S1: The content of phenolic compounds in pure fruit powder, encapsulated fruit powders with maltodextrin, and encapsulated fruit powders with inulin [mg/100 g d.s.].

Author Contributions: Conceptualization, S.L.; prepared of sample, S.L. and E.P.; methodology, S.L. and M.Ś.; writing—original draft preparation, S.L.; writing—editing, S.L.; writing—review, S.L.; project administration, S.L.; funding acquisition, S.L. All authors have read and agreed to the published version of the manuscript.

Funding: This research was supported by Wrocław University of Environmental and Life Sciences; grant name "Innovative scientist", grant number B030/0032/20.

Acknowledgments: The work was created in a leading research team 'Food&Health' (S.L.).

Conflicts of Interest: The authors declare no conflict of interest.

References

1. Bondia-Pons, I.; Aura, A.-M.; Vuorela, S.; Kolehmainen, M.; Mykkänen, H.; Poutanen, K. Rye phenolics in nutrition and health. *J. Cereal Sci.* **2009**, *49*, 323–336. [CrossRef]
2. Banu, I.; Vasilean, I.; Aprodu, I. Effect of Lactic Fermentation on Antioxidant Capacity of Rye Sourdough and Bread. *Food Sci. Technol. Res.* **2010**, *16*, 571–576. [CrossRef]
3. Pejcz, E.; Gil, Z.; Wojciechowicz-Budzisz, A.; Półtorak, M.; Romanowska, A. Effect of technological process on the nutritional quality of naked barley enriched rye bread. *J. Cereal Sci.* **2015**, *65*, 215–219. [CrossRef]
4. Bajerska, J.; Chmurzynska, A.; Mildner-Szkudlarz, S.; Drzymała-Czyż, S. Effect of rye bread enriched with tomato pomace on fat absorption and lipid metabolism in rats fed a high-fat diet. *J. Sci. Food Agric.* **2015**, *95*, 1918–1924. [CrossRef]
5. Bajerska, J.; Mildner-Szkudlarz, S.; Walkowiak, J. Effects of Rye Bread Enriched with Green Tea Extract on Weight Maintenance and the Characteristics of Metabolic Syndrome Following Weight Loss: A Pilot Study. *J. Med. Food* **2014**, *18*, 698–705. [CrossRef]
6. Mildner-Szkudlarz, S.; Zawirska-Wojtasiak, R.; Szwengiel, A.; Pacyński, M. Use of grape by-product as a source of dietary fibre and phenolic compounds in sourdough mixed rye bread. *Int. J. Food Sci. Technol.* **2011**, *46*, 1485–1493. [CrossRef]
7. Juríková, T.; Balla, S.; Sochor, J.; Pohanka, M.; Mlcek, J.; Baron, M. Flavonoid profile of saskatoon berries (*Amelanchier alnifolia* Nutt.) and their health promoting effects. *Molecules* **2013**, *18*, 12571–12586. [CrossRef]
8. Rop, O.; Řezníček, V.; Mlček, J.; Juríková, T.; Sochor, J.; Kizek, R.; Humpolíček, P.; Balík, J. Nutritional values of new Czech cultivars of Saskatoon berries (*Amelanchier alnifolia* Nutt.). *Hortic. Sci.* **2012**, *39*, 123–128. [CrossRef]
9. Lachowicz, S.; Oszmiański, J.; Seliga, Ł.; Pluta, S. Phytochemical Composition and Antioxidant Capacity of Seven Saskatoon Berry (*Amelanchier alnifolia* Nutt.) Genotypes Grown in Poland. *Molecules* **2017**, *22*, 853. [CrossRef]

10. Lachowicz, S.; Wiśniewski, R.; Ochmian, I.; Drzymała, K.; Pluta, S. Anti-Microbiological, Anti-Hyperglycemic and Anti-Obesity Potency of Natural Antioxidants in Fruit Fractions of Saskatoon Berry. *Antioxidants* **2019**, *8*, 397. [CrossRef]
11. Tian, Y.; Puganen, A.; Alakomi, H.-L.; Uusitupa, A.; Saarela, M.; Yang, B. Antioxidant and antibacterial activities of aqueous ethanol extracts of berries, leaves, and branches of berry plants. *Food Res. Int.* **2018**, *106*, 291–303. [CrossRef] [PubMed]
12. Zhao, R.; Khafipour, E.; Sepehri, S.; Huang, F.; Beta, T.; Shen, G.X. Impact of Saskatoon berry powder on insulin resistance and relationship with intestinal microbiota in high fat–high sucrose diet-induced obese mice. *J. Nutr. Biochem.* **2019**, *69*, 130–138. [CrossRef] [PubMed]
13. Ezhilarasi, P.N.; Indrani, D.; Jena, B.S.; Anandharamakrishnan, C. Freeze drying technique for microencapsulation of Garcinia fruit extract and its effect on bread quality. *J. Food Eng.* **2013**, *117*, 513–520. [CrossRef]
14. Vitaglione, P.; Barone Lumaga, R.; Ferracane, R.; Radetsky, I.; Mennella, I.; Schettino, R.; Koder, S.; Shimoni, E.; Fogliano, V. Curcumin Bioavailability from Enriched Bread: The Effect of Microencapsulated Ingredients. *J. Agric. Food Chem.* **2012**, *60*, 3357–3366. [CrossRef]
15. Chávez-Santoscoy, R.A.; Gutiérrez-Uribe, J.A.; Serna-Saldivar, S.O.; Perez-Carrillo, E. Production of maize tortillas and cookies from nixtamalized flour enriched with anthocyanins, flavonoids and saponins extracted from black bean (*Phaseolus vulgaris*) seed coats. *Food Chem.* **2016**, *192*, 90–97. [CrossRef]
16. Morris, C.; Morris, G.A. The effect of inulin and fructo-oligosaccharide supplementation on the textural, rheological and sensory properties of bread and their role in weight management: A review. *Food Chem.* **2012**, *133*, 237–248. [CrossRef]
17. Gawlik-Dziki, U.; Świeca, M.; Dziki, D.; Sęczyk, Ł.; Złotek, U.; Różyło, R.; Kaszuba, K.; Ryszawy, D.; Czyż, J. Anticancer and Antioxidant Activity of Bread Enriched with Broccoli Sprouts. *BioMed Res. Int.* **2014**, *2014*, 608053. [CrossRef]
18. Lachowicz, S.; Michalska, A.; Lech, K.; Majerska, J.; Oszmiański, J.; Figiel, A. Comparison of the effect of four drying methods on polyphenols in saskatoon berry. *LWT* **2019**, *111*, 727–736. [CrossRef]
19. Lachowicz, S.; Michalska-Ciechanowska, A.; Oszmiański, J. The Impact of Maltodextrin and Inulin on the Protection of Natural Antioxidants in Powders Made of Saskatoon Berry Fruit, Juice, and Pomace as Functional Food Ingredients. *Molecules* **2020**, *25*, 1805. [CrossRef]
20. Minekus, M.; Alminger, M.; Alvito, P.; Ballance, S.; Bohn, T.; Bourlieu, C.; Carrière, F.; Boutrou, R.; Corredig, M.; Dupont, D.; et al. A standardised static in vitro digestion method suitable for food – an international consensus. *Food Funct.* **2014**, *5*, 1113–1124. [CrossRef]
21. Oszmiański, J.; Kolniak-Ostek, J.; Lachowicz, S.; Gorzelany, J.; Matłok, N. Effect of dried powder preparation process on polyphenolic content and antioxidant capacity of cranberry (*Vaccinium macrocarpon* L.). *Ind. Crops Prod.* **2015**, *77*, 658–665. [CrossRef]
22. Re, R.; Pellegrini, N.; Proteggente, A.; Pannala, A.; Yang, M.; Rice-Evans, C. Antioxidant activity applying an improved ABTS radical cation decolorization assay. *Free Radic. Biol. Med.* **1999**, *26*, 1231–1237. [CrossRef]
23. Benzie, I.F.F.; Strain, J.J. The Ferric Reducing Ability of Plasma (FRAP) as a Measure of "Antioxidant Power": The FRAP Assay. *Anal. Biochem.* **1996**, *239*, 70–76. [CrossRef] [PubMed]
24. Yen, G.C.; Chen, H.Y. Antioxidant activity of various tea extracts in relation to their antimutagenicity. *J. Agric. Food Chem.* **1995**, *43*, 27–32. [CrossRef]
25. Axelrod, B.; Cheesbrough, T.M.; Laakso, S. LOX from soybeans. *Methods Enzymol.* **1981**, *71*, 441–451.
26. Jakubczyk, A.; Karaś, M.; Złotek, U.; Szymanowska, U. Identification of potential inhibitory peptides of enzymes involved in the metabolic syndrome obtained by simulated gastrointestinal digestion of fermented bean (*Phaseolus vulgaris* L.) seeds. *Food Res. Int.* **2017**, *100*, 489–496. [CrossRef]
27. Sęczyk, Ł.; Świeca, M.; Gawlik-Dziki, U. Effect of carob (*Ceratonia siliqua* L.) flour on the antioxidant potential, nutritional quality, and sensory characteristics of fortified durum wheat pasta. *Food Chem.* **2016**, *194*, 637–642. [CrossRef]
28. Adler-Nissen, J. Determination of the degree of hydrolysis of food protein hydrolysates by trinitrobenzenesulfonic acid. *J. Agric. Food Chem.* **1979**, *27*, 1256–1262. [CrossRef]
29. Tolić, M.-T.; Krbavčić, I.P.; Vujević, P.; Milinović, B.; Jurčević, I.L.; Vahčić, N. Effects of Weather Conditions on Phenolic Content and Antioxidant Capacity in Juice of Chokeberries (*Aronia melanocarpa* L.). *Pol. J. Food Nutr. Sci.* **2017**, *67*, 67–74. [CrossRef]

30. Bajerska, J.; Mildner-Szkudlarz, S.; Podgórski, T.; Oszmatek-Pruszyńska, E. Saffron (*Crocus sativus* L.) Powder as an Ingredient of Rye Bread: An Anti-Diabetic Evaluation. *J. Med. Food* **2013**, *16*, 847–856. [CrossRef]
31. Bakowska-Barczak, A.M.; Kolodziejczyk, P.P. Black currant polyphenols: Their storage stability and microencapsulation. *Ind. Crops Prod.* **2011**, *34*, 1301–1309. [CrossRef]
32. Saénz, C.; Tapia, S.; Chávez, J.; Robert, P. Microencapsulation by spray drying of bioactive compounds from cactus pear (*Opuntia ficus-indica*). *Food Chem.* **2009**, *114*, 616–622. [CrossRef]
33. Cai, Y.Z.; Corke, H. Production and Properties of Spray-dried Amaranthus Betacyanin Pigments. *J. Food Sci.* **2000**, *65*, 1248–1252. [CrossRef]
34. Rodríguez-Roque, M.J.; Rojas-Graü, M.A.; Elez-Martínez, P.; Martín-Belloso, O. Soymilk phenolic compounds, isoflavones and antioxidant activity as affected by *in vitro* gastrointestinal digestion. *Food Chem.* **2013**, *136*, 206–212. [CrossRef] [PubMed]
35. Świeca, M.; Gawlik-Dziki, U.; Dziki, D.; Baraniak, B. Wheat bread enriched with green coffee—*In vitro* bioaccessibility and bioavailability of phenolics and antioxidant activity. *Food Chem.* **2017**, *221*, 1451–1457. [CrossRef]
36. Manzocco, L.; Calligaris, S.; Mastrocola, D.; Nicoli, M.C.; Lerici, C.R. Review of non-enzymatic browning and antioxidant capacity in processed foods. *Trends Food Sci. Technol.* **2000**, *11*, 340–346. [CrossRef]
37. Davidov-Pardo, G.; Moreno, M.; Arozarena, I.; Marín-Arroyo, M.R.; Bleibaum, R.N.; Bruhn, C.M. Sensory and Consumer Perception of the Addition of Grape Seed Extracts in Cookies. *J. Food Sci.* **2012**, *77*, S430–S438. [CrossRef]
38. Kraska, P.; Andruszczak, S.; Kwiecinska-Poppe, E.; Rozylo, K.; Swieca, M.; Palys, E. Chemical composition of seeds of linseed (*Linum usitatissimum* L.) cultivars depending on the intensity of agricultural technology. *J. Elem.* **2016**, *21*. [CrossRef]
39. Złotek, U.; Szychowski, K.A.; Świeca, M. Potential *in vitro* antioxidant, anti-inflammatory, antidiabetic, and anticancer effect of arachidonic acid-elicited basil leaves. *J. Funct. Foods* **2017**, *36*, 290–299. [CrossRef]
40. Yamamoto, S.; Katsukawa, M.; Nakano, A.; Hiraki, E.; Nishimura, K.; Jisaka, M.; Yokota, K.; Ueda, N. Arachidonate 12-lipoxygenases with reference to their selective inhibitors. *Biochem. Biophys. Res. Commun.* **2005**, *338*, 122–127. [CrossRef]
41. Naithani, S.; Saracco, S.A.; Butler, C.A.; Fox, T.D. Interactions among COX1, COX2, andCOX3 mRNA-specific Translational Activator Proteins on the Inner Surface of the Mitochondrial Inner Membrane of *Saccharomyces cerevisiae*. *Mol. Biol. Cell* **2002**, *14*, 324–333. [CrossRef] [PubMed]
42. Jaksevicius, A.; Carew, M.; Mistry, C.; Modjtahedi, H.; Opara, E.I. Inhibitory Effects of Culinary Herbs and Spices on the Growth of HCA-7 Colorectal Cancer Cells and Their COX-2 Expression. *Nutrients* **2017**, *9*, 1051. [CrossRef] [PubMed]
43. Moschona, A.; Liakopoulou-Kyriakides, M. Encapsulation of biological active phenolic compounds extracted from wine wastes in alginate-chitosan microbeads. *J. Microencapsul.* **2018**, *35*, 229–240. [CrossRef] [PubMed]
44. Sujith, K.; Ronald, D.C.; Suba, V. Inhibitory effect of Anacycluspyrethrum extract on acetylcholinesterase enzyme by invitro methods. *Pharmacogn. J.* **2012**, *4*, 31–34. [CrossRef]
45. Zhang, B.; Deng, Z.; Ramdath, D.D.; Tang, Y.; Chen, P.X.; Liu, R.; Liu, Q.; Tsao, R. Phenolic profiles of 20 Canadian lentil cultivars and their contribution to antioxidant activity and inhibitory effects on α-glucosidase and pancreatic lipase. *Food Chem.* **2015**, *172*, 862–872. [CrossRef]
46. Sandberg, J.C.; Björck, I.M.E.; Nilsson, A.C. Effects of whole grain rye, with and without resistant starch type 2 supplementation, on glucose tolerance, gut hormones, inflammation and appetite regulation in an 11–14.5 hour perspective; a randomized controlled study in healthy subjects. *Nutr. J.* **2017**, *16*, 25. [CrossRef]
47. Yousif, A.; Nhepera, D.; Johnson, S. Influence of sorghum flour addition on flat bread *in vitro* starch digestibility, antioxidant capacity and consumer acceptability. *Food Chem.* **2012**, *134*, 880–887. [CrossRef]
48. Karim, Z.; Holmes, M.; Orfila, C. Inhibitory effect of chlorogenic acid on digestion of potato starch. *Food Chem.* **2017**, *217*, 498–504. [CrossRef]

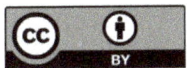

© 2020 by the authors. Licensee MDPI, Basel, Switzerland. This article is an open access article distributed under the terms and conditions of the Creative Commons Attribution (CC BY) license (http://creativecommons.org/licenses/by/4.0/).

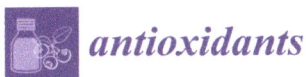

Article

Peptides from Different Carcass Elements of Organic and Conventional Pork—Potential Source of Antioxidant Activity

Paulina Keska [1], Sascha Rohn [2], Michał Halagarda [3] and Karolina M. Wójciak [1,*]

1. Department of Animal Raw Materials Technology, University of Life Sciences in Lublin, 20033 Lublin, Poland; paulina.keska@up.lublin.pl
2. Hamburg School of Food Science, Institute of Food Chemistry, University of Hamburg, 20146 Hamburg, Germany; rohn@chemie.uni-hamburg.de
3. Department of Food Product Quality, Cracow University of Economics, 31510 Kraków, Poland; michal.halagarda@uek.krakow.pl
* Correspondence: karolina.wojciak@up.lublin.pl; Tel.: +48-081-462-3340

Received: 3 August 2020; Accepted: 3 September 2020; Published: 7 September 2020

Abstract: The growing consumer interest in organic foods, as well as, in many cases, the inconclusiveness of the research comparing organic and conventional foods, indicates a need to study this issue further. The aim of the study was to compare the effects of meat origin (conventional vs. organic) and selected elements of the pork carcass (ham, loin, and shoulder) on the meat proteome and the antioxidant potential of its peptides. The peptidomic approach was used, while the ability of antioxidants to scavenge 2,2′-azino-bis-3-ethylbenzthiazoline-6-sulfonic acid (ABTS), to chelate Fe(II) ions, and to reduce Fe(III) was determined. Most peptides were derived from myofibrillary proteins. The meat origin and the element of the pork carcass did not have a significant effect on the proteome. On the other hand, the pork origin and the carcass element significantly affected the iron ion-chelating capacity (Fe(II)) and the reducing power of peptides. In particular, pork ham from conventional rearing systems had the best antioxidant properties in relation to potential antioxidant peptides. This could be a factor for human health, as well as for stabilized meat products (e.g., toward lipid oxidation).

Keywords: antioxidant peptides; element of pork carcasses; spectrometric analysis

1. Introduction

The food consumption pattern has changed over the years. Currently, consumers appreciate foods that, in addition to favorable sensory properties, are characterized by high nutritional value and potential health benefits [1,2]. Therefore, an increasing interest in organic foods can be observed [3,4]. Nonetheless, many consumers still do not believe in the favorable characteristics of organic food products. Moreover, the research findings regarding the extensive, positive effects of the consumption of such foods are not comprehensive enough; in many cases, they are also inconclusive [5–8], which indicates the need to study this issue further.

Meat consumption, although discussed sometimes quite controversially, is a good source of many highly valuable nutrients [9]. Meat has a complex physical structure and chemical composition, highly sensitive to enzymatic activities. Glycolysis and rigor mortis, occurring in the muscles within the first 24 h of slaughtering, are significant processes that can regulate proteolysis and affect the peptide profile of muscle tissue. Proteins involved in these biochemical processes are subject to complex metabolic regulations that significantly contribute to the final quality of the meat. Moreover, the potential resulting peptides not only have nutritional value, but also carry further benefits for human health [10]. Meat-derived peptides have been shown to have antioxidant, antihypertensive, antidiabetic, antimicrobial, opioid, anticoagulant, and other bioactive effects. Regulation of the immune, gastrointestinal, and neurological responses of these bioactive peptides is an important basis for the prevention of noncommunicable diseases such as hypertension, obesity, diabetes, and other metabolic disorders [11]. In addition to nutritional value, natural antioxidants might also be beneficial for stabilizing products with regard to rancidity via lipid peroxidation [12].

Before being released from parent proteins, peptides remain latent and do not show any bioactive effect. Their potential activity is only activated after the release of specific amino-acid sequences, through gastrointestinal digestion or food processing (e.g., drying, curing, fermentation, or enzymatic hydrolysis). The literature data indicate processed meat products as good sources of peptides with biological activity, particularly dry-cured or fermented meats [13–16]. For example, the antiradical activity of protein extracts from dry-cured pork loins over a 12-month period of aging was confirmed. Moreover, antiradical activity was further observed in peptic and pancreatic hydrolysates after simulated gastrointestinal digestion [14]. However, the chemical composition of meat also promotes oxidation processes. Ingredients susceptible to oxidation, i.e., polyunsaturated fatty acids, cholesterol, proteins, and pigments, should be in balance with endogenous antioxidant substances. Endogenous antioxidant systems consist of nonenzymatic compounds such as tocopherols, ascorbic acids, carotenoids, and ubiquinols, as well as enzymes (superoxide dismutase, catalase, and glutathione peroxidase). Furthermore, peptides such as anserine and carnosine have high antioxidant activity, acting as free-radical scavengers and metal-ion chelators. Peptide formation via hydrolytic reactions is the main technique used to create antioxidants from proteins, as the resulting peptides have significantly advanced antioxidant potential compared to intact proteins [17,18].

According to the literature, meat peptides can contribute to maintaining the oxidative stability of meat tissue [18–20]. Lipids are particularly vulnerable to oxidative factors, especially during meat processing. The carbonyl-based compounds known as secondary lipid oxidation products are characterized by cytotoxic and genotoxic properties [17]. In addition to exogenous/added antioxidants or endogenous small-molecular antioxidants (e.g., vitamins), lipid oxidation in meat and meat products can also be inhibited by proteins as a result of biologically designed mechanisms (such as iron-binding proteins and antioxidant enzymes) or via some non-specific mechanisms. The activity of these mechanisms can be intensified when the conformation of proteins is denatured. Previous studies showed that <3.5 kDa peptides have strong antioxidant activity. They can function as inhibitors of lipid oxidation, leading to color change or discoloration during prolonged storage in uncured roasted beef with acid whey [15,21]. Moreover, the role of proteins, as important components of muscle tissue, in developing the sensory profile of meat products was emphasized. Among them, myofibrillar proteins proved to be particularly good flavor precursors, i.e., active peptides and amino acids. The suppressing (sourness and sweetness) and enhancing (salty and umami) role of peptides was also presented in pork meat based on an in silico approach [22]. Apart from improving the shelf-life and organoleptic qualities of meat, controlling lipid-based oxidative degradation contributes to preventing the negative effects of oxidative stress, which is generally caused by the excessive accumulation of reactive oxygen species (ROS). It is an imbalance between the production and accumulation of ROS and endogenous defense mechanisms (e.g., enzymes, vitamins) in cells and tissues. Consequently, the limited capacity of the biological system to detoxify these reactive products can lead to disease-causing pathological conditions. Importantly, according to some literature reports, elevated levels of oxidative stress play a dominant role in initiating many cardiovascular diseases, diabetes mellitus, and other metabolic disorders [23]. Antioxidants are effective in combating the effects of oxidative stress. In this context, digestive amino acids, peptides, and proteins from different food sources can also act as antioxidants to protect cells and organisms from oxidative damage [17,18].

The composition of oxidation-promoting factors and antioxidants may vary between the meat of different animal species [24,25] or gender [26]. In addition, the animal's diet plays a significant role in modifying the concentration of antioxidants or pro-oxidative factors [27–30]. Therefore, different biomolecular compositions of meat from slaughter animals can affect the functionality and use of a particular muscle tissue for specific applications. Thus, it is necessary to know and understand the differences in the biomolecule profiles between different carcass elements of the animal muscles. The understanding of any differences or similarities between them, determined based on the abundance in protein composition and related peptides, can be helpful in achieving this goal. Moreover, the antioxidant potential of peptides from selected elements of organic vs. conventional pork carcasses has not been compared before.

Therefore, the aim of the present study was to investigate the impact of organic and conventional rearing systems on protein stability and peptide formation with regard to their antioxidant activity in pork meat available for consumers. Furthermore, various pork tissues such as ham, loin, and shoulder, in relation to their potential to be used as starting materials for obtaining high-quality functional ingredients or meat products, were characterized.

2. Materials and Methods

2.1. Meat Samples

The research was conducted on organic and conventional pork meat. The material consisted of three elements of pork meat: loin, ham, shoulder. The meat, intended for consumer market, was bought in the same, organically certified slaughterhouse, which enabled the elements to be cut out fresh from the same carcass. Eighteen meat samples (organic and conventional) were selected. The samples were vacuum-packed and transported, in refrigerated conditions, without any exposure of light, directly to the analytical laboratory. The analysis of the samples was carried out 24 h after the slaughter. Before the analysis, the whole-muscle samples were purified by removing external fat and membranes. The experiment was repeated three times. The research aimed at simultaneous verification of all the conditions connected to farming (organic/conventional), as well as their effect on the difference in protein degradation and formation of bioactive peptides with antioxidant activity from meat available for consumers. However, an interview conducted with the manager of the slaughterhouse made it possible to determine the following:

- The pigs were crossbreed (wbp × pbz);
- The first group was reared in conventional stables, while the other group was reared in special stables, arranged according to the Commission Regulation (EC) No. 889/2008 of 5 September 2008 [31], following the detailed rules of Council Regulation (EC) No. 834/2007 [32] on organic production and labeling of organic products with regard to organic production, labeling, and control;
- The conventional rearing system comprised an indoor area of 1 m^2, whereas the organic rearing system had an indoor area with organic saw dust of 1 m^2 and an outdoor area with free ranges of 1 m^2. The conventional stable had a climate control system, and the organic stable had only gravitation ventilation.
- The organic feed consisted exclusively of raw materials from organic farms and was produced directly on the farm. The second group of animals was fed with commercial feeds available for conventional producers. The composition and nutritional value of the compound feed were in line with the pig nutrition standards of the National Research Council [33]. Both conventionally and organically reared animals were given their diets and water ad libitum.
- One day before slaughter, the hogs (weighing approximately 110 kg) were transported to the abattoir, where they were rested overnight with free access to water. The animals were conventionally slaughtered after an electrical stunning.

2.2. Peptide Extraction and LC–MS/MS Identification

The peptides were isolated from the meat samples according to the procedures provided by Mora et al. [13]. Briefly, muscles (15 g) were homogenized with 100 mL of 0.01 N HCl for

5 min. The homogenate was centrifuged (2200 rpm for 20 min at 4 °C). The supernatant was decanted and filtered through glass wool, and then deproteinized by adding three volumes of ethanol and centrifuged, retaining the previously defined conditions. The obtained supernatant was then dried in a vacuum evaporator (Rotavapor R-215, BüchiLabortechnik AG, Flawil, Switzerland). The dried extract was dissolved in 0.01 N HCl, filtered through a 0.45 µM nylon membrane filter (Millipore, Bedford, MA, USA) and stored at −60 °C prior to further use. The peptides were analyzed by liquid chromatography coupled with tandem electrospray mass spectrometry (LC–MS/MS). The samples were concentrated and desalted on an RP-C18 pre-column (Waters Corp., Milford, MA, USA), and further peptide separation was achieved on an RP-C18 nano-Ultra Performance column (Waters) using a 180 min linear acetonitrile gradient (0–35%) at a flow rate of 250 nL·min^{-1}. The outlet of the column was directly connected to a mass spectrometer (Orbitrap Velos, Thermo Fisher Scientific Inc. Waltham, MA, USA). The raw data files were preprocessed using Mascot Distiller software (version 2.4.2.0, Matrix Science Inc., Boston, MA, USA). The obtained peptide masses and their fragmentation pattern were compared with the protein sequence database (UniProt KB, www.uniprot.org) using the Mascot search engine (Mascot Daemon v. 2.4.0, Mascot Server v.2.4.1, Matrix Science, London, UK). The "mammals" option was chosen as the taxonomy constraint parameter. The following search parameters were applied: enzyme specificity, none; peptide mass tolerance, 5 ppm; fragment mass tolerance, 0.01 Da. The protein mass was left unrestricted, and mass values were monoisotopic with a maximum of two missed cleavages allowed. Methylthiolation, oxidation, and carbamidomethylation were set as fixed and variable modifications. The sequences of peptides from unknown original proteins were not listed. The peptide identification was performed using the Mascot search engine (Matrix Science), with a probability-based algorithm. An expected value threshold of 0.05 was used for the analysis (all peptide identifications had less than 0.05% chance of being a random match).

2.3. The Identification of Bioactive Peptides—In Silico Analysis

The peptides identified in meat samples were investigated as a source of bioactive peptides in relation to the information about peptides previously identified in the literature, using the BIOPEP-UWM database (http://www.uwm.edu.pl/biochemia/index.php/pl/biopep; access: December 2019) [34].

2.4. Evaluation of Bioactive (Antioxidant) Peptides—In Vitro Analysis

2.4.1. Ability to Scavenge 2,2′-Azino-bis-3-ethylbenzthiazoline-6-sulfonic Acid (ABTS)

The ability of the extracts obtained to scavenge free radicals was tested using the method of Re et al. [35] with the free-radical ABTS. The degree of reduction of ABTS• was determined spectrophotometrically at 734 nm. The scavenging ability was determined using the following formula:

$$\text{ABTS radical-scavenging activity (\%)} = (1 - A_2/A_1) \times 100,$$

where A_1 is the absorbance of the control sample, and A_2 is the absorbance of the sample.

2.4.2. Ability to Chelate Fe(II) Ions

The study on the ability to chelate Fe(II) ions by compounds contained in sample extracts was conducted according to the method of Decker and Welch [36]. The absorbance of the colored complex was measured spectrophotometrically at 562 nm.

$$\text{Fe(II)-chelating activity (\%)} = (1 - A_2/A_1) \times 100,$$

where A_1 is the absorbance of the control sample, and A_2 is the absorbance of the sample.

2.4.3. Fe(III) Reduction Power (FRAP)

The FRAP method according to Oyaizu [37] involves the reduction of the reagent (Fe(III)) in stoichiometric excess relative to antioxidants. A spectrophotometric method with measurements at 700 nm was used. A higher absorbance value indicates a higher ability to reduce the test substance.

2.5. Statistical Analysis

Statistical analysis was carried out using Statistica 13.1 (StatSoft, Cracov, Poland) and Microsoft Office Excel 2013 software. Based on a two-factor analysis of variance (meat element, rearing system), homogeneous groups were separated using the Tukey test. The differences were considered statistically significant at $p < 0.05$. All of the data were presented as mean ± standard error. In the case of multidimensional analyses, a hierarchical grouping of data based on identified peptides was performed, and the results were presented as a heat map and dendrogram, using the Ward method and Euclidean distance. Data were normalized prior to the analysis.

3. Results

3.1. Protein Degradation and Peptide Formation

In this study, organic vs. conventional pork and the culinary element of the pork carcass (ham, loin, or shoulder) were compared, taking into account protein stability and peptide formation. Potential differences in the abundance of endogenous peptides were evaluated with an LC–MS-based peptidomic approach. In total, 4178 peptide sequences were identified. The analyses were performed in triplicate, and only the sequences present in three independent replicates were selected for further analysis. Eventually, 646 peptides were chosen for the subsequent stages of the analysis.

The distribution of identified peptides with regard to their protein origin is shown in Figure 1. A diverse number of protein fragments were identified, with no clear tendency depending on the type of muscle. Nevertheless, Picard et al. demonstrated a relationship between the protein profile and the muscle type [38]. The authors revealed relationships between proteins differing in contractile and metabolic properties (acting as biomarkers of tenderness and intramuscular fat content) compared in five bovine muscles [38]. According to Picard and Gagaou, a muscle-type effect depends on the biological function of proteins [39]. The authors emphasized that, in longissimus thoracis muscle, tenderness-related proteins mainly correspond to contractile, structural, and heat-shock proteins, while, in semitendinosus muscle, the tenderness-related proteins are mainly involved in metabolism. In the present study, the rearing system did not affect the protein profile distinctly. This observation is consistent with descriptions by Picard et al., who reported that the abundance of very few proteins from bovine meats was modified by rearing practices [40]. Moreover, factors associated with diet composition had weak effects on protein abundances determined by proteomics [39]. These data indicate that the impact of rearing practices on the proteome is muscle-type-dependent. As expected, several significant proteins were identified. Protein chains were degraded to produce a large number of different peptides, which confirmed proteolytic activity postmortem.

The highest diversity of proteins as peptide precursors was obtained in organically produced shoulder meat, where the highest percentage of the most different proteins (named "other" according to the designations in Figure 1) was classified. The protein generating the highest number of peptides was nebulin (in order, conventionally produced shoulder meat (44.26%) > conventional loin (37.85%) > organic loin (28.68%) > organic ham (20.74%) > conventional ham (6.58%)). Other myofibrillar proteins, especially structural proteins such as desmin, titin, or troponin were also the main sources of peptides in the analyzed meat samples (Figure 1). According to the literature, myosin, nebulin, actin, tropomyosin, tropomodulin, and troponin (assigned a role in stabilizing and determining highly ordered muscle structure), and nebulin, tropomyosin, and tropomodulin ("protein rulers" to precisely regulate the connection of myosin and actin fibers) are very sensitive to proteolysis [41].

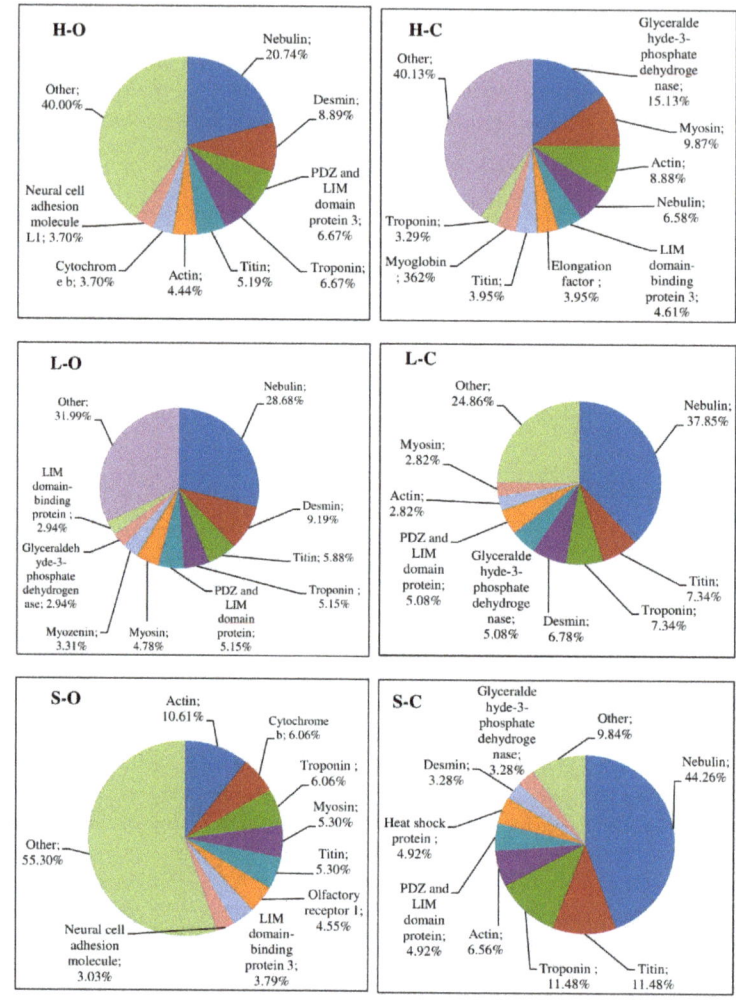

Figure 1. Distribution in percentages of identified peptides according to the origin of proteins in the analyzed muscle tissue (abbreviations: H-O: organic ham, L-O: organic loin, S-O: organic shoulder, H-C: conventional ham, L-C: conventional loin, S-C: conventional shoulder).

Previous studies of postmortem protein degradation in pig muscle, using peptide profiling and amino-acid sequence analysis of protein fragments, showed that fragments of myofibrillary protein primarily undergo postmortem degradation, before severe deterioration catalyzed by cathepsins takes place. Taylor et al. reported that nebulin, titin, vinculin, and desmin are significantly degraded within three days of death in the semimembranosus muscle, which is consistent with the present report [42]. Furthermore, Huff Lonergan reported the postmortem μ-calpain-induced degradation of titin, nebulin, filamin, desmin, and troponin-T from bovine longissimus thoracis [43,44]. Sarcoplasmic proteins (among others, glyceraldehyde-3-phosphate dehydrogenase, myosin, and PDZ (PSD95, Dig, ZO-1) and LIM (Lin11, Isl-, Mec-3) domain protein-3) gave smaller amounts of peptides relative to myofibrillary proteins (Figure 1). Previous studies consistently showed that myofibrillar proteins were more easily hydrolyzed than sarcoplasmic proteins during postmortem meat tenderization.

Nevertheless, sarcoplasmic protein fragments similar to those from the present study were also reported as occurring in tenderization processes [45,46].

Various methods of analyzing meat tissue were presented in the literature, regarding the presence of tissue-specific proteins, as well as their proteolysis or denaturation due to storage and processing. As an example, Sarah et al. discovered porcine-specific peptides as potential markers for meat species using LC–QTOF-MS [47]. In addition, Kim et al. [48] proposed a proteomic method for the authentication of meat species such as raw beef, pork, and poultry (chicken and duck), using a protein-based approach, including one-dimensional (1D) gel electrophoretic separation and LC–MS/MS analysis. The authors showed that troponin I, enolase 3, 1-lactate dehydrogenase, and triose phosphate isomerase may be useful markers for distinguishing mammalian meat from poultry [48]. They also emphasized that species-specific peptides determined by LC–MS/MS allow each species to be identified independently from the same protein. Furthermore, Mi et al. [49] defined the differences between Tibetan and Duroc (Landrace × Yorkshire) pork, using a label-free quantitative proteomics approach. Therefore, in the present study, an attempt was made to assess whether specific peptides show a difference between different elements of pork carcasses, but from the same species. The impact of conventional or organic pork origin was also considered. The general aim of this approach consisted of profiling the changes in peptide composition. The final peptide composition was identified, and, among the selected peptides, only five identical peptides from muscle tissue proteins occurred in each variant analyzed (Table 1), suggesting large differences in the peptide profiles.

Table 1. Peptide sequences identified in all analyzed samples.

Lp	Sequence [1]	Protein	Position [2]
1	R.VREPVISAVEQTAQR.T	Titin	[438–452]
2	T.IEPDAVHIKAAKDAYK.V	Nebulin	[5535–5550]
3	E.EAPPPPAEVHEVHEEVH.E	Troponin T, fast skeletal muscle	[21–38]
4	W.ITKQEYDEAGPSIVHRK.C	Actin, alpha-skeletal muscle	[358–375]
5	M.WITKQEYDEAGPSIVHRK.C		[357–375]

[1] The period indicates cutting points; [2] position in parental protein.

A qualitative comparison of the unique and common peptides identified in the three muscle types is shown in the Venn diagrams (Figure 2). The analyzed samples had a different peptide profile, depending on the meat origin (conventional vs. organic). The obtained LC–MS/MS spectra made it possible to identify the peptides characteristic for conventional (Table 2) or organic (Table 3) meat.

In addition, the samples collected from different elements of pork carcasses had a different peptide profile (Tables S1–S3, Supplementary Materials). The highest diversity of peptides was obtained for ham samples, characterized by the highest number of individual sequences (105 peptides and 261 peptides for organic ham and conventional ham, respectively) with a low number of common sequences (i.e., 33 peptides). The most similar analysis results were obtained for loins, for which 93 common peptide sequences were determined. Considering the pork origin (organic vs. conventional), there was no clear trend in the number of peptides. A higher variety of peptides, characteristic for the element of pork carcasses, was noted for the organic meat samples (organic loin, 166 peptides; organic shoulder, 64 peptides), while the smallest number of specific sequences (typical for these samples only) was obtained for organic ham (i.e., 51 peptides).

Table 2. List of peptide sequences common for conventional meat. ACE: angiotensin-I converting enzyme; DPP: dipeptidyl peptidase.

	Sequence [1]	Protein	Position [2]	ACE Inhibitor	DPP-IV Inhibitor	Stimulating [3]	Antioxidant
1	R.VREPVISAVEQTAQR.T	Titin	[438–452]	VR, VE, AV	EP, TA, VR, AV, PV, QT, VE, VI	-	-
2	S.VVDTPEIIHAQQVKN.L [4]	Nebulin	[6063–6077]	VK, EI, TP	VV, HA, TP, EI, IH, II, QQ, QV, VD, VK,	II	-
3	T.IEPDAVHIKAAKDAYK.V [5]	Nebulin	[5525–5540]	AV, AA, DA(2) [6], YK, KA, IE, AV, IEP	KA, EP, AA, AV, AY, HI, VH, YK	-	AY, KD
4	Q.IRKETEKAFVPKVVIS.A [7]	Titin	[512–527]	IR, AF, VP, KA, TE, EK, KE, VPK, FVP	KA, VP, VV, EK, AF, ET, IR, KE, KV, PK, RK, TE, VI	-	IR
5	E.EAPPPPAEVHEVHEEVH.E [8]	Troponin T, fast skeletal muscle	[22–38]	AP, EA, EV(3), EAP, PPP(2)	PPPP, PPP(3), AP, PA, AE, EV(3), HE(2), VH(2)	EE	-
6	M.ARVREPVISAVEQTAQR.T [9]	Titin	[436–452]	VR, AR, VE, AV, RVR	EP, TA, VR, AV, PV, QT, VE, VI	-	-
7	T.IETRDGEVVSEATQQQH.E [10]	Desmin	[452–468]	GE, EA, DG, IE, EV, TQ,	VV, AT, ET, EV, GE, QH, QQ(2), TQ, TR, VS,	SE	-
8	W.ITKQEYDEAGPSIVHRK.C [11]	Actin, alpha-skeletal muscle	[359–375]	GP, AG, EA, EY, AGP	GP, AG, EY, HR, PS, QE, RK, SI, TK, VH, YD	IV	-
9	N.FTSVVDTPEIIHAQQVKN.L [12]	Nebulin	[6060–6077]	VK, EI, TP	VV, HA, TP, EI, HI, II, QQ, QV, SV, TS, VD, VK	II	-
10	N.YKADLKDLSKKGYDLKTD.A [13]	Nebulin	[1052–1069]	GY, KG, YK, KA, LR	KA, AD, GY, KG, KK, SK, TD, YD, YK	-	KD, LK
11	M.WITKQEYDEAGPSIVHRK.C [14]	Actin, alpha-skeletal muscle	[358–375]	GP, AG, EA, EY, AGP	GP, WI, AG, EY, HR, PS, QE, RK, SI, TK, VH, YD	IV	-
12	A.AVDMARVREPVISAVEQTAQR.T [15]	Titin	[432–452]	VR, AR, VE, AV(2), DM, RVR	MA, EP, TA, VR, AV(2), PV, QT, VD, VE, VI	-	-
13	LYKEDVSPGTAJGKTPEMMRVKQTQDH.I [16]	Nebulin	[6154–6179]	VK, IG, GK, GT, PG, YK, TQ, KE, AI, TP, MM, VSP	TP, SP, TA, KE, KT, MM, MR, PG, QD, QT, TQ, VK, VS, YK	-	MM

[1] Periods indicate cutting points; [2] position in parental protein; [3] stimulating vasoactive substance release or glucose uptake-stimulating peptide; [4] other activity: DPP-III inhibitor, IH, PE; [5] other activity: DPP-III inhibitor, YK, DA (2) 6, KA; [6] the number in parentheses indicates the number of identified peptides if more than one; [7] other activity: CaMPDE (calmodulin-dependent phosphodiesterase) inhibitor and renin inhibitor, IR; DPP-III inhibitor, KA; [8] other activity: dipeptidyl carboxypeptidase inhibitor, PPPA; [9] other activity: DPP-III inhibitor, RV; [10] other activity: DPP-III inhibitor, GE; [11] other activity: antiamnestic (prolyl endopeptidase inhibitor) and antithrombotic, GP; regulating stomach mucosal membrane activity, GP; [12] other activity: DPP-III inhibitor, PE; rennin inhibitor, FT; [13] other activity: bacterial permease ligand, KK; DPP-III inhibitor, LR, YK, KA; rennin inhibitor, LR; [14] other activity: antiamnestic (prolyl endopeptidase inhibitor), antithrombotic, and regulating stomach mucosal membrane activity, GP; [15] other activity: DPP-III inhibitor, RV; [16] other activity: antiamnestic (prolyl endopeptidase inhibitor), antithrombotic, and regulating stomach mucosal membrane activity, PG; DPP-III inhibitor, MR, YK, RV, PE.

Table 3. List of peptide sequences common for organic meat.

	Sequence [1]	Protein	Position [2]	ACE Inhibitor	DPP-IV Inhibitor	Stimulating [4]	Antioxidant
1	VIIIIIIIII	Killer cell immunoglobulin-like receptor	[341–349]	-	II (9) [3]	II (9)	-
2	A.IIIL.LLLLLL	Neural cell adhesion molecule	[1132–1142]	IL(2)	LL(4), IL, IL(2), LI(2)	LLL(2), IL(2), LI(2), II, LL(4)	-
3	IIIILILLIL.C	Neural cell adhesion molecule	[1133–1143]	IL(3)	LL(4), IL(3), LI(2)	LLL(2), IL(3), LI(2), LL(4)	-
4	S.ILILLIILLLH	Cytochrome b	[297–307]	IL(3)	LL(3), IL, IL(3), LI(2)	LLL(1), IL(3), LI(2), IL, LL(3)	-
5	VIL.LLLLLLL.F	Leukocyte immunoglobulin-like receptor subfamily B	[469–479]	IL(2)	LL(5), IL(2), LI(2)	LLL(4), IL(2), LI(2), LL(5)	-
6	F.LIL.LLLLL.V	Cadherin-1	[731–741]	IL(2)	LL(5), IL(2), LI(2)	LLL(4), IL(2), LI(2), LL(5)	-
7	G.LLILLLLLLL	Cytochrome b	[232–241]	IL(2)	LL(5), IL(2), LI(2)	LLL(3), IL(2), LI(2), LL(5)	-
8	A.LLLIL.ILLL.V	Cytochrome b	[233–242]	IL(2)	LL(3), IL(2), LI(2)	LLL(3), IL(2), LI(2), LL(5)	-
9	H.LLLLLLIIL.T	Myeloma-overexpressed gene protein	[302–311]	IL(2)	LL(5), II(2), IL, LI	LLL(4), IL, LL, II(2), LL(5)	-
10	C.LLLLLLLIL.R	Ephrin	[186–195]	IL	LLL(6), IL, LI, LL(7)	LL(7), IL, LI	-
11	P.PPPAEVHEVHEEVH.E [5]	Troponin T, fast skeletal muscle	[25–38]	EV(3), PP(2), PPP	PP(2), PA, AE, EV(3), HE(2), VH(3)	EE	-
12	R.VREPVI.SAVEQTAQR.T	Titin	[437–452]	VR, VE, AV	EP, TA, VR, AV, PV, QT, VE, VI	-	-
13	S.VNVDYSK.LKKEGPDF [6]	Cytochrome c oxidase subunit NDUFA4	[68–82]	GP, BG, KE, KE, DY, DF	GP, EG, KE, KK, NV, SK, VD, VN, YS	-	LK
14	T.IEPDAVHIKAAKDAYK.V [7]	Nebulin	[5525–5540]	AY, AA, DA(2), YK, KA, IE, IEP, AV	KA, KD, AA, AV, AV, HI, VH, YK,	-	AY, KD
15	E.APPPAEVHEVHEEVH.E [8]	Troponin T, fast skeletal muscle	[23–38]	AP, EV(3), PP(3)	PPPP, PPP(3), AP, PA, AE, EV(3), HE(2), VH(3)	EE	-
16	L.TKQEYDEAGPSIVHRK.C [9]	Actin, alpha-skeletal muscle	[360–375]	GP, AG, EA, EY, AGP	GP, AG, EY, HR, PS, QE, RK, SL, TK, VH, YD	IV	-
17	L.KVSILAAIDEASKKLNAQ [10]	Apolipoprotein A-I	[248–265]	LAA, LA, AA, EA, KL, LN, AI, IL	LA, AA, AS, IL, KK, KV, LN, NA, SK, VS	IL	-
18	E.EAPPPAEVHEVHEEVH.E [11]	Troponin T, fast skeletal muscle	[22–38]	AP, EA, EV(3), PP(3), EAP, PPP(2)	PPPP, PP(3), AP, PA, AE, EV, HE, VH	EE	-
19	E.KAKDIEHAKKVSQQVSK.V [12]	Nebulin	[153–169]	AKK, KA, IE	KA, HA, EH, KK, KV, QQ, QV, SK, VS(2), KA	-	KD
20	W.ITKQEYDEAGPSIVHRK.C [13]	Actin, alpha-skeletal muscle	[359–375]	GP, AG, EA, EY, AGP	GP, AG, EY, HR, PS, QE, RK, SL, TK, VH, YD	IV	-
21	I.SKQEYDESGPSIVHRK [14]	POTE ankyrin domain family member F	[358–375]	GP, SG, EY, SGP	GP, ES, EY, HR, PS, QE, RK, SL, SK, VH, YD	IV	-
22	M.IWITKQEYDEAGPSIVHRK.C [15]	Actin, alpha-skeletal muscle	[358–375]	GP, AG, EA, EY, AGP	GP, WI, AG, EY, HR, PS, QE, RK, SL, TK, VH, YD	IV	-
23	L.KPRPPPPAPPKEDVKEKIFQ.L [16]	Titin	[11804–11836]	PR, VK, RP, AP, IF, PAP, PPK, KP, PP(6), EK, KE(2), PAPFK, RPF, FQ, PPP(4)	PPP(3), PP(6), AP, PA, RP, KP, EK, FQ, KE(2), KI, PK, VK, PR,	-	KP

[1] Periods indicate cutting points; [2] position in parental protein; [3] the number in parentheses indicates the number of identified peptides if more than one; [4] stimulating vasoactive substance release or glucose uptake-stimulating peptide; [5] other activity: dipeptidyl carboxypeptidase inhibitor, PPPA; [6] other activity: antiamnestic (prolyl endopeptidase inhibitor) and antithrombotic, GP; regulating, DY, GP; bacterial permease ligand, KK; [7] other activity: DPP-III inhibitor, YK, DA (2), KA; [8] other activity: dipeptidyl carboxypeptidase inhibitor, PPPA; [9] other activity: antiamnestic (prolyl endopeptidase inhibitor), antithrombotic, and regulating, GP; [10] other activity: bacterial permease ligand, KK; activating ubiquitin-mediated proteolysis, LA; DPP-III inhibitor, LA; [11] other activity: dipeptidyl carboxypeptidase inhibitor, PPPA; [12] other activity: bacterial permease ligand, KK; [13] other activity: antiamnestic (prolyl endopeptidase inhibitor), antithrombotic, and regulating stomach mucosal membrane activity, GP; [14] other activity: antiamnestic (prolyl endopeptidase inhibitor), antithrombotic, and regulating stomach mucosal membrane activity, GP; [15] other activity: antiamnestic (prolyl endopeptidase inhibitor), antithrombotic, and regulating stomach mucosal membrane activity, GP; [16] other activity: antithrombotic, PPK; dipeptidyl carboxypeptidase inhibitor, PPPA, PPAP.

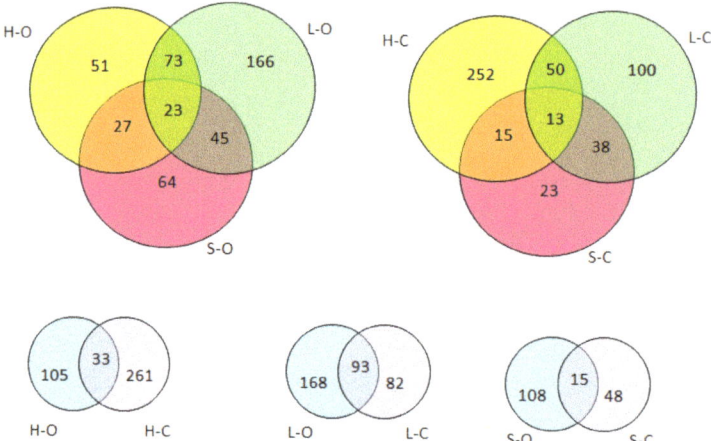

Figure 2. Venn diagram showing number of peptides obtained in the pork meat tissue (abbreviations: H-O: organic ham, L-O: organic loin, S-O: organic shoulder, H-C: conventional ham, L-C: conventional loin, S-C: conventional shoulder).

The resulting dataset was also used to assess the similarity between the samples, using multidimensional hierarchical clustering of objects. For data visualization, a heat map with a color scale was introduced to encode existing values from the smallest to the largest (a higher color intensity at each scale represents a higher change in the number of each place). The highest intensity of green color (and, hence, the smallest abundance of given peptide sequences) was characterized for conventional ham and organic loin, which corresponds to the results presented in Figure 2. These batches contained the largest number of individual, characteristic peptide sequences. The highest values marked on the heat map in red were obtained for conventional shoulder, followed by organic ham and organic shoulder, indicating the smallest diversity of peptide sequences among all analyzed variants. These assays simultaneously formed a common cluster on the dendrogram shown in Figure 3.

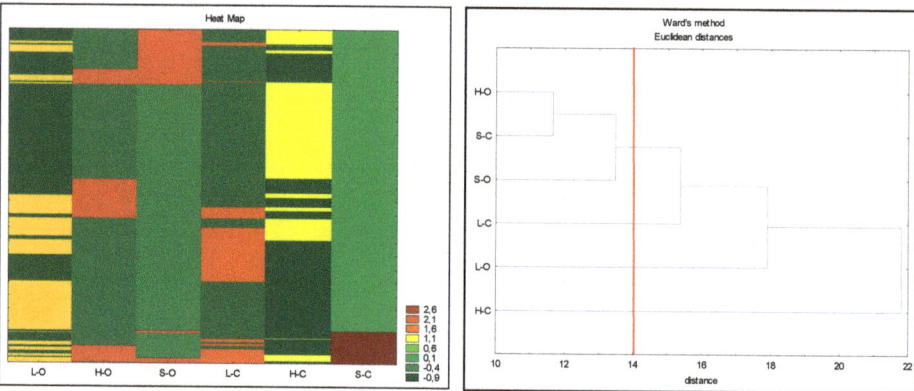

Figure 3. Heat map of abundance levels (**left**) and dendrogram (**right**) obtained as a result of hierarchical clustering based on proteomic data. The changes in abundance of statistically significant ($p < 0.05$) spots among meat tissue models were analyzed. Fold change: negative values (decreasing abundance), 0 (no differences), positive values (increasing abundance); abbreviations: H-O: organic ham, L-O: organic loin, S-O: organic shoulder, H-C: conventional ham, L-C: conventional loin, S-C: conventional shoulder.

Differences in the peptide content between particular muscle types may probably result from their chemical composition. Oxidative muscles generally contain more lipids than glycolytic muscles. As reported by Bonnet et al., the abundance of myosine-1- or triosephosphate isomerase was appropriately distinguished between the lean or fat muscle groups observed, when using proteomics [50]. Bazile et al. identified proteins with abundance differing depending on carcass and muscular dispositions in longissimus thoracis from cows [51]. Seven proteins involved in glycolysis or gluconeogenesis were the least abundant, while 14 proteins related to oxidative metabolism, slow-type muscle, or retinoic acid metabolism were the most abundant in the high-adiposity group.

3.2. Antioxidant Properties of Peptides—In Silico Analysis

In this study, peptides were identified with high precision and a mass tolerance lower than 5 ppm. The length of identified peptides ranged from 7–50 amino acids (50 amino acids: only one peptide from creatine kinase at chain position 331–381, M-type; Uniprot ID Q5XLD3, data not shown). The number and type of peptide sequences were compared depending on the type of carcass element and rearing system, and the results are presented graphically in Figures 4 and 5.

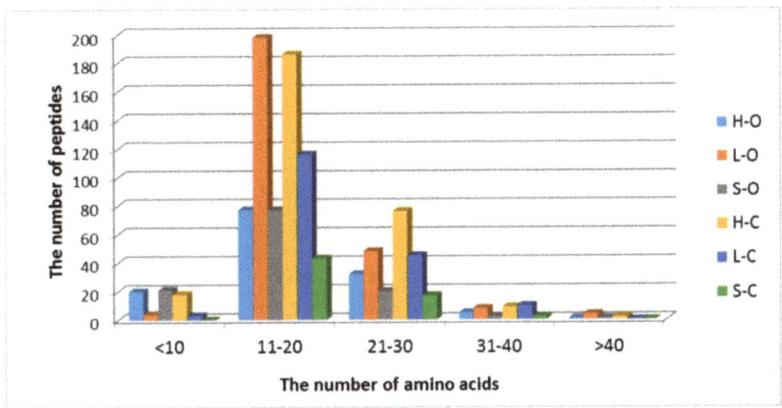

Figure 4. The distributions of peptides based on their molecular weight (abbreviations: H-O: organic ham, L-O: organic loin, S-O: organic shoulder, H-C: conventional ham, L-C: conventional loin, S-C: conventional shoulder).

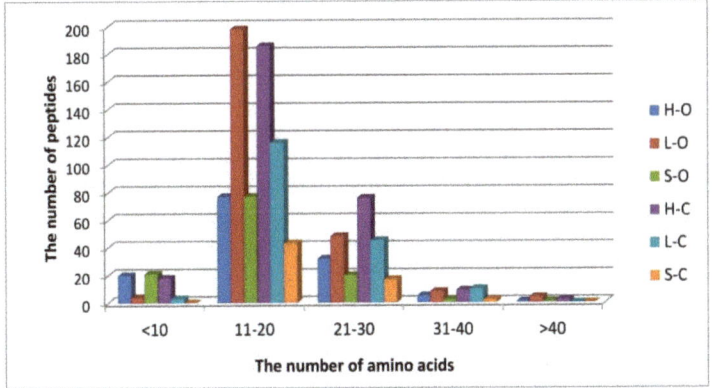

Figure 5. The distributions of peptides based on their number of amino-acid residues (abbreviations: H-O: organic ham, L-O: organic loin, S-O: organic shoulder, H-C: conventional ham, L-C: conventional loin, S-C: conventional shoulder).

Short-chain peptides had higher antioxidant activity than their proteins and polypeptides of origin, as also suggested by Zhu et al. [52]. A common feature of antioxidant peptides is 4–16 amino acids and a molecular weight of about 400–2000 Da [19]. In the present study, sequences predominantly contained 11–20 amino acids (Figure 4), with a molecular weight ranging from 1500 to 2000 Da (Figure 5).

The obtained peptide sequences were evaluated with regard to a potential biological activity using an in silico approach. In particular, the antioxidant potential properties of peptides were considered. To reduce the search area, peptides common for the muscle types tested (Supplementary Materials) and the meat origin (conventional vs. organic; Tables 2 and 3, respectively) were selected for further analysis.

The main purpose of the in silico approach was to determine the antioxidant capacity of meat peptides. However, among the analyzed sequences, low levels of antioxidant peptides were recognized. Only a few peptide sequences, such as dipeptides (AY, AH, EL, HH, HL, KD, IR, KP, LK, LY, LH, MM, SE, TW, WY, VY) and tripeptides (LHV, IKK, VKL, VKV, PEL, PHQ, SDF, FVP, GAA, GAH), as well as one four-amino acid sequence (YVGD) were found. Their location and source of origin are presented in Tables 3 and 4, Tables S1–S3. Nevertheless, in this study, peptides acting as a potential antioxidant were obtained primarily from myofibrillar proteins (nebulin and rarely titin, regardless of the rearing system applied). Kęska and Stadnik [14] indicated higher values of the in vitro antioxidant activity of myofibrillar proteins compared to water-soluble (sarcoplasmic) proteins in the ABTS test in dry-cured pork loin. These results are in line with the previous observations that the total number of bioactive peptides predicted to be released after in silico pepsin or pancreatin hydrolysis of selected porcine myofibrillar proteins ranged from six peptides for troponin C, skeletal muscle troponin C (TNNC2) to 112 for myosin-2 Myosin-2 (MYH2), preceded by nebulin (NEB) with 109 peptides per protein molecule. Of these, 1, 13, and 11 two- or three amino-acid peptides with antioxidant properties were observed (for TNNC2, MYH2, and NEB, respectively) [20].

Table 4. The antioxidant properties of peptides based on in vitro analysis. ABTS: 2,2′-azino-bis-3-ethylbenzthiazoline-6-sulfonic acid; FRAP: Fe(III) reduction power.

Antioxidant Properties		Ham	Loin	Shoulder	Rearing System (A)	Meat Element (B)	A × B
ABTS assay [%]	O	39.80 ± 3.11 [Aa]	41.89 ± 3.48 [Aa]	33.92 ± 3.97 [Ab]	NS	***	***
	C	41.51 ± 3.21 [Ba]	38.06 ± 2.69 [Bb]	34.19 ± 1.71 [Ac]			
Fe(II) assay [%]	O	12.91 ± 2.01 [Aa]	13.49 ± 1.60 [Aa]	13.24 ± 2.50 [Aa]	***	*	**
	C	17.37 ± 1.41 [Ba]	14.77 ± 1.73 [Ab]	14.72 ± 1.37 [Ab]			
FRAP assay	O	0.567 ± 0.024 [Aa]	0.653 ± 0.028 [Ab]	0.606 ± 0.011 [Ac]	***	***	**
	C	0.742 ± 0.058 [Ba]	0.767 ± 0.036 [Ba]	0.767 ± 0.039 [Ba]			

Abbreviations: O: organic rearing, C: conventional rearing. The results are presented as mean ± SD (standard deviation); [a–c] means in the same row with different letters differ significantly ($p < 0.05$); [A, B] means in the same column with different letters differ significantly ($p < 0.05$); NS, not significant; * $p < 0.05$, ** $p < 0.01$, *** $p < 0.001$.

Some food-derived peptides were reported to be multifunctional, because they can provide two or more health-promoting effects. As shown in Tables 2 and 3, the analyzed peptides may have more than one bioactivity, mainly acting as dipeptidyl peptidase-IV (DPP-IV) and angiotensin-I converting enzyme (ACE-I) inhibitors. Both groups of biologically active peptides can act against the effects of non-communicable diseases. The DPP-IV inhibitors belonging to one of these groups are involved in the regulation of blood glucose levels and are, therefore, strong antidiabetic agents. A similar bioactive action attributed also to another group of peptides termed "glucose uptake-stimulating peptides" was detected in this study. In turn, the ACE-I inhibitor, by inhibiting the conversion of angiotensin, reduces the negative effects of hypertension. All peptides analyzed in this study can act as DPP-IV inhibitors as well as ACE-I inhibitors (except for one peptide sequence (V.IIIIIIIIII.I), as shown in Table 3). As an example, based on the in silico analysis, dipeptide AY has antioxidant, cardioprotective, and antidiabetic effects. In addition, the potential of proteins as precursors of dipeptidyl peptidase-III (DPP III) inhibitors was also noted. The peptidase with DPP-III-inhibiting activity has a high affinity for cleavage of opioid peptides such as endomorphins and encephalin. These opioid peptides regulate a variety of physiological functions, such as signal transduction, gastrointestinal motility, immune and hormonal functions, and pain modulation.

According to the report by Khaket et al. [53], the β-subunit of chicken hemoglobin and annexin A5 showed a high inhibitory potential for DPP-III in in silico studies. However, as noted by Galleo et al. [16], only a few studies identified peptides that inhibit DPP-III from meat proteins. Therefore, the information gathered in this study regarding pork as a potential source of DPP-III is of particular interest. The presence of these biopeptides was identified in nebulin (YK, DA, KA, IH, PE, LR MR, RV), as well as in astitin (RV) and desmin (GE) (Tables 2 and 3). Furthermore, several peptides with biologically active properties, such as renin inhibition, calmodulin-dependent phosphodiesterase (CaMPDE) inhibition, dipeptidyl carboxypeptidase inhibition, antiamnestic and antithrombotic activity, regulation of the stomach mucosal membrane activity, bacterial permease ligand ability, and activation of ubiquitin-mediated proteolysis, were reported in unique biopeptides (Tables 2 and 3).

3.3. Antioxidant Properties of Peptides—In Vitro Analysis

The effectiveness of antioxidant compounds depends on various mechanisms. Consequently, a single test cannot cover all of the different modes of action of different food systems, especially in complex tissues such as meat. Therefore, three different tests were used to assess the differences between conventional and organic meats, as well as between selected pork elements. The variance analysis indicated that all of the effects of the rearing system or muscle type on the total antioxidant activity were significant ($p < 0.05$). The obtained values of radical-scavenging activity measured by the ABTS test were similar, ranging from 41.89% for organic loin to 33.92% for organic shoulder. The rearing method did not significantly affect the radical-scavenging activity of peptides in the ABTS test. This observation is also consistent with other descriptions in the literature, where meat extracts were also analyzed [27,28]. However, the meat origin (organic vs. conventional) and the carcass element significantly affected the iron-ion-chelating capacity (Fe(II)) and the reducing power. Descalzo et al. [54] reported that meat samples from animals reared on pasture had a higher content of antioxidant vitamins (α-tocopherol, β-carotene, and ascorbic acid) than the meat obtained from grain-fed animals. This observation became the basis for estimating the antioxidant potential of meat samples from various feeding systems. The authors further showed that the pasture rearing system had a greater reduction potential than in the case of grain-fed animal samples according to the FRAP assessment; however, there were no differences between these groups in the ABTS test. Importantly, the results indicated the non-enzymatic antioxidants as a cause of differences in antioxidant properties in the samples of meat from animals reared on pasture or fed on grains [28].

As presented in Table 4, the antioxidant properties were higher in the conventional meat samples, while the largest differences were noted in ham samples, i.e., 4.46% for the iron chelate efficiency ($p < 0.05$) and $\Delta A_{700} = 0.175$ for reducing power activity ($p < 0.05$). Based on the results of the FRAP tests, the smallest differences between organic and conventional pork were noted for shoulder batches.

To better understand how the carcass elements (ham, loin, or shoulder) collected from animals from a conventional or organic farming system were associated with the presence of antioxidant peptides, the changes in their antioxidant properties were quantified using various tests. By means of hierarchical clustering, the peptides were grouped according to their antioxidant trends. The hierarchical cluster analysis (HCA) was used in this study to calculate the multidimensional Euclidian distances between the observations (antioxidant activity). Using a stepwise algorithm (Ward's linkage criterion), observations behaving similarly across the initial variables were linked, and the results were graphically shown in a clustering tree (Figure 6).

The groups of observations behaving similarly were gathered in clusters. The derived dendrogram made it possible to distinguish three groups: cluster 1, organic loins and conventional ham; cluster 2, organic ham and conventional loins; cluster 3, organic and conventional shoulders (the most separated group). As observed in this study, conventional ham and organic loin were characterized by the highest variety of peptides. This confirms the hypothesis that the quantity and quality of peptides determine their contribution to act as additional antioxidant compounds against oxidation. On the basis of the results obtained, it can be stated that the antioxidant activity of peptides from pig muscles corresponds to their specific (individual) sequences.

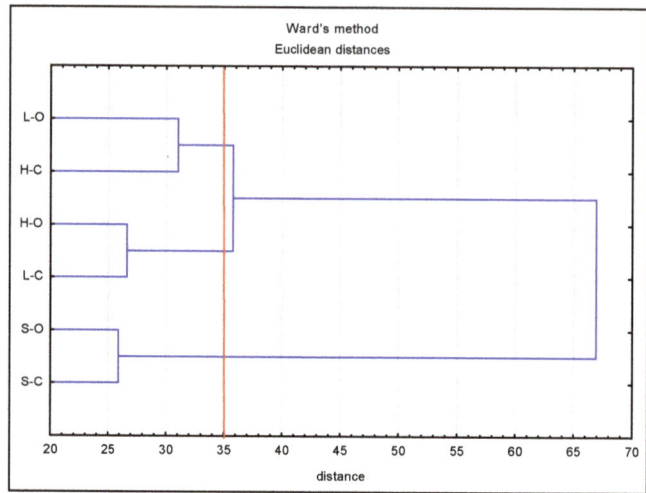

Figure 6. Dendrogram resulting from Ward's method of hierarchical cluster analysis of antioxidant activity.

As the role of food-derived antioxidants is significant, research on them is still widely carried out. Despite the fact that studies on living organisms are important in verifying the biological properties of peptides, there are little data on the direct antioxidant potential of food peptides on cell biology at the living organism level. So far, there have only been a few studies on food-origin antioxidant peptides in animal models. The administration of egg-white hydrolysate to spontaneously hypertensive rats for 17 weeks was shown to improve plasma antioxidant properties [55]. In turn, Ebaid et al. [56] showed that administering 100 mg/kg body weight of whey protein to streptozotocin-induced diabetic rats reduced several indicators of oxidative stress, such as malondialdehyde, nitric oxide, and ROS levels, while it also reduced proinflammatory cytokines and increased the level of glutathione [56]. Cellular assays are more commonly used as indirect methods to assess the protective effect of antioxidants against oxidative stressors and to elucidate the mechanism of action of peptides in cells. Thus, Katayama, Xu, Fan, and Mine, using human intestinal epithelial cells (Caco-2) as an intestinal epithelia model, reported that oligophosphopeptides derived from hen egg yolk exert an antioxidant effect, causing the upregulation of glutathione-induced biosynthesis accompanied by increased glutathione reductase activity [57]. This observation was also accompanied by inhibition of the production of proinflammatory cytokines, contributing to antioxidative protection against hydrogen peroxide-induced damage in Caco-2 cells. Moreover, the antioxidant peptide from fish skin gelatin hydrolysate increased the expression of cellular antioxidant enzymes (catalase, superoxide dismutase, and glutathione peroxidase) in human hepatoma (Hep3B) cells [58]. Numerous reports showed that food-derived peptides can retain antioxidant activity in simulating gastrointestinal digestion and then retain their properties in further studies of the cellular pathway (as a simulated uptake step) in the Caco-2 cell monolayer [59–61]. Research results confirmed that peptides from food can cross the gastrointestinal barrier and exert antioxidant effects. Thus, upon oral ingestion of peptide-rich foods, such as meat, different in vivo antioxidant efficacy can be produced.

4. Conclusions

The obtained results indicate some influence of the meat origin (organic vs. conventional) on the health characteristics of pork. Moreover, an in-depth mapping of the peptidome of pig carcass elements obtained from these two farming methods provides (at the molecular level of the protein) important information on how the peptide profile is being shaped. Based on the LC–MS/MS analysis of the different carcass elements, myofibrillar proteins (such as nebulin, titin, or desmin) were identified as the main sources of peptides. However, the meat origin (organic vs. conventional), as well as the element of the pork carcass (ham, loin, or shoulder), did not have a significant effect on the proteome. On the other hand, the pork origin and the carcass element significantly affected the iron-ion-chelating capacity (Fe(II)) and the reducing power of peptides. In particular, pork ham from the conventional rearing system, which had the best antioxidant properties due to the presence of peptides, can be recommended for daily consumption to people who care about their health. Analyses also showed that this meat element may be a source of peptides that support the treatment of noncommunicable diseases such as hypertension and diabetes, but additional research is needed to further confirm this aspect.

Supplementary Materials: The following are available online at http://www.mdpi.com/2076-3921/9/9/835/s1, Table S1. The list of peptide sequences common for conventional and organic ham; Table S2. The list of peptide sequences common for conventional and organic loins; Table S3. The list of peptide sequences common for conventional and organic shoulders.

Author Contributions: Conceptualization, K.M.W. and P.K.; methodology, P.K.; formal analysis, M.H., K.M.W., and P.K.; investigation, K.M.W., S.R., M.H., and P.K.; writing—original draft preparation, P.K.; writing—review and editing, K.M.W., P.K., M.H., and S.R. All authors have read and agreed to the published version of the manuscript.

Funding: This project was financed under the program of the Minister of Science and Higher Education (Poland) under the name "Regional Initiative of Excellence" in 2019–2022, project number 029/RID/2018/19, funding amount 11 927 330.00 PLN.

Conflicts of Interest: The authors declare no conflict of interest.

References

1. Halagarda, M. Decomposition analysis and consumer research as essential elements of the new food product development process. *Br. Food J.* **2017**, *119*, 511–526. [CrossRef]
2. Halagarda, M.; Kędzior, W.; Pyrzyńska, E. Nutritional Value and Potential Chemical Food Safety Hazards of Selected Traditional and Conventional Pork Hams from Poland. *J. Food Qual.* **2017**, *2017*, 9037016. [CrossRef]
3. Yadav, R.; Pathak, G.S. Intention to purchase organic food among young consumers: Evidences from a developing nation. *Appetite* **2016**, *96*, 122–128. [CrossRef] [PubMed]
4. IFOAM Organics International. IFOAM—Organics International. 2016. Available online: https://www.ifoam.bio/ (accessed on 4 November 2019).
5. Dangour, A.D.; Allen, E.; Lock, K.; Uauy, R. Nutritional composition and health benefits of organic foods—Using systematic reviews to question the available evidence. *Indian J. Med. Res.* **2010**, *131*, 478–480. [PubMed]
6. Dangour, A.D.; Lock, K.; Hayter, A.; Aikenhead, A.; Allen, E.; Uauy, R. Nutrition-related health effects of organic foods: A systematic review. *Am. J. Clin. Nutr.* **2010**, *92*, 203–210. [CrossRef] [PubMed]
7. Komprda, T. Comparison of quality and safety of organic and conventional foods. *Chemickélisty* **2009**, *103*, 729–732.
8. Schulzová, V.; Hajšlová, J.; Botek, P.; Peroutka, R. Furanocoumarins in vegetables: Influence of farming system and other factors on levels of toxicants. *J. Sci. Food Agric.* **2007**, *87*, 2763–2767. [CrossRef]
9. Zhao, Y.; Wang, D.; Yang, S. Effect of organic and conventional rearing system on the mineral content of pork. *Meat Sci.* **2016**, *118*, 103–107. [CrossRef]
10. De Smet, S.; Vossen, E. Meat: The balance between nutrition and health. *A review. Meat Sci.* **2016**, *120*, 145–156. [CrossRef]
11. Cicero, A.F.; Fogacci, F.; Colletti, A. Potential role of bioactive peptides in prevention and treatment of chronic diseases: A narrative review. *Br. J. Pharm.* **2017**, *174*, 1378–1394. [CrossRef]

12. Falowo, A.B.; Fayemi, P.O.; Muchenje, V. Natural antioxidants against lipid–protein oxidative deterioration in meat and meat products: A review. *Food Res. Int.* **2014**, *64*, 171–181. [CrossRef] [PubMed]
13. Mora, L.; Sentandreu, M.A.; Toldrá, F. Identification of small troponin T peptides generated in dry-cured ham. *Food Chem.* **2010**, *123*, 691–697. [CrossRef]
14. Kęska, P.; Stadnik, J. Stability of antiradical activity of protein extracts and hydrolysates from dry-cured pork loins with probiotic strains of LAB. *Nutrients* **2018**, *10*, 521. [CrossRef] [PubMed]
15. Wójciak, K.M.; Kęska, P.; Okoń, A.; Solska, E.; Libera, J.; Dolatowski, Z.J. The influence of acid whey on the antioxidant peptides generated to reduce oxidation and improve colour stability in uncured roast beef. *J. Sci. Food Agric.* **2018**, *98*, 3728–3734. [CrossRef]
16. Gallego, M.; Mora, L.; Toldrá, F. The relevance of dipeptides and tripeptides in the bioactivity and taste of dry-cured ham. *Food Prod. Process. Nutr.* **2019**, *1*, 2. [CrossRef]
17. Jiang, J.; Xiong, Y.L. Natural antioxidants as food and feed additives to promote health benefits and quality of meat products: A review. *Meat Sci.* **2016**, *120*, 107–117. [CrossRef] [PubMed]
18. Sohaib, M.; Anjum, F.M.; Sahar, A.; Arshad, M.S.; Rahman, U.U.; Imran, A.; Hussain, S. Antioxidant proteins and peptides to enhance the oxidative stability of meat and meat products: A comprehensive review. *Int. J. Food Prop.* **2017**, *20*, 2581–2593. [CrossRef]
19. Liu, R.; Xing, L.; Fu, Q.; Zhou, G.H.; Zhang, W.G. A review of antioxidant peptides derived from meat muscle and by-products. *Antioxidants* **2016**, *5*, 32. [CrossRef]
20. Kęska, P.; Stadnik, J. Porcine myofibrillar proteins as potential precursors of bioactive peptides–An in silico study. *Food Funct.* **2016**, *7*, 2878–2885. [CrossRef]
21. Kęska, P.; Wójciak, K.M.; Stadnik, J. Effect of Marination Time on the Antioxidant Properties of Peptides Extracted from Organic Dry-Fermented Beef. *Biomolecules* **2019**, *9*, 614. [CrossRef]
22. Kęska, P.; Stadnik, J. Taste-active peptides and amino acids of pork meat as components of dry-cured meat products: An in-silico study. *J. Sens. Stud.* **2017**, *32*, e12301. [CrossRef]
23. Willcox, J.K.; Ash, S.L.; Catignani, G.L. Antioxidants and prevention of chronic disease. *Crit. Rev. Food Sci. Nutr.* **2004**, *44*, 275–295. [CrossRef] [PubMed]
24. Hernández, P.; Zomeno, L.; Ariño, B.; Blasco, A. Antioxidant, lipolytic and proteolytic enzyme activities in pork meat from different genotypes. *Meat Sci.* **2004**, *66*, 525–529. [CrossRef]
25. Cabrera, M.C.; Saadoun, A. An overview of the nutritional value of beef and lamb meat from South America. *Meat Sci.* **2014**, *98*, 435–444. [CrossRef]
26. Ntawubizi, M.; Raes, K.; De Smet, S. Genetic parameter estimates for plasma oxidative status traits in slaughter pigs. *J. Anim. Sci.* **2020**, *98*, skz378. [CrossRef]
27. Gatellier, P.; Mercier, Y.; Renerre, M. Effect of diet finishing mode (pasture or mixed diet) on antioxidant status of Charolais bovine meat. *Meat Sci.* **2004**, *67*, 385–394. [CrossRef]
28. Descalzo, A.M.; Rossetti, L.; Grigioni, G.; Irurueta, M.; Sancho, A.M.; Carrete, J.; Pensel, N.A. Antioxidant status and odour profile in fresh beef from pasture or grain-fed cattle. *Meat Sci.* **2007**, *75*, 299–307. [CrossRef]
29. Nian, Y.; Allen, P.; Harrison, S.M.; Brunton, N.P.; Prendiville, R.; Kerry, J.P. Fatty acid composition of young dairy bull beef as affected by breed type, production treatment, and relationship to sensory characteristics. *Anim. Prod. Sci.* **2019**, *59*, 1360–1372. [CrossRef]
30. Xu, X.; Chen, X.; Chen, D.; Yu, B.; Yin, J.; Huang, Z. Effects of dietary apple polyphenol supplementation on carcass traits, meat quality, muscle amino acid and fatty acid composition in finishing pigs. *Food Funct.* **2019**, *10*, 7426–7434. [CrossRef]
31. Commission Regulation (EC) No 889/2008 of 5 September 2008 Laying down Detailed Rules for the Implementation of Council Regulation (EC) No 834/2007 on Organic Production and Labelling of Organic Products with Regard to Organic Production, Labelling and Control. Available online: https://eur-lex.europa.eu/legal-content/EN/TXT/?uri=CELEX%3A32008R0889 (accessed on 7 December 2019).
32. Council Regulation (EC) No 834/2007 of 28 June 2007 on organic production and labelling of organic products and repealing Regulation (EEC) No 2092/91. Available online: https://eur-lex.europa.eu/legal-content/EN/TXT/?uri=celex%3A32007R0834 (accessed on 7 December 2019).
33. National Research Council. *Nutrient Requirements of Swine*; Tenth Revised Edition; The national Academies Press: Washington, DC, USA, 1998.
34. BIOPEP-UWM Database. Available online: http://www.uwm.edu.pl/biochemia/index.php/pl/biopep (accessed on 14 December 2019).

35. Re, R.; Pellegrini, N.; Proteggente, A.; Pannala, A.; Yang, M.; Rice-Evans, C. Antioxidant activity applying an improved ABTS radical cation decolorization assay. *Free Radic. Biol. Med.* **1999**, *26*, 1231–1237. [CrossRef]
36. Decker, E.A.; Welch, B. Role of ferritin as a lipid oxidation catalyst in muscle food. *J. Agric. Food Chem.* **1990**, *38*, 674–677. [CrossRef]
37. Oyaizu, M. Studies on products of browning reaction: Antioxidative activity of products of browning reaction. *Jpn. J. Nutr.* **1986**, *44*, 307–315. [CrossRef]
38. Picard, B.; Gagaoua, M.; Al-Jammas, M.; De Koning, L.; Valais, A.; Bonnet, M. Beef tenderness and intramuscular fat proteomic biomarkers: Muscle type effect. *Peer J.* **2018**, *6*, e4891. [CrossRef] [PubMed]
39. Picard, B.; Gagaoua, M. Meta-proteomics for the discovery of protein biomarkers of beef tenderness: An overview of integrated studies. *Food Res. Int.* **2019**, *127*, 108739. [CrossRef] [PubMed]
40. Picard, B.; Gagaoua, M.; Al Jammas, M.; Bonnet, M. Beef tenderness and intramuscular fat proteomic biomarkers: Effect of gender and rearing practices. *J. Proteom.* **2019**, *200*, 1–10. [CrossRef] [PubMed]
41. Zhou, C.Y.; Wang, C.; Tang, C.B.; Dai, C.; Bai, Y.; Yu, X.B.; Li, C.B.; Xu, X.L.; Zhou, G.H.; Cao, J.X. Label-free proteomics reveals the mechanism of bitterness and adhesiveness in Jinhua ham. *Food Chem.* **2019**, *297*, 125012. [CrossRef]
42. Taylor, R.G.; Geesink, G.H.; Thompson, V.F.; Koohmaraie, M.; Goll, D.E. Is Z-disk degradation responsible for postmortem tenderization? *J. Anim. Sci.* **1995**, *73*, 1351–1367. [CrossRef]
43. Huff-Lonergan, E.; Mitsuhashi, T.; Beekman, D.D.; Parrish, F.C., Jr.; Olson, D.G.; Robson, R.M. Proteolysis of specific muscle structural proteins by μ-calpain at low pH and temperature is similar to degradation in postmortem bovine muscle. *J. Anim. Sci.* **1996**, *74*, 993–1008. [CrossRef]
44. Huff-Lonergan, E.; Mitsuhashi, T.; Parrish, F.C., Jr.; Robson, R.M. Sodium dodecyl sulfate-polyacrylamide gel electrophoresis and western blotting comparisons of purified myofibrils and whole muscle preparations for evaluating titin and nebulin in postmortem bovine muscle. *J. Anim. Sci.* **1996**, *74*, 779–785. [CrossRef]
45. Ladrat, C.; Verrez-Bagnis, V.; Noël, J.; Fleurence, J. In vitro proteolysis of myofibrillar and sarcoplasmic proteins of white muscle of sea bass (*Dicentrarchus labrax* L.): Effects of cathepsins B, D and L. *Food Chem.* **2003**, *81*, 517–525. [CrossRef]
46. Li, M.; Li, Z.; Li, X.; Xin, J.; Wang, Y.; Li, G.; Wu, L.; Shen, Q.W.; Zhang, D. Comparative profiling of sarcoplasmic phosphoproteins in ovine muscle with different color stability. *Food Chem.* **2018**, *240*, 104–111. [CrossRef] [PubMed]
47. Sarah, S.A.; Faradalila, W.N.; Salwani, M.S.; Amin, I.; Karsani, S.A.; Sazili, A.Q. LC–QTOF-MS identification of porcine-specific peptide in heat treated pork identifies candidate markers for meat species determination. *Food Chem.* **2016**, *199*, 157–164. [CrossRef] [PubMed]
48. Kim, G.D.; Seo, J.K.; Yum, H.W.; Jeong, J.Y.; Yang, H.S. Protein markers for discrimination of meat species in raw beef, pork and poultry and their mixtures. *Food Chem.* **2017**, *217*, 163–170. [CrossRef] [PubMed]
49. Mi, S.; Li, X.; Zhang, C.H.; Liu, J.Q.; Huang, D.Q. Characterization and discrimination of Tibetan and Duroc×(Landrace× Yorkshire) pork using label-free quantitative proteomics analysis. *Food Res. Int.* **2019**, *119*, 426–435. [CrossRef] [PubMed]
50. Bonnet, M.; Soulat, J.; Bons, J.; Léger, S.; De Koning, L.; Carapito, C.; Picard, B. Quantification of biomarkers for beef meat qualities using a combination of Parallel Reaction Monitoring-and antibody-based proteomics. *Food Chem.* **2020**, *317*, 126376. [CrossRef] [PubMed]
51. Bazile, J.; Picard, B.; Chambon, C.; Valais, A.; Bonnet, M. Pathways and biomarkers of marbling and carcass fat deposition in bovine revealed by a combination of gel-based and gel-free proteomic analyses. *Meat Sci.* **2019**, *156*, 146–155. [CrossRef]
52. Zhu, C.Z.; Zhang, W.G.; Zhou, G.H.; Xu, X.L.; Kang, Z.L.; Yin, Y. Isolation and identification of antioxidant peptides from Jinhua ham. *J. Agric. Food Chem.* **2013**, *61*, 1265–1271. [CrossRef]
53. Khaket, T.P.; Redhu, D.; Dhanda, S.; Singh, J. In silico evaluation of potential DPP-III inhibitor precursors from dietary proteins. *Int. J. Food Prop.* **2015**, *18*, 499–507. [CrossRef]
54. Descalzo, A.M.; Insani, E.M.; Biolatto, A.; Sancho, A.M.; Garcia, P.T.; Pensel, N.A.; Josifovich, J.A. Influence of pasture or grain-based diets supplemented with vitamin E on antioxidant/oxidative balance of Argentine beef. *Meat Sci.* **2005**, *70*, 35–44. [CrossRef]

55. Manso, M.A.; Miguel, M.; Even, J.; Hernández, R.; Aleixandre, A.; López-Fandiño, R. Effect of the long-term intake of an egg white hydrolysate on the oxidative status and blood lipid profile of spontaneously hypertensive rats. *Food Chem.* **2008**, *109*, 361–367. [CrossRef]
56. Ebaid, H.; Salem, A.; Sayed, A.; Metwalli, A. Whey protein enhances normal inflammatory responses during cutaneous wound healing in diabetic rats. *Lipids Health Dis.* **2011**, *10*, 1–10. [CrossRef] [PubMed]
57. Katayama, S.; Xu, X.; Fan, M.Z.; Mine, Y. Antioxidative stress activity of oligophosphopeptides derived from hen egg yolk phosvitin in Caco-2 cells. *J. Agric. Food Chem.* **2006**, *54*, 773–778. [CrossRef] [PubMed]
58. Mendis, E.; Rajapakse, N.; Kim, S.K. Antioxidant properties of a radical-scavenging peptide purified from enzymatically prepared fish skin gelatin hydrolysate. *J. Agric. Food Chem.* **2005**, *53*, 581–587. [CrossRef] [PubMed]
59. Picariello, G.; Iacomino, G.; Mamone, G.; Ferranti, P.; Fierro, O.; Gianfrani, C.; Di Luccia, A.; Addeo, F. Transport across Caco-2 monolayers of peptides arising from in vitro digestion of bovine milk proteins. *Food Chem.* **2013**, *139*, 203–212. [CrossRef] [PubMed]
60. Xie, N.; Liu, S.; Wang, C.; Li, B. Stability of casein antioxidant peptide fractions during in vitro digestion/Caco-2 cell model: Characteristics of the resistant peptides. *Eur. Food Res. Technol.* **2014**, *239*, 577–586. [CrossRef]
61. Xie, N.; Wang, B.; Jiang, L.; Liu, C.; Li, B. Hydrophobicity exerts different effects on bioavailability and stability of antioxidant peptide fractions from casein during simulated gastrointestinal digestion and Caco-2 cell absorption. *Food Res. Int.* **2015**, *76*, 518–526. [CrossRef]

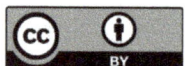 © 2020 by the authors. Licensee MDPI, Basel, Switzerland. This article is an open access article distributed under the terms and conditions of the Creative Commons Attribution (CC BY) license (http://creativecommons.org/licenses/by/4.0/).

MDPI
St. Alban-Anlage 66
4052 Basel
Switzerland
Tel. +41 61 683 77 34
Fax +41 61 302 89 18
www.mdpi.com

Antioxidants Editorial Office
E-mail: antioxidants@mdpi.com
www.mdpi.com/journal/antioxidants

www.ingramcontent.com/pod-product-compliance
Lightning Source LLC
LaVergne TN
LVHW070252100526
838202LV00015B/2210